Liver Cancer and Phytomedicine

Chemoprevention, Chemo Sensitization and Chemotherapy Strategies

Liver Cancer and Phytomedicine

Chemoprevention, Chemo Sensitization and Chemotherapy Strategies

editors

Lekshmi R Nath
Amrita Vishwa Vidyapeetham, India

Gautam Sethi
National University of Singapore, Singapore

B S Vinod
Sree Narayana College, India

World Scientific

NEW JERSEY • LONDON • SINGAPORE • BEIJING • SHANGHAI • HONG KONG • TAIPEI • CHENNAI • TOKYO

Published by

World Scientific Publishing Co. Pte. Ltd.
5 Toh Tuck Link, Singapore 596224
USA office: 27 Warren Street, Suite 401-402, Hackensack, NJ 07601
UK office: 57 Shelton Street, Covent Garden, London WC2H 9HE

British Library Cataloguing-in-Publication Data
A catalogue record for this book is available from the British Library.

LIVER CANCER AND PHYTOMEDICINE
Chemoprevention, Chemo Sensitization and Chemotherapy Strategies

ISBN 978-981-12-9331-3 (hardcover)
ISBN 978-981-12-9332-0 (ebook for institutions)
ISBN 978-981-12-9333-7 (ebook for individuals)

For any available supplementary material, please visit
https://www.worldscientific.com/worldscibooks/10.1142/13843#t=suppl

Typeset by Stallion Press
Email: enquiries@stallionpress.com

Printed in Singapore

https://doi.org/10.1142/9789811293320_fmatter

Preface

The global burden of primary liver cancer is increasing substantially, causing one major cause of cancer death in recent years. Conventional cancer chemotherapy is ineffective against liver cancer and exacerbates side effects. Even the clinical use of therapies such as sorafenib is declining nowadays due to the emergence of drug resistance. Natural products are well known for their wide range of pharmacological activities. Phytomedicine can be the best lead for the emerging concept of multidrug multi-target against liver cancer. *Phytomedicine can be defined as herbal medicine with therapeutic and healing properties.* This book provides an overview of the potential of phytomedicine in three aspects of cancer management: prevention, sensitization, and therapy, along with recent advancements in research associated with gut microbiota and immunotherapy. This book also addresses the challenges in the clinical translation of phytochemicals and further their development as phytonanomedicine.

The book explores herbal medicine with therapeutic effects, namely "Phytomedicine," emerging as a plausible therapeutic agent for treating hepatocellular carcinoma (HCC), emphasizing their mode of action focusing on tumor microenvironment (TME). It describes evidence based on *in vitro* experiments and studies involving animal models and humans to support the potential chemopreventive and therapeutic effects of diverse phytochemicals in liver cancer. Chemo resistance is the major problem in the management of hepatocellular carcinoma. The following chapter discusses some plant-derived compounds that show a chemo-sensitization effect in HCC. The subsequent chapter provides an in-depth analysis of the emerging role of phytomedicine in combating liver cancer, emphasizing phytochemical inhibitors of the mammalian target of the rapamycin (mTOR) pathway. Phytochemicals significantly affect both pathogenic and non-pathogenic microorganisms, and the following chapter will cover the effects on the gut-microbiota-associated with liver cancer. The role of plant-derived products in emerging areas of immunotherapy is also given importance. Still, the utility of phytomedicine has been limited by low water solubility, poor bioavailability, poor cell penetration, hepatic disposition, a narrow therapeutic index, and quick absorption by normal tissues. Therefore, there is ongoing research into nanoparticle-based delivery systems to enhance therapeutic effectiveness. Nanobiotechnology employs nanoparticles for the safe and efficient administration of drugs based on the tumor's unique characteristics. Large-scale controlled clinical trials are needed to validate their efficacy, adverse effects, and safety before clinical practice. This comprehensive book can be helpful for students and researchers in life science, biotechnology, and pharmacy working in plant-derived liver cancer therapeutics.

https://doi.org/10.1142/9789811293320_fmatter

Contents

https://doi.org/10.1142/9789811293320_0001

Chapter 1

Phytochemicals Targeting Tumor Microenvironment in Hepatocellular Carcinoma

Sruti C and Chithra JS*

Aster Research Foundation, Research and Innovation,
Dr Moopen's Medical College, Naseera Nagar,
Meppadi P.O. Wayanad, Kerala - 673577, India.

Table of Contents:

*Corresponding author: E-mail address: chithra.js@drmoopensmc.ac.in, jschithra@gmail.com; Email ID of co-author: srutisree2258@gmail.com

Abbreviations:

Bregs — Regulatory B cells
CAFs — Cancer-associated fibroblasts
CDK — Cyclin dependent kinases
CDKIs — Cyclin dependent kinase inhibitors
CSCs — Cancer stem cells
CSN5 — COP9 signalosome subunit 5
CTNNB1 — Catenin beta 1
ECM — Extracellular matrix
EGCG — Epigallocatechin gallate
EGF — Epidermal growth factor
EGFR — Epidermal growth factor receptor
EMT — Epithelial-mesenchymal transition
ERK — Extracellular signal-regulated kinase
FDA — US Food and Drug Administration
FGF — Fibroblast growth factor
HBV — Hepatitis B virus
HCC — Hepatocellular carcinoma
HCV — Hepatitis C virus
HGF — Hepatocyte growth factor
HSCs — Hepatic stellate cells
IFN — Interferon
IGF — Insulin-like growth factor
IGFR — Insulin-like growth factor receptor
IL-10 — Interleukin 10
IL-6 — Interleukin 6
JAK/STAT — Janus kinase/signal transducers and activators of transcription
MAPK/MEK — Mitogen-activated protein kinase
MDSCs — Myeloid-derived suppressor cells

MET — Mesenchymal epithelial transition
mTOR — Mammalian target of rapamycin
N K cells — Natural killer cells
NF-kB — Nuclear factor kappa B
Nrf2 — Nuclear factor erythroid 2-related factor 2
OS — Oxidative stress
P13k — Phosphoinositide 3-kinase
PDGF — Platelet-derived growth factor
PTEN — Phosphatase and TENsin homolog
RAF — Rapidly accelerated fibrosarcoma
RAS — Rat sarcoma
ROS — Reactive Oxygen Species
TAECs — Tumor-associated endothelial cells
TAMs — Tumor-associated macrophages
TANs — Tumor-associated neutrophils
TGF — Transforming growth factor
TLR4 — Toll-like receptor 4
TME — Tumor microenvironment
TNF — Tumor necrosis factor
TP53 — Tumor protein 53
Tregs — Regulatory T cells
VEGF — Vascular endothelial growth factor
VEGFR — Vascular endothelial growth factor receptor

Abstract

High throughput sequencing and omics technologies have transformed our understanding of the pathophysiology of cancer, providing new insights into the tumor microenvironment and the significance thereof in cancer regression. Hepatocellular carcinoma (HCC) still remains a lethal disease even after decades of cancer research providing promising results, primarily due to the complex tumor microenvironment (TME). Targeting the dynamic interactions of cancer cells with their environment along with the conventional therapeutics is considered a reliable approach for better prognosis in HCC patients. Novel and effective treatment approaches are being designed to target the intricate system of TME in HCC, including immune-therapeutics and combinatorial therapies. The quest for new strategies and novel chemoprevention agents to complement current treatment modalities for enhancing efficiency has advanced the development of phytochemicals as prophylactics and therapeutic agents. Phytochemicals emerging as plausible therapeutic agents for the treatment of HCC are described in this chapter with special emphasis on their mode of action, focusing on TME.

1. Introduction

Liver cancer, being the sixth most common cancer and the third leading cause of cancer-related death, remains a major health challenge due to rapid increase in its rate of incidence and mortality [1, 2]. Hepatocellular carcinoma (HCC) is the predominant histological type among primary liver cancers, making up 90% of cases, and its occurrence differs based on geographical locations [3, 4]. The main risk factors for the development of HCC are widely recognized. These factors encompass chronic liver damage resulting from fibrosis and inflammation, infections like hepatitis B or C, metabolic syndrome, exposure to aflatoxin B and alcohol consumption [5]. For HCC patients in the early stages, surgery has been a gold-standard treatment which is often complemented by radiofrequency ablation (RFA) or trans-arterial chemoembolization (TACE). However, in the case of advanced disease, therapy options are limited due to disease relapse and metastasis [6]. Studies have shown that systemic drug treatment using sorafenib and lenvatinib on patients with unresectable HCC was not curative but useful in curbing cancer progression or to increase life expectancy [7–9]. Chemo-resistance, untargeted tissue damage and other side effects including immunosuppression, low red blood cell count, and so on are developed in these patients over time [10–14]. Moreover, in HCC, a complex tumor microenvironment (TME) is formed causing major challenges to treatment modalities.

The concept of the tumor microenvironment has evolved, recognizing that cancer behavior is influenced not only by the genetics of the tumor cells but also by the immediate surrounding, which is essential for tumor cell growth, proliferation, metastasis as well as survival. The TME is a dynamic system primarily regulated by inflammatory cells including cancer cells, stromal tissue (immune cells, fibroblasts, myo-fibroblasts, cytokines, and vascular tissue), and the surrounding extracellular matrix [15, 16]. Given the crucial role of the TME in HCC tumorigenesis, immune evasion and resistance to treatment, there is a growing interest in exploring strategies to target the TME [2]. Significance of tumor microenvironment (TME) in the dynamic regulation of cancer progression with an influence on the therapeutic outcomes has been extensively studied whereby several therapies targeting the various components of TME have been developed in recent years [17, 18]. In recent years, the increasing complexity of the tumor microenvironment (TME) has become evident, resulting in a lack of effective therapeutic choices and a trend toward late diagnosis. This underscores the pressing necessity to discover new prognostic and therapeutic agents in the context of hepatocellular carcinoma (HCC) [19, 20].

Recently, phytochemicals have gained immense attention as promising anticancer agents due to the versatility to target multimodal oncogenic pathways as well as to induce cell cycle arrest and apoptosis [21, 22]. Phytochemicals have demonstrated their effectiveness in reducing the primary characteristics of cancer, including proliferation, migration, and invasion. They achieve this by promoting apoptosis, and regulating the metastasis of HCC mainly by targeting crucial molecular markers involved in these biological processes [23]. Moreover, phytochemicals with multimodal targeting abilities are recently being explored for reprogramming TME and thereby modulating the therapeutic response in HCC. This chapter provides an overview of the following aspects related to HCC: (i) The tumor microenvironment of HCC, including its components and the dynamic interactions between the tumor cells and TME, (ii) Current and emerging targeted therapies for HCC with a particular focus on their impact on the TME, and (iii) The use of phytochemicals in drug discovery and their effects on modulating the TME.

2. Tumor Microenvironment of HCC

Tumor microenvironment serves as a microsystem that facilitates the survival and progression of cancer cells by constant regulation of cellular metabolism, genetic, and epigenetic factors [24]. The tumor microenvironment of HCC contains cancer cells and stromal cells, including fibroblasts, endothelial cells, macrophages, and lymphocytes with each of these cell types playing a unique function in the occurrence as well as progression of HCC [25–27]. Also, the extracellular matrix that complements the immune as well as non-immune components of the TME and brings about a collective effect on HCC progression.

2.1. *Cellular components of TME in HCC*

TME being an intricate environment is composed of both cellular and non-cellular components which work in a co-ordinated manner along with the extracellular matrix in various stages of HCC development, proliferation, migration as well as its progression. Major cell types in HCC TME include hepatic stellate cells (HSCs), myeloid-derived suppressor cells (MDSCs), cancer-associated fibroblasts (CAFs), tumor-associated macrophages (TAMs), tumor-associated neutrophils (TANs), immune, and endothelial cells.

Hepatic Stellate Cells (HSCs) are associated with collagen production in liver and their activation due to liver injuries leading to excessive ECM production causing hepatic fibrosis [28, 29]. The roles of HSCs in HCC are intricate and varied. Some researchers propose that HSCs act as tumor suppressors in HCC, while others argue that they contribute to tumor growth by promoting processes such as tumor angiogenesis, invasion, metastasis and immune modulation [30]. When activated, HSCs have the capacity to enhance the malignant characteristics of HCC through the activation of key signaling pathways, including NF-kB and extracellular regulated protein kinases (ERK) [31]. Clinical studies have indicated that HSCs are linked to HCC recurrence and are associated with poor survival rates [32, 33].

Myeloid-derived suppressor cells (MDSCs) exist as a heterogeneous population of immature myeloid cells and play a crucial role in suppressing the anti-tumor immune responses in patients [34, 35]. In the context of HCC, MDSCs have been found to exert potent immunosuppressive effects by inhibiting effector T cells, reducing the cytotoxicity of natural killer (NK) cells, and amplifying immune checkpoint signaling through various mechanisms [36]. Additionally, MDSCs impede the infiltration of immune cells into tumor sites, allowing tumor cells to evade immune surveillance [37].

Cancer-associated fibroblasts (CAFs) are a group of fibroblastic cells that interact closely with cancerous cells [38]. Recent studies revealed that CAFs possess tumor-promoting function even though there have been studies on its tumor-suppressing role [39]. CAFs impact the progression of HCC by promoting cell epithelial-to-mesenchymal transition (EMT) through the activation of specific pathways and facilitating metastasis [40–42]. CAFs have the capacity to accelerate tumor growth by producing growth factors, cytokines and chemokines [43–45]. CAFs often engage in communication with both immune and non-immune cells, contributing to the intricate mechanisms of HCC progression by shaping the tumor microenvironment and supporting cancer growth.

Tumor-associated macrophages (TAMs) found within the tumor stroma tend to possess both pro-tumoral and anti-tumoral roles based on their polarization to M1 or M2 phenotype [46]. In HCC, macrophages have a natural tendency to polarize into M2 type whose high levels are associated with a more aggressive phenotype [47]. TAMs play a role in tumor angiogenesis and metastasis by producing cytokines that facilitate these processes [48]. They are also involved in promoting immune suppression by inducing the infiltration of regulatory T cells into tumor tissues [49, 50]. Notably, TAMs have been associated with resistance to both sorafenib treatment and anti-PD-L1 therapy, highlighting their potential as a therapeutic target in HCC [51–53].

Tumor-associated neutrophils (TANs) can take on either N1 (anti-tumoral) or N2 (pro-tumoral) phenotypes, a determination influenced by factors like the presence of TGF-β [54, 55]. An increase in the intra-tumoral neutrophil count is linked to lower rates of recurrence-free survival and overall survival among HCC patients [56]. The interactions between neutrophils and other immune cells within the tumor microenvironment hold significant importance. Neutrophils play a role in advancing HCC progression and promoting sorafenib resistance by recruiting macrophages, Treg cells, and NK cells [57, 58].

Regulatory T cells (Tregs) are a dominant type of tumor-infiltrating T cells known for their role in immune suppression and inflammation control, which hinders anti-tumor immune responses [59]. Tregs contribute to HCC invasion through TGF-β1induced EMT and also play a role in mediating sorafenib resistance [60]. Consequently, blocking Tregs has the potential to overcome sorafenib resistance and enhance HCC sensitivity to immunotherapy [61, 62]. High levels of infiltrating **regulatory B cells** (Bregs) are linked to advanced disease stages, recurrence and lower survival rates among HCC patients [63]. **Th17 cells**, a subset of $CD4^+$ lymphocytes, have been observed to increase concurrently with Tregs and Bregs in the peripheral circulation and tumor tissues of HCC patients. Clinical data indicate that elevated levels of Th17 cells within the tumor-stromal region are associated with poor survival and a higher likelihood of post-operative recurrence [64, 65].

Tumor-associated endothelial cells (TAECs) are involved in endothelial cell survival, proliferation, mobilization, invasion in tumors and tumor neo-vasculature [66, 67]. In HCC, TAECs facilitate accelerated cell cycle, enhanced migratory capabilities and over-expression of CD105 and TGF-β1 along with angiogenic surface receptors, such as VEGFR, EGFR, and CXCL12, rendering tumor angiogenesis and resistance to chemotherapeutic drugs [68, 69].

2.2. *Non-cellular components of TME in HCC*

Non-cellular components of TME include ECM proteins, enzymes, growth factors, cytokines, and chemokines which possess a significant impact on HCC progression and prognosis. **Extracellular matrix** (ECM) contains proteoglycans, including heparin sulfate, chondroitin sulfate, and keratin sulfate, which act as binding receptors for a range of growth factors, cytokines and chemokines influencing various physiological and pathological processes [70, 71]. Collagen, the most abundant ECM protein plays a dual role as both a barrier to tumor metastasis and a substrate for tumor movement. Another ECM component, Laminin, is involved in various biological functions such as cell adhesion, growth, migration and angiogenesis [72].

A complex array of cytokines that are characteristic of the HCC microenvironment plays a pivotal role in tumor evolution. Changes in cytokine expressions are often studied to formulate different treatment regimens. In HCC, higher levels of **Interleukin**-6 (IL-6) are found in patients with advanced HCC, and their elevated levels are related to lower overall survival as well as higher chances of relapsing [73, 74].

Transforming growth factors (TGF-α and TGF-β) are involved in the process of hepato-carcinogenesis. Upregulation of TGF-α due to liver damage results in its elevated levels, leading to tissue regeneration, hepatocyte dysplasia, proliferation and eventually the development of HCC [75]. TGF-β is highly involved in various inflammatory processes whereby they promote tissue repair and inhibit leukocyte activation as well as infiltration [76]. In early stages of cancer, TGF-β acts as a tumor suppressor by promoting cytostasis and apoptosis. However, it also plays a role in facilitating pro-tumorigenic processes such as inducing EMT, invasion, metastasis and angiogenesis [77]. **Interleukin 10** (IL 10) is recognized as a potent anti-inflammatory cytokine. Clinical studies have shown that elevated levels of IL-10 in HCC patients are linked to poor prognosis and unfavorable clinical outcomes, making it a negative prognostic factor [78–80]. **Tumor necrosis factor** (TNF) is found to have serious implications in HCC as it can induce various biological responses in liver, including hepatocyte apoptosis, necrosis, inflammation as well as regeneration. Hence, TNF plays a multi-faceted role in HCC development and progression as polymorphisms in its genes are linked to the risk of HCC [81].

Molecular Signaling in TME of HCC

The aberrant molecular signaling pathways in the cells of HCC TME are crucial in hepato-carcinogenesis due to the regulatory role in TME maintenance and anti-tumor immunity. The primary pathways involved in HCC pathogenesis can be categorized into three groups — (i) Pathways associated with cell differentiation, including Wnt, Hedgehog, and Notch pathways, (ii) Pathways related to angiogenesis such as vascular endothelial growth factor (VEGF) pathway, and (iii) Pathways that regulate the signaling of growth factors like fibroblast growth factor (FGF), hepatocyte growth factor (HGF/MET), insulin-like growth factor (IGF), epidermal growth factor (EGF) and platelet-derived growth factor (PDGF) [82–84]. The EGF/EGFR pathway mainly regulates the release of inflammatory meditators and is engaged in extensive cross-talks with other signaling pathways that contribute to tumor progression. Aberrant IGF/IGFR pathway in HCC confers stemness to cancer cells and drives tumor progression and drug resistance while HGF/c-MET pathway induces EMT and is actively involved in tumor growth, invasion and angiogenesis. Wnt signaling regulates angiogenic factors and induces endothelial cell proliferation leading to angiogenesis in HCC. Wnt activation also regulates tumor immunity in HCC via NKT cell activation and M2 macrophage polarization [85]. In highly vascular tumors like HCC, VEGF and angiopoetins are key players in promoting and maintaining neo-angiogenesis.

TME and the complex interactions among its components play a vital role in HCC development as discussed. Often traditional therapies fail to treat HCC due to the complexity of the TME, emphasizing the need for novel therapeutic approaches.

3. Targeted Therapies for HCC

Current treatment modalities often fall short in effectively addressing the multiple critical factors associated with cancer progression, including angiogenesis, uncontrolled cell division, and metastasis. Moreover, the intricate tumor microenvironment (TME) significantly contributes to HCC progression and resistance to standard treatments. Therefore, there is a need for ongoing research to create new therapeutic agents and treatment strategies for combating HCC. In the following section, we will explore the emerging targeted therapies for HCC and the areas of active research that hold promise in this complex clinical context.

3.1. *Molecular targets*

Enhancing our comprehension of the numerous molecular mechanisms driving tumor initiation and advancement is crucial for the creation of innovative pharmacological treatments. In recent years, multiple molecular-targeted agents have undergone assessment in clinical trials for advanced HCC.

3.1.1. *Targeting signaling molecules*

Several molecular-targeted agents have been developed for the treatment of advanced HCC, and these agents are expected to restore control over various pathways, thereby preventing the uncontrolled growth and metastasis of tumor cells. As an illustration, Sorafenib, a multiple kinase inhibitor that acts on growth factor receptors including VEGFR and platelet-derived growth factor receptor (PDGFR), has been established as the primary treatment for advanced, non-resectable HCC. Nevertheless, approximately 50% of patients develop resistance to this therapy, and this resistance is likely linked to the tumor microenvironment (TME) which includes immune cells associated with the tumor, such as TANs [57, 86]. Other multi-kinase inhibitors used in HCC include cediranib (inhibitor of VEGFR,

PDGF-β, and c-KIT), sunitinib (inhibits VEGFR and PDGFR), linifarnib (inhibits VEGFR and PDGFR), vatalanib (inhibits VEGFR, PDGFR, and c-KIT), and brivanib (inhibitor of VEGFR and FGFR). Other classes of drugs include the EGFR inhibitors such as erlotinib, gefitinib, cetuximab, and lapatinib; VEGF inhibitors such as bevacizumab and ramucirumab; MET inhibitor-tivantinib; mTOR inhibitor-everolimus and intracellular signaling inhibitors such as selumetinib (inhibits Raf-MEK-ERK signaling pathway) and bortezomib (regulates NF-κB-mediated anti-apoptotic signaling). The challenges of these drugs include lack of efficacy and unpalatable toxicity. Hence, identifying the key molecules/receptors/signaling pathways and assessing their relevance as potential therapeutics with emphasis on TME has been a great challenge for researchers.

3.1.2. *Targeting complement system*

The complement system acts as a bridge connecting innate and adaptive immunity, making it an essential component in the functioning of the immune system [87]. Reduced levels of complement components or over-activation of these components can lead to tumor initiation and progression [88]. Complements are also the key players in tumor metastasis whereby they bring about a change in the metastasis niche [89]. The complement system can function as an innate immunity modulator as well as regulates secondary immune cell activities. Hence, in cancer cells, blocking the activation of various complement components can result in improved tumor immunotherapy efficacy [90]. C5aR1 inhibitors have been investigated as part of combination therapies with paclitaxel or temozolomide in melanoma, colon cancer and glioblastoma [91, 92]. While complement combination therapy has been explored in these cancers, it has not yet been used as a treatment option for liver cancer. Currently, clinical trials are evaluating the effectiveness of anti-C5 antibodies like Eculizumab, which target C5a generation, and the use of receptor antagonists such as PMX-53 to block C4a-C5aR interactions. Additionally, inhibitors such as POT-4 and compostatin can target other components of the complement cascade, including C3 and C3a/C3b [93]. Inhibiting complement components in HCC may help prevent vascular invasion and potentially reduce the formation of immunosuppressive microenvironments by inhibiting immune suppressor cells like M2-like TAMs and TANs. Researchers are exploring various molecules within the complement system as potential therapeutic targets to improve the survival of HCC patients.

3.2. *Cellular targets*

Enhanced and comprehensive cellular and molecular profiling of the tumor microenvironment (TME) is crucial, as it plays a pivotal role in the initiation and advancement of HCC. The TME in HCC is marked by intricate interconnections between tumor cells and various cell types. It encompasses a diverse array of immune cells, CAFs, and endothelial cells that support cell proliferation, angiogenesis, and immune evasion. The immune system maintains close interactions with tumors across the entire spectrum of disease development, from initial stages to metastasis. Consequently, these intricate interactions between the immune system and cancer cells can either promote or hinder tumor growth and progression.

3.2.1. *Targeting immune cells*

Tumor-associated immune cells can be placed under two categories: tumor-promoting and tumor-antagonistic immune cells that work in a co-ordinated manner at different stages of tumor formation. Immunotherapy, that targets immune cells within or outside of the TME, is a promising choice in HCC treatment due to high specificity and low side effects. Various forms of immune cell therapies are currently being assessed for their effectiveness in treating cancer. These therapies encompass immune-modulating approaches, the use of cytokines like interferons (IFN) and interleukins (IL), as well as treatments involving lymphokine-activated killer (LAK) and Cytokine-induced killer (CIK) cells. Research studies have indicated that immune cell therapy, whether administered as a standalone treatment or in conjunction with procedures like RFA or trans-arterial chemoembolization (TACE), results in reduced recurrence and improved overall survival rates for patients [94, 95]. Additionally, novel treatment strategies for HCC are being explored, including gene-modified T cell therapies such as CAR-T or TCR-T cell therapies.

3.2.2. *Targeting cancer stem cells*

Cancer stem cells (CSCs) represent a minority of cells within the tumor that exhibit characteristics such as slow cycling, self-renewal capacity and the capability to initiate the formation of new tumors [96]. CSCs are known for their properties to promote tumorigenesis, metastasis, recurrence as well as therapy resistance in tumors. There exists a constant interactive network between CSCs and TME which together form a dynamic system that fosters the generation and maintenance of CSCs [97]. Extensive research has provided evidence that CSCs contribute to HCC by conferring properties such as proliferation, invasion and recurrence. It has been recently reported that inhibiting the self-renewal properties of CSCs, targeting their metabolism or modifying the cancer niche in which they reside can be an excellent method for cancer prevention [98, 99]. Researchers are approaching CSCs form various angles, with a focus on CSC markers like CD40 and CD90 for drug targeting [100]. Some potential therapeutic strategies for HCC based on CSC targeting include: (i) Developing CSC vaccines for immunotherapy, (ii) Inducing CSC differentiation after chemotherapy and radiotherapy, (iii) Stimulating quiescent CSCs to enter the cell cycle, and (iv) Micro/nano-targeting of CSCs.

Specific phytochemicals have been identified as regulators or inhibitors of the self-renewal mechanisms of CSCs. They achieve this by targeting key signaling pathways such as hedgehog, notch, and Wnt/β-Catenin, which are responsible for conferring stemness properties to CSCs [96]. Notable phytochemicals in this area includes: (i) Curcumin, known for the regulation of normal stem cells where they inhibit CSC growth by targeting their self-renewal pathways, (ii) Genistein, an isoflavone having the potential to reduce CSC proliferation, (iii) Epigallocatechin gallate (EGCG) found in abundance in green tea influences self-renewal pathways and also contributes to regulation of normal stem cells, (iv) Resveratrol and Lycopene found in red grapes, berries, and tomatoes respectively possess functions of reducing CSC growth and influencing CSC self-renewal, and (v) Piperine, a compound in black pepper, has been shown to play a role in controlling the self-renewal mechanisms of CSCs [107].

Various bioactive compounds and specific dietary strategies are currently under investigation to regulate cancer cell metabolism and enhance traditional cancer approaches. Nutrients such as iron, sulfur, vitamin B complex, cysteine, manganese, and magnesium have been identified as factors that impact the functionality and biogenesis of mitochondrial enzymes. Plant-based diets rich in vitamins and minerals have the potential to mitigate mitochondrial damage associated with cancer cell proliferation [101]. Therefore, targeting the unique CSC metabolism and disrupting key metabolic enzymes with the help of nutritional interventions are providing promising options for developing novel cancer therapies.

CSCs tend to inhabit specialized microenvironments within tumors that support their survival, proliferation and self-renewal as well [102–106]. Plant-derived bioactive compounds offer a promising avenue for regulating these CSC niches by targeting the signaling pathways responsible for maintaining the tumor microenvironment. These compounds disrupt the conditions in the CSC niche, rendering it less conducive for CSC growth and tumor progression. Phytochemicals are well-known for their anti-oxidant and anti-inflammatory properties, which have demonstrated effectiveness in inhibiting CSC growth, metabolism and the TME. Therefore, their consumption in substantial amounts through dietary sources is strongly recommended to reduce the risk of developing cancer [107].

4. Phytochemicals as Therapeutic Agents in HCC

Currently available therapeutic approaches includes surgical removal or radiation with high-risk factors such as drug resistance, toxicity, and relapsing chances. This underscores the importance of focusing on therapies that are less toxic, cost-effective and associated with a lower risk of cancer recurrence [108, 109]. Phytochemicals derived from natural sources are being continuously investigated for their potential to target cancer cells through various mechanisms [110]. Some notable phytochemicals that have demonstrated diverse functions in disrupting the interactions between the tumor microenvironment and cancer cells include resveratrol, genistein, plumbagin, curcumin, epigallocatechin gallate (EGCG), and more. Various plant-derived compounds that affect the signaling pathways in HCC are enlisted in Table 1.

Several other phytochemicals have also exhibited anticancer properties, including rhein [145], luteolin [146], quercetin [147], silibinin [148], artemisinin and its derivatives [149], and more. These compounds are currently undergoing clinical trials to assess their potential as potent therapeutic agents for the treatment of HCC.

4.1. *Regulation of molecular targets in TME by phytochemicals*

Phytochemicals exert a TME modulatory effect by not only disrupting the crosstalk between the tumor microenvironment (TME) and cancer cells but also by influencing the molecular pathways of non-cancer cells in close proximity to cancer cells, thereby limiting their support for cancer cells. For example, ALDE can prevent NF-kB translocation and MAPK activation and also stabilize Nrf2 expression [143]. Resveratrol is involved in inhibiting the PDGF signaling pathway [125–128]. Plumbagin inhibits the P13K/Akt signaling pathway in HCC [140]. Silibinin targets downstream activities of NF-kB by blocking its binding to DNA [148]. Curcumin's key feature is the suppression of mTOR and NF-kB through the targeting of the P13/Akt/IkBα signaling pathway [112–115]. Luteolin hinders the STAT6 pathway, whereas artemisinin derivatives focus on inhibiting the TGF-β pathway [146]. Quercetin has been reported to inhibit the P13/Akt signaling pathway in liver epithelial cells [147], and rhein can inhibit the sonic hedgehog and Akt signaling pathway [145] (Figure 1).

Table 1: List of potent phytochemicals with anticancer properties

Phytochemical	Source	Medicinal Properties	Clinical Implications	References
Curcumin 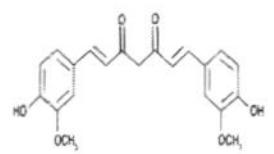	*Curcuma longa* (Turmeric)	Anti-oxidant and anti-inflammatory effects	➢ Suppress NF-kB and mTOR via targeting the P13/Akt/IkBα signaling pathway. ➢ Inhibition of hedgehog pathway. ➢ Inhibition of hypoxia-induced EMT formation. ➢ Inhibits CSN5, thereby blocking TNF-α induced immunosuppression.	[110–115]
Epigallocatechin Gallate (EGCG) 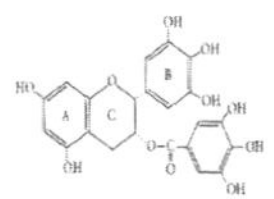	*Camellia sinensis* (Green tea)	Anti-oxidant effects, cancer chemoprevention, reduction of inflammatory responses	➢ Suppresses cell proliferation by either inhibiting ERalpha36 or by obstructing the P13K/Akt and MAPK/ERK pathways. ➢ Initiates apoptosis by activating caspase-3 and through the feedback loop involving ERα36, EGFR and Her-2.	[116–124]
Resveratrol 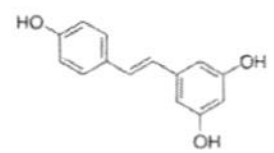	*Vitis vinifera*(grapes) *Arachis hypogaea* (peanuts)	Anti-oxidative, anti-carcinogenic, anti-viral, phtyoestrogenic and anti-tumor properties	➢ Inhibition of cell growth by inhibition of metabolic phenotypes that support anaerobic growth. ➢ Inhibition of angiogenesis by reducing the expression of VEGF through blocking HIF-1α.	[125–137]

(*Continued*)

Table 1: (*Continued*)

Phytochemical	Source	Medicinal Properties	Clinical Implications	References
Plumbagin 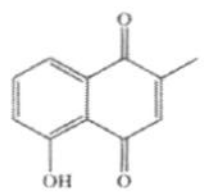	Plumbago species	Antimicrobial effects	➢ Preventing the P13K/Akt pathway activation induced by various pro-angiogenic factors secreted by tumor cells inhibits several characteristics of endothelial cells, including migration, tube formation and microvessel density.	[138–140]
Genistein 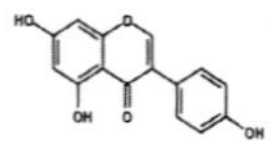	Soybeans	Anti-inflammatory effects, anti-tumor properties	➢ Halting tumor growth by causing cell cycle arrest at the G0/G1 and G2/M phases. ➢ Facilitating apoptosis and enhancing the expression of phosphor-AMPK.	[141, 142]
ALDE is ethanolic extract from root of Saussurea (Aucklandia) lappa Clarke, containing 1–2.5% purified oils and a high concentration of sesquiterpenoid compounds such as costunolide.	*Saussurea costus*	Analgesic properties, anti-inflammatory activity	➢ Stabilizing Nrf2 expression through NF-kB translocation and MAPK activation. ➢ Reducing angiogenesis and impeding the progression of tumors.	[143, 144]

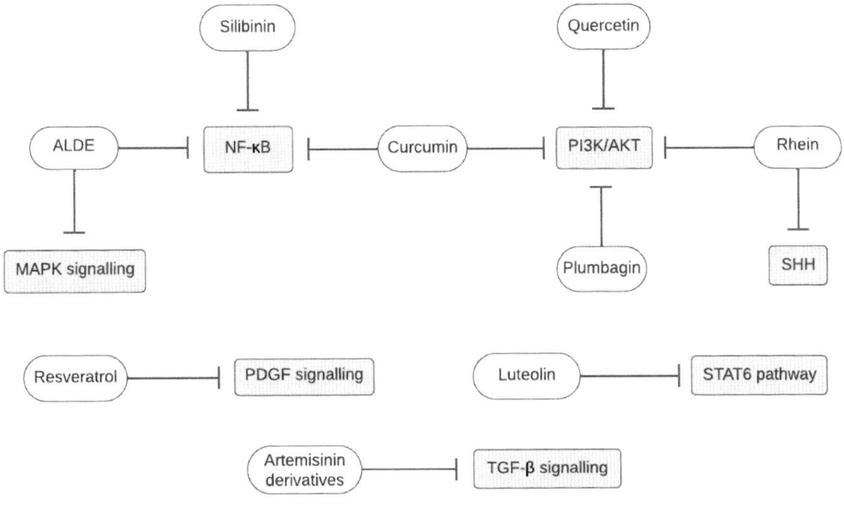

Figure 1: Signaling pathways targeted by phytochemicals in HCC: ALDE inhibits NF-κB signaling pathway via stabilization of Nrf2, preventing nuclear translocation of NF-κB. Silibinin regulates NF-κB signaling by inhibiting its binding to DNA. Curcumin suppresses both NF-κB signaling and PI3K/AKT/IκBα signaling pathway along with mTOR. Plumbagin and Quercetin also target PI3K/AKT signaling. Rhein regulates both AKT and SHH pathways. ALDE prevents MAPK activation. PDGF signaling, STAT6 pathway and TGF-β signaling are inhibited by resveratrol, luteolin and derivatives of artemisinin, respectively. ALDE, *Aucklandia lappa* Decne; MAPK, mitogen-activated protein kinase; NF-κB, nuclear factor kappa B; Nrf2, nuclear factor erythroid 2-related factor 2; PDGF, platelet-derived growth factor; PI3K/AKT, phosphoinositide 3-kinase/protein kinase B; STAT6, signal transducer and activator of transcription 6; SHH, sonic hedgehog; TGF-β, transforming growth factor beta.

4.2. *Regulation of oxidative stress in TME by phytochemicals*

Oxidative stress (OS) occurs when the body receives signals of danger from either internal or external sources, resulting in oxidative damage of DNA and abnormal protein expression. This state of vulnerability makes the body susceptible to various diseases, including cancer. Liver carcinogenesis is influenced by factors such as HCV/HBV infection, non-alcoholic fatty liver disease and alcohol abuse. Recently, there has been growing interest in the relationship between HCC and OS, with a focus on cellular and molecular mechanisms [150]. OS plays a role in three main stages of cancer development — initiation, promotion and progression. During the initiation phase, OS leads to mutations in oncogenes and tumor suppressor genes [151, 152]. During the promotion phase, clonal expansion of transformed or initiated cells is regulated by reactive oxygen species (ROS). In this phase, various signaling pathways including RAS-MEK/ERK ½, P13K/AKT, Keap1-Nrf2-ARE, JAK/STAT, and NF-kB are disrupted, and enzymatic activities are lost due to the oxidation of cysteine and methionine residues by ROS [153]. Lastly, elevated levels of ROS gear up the progression phase by generating genomic instability which in turn increases the metastatic potential of tumor cells.

Anticancer drugs disrupt the redox balance by generating ROS, which can induce programmed cell death and kill cancer cells. However, prolonged exposure to these drugs can lead to drug-induced resistance, causing initially drug-sensitive cancer cells to become drug-resistant [154]. ROS, due to their reactive nature, can modify the structure and function of various proteins, subsequently affecting the functions of receptors in downstream signaling cascades involved in cancer. Therefore, it is essential to analyze the specific effects of ROS in the context of phytochemical-mediated anticancer activity and conduct more in-depth studies on the mechanisms affecting drug efficacy for future development of cancer drugs. On the other hand, targeting the dynamic properties of the tumor microenvironment (TME) by focusing on the mechanisms involving cancer-associated stromal cells provides an approach for anticancer therapy. Identifying critical pathways that trigger anti-tumor responses and maintaining a certain level of OS in cancer cells can improve therapeutic efficacy, ultimately leading to long-term patient survival [155, 156].

Traditional medicinal plants, dietary vegetables and fruits have emerged as valuable sources of anticancer treatments that help maintain optimal body homeostasis [155, 156]. Therefore, a combination of therapy involving phytochemicals that induce the production of ROS in cancer cells and anticancer drugs, can reactivate the signaling pathways initially targeted by chemotherapeutic agents. This approach can result in an additive or synergistic effect that helps suppress tumor resistance or recurrence. [157]. Specific phyto-extracts or phyto-agents demonstrate anticancer effects by disrupting the tumor-stromal microenvironment through ROS-induced OS [158–161]. Additionally, the anti-inflammatory properties of phytochemicals or phytoextracts offer a promising option for treating cancer-related inflammation and other inflammatory disorders, without causing the side effects often associated with anticancer drugs in patients.

For instance, broccoli sprout juice has demonstrated its capacity to protect the integrity of the intestinal barrier in a human intestinal cell model of gut inflammation. Berberine and mistletoe have shown potential cardioprotective properties by mitigating the cardiotoxic effects induced by chemotherapy drugs like doxorubicin or cyclophosphamide. Furthermore, piperine has the ability to prevent diarrhea by reducing excessive secretion of intestinal chloride, while green tea polyphenols can effectively regulate inflammation in the intestines.

4.3. *Regulation of immune cells in TME by phytochemicals*

Various natural substances derived from plants or nutrients like flavonoids, omega-3 fatty acids, vitamin C and zinc are believed to have the potential to boost the immune system. However, their precise roles as immune-strengthening agents or their ability to effectively combat inflammation and inhibit tumor development are not strongly supported by human studies [162–165]. Often, these alternative or complementary agents are not rigorously evaluated using established clinical outcomes, which are essential for gaining a better understanding of how nutritional components and phytochemicals can enhance the immune system's ability to eliminate tumors or hinder the immune evasion strategies of tumors. While some dietary supplements have shown the capacity to enhance the ability of NK cells to identify and destroy malfunctioning cells, such as infected or cancerous cells, these studies have not been extensively examined whether they increase the production of cytokines like IFN and TNF by T cells or reduce the secretion of immune-suppressive factors by tumors. Recent evidence also suggests that consuming dietary supplement doses significantly higher than normal nutrient exposures can be potentially harmful, and their use during cancer is strongly discouraged [166]. Certain dietary supplements have demonstrated the potential to aid NK cells in recognizing dysfunctional cells like cancerous or infected cells [166, 167]. Nevertheless, these alternative or complementary agents are still being studied, with the goal of establishing a standardized set of clinical outcomes. These outcomes are crucial for comprehending how these nutritional supplements or phytochemicals can enhance the body's ability to eliminate tumor cells and prevent immune evasion mechanisms employed by cancers.

5. Challenges, Opportunities, and Limitations

Extensive research over the past decades has explored the potential anticancer properties of phytochemicals, which are compounds found in dietary and medicinal plants. However, their clinical applications have been hindered by issues such as poor aqueous solubility and low retention in the body. Consequently, there is an urgent need for new pharmacological options. Phytochemicals have emerged as promising candidates for anticancer agents and chemotherapy adjuvants, supported by evidence of their molecular mechanisms, quality, safety and efficacy. Current strategies for evaluating the anticancer properties of phytochemicals focus on four key aspects: (1) regulation of cell cycle and apoptosis, (2) addressing drug resistance in cancer cells, (3) targeting specific molecular pathways involved in metastasis and carcinogenesis, and (4) anti-OS and anti-inflammatory activities. It is essential to give scientific attention to phytochemicals by continuously assessing their beneficial effects and their potential to combat HCC. However, it is important to note that around 80% of compounds fail in clinical trials due to lack of evidence regarding their bioavailability, efficacy and unforeseen toxicity to normal cells. While substantial data is required to validate these phytochemicals for clinical treatment, the foundation in this field appears promising.

6. Future Perspectives

Phytochemicals play a significant role in enhancing the anticancer effects, especially when combined with various chemotherapeutic agents. However, further research is needed to fully understand the detailed mechanisms by which phytochemicals modulate the tumor microenvironment (TME). This understanding is crucial for a successful transition from pre-clinical to clinical approaches, resulting in therapeutic compounds with high efficacy and stability. To harness the therapeutic potential of these compounds, there should be a strong focus on precisely identifying their targets within the TME. This means understanding how phytochemicals specifically interact with components such as tumor-associated macrophages or other cells residing in the TME, while minimizing off-target effects. In-depth investigations into molecular targets in different tissues and tumor types, coupled with studies on cellular signaling mechanisms *in vitro* and *in vivo* using animal models, are essential. Ultimately, this research will pave the way for the clinical application of phytochemicals in cancer prevention and the suppression of tumor initiation and metastasis. The use of predictive non-clinical and pre-clinical models, along with cutting-edge technologies like organ-on-a-chip systems that closely mimic human physiology, is vital for assessing the pharmacokinetics, pharmodynamics, efficacy, and safety of therapeutic phytochemicals. These approaches will help bring us closer to realizing the full potential of phytochemicals in cancer treatment.

7. Conclusion

HCC is a fast-growing and often lethal disease with limited treatment options. Thankfully, phytochemical compounds offer a promising avenue for HCC treatment, given their effectiveness, feasibility and compatibility with existing therapies. However, there are several challenges associated with the use of phytochemicals in HCC treatment. These challenges include primarily relying on *in vitro* studies, issues related to statistical power and population size, dosing concerns, and the need to assess the efficacy and potency of phytochemicals concerning their absorption, bioavailability and clearance in the body. Additionally, the lack of standardization techniques hinders the progression of many compounds into clinical studies. Despite these obstacles, phytochemicals have the potential to serve as alternative or complementary therapies alongside existing HCC chemotherapies. More research and focused evaluation are necessary to unlock their full potential and combat HCC effectively.

Acknowledgments

The authors thank Ms. Roshna Jose for helping with the illustration work.

References

1. Sung H, Ferlay J, Siegel RL, Laversanne M, Soerjomataram I, Jemal A, Bray F. Global cancer statistics 2020: GLOBOCAN estimates of incidence and mortality worldwide for 36 cancers in 185 countries. *Cancer J Clin.* 2021 May;71(3):209–249.
2. Huang Y, Wang T, Yang J, Wu X, Fan W, Chen J. Current strategies for the treatment of hepatocellular carcinoma by modulating the tumor microenvironment via nano-delivery systems: A review. *Int J Nanomed.* 2022;17:2335–2352.
3. Llovet JM, Kelley RK, Villanueva A, Singal AG, Pikarsky E, Roayaie S, et al. Hepatocellular carcinoma. *Nat Rev Dis Primers.* 2021;7:6. http://doi.org/10.1038/s41572-020-00240-3
4. Nishida N, Kudo M. Oncogenic signal and tumor microenvironment in hepatocellular carcinoma. *Oncology.* 2017;93(Suppl 1):160–164. http://doi.org/10.1159/000481246.
5. Jindal A, Thadi A, Shailubhai K. Hepatocellular carcinoma: Etiology and current and future drugs. *J Clin Exp Hepatol.* 2019;9(2):221–232. http://doi.org/10.1016/j.jceh.2019.01.004.
6. Stotz M, Gerger A, Haybaeck J, Kiesslich T, Bullock MD, Pichler M. Molecular targeted therapies in hepatocellular carcinoma: Past, present and future. *Anticancer Res.* 2015;35(11):5737–5744.

7. Spallanzani A, Orsi G, Andrikou K, Gelsomino F, Rimini M, Riggi L, Cascinu S. Lenvatinib as a therapy for unresectable hepatocellular carcinoma. *Expert Rev Anticancer Ther.* 2018;18:1069–1076.
8. Llovet JM, Ricci S, Mazzaferro V, Hilgard P, Gane E, Blanc JF, et al. Sorafenib in advanced hepatocellular carcinoma. *N Engl J Med.* 2008;359:378–390.
9. Rimassa L, Pressiani T, Merle P. Systemic treatment options in hepatocellular carcinoma. *Liver Cancer.* 2019;8:427–446.
10. Zheng A, Chevalier N, Calderoni M, Dubuis G, Dormond O, Ziros PG, Sykiotis GP, Widmann C. CRISPR/Cas9 genome-wide screening identifies KEAP1 as a sorafenib, lenvatinib, and regorafenib sensitivity gene in hepatocellular carcinoma. *Oncotarget.* 2019;10:7058–7070.
11. Ao J, Chiba T, Shibata S, Kurosugi A, Qiang N, Ma Y, et al. Acquisition of mesenchymal-like phenotypes and overproduction of angiogenic factors in lenvatinib-resistant hepatocellular carcinoma cells. *Biochem Biophys Res Commun.* 2021;549:171–178.
12. Tang W, Chen Z, Zhang W, Cheng Y, Zhang B, Wu F, et al. The mechanisms of sorafenib resistance in hepatocellular carcinoma: Theoretical basis and therapeutic aspects. *Signal Transduct Target Ther.* 2020;5:87.
13. Habib A, Desai K, Hickey R, Thornburg B, Lewandowski R, Salem R. Locoregional therapy of hepatocellular carcinoma. *Clin Liver Dis.* 2015;19:401–420.
14. Sangro B, Iñarrairaegui M, Bilbao JI. Radioembolization for hepatocellular carcinoma. *J Hepatol.* 2012;56:464–473.
15. Mbeunkui F, Johann DJ. Cancer and the tumor microenvironment: A review of an essential relationship. *Cancer Chemother Pharmacol.* 2009;63: 571–582.
16. Witz IP, Levy-Nissenbaum O. The tumor microenvironment in the post-PAGET era. *Cancer Lett.* 2006;242:1–10.
17. Junttila MR, de Sauvage FJ. Influence of tumour micro-environment heterogeneity on therapeutic response. *Nature.* 2013;501:346–354.
18. Quail DF, Joyce JA. Microenvironmental regulation of tumor progression and metastasis. *Nat Med.* 2013;19:1423–1437.

19. Salmon H, Remark R, Gnjatic S, Merad M. Host tissue determinants of tumour immunity. *Nat Rev Cancer.* 2019;19:215–227.
20. Lang H, Sotiropoulos GC, Domland M, Fruhauf NR, Paul A, Husing J, Malago M, Broelsch CE. Liver resection for hepatocellular carcinoma in non-cirrhotic liver without underlying viral hepatitis. *Br J Surg.* 2005;92(2):198–202.
21. Mohapatra P, Singh P, Singh D, Sahoo S, Sahoo SK. Phytochemical based nanomedicine: A panacea for cancer treatment, present status and future prospective. *OpenNano.* 2022;7:100055.
22. Rizwanullah M, Amin S, Mir SR, Fakhri KU, Rizvi MMA. Phytochemical based nanomedicines against cancer: Current status and future prospects. *J Drug Target.* 2018;26(9):731–752.
23. Rodriguez S, Skeet K, Mehmetoglu-Gurbuz T, Goldfarb M, Karri S, Rocha J, et al. Phytochemicals as an alternative or integrative option, in conjunction with conventional treatments for hepatocellular carcinoma. *Cancers.* 2021;13(22):5753.
24. Hernandez-Gea V, Toffanin S, Friedman SL, Llovet JM. Role of the microenvironment in the pathogenesis and treatment of hepatocellular carcinoma. *Gastroenterology.* 2013;144:512–527. http://doi.org/10.1053/j.gastro.2013.01.002.
25. Birgani MT, Carloni V. Tumor microenvironment, a paradigm in hepatocellular carcinoma progression and therapy. *Int J Mol Sci.* 2017;18:(2):405. http://doi.org/10.3390/ijms18020405.
26. Leonardi GC, Candido S, Cervello M, Nicolosi D, Raiti F, Travali S, et al. The tumor microenvironment in hepatocellular carcinoma. *Int J Oncol.* 2012;40(6):1733–1747. http://doi.org/10.3892/ijo.2012.1408.
27. Yang JD, Nakamura I, Roberts LR. The tumor microenvironment in hepatocellular carcinoma: Current status and therapeutic targets. *Semin Cancer Biol.* 2011;21(1):35–43. http://doi.org/10.1016/j.semcancer.2010.10.007.
28. Tsuchida T, Friedman SL. Mechanisms of hepatic stellate cell activation. *Nat Rev Gastroenterol Hepatol.* 2017;14:397–411. http://doi.org/10.1038/nrgastro.2017.38.
29. Yan Y, Zeng J, Xing L, Li C. Extra- and intra-cellular mechanisms of hepatic stellate cell activation. *Biomedicines.* 2021;9:1014. http://doi.org/10.3390/biomedicines9081014.

30. Mogler C, Konig C, Wieland M, Runge A, Besemfelder E, Komljenovic D, et al. Hepatic stellate cells limit hepatocellular carcinoma progression through the orphan receptor endosialin. *EMBO Mol Med.* 2017;9:741–749. http://doi.org/10.15252/emmm.201607222.
31. Amann T, Bataille F, Spruss T, Muhlbauer M, Gabele E, Scholmerich J, et al. Activated hepatic stellate cells promote tumorigenicity of hepatocellular carcinoma. *Cancer Sci.* 2009;100:646–653. http://doi.org/10.1111/j.1349-7006.2009.01087.x.
32. Ji J, Eggert T, Budhu A, Forgues M, Takai A, Dang H, et al. Hepatic stellate cell and monocyte interaction contributes to poor prognosis in hepatocellular carcinoma. *Hepatology.* 2015;62:481–495. http://doi.org/10.1002/hep.27822.
33. Zhang DY, Goossens N, Guo J, Tsai MC, Chou HI, Altunkaynak C, et al. A hepatic stellate cell gene expression signature associated with outcomes in hepatitis C cirrhosis and hepatocellular carcinoma after curative resection. *Gut.* 2016;65:1754–1764. http://doi.org/10.1136/gutjnl-2015-309655.
34. Ma T, Renz BW, Ilmer M, Koch D, Yang Y, Werner J, et al. Myeloid-derived suppressor cells in solid tumors. *Cells.* 2022;11:310. http://doi.org/10.3390/cells11020310.
35. Tcyganov E, Mastio J, Chen E, Gabrilovich DI. Plasticity of myeloid-derived suppressor cells in cancer. *Curr Opin Immunol.* 2018;51:76–82. http://doi.org/10.1016/j.coi.2018.03.009.
36. Srivastava MK, Sinha P, Clements VK, Rodriguez P, Ostrand-Rosenberg S. Myeloid-derived suppressor cells inhibit T-cell activation by depleting cystine and cysteine. *Cancer Res.* 2010;70:68–77. http://doi.org/10.1158/0008-5472.CAN-09-2587.
37. Liu M, Zhou J, Liu X, Feng Y, Yang W, Wu F, et al. Targeting monocyteintrinsic enhancer reprogramming improves immunotherapy efficacy in hepatocellular carcinoma. *Gut.* 2020;69:365–379. http://doi.org/10.1136/gutjnl-2018-317257.
38. Ganguly D, Chandra R, Karalis J, Teke M, Aguilera T, Maddipati R, et al. Cancer-associated fibroblasts: Versatile players in the tumor microenvironment. *Cancers.* 2020;12:2652. http://doi.org/10.3390/cancers1209265.

39. Liu T, Zhou L, Li D, Andl T, Zhang Y. Cancer-associated fibroblasts build and secure the tumor microenvironment. *Front Cell Dev Biol.* 2019;7:60. http://doi.org/10.3389/fcell.2019.00060.
40. Jia C, Wang G, Wang T, Fu B, Zhang Y, Huang L, et al. Cancer-associated fibroblasts induce epithelial-mesenchymal transition Via the transglutaminase 2-dependent IL-6/Il6r/STAT3 axis in hepatocellular carcinoma. *Int J Biol Sci.* 2020;16:2542–2558. http://doi.org/10.7150/ijbs.45446.
41. Bhowmick NA, Neilson EG, Moses HL. Stromal fibroblasts in cancer initiation and progression. *Nature.* 2004;432:332–337. http://doi.org/10.1038/nature03096.
42. Xu H, Zhao J, Li J, Zhu Z, Cui Z, Liu R, et al. Cancer associated fibroblast derived CCL5 promotes hepatocellular carcinoma metastasis through activating HIF1α/ZEB1 axis. *Cell Death Dis.* 2022;13:478. http://doi.org/10.1038/s41419-022-04935-1.
43. Lin ZY, Chuang YH, Chuang WL. Cancer-associated fibroblasts up-regulate CCL2, CCL26, IL6 and LOXL2 genes related to promotion of cancer progression in hepatocellular carcinoma cells. *BioMed Pharmacother.* 2012;66:525–529. http://doi.org/10.1016/j.biopha.2012.02.001.
44. Liu F, Zhang W, Yang F, Feng T, Zhou M, Yu Y, et al. Interleukin-6-stimulated progranulin expression contributes to the malignancy of hepatocellular carcinoma cells by activating mTOR signaling. *Sci Rep.* 2016;6:21260. http://doi.org/10.1038/srep21260.
45. Affo S, Yu LX, Schwabe RF. The role of cancer-associated fibroblasts and fibrosis in liver cancer. *Annu Rev Pathol.* 2017;12:153–186. http://doi.org/10.1146/annurevpathol-052016-10032.
46. Cassetta L, Pollard JW. Tumor-associated macrophages. *Curr Biol.* 2020;30:R246–R248. http://doi.org/10.1016/j.cub.2020.01.031.
47. Dong P, Ma L, Liu L, Zhao G, Zhang S, Dong L, et al. CD86^{+}/CD206^{+}, diametrically polarized tumor-associated macrophages, predict hepatocellular carcinoma patient prognosis. *Int J Mol Sci.* 2016;17:320. http://doi.org/10.3390/ijms17030320.
48. Fu LQ, Du WL, Cai MH, Yao JY, Zhao YY, Mou XZ. The roles of tumor associated macrophages in tumor angiogenesis and metastasis.

Cell Immunol. 2020;353:104119. http://doi.org/10.1016/j.cellimm.2020.104119.

49. Zhou J, Ding T, Pan W, Zhu LY, Li L, Zheng L. Increased intratumoral regulatory T cells are related to intratumoral macrophages and poor prognosis in hepatocellular carcinoma patients. *Int J Cancer.* 2009;125:1640–1648. http://doi.org/10.1002/ijc.24556.
50. Sung PS. Crosstalk between tumor-associated macrophages and neighboring cells in hepatocellular carcinoma. *Clin Mol Hepatol.* 2021;28:333–350. http://doi.org/10.3350/cmh.2021.030.
51. Wu Q, Zhou W, Yin S, Zhou Y, Chen T, Qian J, et al. Blocking triggering receptor expressed on myeloid cells-1-Positive tumor-associated macrophages induced by hypoxia reverses immunosuppression and anti-programmed cell death ligand 1 resistance in liver cancer. *Hepatology.* 2019;70:198–214. http://doi.org/10.1002/hep.30593.
52. Zhang W, Zhu XD, Sun HC, Xiong YQ, Zhuang PY, Xu HX, et al. Depletion of tumor-associated macrophages enhances the effect of sorafenib in metastatic liver cancer models by antimetastatic and antiangiogenic effects. *Clin Cancer Res.* 2010;16:3420–3430. http://doi.org/10.1158/1078-0432.CCR-09-2904.
53. Dong N, Shi X, Wang S, Gao Y, Kuang Z, Xie Q, et al. M2 macrophages mediate sorafenib resistance by secreting HGF in a feed-forward manner in hepatocellular carcinoma. *Br J Cancer.* 2019;121:22–33. http://doi.org/10.1038/s41416-019-0482-x.
54. Kalafati L, Mitroulis I, Verginis P, Chavakis T, Kourtzelis I. Neutrophils as orchestrators in tumor development and metastasis formation. *Front Oncol.* 2020;10:581457. http://doi.org/10.3389/fonc.2020.581457.
55. Fridlender ZG, Sun J, Kim S, Kapoor V, Cheng G, Ling L, et al. Polarization of tumor-associated neutrophil phenotype by TGF-beta: "N1" versus "N2" tan. *Cancer Cell.* 2009;16:183–194. http://doi.org/10.1016/j.ccr.2009.06.017.
56. Li YW, Qiu SJ, Fan J, Zhou J, Gao Q, Xiao YS, et al. Intratumoral neutrophils: A poor prognostic factor for hepatocellular carcinoma following resection. *J Hepatol.* 2011;54:497–505. http://doi.org/10.1016/j.jhep.2010.07.044.
57. Zhou S-L, Zhou Z-J, Hu Z-Q, Huang X-W, Wang Z, Chen E-B, et al. Tumor-associated neutrophils recruit macrophages and t-regulatory

cells to promote progression of hepatocellular carcinoma and resistance to Sorafenib. *Gastroenterology.* 2016;150:1646–1658.e17.

58. Sun R, Xiong Y, Liu H, Gao C, Su L, Weng J, et al. Tumor-associated neutrophils suppress antitumor immunity of NK cells through the PD-L1/PD-1 axis. *Transl Oncol.* 2020;13:100825. http://doi.org/10.1016/j.tranon.2020.100825.
59. Stockis J, Roychoudhuri R, Halim TYF. Regulation of regulatory T cells in cancer. *Immunology.* 2019;157:219–231. http://doi.org/10.1111/imm.13064.
60. Han Y, Yang Y, Chen Z, Jiang Z, Gu Y, Liu Y, et al. Human hepatocellular carcinoma-infiltrating $CD4^+CD69^+Foxp3^-$ regulatory T cell suppresses T cell response via membrane-bound TGF-β1. *J Mol Med (Berl).* 2014;92:539–550. http://doi.org/10.1007/s00109-014-1143-4.
61. Shi C, Chen Y, Chen Y, Yang Y, Bing W, Qi J. $CD4^+$ $Cd25^+$ regulatory T cells promote hepatocellular carcinoma invasion Via TGF-Beta1-Induced epithelial-mesenchymal transition. *Onco Targets Ther.* 2019;12:279–289. http://doi.org/10.2147/OTT.S172417.
62. Gao Y, You M, Fu J, Tian M, Zhong X, Du C, et al. Intratumoral stem-like $CCR4^+$ regulatory T cells orchestrate the immunosuppressive microenvironment in HCC associated with hepatitis B. *J Hepatol.* 2022;76:148–159. http://doi.org/10.1016/j.jhep.2021.08.029.
63. Ye L, Zhang Q, Cheng Y, Chen X, Wang G, Shi M, et al. Tumor-derived exosomal HMGB1 fosters hepatocellular carcinoma immune evasion by promoting $TIM\text{-}1^+$ regulatory B cell expansion. *J Immunother Cancer.* 2018;6:145. http://doi.org/10.1186/s40425-018-0451-6.
64. Wang W, Wang Z, Qin Y, Tang G, Cai G, Liu Y, et al. Th17, synchronically increased with T_{regs} and B_{regs}, promoted by tumour cells via cell-contact in primary hepatic carcinoma. *Clin Exp Immunol.* 2018;192:181–192. http://doi.org/10.1111/cei.13094.
65. Zhang JP, Yan J, Xu J, Pang XH, Chen MS, Li L, et al. Increased intratumoral IL-17-Producing cells correlate with poor survival in hepatocellular carcinoma patients. *J Hepatol.* 2009;50:980–989. http://doi.org/10.1016/j.jhep.2008.12.03.

66. Tsai CN, Yu SC, Lee CW, Pang JS, Wu CH, Lin SE, et al. SOX4 activates CXCL12 in hepatocellular carcinoma cells to modulate endothelial cell migration and angiogenesis *in vivo*. *Oncogene*. 2020;39: 4695–4710. http://doi.org/10.1038/s41388-020-1319-z.
67. Dai W, Wang Y, Yang T, Wang J, Wu W, Gu J. Downregulation of exosomal CLEC3B in hepatocellular carcinoma promotes metastasis and angiogenesis via AMPK and VEGF signals. *Cell Commun Signal*. 2019;17:113. http://doi.org/10.1186/s12964-019-0423-6.
68. Benetti A, Berenzi A, Gambarotti M, Garrafa E, Gelati M, Dessy E, et al. Transforming growth factor-Beta1 and CD105 promote the migration of hepatocellular carcinoma-derived endothelium. *Cancer Res*. 2008;68:8626–8634. http://doi.org/10.1158/0008-5472.CAN-08-121.
69. Xiong YQ, Sun HC, Zhang W, Zhu XD, Zhuang PY, Zhang JB, et al. Human hepatocellular carcinoma tumor-derived endothelial cells manifest increased angiogenesis capability and drug resistance compared with normal endothelial cells. *Clin Cancer Res*. 2009;15:4838–4846. http://doi.org/10.1158/1078-0432.CCR-08-2780.
70. Huang J, Zhang L, Wan D, Zhou L, Zheng S, Lin S, et al. Extracellular matrix and its therapeutic potential for cancer treatment. *Signal Transduct Target Ther*. 2021;6:153. http://doi.org/10.1038/s41392-021-00544-0.
71. Popova NV, Jucker M. The functional role of extracellular matrix proteins in cancer. *Cancers*. 2022;14:238. http://doi.org/10.3390/cancers14010238.
72. Wu SD, Ma YS, Fang Y, Liu LL, Fu D, Shen XZ. Role of the microenvironment in hepatocellular carcinoma development and progression. *Cancer Treat Rev*. 2012;38:218–225. http://doi.org/10.1016/j.ctrv.2011.06.010.
73. Kao J-T, Lai H-C, Tsai S-M, Lin P-C, Chuang P-H, Yu C-J, et al. Rather than interleukin-27, interleukin-6 expresses positive correlation with liver severity in naïve hepatitis B infection patients. *Liver Int*. 2012;32:928–936.
74. Lai S-C, Su Y-T, Chi C-C, Kuo Y-C, Lee K-F, Wu Y-C, et al. DNMT3b/OCT4 expression confers sorafenib resistance and poor prognosis of hepatocellular carcinoma through IL-6/STAT3 regulation. *J Exp Clin Cancer Res*. 2019;38:474.

75. Zhang J, Wang W-L, Li Q, Qiao Q. Expression of transforming growth factor-alpha and hepatitis B surface antigen in human hepatocellular carcinoma tissues and its significance. *World J Gastroenterol.* 2004;10:830–833.
76. Marino M, Scuderi F, Mannella F, Bartoccioni E. TGF-B1 and IL-10 modulate IL-1β-Induced membrane and soluble ICAM-1 in human myoblasts. *J Neuroimmunol.* 2003;134:151–157.
77. Gonzalez-Sanchez E, Vaquero J, Férnandez-Barrena MG, Lasarte JJ, Avila MA, Sarobe P, et al. The TGF-β pathway: A pharmacological target in hepatocellular carcinoma? *Cancers.* 2021;13:3248.
78. Shakiba E, Ramezani M, Sadeghi M. Evaluation of serum interleukin-6 levels in hepatocellular carcinoma patients: A systematic review and meta-analysis. *Clin Exp Hepatol.* 2018;4:182–190.
79. Chau GY, Wu CW, Lui WY, Chang TJ, Kao HL, Wu LH, et al. Serum interleukin-10 but not interleukin-6 is related to clinical outcome in patients with resectable hepatocellular carcinoma. *Ann Surg.* 2000;231:552–558.
80. Shakiba E, Ramezani M, Sadeghi M. Evaluation of serum interleukin-10 levels in hepatocellular carcinoma patients: A systematic review and meta-analysis. *Clin Exp Hepatol.* 2018;4:35–40.
81. Tiegs G, Horst AK. TNF in the liver: Targeting a central player in inflammation. In: *Seminars in Immunopathology.* Springer: Berlin/Heidelberg, Germany, 2022.
82. Dimri M, Satyanarayana A. Molecular signaling pathways and therapeutic targets in hepatocellular carcinoma. *Cancers.* 2020;12(2):491.
83. Kudo M. Signaling pathway and molecular-targeted therapy for hepatocellular carcinoma. *Dig Dis.* 2011;29(3):289–302.
84. Dhanasekaran R, Bandoh S, Roberts LR. Molecular pathogenesis of hepatocellular carcinoma and impact of therapeutic advances. *F1000Res.* 2016:5;F1000.
85. Wang K, Qiu X, Zhao Y, Wang H, Chen L. The Wnt/β-catenin signaling pathway in the tumor microenvironment of hepatocellular carcinoma. *Cancer Biol Med.* 2022;19(3):305.
86. Marisi G, Cucchetti A, Ulivi P, Canale M, Cabibbo G, Solaini L, et al. Ten years of sorafenib in hepatocellular carcinoma: Are there any predictive and/or prognostic markers? *World J Gastroenterol.* 2018;24:4152–4163.

87. West EE, Kunz N, Kemper C. Complement and human T cell metabolism: Location, location, location. *Immunol Rev.* 2020;295:68–81.
88. Roumenina LT, Daugan MV, Petitprez F, Sautes-Fridman C, Fridman WH. Context-dependent roles of complement in cancer. *Nat Rev Cancer.* 2019;19:698–715.
89. Seol HS, Lee SE, Song JS, Rhee JK, Singh SR, Chang S, Jang SJ. Complement proteins C7 and CFH control the stemness of liver cancer cells via LSF-1. *Cancer Lett.* 2016;372:24–35.
90. Holers VM. Complement and its receptors: New insights into human disease. *Annu Rev Immunol.* 2014;32:433–459.
91. Zha H, Han X, Zhu Y, Yang F, Li Y, Li Q, Guo B, Zhu B. Blocking C5aR signaling promotes the anti-tumor efficacy of PD-1/PD-L1 blockade. *Oncoimmunology.* 2017;6:e1349587. http://doi.org/10.1080/2162402X.2017.1349587.
92. Li Z, Meng X, Wu P, Zha C, Han B, Li L, et al. Glioblastoma cell-derived lncRNA-containing exosomes induce microglia to produce complement C5, promoting chemotherapy resistance. *Cancer Immunol Res.* 2021;9:1383–1399. http://doi.org/10.1158/2326-6066.CIR-21-0258.
93. Ricklin D, Lambris JD. Complement-targeted therapeutics. *Nat Biotechnol.* 2007;25(11):1265–1275. http://doi.org/10.1038/nbt1342.
94. Lee JH, Lim YS, Yeon JE, Song TJ, Yu SJ, Gwak GY, et al. Sustained efficacy of adjuvant immunotherapy with cytokine-induced killer cells for hepatocellular carcinoma: An extended 5-year follow-up. *Cancer Immunol Immunother.* 2019;68(1):23–32.
95. Lee JH, Lim YS, Yeon JE, Song TJ, Yu SJ, Gwak GY, et al. Adjuvant immunotherapy with autologous cytokine-induced killer cells for hepatocellular carcinoma. *Gastroenterology.* 2015;148(7):1383–1391 e1386.
96. Visvader JE, Lindeman GJ. Cancer stem cells in solid tumours: Accumulating evidence and unresolved questions. *Nat Rev Cancer.* 2008;8:755–768. http://doi.org/10.1038/nrc2499.
97. Sun HR, Wang S, Yan SC, Zhang Y, Nelson PJ, Jia HL, et al. Therapeutic strategies targeting cancer stem cells and their microenvironment. *Front Oncol.* 2019;9:1104.
98. Ristow M. Oxidative metabolism in cancer growth. *Curr Opin Clin Nutr Metab Care.* 2006;9:339–345.

99. Zhang G, Yang P, Guo P, Miele L, Sarkar FH, Wang Z, et al. Unraveling the mystery of cancer metabolism in the genesis of tumor-initiating cells and development of cancer. *Biochim Biophys Acta.* 2013;1836:49–59.
100. Yoshida M, Yamashita T, Okada H, Oishi N, Nio K, Hayashi T, et al. Sorafenib suppresses extrahepatic metastasis de novo in hepatocellular carcinoma through inhibition of mesenchymal cancer stem cells characterized by the expression of CD90. *Sci Rep.* 2017;71:11292. http://doi.org/10.1038/s41598-017-11848-z.
101. Forbes-Hernández TY, Giampieri F, Gasparrini M, Mazzoni L, Quiles JL, Alvarez-Suarez JM, Battino M. The effects of bioactive compounds from plant foods on mitochondrial function: A focus on apoptotic mechanisms. *Food Chem Toxicol.* 2014;68:154–182.
102. Benito J, Zeng Z, Konopleva M, Wilson WR. Targeting hypoxia in the leukemia microenvironment. *Int J Hematol Oncol.* 2013;2(4):279–288.
103. Catalano V, Turdo A, Di Franco S, Dieli F, Todaro M, Stassi, G. Tumor and its microenvironment: A synergistic interplay. In: *Seminars in Cancer Biology* (Vol. 23, pp. 522–532). Academic Press, 2013.
104. Hjelmeland AB, Wu Q, Heddleston JM, Choudhary GS, MacSwords J, Lathia JD, et al. Acidic stress promotes a glioma stem cell phenotype. *Cell Death Differ.* 2011;18(5):829–840.
105. Mao Q, ZhangY, Fu X, Xue J, Guo W, Meng M, et al. A tumor hypoxic niche protects human colon cancer stem cells from chemotherapy. *J Cancer Res Clin Oncol.* 2013;139:211–222.
106. Vera-Ramirez L, Ramirez-Tortosa M, Perez-Lopez P, Granados-Principal S, Battino M, Quiles JL. Long-term effects of systemic cancer treatment on DNA oxidative damage: The potential for targeted therapies. *Cancer Lett.* 2012;327(1–2):134–141.
107. Pistollato F, Giampieri F, Battino, M. The use of plant-derived bioactive compounds to target cancer stem cells and modulate tumor microenvironment. *Food Chem Toxicol.* 2015;75:58–70.
108. Choudhari AS, Mandave PC, Deshpande M, Ranjekar P, Prakash O. Phytochemicals in cancer treatment: From preclinical studies to clinical practice. *Front Pharmacol.* 2019;10:1614. https:// doi.org/10.3389/fphar.2019.01614.

109. Block KI, Gyllenhaal C, Lowe L, Amedei A, Amin ARMR, Amin A, et al. Designing a broad-spectrum integrative approach for cancer prevention and treatment. *Semin Cancer Biol.* 2015;35(Suppl):S276–S304. https://doi.org/10.1016/j.semcancer.2015.09.007.
110. Zubair H, Azim S, Ahmad A, Khan MA, Patel GK, Singh S, Singh, AP. Cancer chemoprevention by phytochemicals: Nature's healing touch. *Molecules.* 2017;22(3):395. https://doi.org/10.3390/molecules22030395.
111. Hewlings SJ, Kalman DS. Curcumin: A review of its effects on human health. *Foods.* 2017;6(10):92. https://doi.org/10.3390/foods6100092.
112. Stanic Z. Curcumin, a compound from natural sources, a true scientific challenge — A review. *Plant Foods Hum Nutr.* 2017;72(1):1–12. https://doi.org/10.1007/s11130-016-0590-1.
113. Chen SS, Michael A, Butler-Manuel SA. Advances in the treatment of ovarian cancer: A potential role of anti-inflammatory phytochemicals. *Dis Med.* 2012;13(68):7–17.
114. Cao L, Xiao X, Lei J, Duan W, Ma Q, Li W. Curcumin inhibits hypoxia-induced epithelialmesenchymal transition in pancreatic cancer cells via suppression of the hedgehog signaling pathway. *Oncol Rep.* 2016;35(6):3728–3734. https://doi.org/10.3892/or.2016.4709.
115. Shehzad A, Lee YS. Molecular mechanisms of curcumin action: signal transduction. *Biofactors.* 2013 Jan;39(1):27–36.
116. Nagle DG, Ferreira D, Zhou YD. Epigallocatechin-3-gallate (EGCG): chemical and biomedical perspectives. *Phytochemistry.* 2006;67(17):1849–55.
117. Tang Y, Cao J, Cai Z, An H, Li Y, Peng Y, et al. Epigallocatechin gallate induces chemopreventive effects on rats with diethylnitrosamine-induced liver cancer via inhibition of cell division cycle 25A. *Mol Med Rep.* 2020;22:3873–3885.
118. Bimonte S, Albino V, Piccirillo M, Nasto A, Molino C, Palaia R, Cascella M. Epigallocatechin-3-gallate in the prevention and treatment of hepatocellular carcinoma: experimental findings and translational perspectives. *Drug Des Devel Ther.* 2019;12:611–21.
119. Chen L, Ye HL, Zhang G, Yao WM, Chen XZ, Zhang FC, Liang G. Autophagy inhibition contributes to the synergistic interaction between

EGCG and doxorubicin to kill the hepatoma Hep3B cells. *PLOS ONE*. 2014;9:e85771.

120. Sojoodi M, Wei L, Erstad DJ, Yamada S, Fujii T, Hirschfield H, et al. Epigallocatechin gallate induces hepatic stellate cell senescence and attenuates development of hepatocellular carcinoma. *Cancer Prev. Res.* 2020;13:497–508.
121. Liao S, Lin J, Liu J, Chen T, Xu M, Zheng J. Chemoprevention of elite tea variety CFT-1 rich in EGCG against chemically induced liver cancer in rats. *Food Sci Nutr*. 2019;7:2647–2665.
122. Agioutantis PC, Kotsikoris V, Kolisis FN, Loutrari H. RNA-seq data analysis of stimulated hepatocellular carcinoma cells treated with epigallocatechin gallate and fisetin reveals target genes and action mechanisms. *Comput Struct Biotechnol J*. 2020;18:686–695.
123. Kang Q, Tong Y, Gowd V, Wang M, Chen F, Cheng KW. Oral administration of EGCG solution equivalent to daily achievable dosages of regular tea drinkers effectively suppresses miR483-3p induced metastasis of hepatocellular carcinoma cells in mice. *Food Funct*. 2021;12:3381–3392.
124. Yang H, Wang M, Sun H, Zhu S, Jin J. Synergetic effect of EP1 receptor antagonist and (-)-epigallocatechin-3-gallate in hepatocellular carcinoma. *Pharmacology*. 2019;104:267–275.
125. Burns J, Yokota T, Ashihara H, Lean ME, Crozier A. Plant foods and herbal sources of resveratrol. *J Agric Food Chem*. 2002;50(11):3337–3340. https://doi.org/10.1021/jf0112973.
126. Gambini, J, Ingles M, Olaso G, Lopez-Grueso R, Bonet-Costa V, Gimeno-Mallench L, et al. Properties of resveratrol: *In vitro* and *in vivo* studies about metabolism, bioavailability, and biological effects in animal models and humans. *Oxid Med Cell Longev*. 2015;2015:837042. https://doi.org/10.1155/2015/837042.
127. Al-Ani B. Resveratrol inhibits proteinase-activated receptor-2-induced release of soluble vascular endothelial growth factor receptor-1 from human endothelial cells. *EXCLI J*. 2013;12:598–604.
128. Zhang Q, Huang H, Zheng F, Liu H, Qiu F, Chen Y, Liang CL, Dai Z. Resveratrol exerts antitumor effects by downregulating CD8. *Oncoimmunology*. 2020;9:1829346.

129. Malhotra A, Bath S, Elbarbry F. An organ system approach to explore the antioxidative, anti-inflammatory, and cytoprotective actions of resveratrol. *Oxid Med Cell Longev.* 2015;2015:803971.
130. Aja I, Ruiz-Larrea MB, Courtois A, Krisa S, Richard T, Ruiz-Sanz JI. Screening of natural stilbene oligomers from *Vitis vinifera* for anticancer activity on human hepatocellular carcinoma cells. *Antioxidants.* 2020;9:469.
131. Dai H, Li M, Yang W, Sun X, Wang P, Wang X, et al. Resveratrol inhibits the malignant progression of hepatocellular carcinoma via MARCH1-induced regulation of PTEN/AKT signaling. *Aging.* 2020;12:11717–11731.
132. Rawat D, Chhonker SK, Naik RA, Koiri RK. Modulation of antioxidant enzymes, SIRT1 and NF-κB by resveratrol and nicotinamide in alcohol-aflatoxin B1-induced hepatocellular carcinoma. *J Biochem Mol Toxicol.* 2021;35:e22625.
133. Bishayee A, Barnes KF, Bhatia D, Darvesh AS, Carroll RT. Resveratrol suppresses oxidative stress and inflammatory response in diethylnitrosamine-initiated rat hepatocarcinogenesis. *Cancer Prev Res.* 2010;3:753–763.
134. Dai W, Wang F, Lu J, Xia Y, He L, Chen K, et al. By reducing hexokinase 2, resveratrol induces apoptosis in HCC cells addicted to aerobic glycolysis and inhibits tumor growth in mice. *Oncotarget.* 2015;6:13703–13717.
135. Karabekir SC, Özgörgülü A. Possible protective effects of resveratrol in hepatocellular carcinoma. *Iran J Basic Med Sci.* 2020;23:71–78.
136. Rahman M, Almalki WH, Afzal O, Alfawaz Altamimi AS, Kazmi I, Al-Abbasi FA, et al. Cationic solid lipid nanoparticles of resveratrol for hepatocellular carcinoma treatment: Systematic optimization, in vitro characterization and preclinical investigation. *Int J Nanomed.* 2020;15:9283–9299.
137. Jagwani S, Jalalpure S, Dhamecha D, Jadhav K, Bohara R. Pharmacokinetic and pharmacodynamic evaluation of resveratrol loaded cationic liposomes for targeting hepatocellular carcinoma. *ACS Biomater Sci Eng.* 2020;6:4969–4984.
138. Hafeez BB, Zhong W, Fischer JW, Mustafa A, Shi X, Meske L, Verma AK. Plumbagin, a medicinal plant (*Plumbago zeylanica*)-derived

1,4-naphthoquinone, inhibits growth and metastasis of human prostate cancer PC-3M-luciferase cells in an orthotopic xenograft mouse model. *Mol Oncol.* 2013;7(3):428–439. https://doi.org/10.1016/j.molonc.2012.12.001.

139. Nair SV, Baranwal G, Chatterjee M, Sachu A, Vasudevan AK, Bose C, Banerji A, Biswas R. Antimicrobial activity of plumbagin, a naturally occurring naphthoquinone from *Plumbago rosea*, against *Staphylococcus aureus* and *Candida albicans. Int J Med Microbiol.* 2016;306(4):237–248. https://doi.org/10.1016/j.ijmm.2016.05.004.
140. Wei YF, Yang QI, Zhang Y, Zhao TJ, Liu XM, Zhong J, et al. Plumbagin restrains hepatocellular carcinoma angiogenesis by suppressing the migration and invasion of tumor-derived vascular endothelial cells. *Oncotarget.* 2017;8(9):15230–15241. https://doi.org/10.18632/oncotarget.14774.
141. Gu Y, Zhu CF, Iwamoto H, Chen JS. Genistein inhibits invasive potential of human hepatocellular carcinoma by altering cell cycle, apoptosis, and angiogenesis. *World J Gastroenterol.* 2005;11:6512–6517.
142. Tong Y, Wang M, Huang H, Zhang J, Huang Y, Chen Y, Pan H. Inhibitory effects of genistein in combination with gefitinib on the hepatocellular carcinoma Hep3B cell line. *Exp Ther Med.* 2019;18: 3793–3800.
143. Lim JS, Lee SH, Lee SR, Lim H-J, Roh Y-S, Won EJ, et al. Inhibitory effects of Aucklandia lappa Decne. Extract on inflammatory and oxidative responses in LPS-treated macrophages. *Molecules.* 2020;25(6):1336. http://doi.org/10.3390/molecules25061336.
144. Rahman Md. A, Dhar DK, Yamaguchi E, Maruyama S, Sato T, et al. Coexpression of inducible nitric oxide synthase and COX-2 in hepatocellular carcinoma and surrounding liver. *Clin Cancer Res.* 2001;7(5):1325–1332. http://clincancerres.aacrjournals.org/content/7/5/1325.
145. Tsang SW, Zhang H, Lin C, Xiao H, Wong M, Shang H, et al. Rhein, a natural anthraquinone derivative, attenuates the activation of pancreatic stellate cells and ameliorates pancreatic fibrosis in mice with experimental chronic pancreatitis. *PLoS One.* 2013;8(12):e82201. https://doi.org/10.1371/journ al.pone.0082201.

146. Lin Y, Shi R, Wang X, Shen HM. Luteolin, a flavonoid with potential for cancer prevention and therapy. *Curr Cancer Drug Targets.* 2008;8(7): 634–646. https://doi.org/10.2174/156800908786241050.
147. Anand David AV, Arulmoli R, Parasuraman S. Overviews of biological importance of quercetin: A bioactive flavonoid. *Pharmacogn Rev.* 2016;10(20):84–89. https://doi.org/10.4103/0973-7847.194044.
148. Wing Ying Cheung C, Gibbons N, Wayne Johnson D, Lawrence Nicol D. Silibinin-a promising new treatment for cancer. *Anti-Cancer Agents in Medicinal Chemistry (Formerly Curr Med Chem Anticancer Agents).* 2010;10(3):186–95.
149. Wang J, Zhang J, Shi Y, Xu C, Zhang C, Wong YK, Lee YM, Krishna S, He Y, Lim TK, Sim W, Hua Z-C, Shen H-M, Lin Q. Mechanistic investigation of the specific anticancer property of artemisinin and its combination with aminolevulinic acid for enhanced anticolorectal cancer activity. *ACS Cent Sci.* 2017;3(7):743–750. https://doi.org/10.1021/acscentsci.7b00156.
150. Wang Z, Li Z, Ye Y, Xie L, Li W. Oxidative stress and liver cancer: Etiology and therapeutic targets. *Oxid Med Cell Longev.* 2016;2016: 7891574.
151. Toyokuni S. Novel aspects of oxidative stress-associated carcinogenesis. *Antioxid Redox Signal.* 2006;8(7–8):1373–1377.
152. Reuter S, Gupta SC, Chaturvedi MM, Aggarwal BB. Oxidative stress, inflammation, and cancer: How are they linked?. *Free Radic Biol Med.* 2010;49(11):1603–1616.
153. Simon AR, Rai U, Fanburg BL, Cochran BH. Activation of the JAK-STAT pathway by reactive oxygen species. *Am J Physiol Cell Physiol.* 1998;275(6):C1640–C1652.
154. Miki H, Funato Y. Regulation of intracellular signalling through cysteine oxidation by reactive oxygen species. *J Biochem.* 2012;151:255–261.
155. Singh TU, Lingaraju MC, Garg G, Sharma M, Parida S, Kumar D. Phytocompounds-Based Approaches to Combat Oxidative Stress in Cancer. In *Handbook of Oxidative Stress in Cancer: Mechanistic Aspects* 2021; 1–15. Singapore: Springer Singapore.
156. Agbarya A, Ruimi N, Epelbaum R, Ben-Arye E, Mahajna J. Natural products as potential cancer therapy enhancers: A preclinical update.

SAGE Open Med. 2014;2:2050312114546924. http://doi.org/10.1177/2050312114546924.

157. Apaya MK, Chang MT, Shyur LF. Phytomedicine polypharmacology: Cancer therapy through modulating the tumor microenvironment and oxylipin dynamics. *Pharmacol Ther.* 2016;162:58–68.
158. Lee WL, Shyur LF. Deoxyelephantopin impedes mammary adenocarcinoma cell motility by inhibiting calpain-mediated adhesion dynamics and inducing reactive oxygen species and aggresome formation. *Free Radic Bio Med.* 2012;52:1423–1436.
159. Huang CC, Lo CP, Chiu CY, Shyur LF. Deoxyelephantopin, a novel multifunctional agent, suppresses mammary tumour growth and lung metastasis and doubles survival time in mice. *Br J Pharmacol.* 2010;159:856–871.
160. Feng JH, Nakagawa-Goto K, Lee KH, Shyur LF. A novel plant sesquiterpene lactone derivative, DETD-35, suppresses BRAFV600E mutant melanoma growth and overcomes acquired vemurafenib resistance in mice. *Mol Cancer Ther.* 2016;15:1163–1176.
161. Nakagawa-Goto K, Chen JY, Cheng YT, Lee W-L, Takeya M, Saito Y, et al. Novel sesquiterpene lactone analogues as potent anti-breast cancer agents. *Mol Oncol.* 2016;10:921–937.
162. Middleton Jr E, Kandaswami C. Effects of flavonoids on immune and inflammatory cell functions. *Biochem Pharmacol.* 1992;43:1167–1179.
163. Calder PC. Immunomodulation by omega-3 fatty acids. *Prostaglandins Leukot Essent Fatty Acids.* 2007;77:327–335.
164. Dardenne M. Zinc and immune function. *Eur J Clin Nutr.* 2002;56:520–523.
165. Calder PC, Kew S. The immune system: A target for functional foods? *Br J Nutr.* 2002;88:S165–S176.
166. Kodama N, Komuta K, Nanba H. Effect of Maitake (*Grifola frondosa*) D-fraction on the activation of NK cells in cancer patients. *J Med Food.* 2003;6:371–377.
167. Hughes DA. Dietary carotenoids and human immune function. *Nutrition.* 2001;10:823–827.

https://doi.org/10.1142/9789811293320_0002

Chapter 2

Phytochemicals in Liver Cancer Prevention

Shelmi Antony[1], Nisha N C[2] and Jayesh Antony[3*]

[1]*Assistant Professor in Zoology, Assumption College Autonomous, Changanassery, Kerala, India*
[2]*Assistant Professor in Botany, Assumption College Autonomous, Changanassery, Kerala, India*
[3*]*Assistant Professor in Zoology, St Thomas College Autonomous Palai, Kottayam, Kerala, India*

Table of Contents

*Corresponding author: E-mail address: jayesha.zoo@stcp.ac.in

Abbreviations

WHO — World Health Organization
HCC — Hepatocellular carcinoma
HCV — Hepatitis C virus
NASH — Non-alcoholic steatohepatitis
NAFLD — Non-alcoholic fatty liver disease (NAFLD)
AAT — Alpha 1-antitrypsin
HDV — Hepatitis D virus
HBV — Hepatitis B virus
HIV — Human immunodeficiency virus
SREBP — Sterol regulatory element-binding protein
PPAR — Peroxisome proliferator-activated receptor γ
VEGF — Vascular endothelial growth factor
EGF — Epidermal growth factor
HGF — Hepatocyte growth factor
JAK — Janus kinase
ALD — Alcoholic liver disease
RFA — Radio frequency ablation
PEIT — Percutaneous ethanol injection

TACE — Transarterial chemoembolization
MTT — Molecular targeted therapy
EPI — Expanded program of immunization
AFB1 — Aflatoxin B1
IFN — Interferon
HMG-CoA — 3-hydroxy-3-methylglutaryl coenzyme A
$[Ca]^{++}$ — Calcium ion
2-AAF — 2-Acetyl amino fluorene
CYP 2E1 — Cytochrome p450 2E1
AAD — 7-amino actinomycin D
ACP — Acid phosphatase
ADMET — Absorption, distribution, metabolism, excretion, and toxicity
ADP — Adenosyl diphosphate
AFP — Alpha-fetoprotein
AH109A — Liver carcinoma cell line
AIF — Allograft inflammatory factor
Akt — Protein kinase B
ALP — Alkaline phosphatase
ALT — Alanine aminotransferase
AMPK — AMP-activated kinase
AP-1 — Activator protein 1
Apaf-1 — Apoptotic protease activating factor-1
AST — Aspartate aminotransferase
ATG — Autophagy related
ATG5 — Autophagy protein 5
ATG7 — Autophagy protein 7
ATM — Ataxia telangiectasia mutated
ATPase — Adenosine tri phosphatase
B6C3F1 — A hybrid mouse
Bad — Bcl-2 associated agonist of cell death
Bak — B-cell lymphoma 2 antagonistic/killer
BALB/c — Inbred mice strain
Bax — Bcl-2-associated X
Bcl-2 — B-cell lymphoma 2
Bcl-XL — B-cell lymphoma extra large

BEL — Hepatic cancer cell line
BEL-7402 — Hepatic cancer cell line
BHA — Butylated hydroxyanisole
BHC — Benzene hexachloride
Bim — BCL-2-interacting mediator
BiP — Binding immunoglobulin protein
BSG — Breast Safeguard
C3H/He mice — Mouse strain
Caco-2 — Cancer coli
CAT — Catalase
CCl 4 — Carbon tetra chloride
CD — Conjugated dienes
CD-1 mice — Albino outbred mouse strain
CDC2 — Cyclin-dependent kinase 1
Cdc25A — Cell division cycle 25 A
Cdk2 — Cyclin-dependent kinase 2
Cdk4 — Cyclin-dependent kinase 4
CEA — Carcinoembryonic antigen
c-Fos — Proto-oncogene transcription factor subunit
CHOP — C/EBP homologous protein
CIP1 — Cyclin-dependent kinase inhibitor
c-Jun — Oncogenic transcription factor
c-Myc — Cellular myelocytomatosis
COX2 — Cyclooxygenase 2
Cqn — Chloroquine
CX32 — Connexin 32
Cx43 — Connexin 43
CYP2E1 — Cytochrome P450 family 2 subfamily E member 1
CYP2J2 — Cytochrome P450 family 2 subfamily J member 2
Cyt c — Cytochrome C
DAB — 3′-methyl-4-dimethyl aminoazobenzene
DEN — Diethylnitrosamine
DENA — Diethylnitrosamine
DNA — Deoxyribonucleic acid
DNMT1 — DNA methyltransferase 1
DPPH — 2,2-diphenyl-1-picrylhydrazyl

DR3 — Death receptor 3
E2F — E2 transcription factor
EMT — Epithelial-mesenchymal transition
Endo G — Endonuclease G
ER — Endoplasmic reticulum
ERK — Extracellular signal-related kinases
ERK1/2 — Extracellular signal-related kinases 1/2
F344 — Fischer 344
FADD — Fas-associated protein with death domain
Fas — First apoptosis signal
FasL — First apoptosis signal ligand
FDA — Food and Drug administration
FIE — *Fumaria indica* extract
FOXO3 — Forkhead box protein O1
FSCN1 — Fascin-1
G. resinaceum — *Ganoderma resinaceum*
G-6-Pase — Glucose-6-phosphatase
G6PD — Glucose-6-phosphatase dehydrogenase
GADD153 — Growth arrest and DNA damage inducible gene 153
GC/MS — Gas chromatography/mass spectrometry
GF2 — Ginsenoside F2
GGT — Gamma-glutamyl transferase
GJIC — Gap junctional intercellular communication
GLI1 — glioma-associated oncogene-1
GME — *Garcinia mangostana* fruit extract
GPX — Glutathione peroxidase
GR — *Ganoderma resinaceum*
GRP I and GRP II — *G. resinaceum* polysaccharide-rich fractions
GRP78 — *G. resinaceum* polysaccharide 78
GSH — Glutathione
GSH — reducing glutathione
GST — Glutathione S-transferase
GSTp — Glutathione S-transferase p
GT — Glutamyl transferse
H4IIE — Liver carcinoma cell line
HA22T — Liver carcinoma cell line

HCCLM3 — Human hepatoma cell line
HCCLM6 — Human hepatoma cell line
HDAC-1 — Histone deacetylases
HeLa — Cervical cancer cell line
HeN — Human serous ovarian adenocarcinoma
Hep3B — Human hepatoma cell line integrated with hepatitis B virus genome
HepG2 — Human hepatoma
HepT — Liver cancer cell line
HepT1 — Liver cancer cell line
HIF-1α — Hypoxia-inducible factor 1-alpha
HIF-1a — Hypoxia-inducible factor 1-alpha
HLE — Hepatoma cell line
HMG-CoA — β-hydroxy β-methylgluraryl Coenzyme A
HO-1 — Heme oxygenase 1
HP — Lipid hydroperoxides
HPLC — High pressure liquid chromatography
HSP105 — Hispidin 105
HSP70 — Heat shock protein 70
HSP90 — Heat shock protein 90
HSPA1A — Heat shock protein family A
HSPA8 — Heat shock cognate protein
HUH6 — Human hepatoma cell line
HuH-7 — Human hepatoma cell line
HUVEC — Human umbilical vein endothelial cells
ICAM-1 — Intercellular adhesion molecule 1
IGF-1R — Insulin-like growth factor receptor
IH-901 — 20-O-beta-D-glucopyranosyl-20(S)-protopanaxadiol
IR — Infra red
IRE-1 — Inositol-requiring enzyme type 1
JAK2 — Janus kinase 2
JNK — c-Jun NH_2 terminal kinase
K^+ — Potassium ion
Ki67 — Nuclear non-histone protein

LC3 II — Lapidated microtubule-associated protein 1A/1B light chain 3
LDH — Lactate dehydrogenase
LM6 — Hepatocellular carcinoma LM6 cell line
LO2 — Human fetal hepato cell line
LPO — Lipid peroxidation
M phase — Mitotic phase
M6P — Mannose 6-phosphate
MADLI/MS — Matrix-assisted laser desorption ionization/mass spectrometry
MAPKs — Mitogen-activated protein kinase
MDA — Malonyl dialdehyde
MDA-MB 231 — Breast cancer cell line or M.D. Anderson Metastasis Breast cancer cell line
Met-capsaicin — Metformin-capsaicin
Mg^{2+} — Magnesium ion
MH1C1 — Cancer cell line
MHCC-97H — Highly potential metastatic hepatocellular carcinoma cell line
MHCC-97L — Highly potential metastatic hepatocellular carcinoma cell line
MiR-122 — MicroRNA 122
MMP-9 — Matrix metalloproteinase-9
MMPs — Matrix metalloproteinases
mRNA — Messenger ribonucleic acid
mTOR — Mammalian target of rapamycin
MTT — 3-[4,5-dimethylthiazol-2-yl]-2,5 diphenyl tetrazolium bromide]
ND1 — NADH-ubiquinone oxidoreductase chain 1
NDEA — N-nitrosodiethylamine
NF-B — Nuclear factor-kappaB
NF-κB — Nuclear factor-κB
NNM — N-Nitrosomorphine
NO_2 — Nitric oxide
NOX-1 — NADPH-oxidase 1

NPC1L1 — Niemann–Pick type C1-like 1
NQO1 — Quinone oxidoreductase 1
Nrf2 — Nuclear factor E2-related factor 2
O. fragrans — *Osmanthus fragrans*
OCT — Ornithine carbamoyl transferase
P13K — Phosphoinositide 3-kinase
P21 — Tumor protein 21
P21WAF1 — Cyclin-dependent kinase inhibitor
P27kip1 — Cyclin-dependent kinase inhibitor
P38 — Mitogen-activated protein kinases
P450 — Cytochrome P450
P53 — Tumor protein 53
P65 — Transcription factor p65
p73 — Tumor protein
p-AKT — Protein kinase B (AK strain transforming protein)
PAR — Protease-activated receptors
PARP1 — Poly [ADP-ribose] polymerase 1
PB — Phenobarbital
PC — Protein carbonylation
PCC — Protein carbonyl content
PCNA — Proliferating cell nuclear antigen
PGC1 — Peroxisome proliferator-activated receptor gamma coactivator
PI3K — Phosphatidylinositol 3-kinase
pJNK — Phosphorylated Jun N-terminal kinase
PLC/PRF — (Alexander) Hepatoma Cell line
Pp38 — Mitogen-activated protein kinases
pPERK — Phosphorylated extra cellular signal regulated kinase
PPF — Porphyrin-based paddle-wheel framework
pRB — Retinoblastoma protein
pSTAT3 — Signal transducer and activator of transcription 3 protein
PTCH1 — Patched protein 1
PTEN — phosphatase and tensin homolog
RECK — Reversion-inducing cysteine-rich protein with Kazal motifs

R-HepG2 — Hepatic tumor cell line
RNA — Ribonucleic acid
ROS — Reactive oxygen species
SDH — Sorbitol dehydrogenase
Ser473 — Serine 473
SFN — Sulforaphane (1-isothioyanato-4-(methyl-sulfinyl) butane)
SGOT — Serum glutamic oxaloacetic transaminase
SGPT — Serum glutamic pyruvic transaminase
SK-Hep-1 — Human hepatic adenocarcinoma cell line
SK-Hep-2 — Human hepatic adenocarcinoma cell line
SMMC — Human hepatoma cell line
SMMC7721 — Human hepatoma cell line
SOD — Superoxide dismutase
sp. — Species
SP-1 — Specificity protein 1
STAT3 — Signal transducer and activator of transcription 3
SW480 — Colorectal cancer cell line
TBARS — Thiobarbituric acid reactive substance
tBid — Truncated proapoptotic Bcl-2 protein
TBL — Total bilirubin level
TGF-β1 — Transforming growth factor beta-1
THLE-2 — Liver cancer cell line
TIMP-2 — Tissue inhibitor metalloproteinase-2
TNF — Tumor necrosis factor
TRAIL — TNF related apoptosis inducing ligand
u-PA — Urokinase plasminogen activator
var. — variety
Vav — Guanine nucleotide exchange factor
VEGFR1 — Vascular endothelial growth factor receptor-1
Vit A — Vitamin A
Vit E — Vitamin E
viz — namely
Wnt — Wingless and Int-1
WR — Wistar

XIAP — X-linked inhibitor of apoptosis protein
IκBα — Nuclear factor-kappa B inhibitor

Abstract

Globally liver cancer, specifically hepatocellular carcinoma (HCC), continues to be a significant cause of mortality, despite considerable progress in the field of medicine. Liver cancer patients are facing a shortage problem of treatment options, which forces to explore novel preventive and control methods. These preventive methods and effective therapeutic approaches are reasonable and decisive in the fight against this disease. Both dietary and non-dietary phytochemicals in nature exhibit significant potential in preventing and treating various cancers, including HCC. Chemoprevention is an effective strategy to decelerate or reverse disease occurrence and progression by administering naturally occurring and/or synthetic compounds. Phytochemicals, derived from fruits, vegetables, nuts, and spices, are notable for their capacity to selectively kill tumor cells and suppress carcinogenesis in preclinical animal models. A large number of these plant-derived substances have demonstrated their efficacy in preventing or delaying cancer development in several high-risk populations. This chapter reveals evidences based on *in vitro* and *in vivo* experiments (involving animal models and humans) which support potential chemopreventive and therapeutic effects of diverse phytochemicals in liver cancer.

1. Introduction

Cancer is one of the leading causes of the mortality and morbidity affecting various organs in the body [1]. According to WHO (World Health Organization), the death rate due to cancer will raise up to 29.4 million cases annually on a global scale [2]. Liver is responsible for all crucial vital functions of the body like removing various blood toxins, maintaining bioenergetics, responsible for bile secretion and cellular metabolism [3–5]. So maintaining a healthy liver is crucial for general health and overall wellness. Overconsumption of drugs and alcohol, modern lifestyle patterns, and consumption of various unsanitary nutritional supplements induce strain and damage to the liver [6, 7]. As per surveillance reports from the World Health Organization (WHO), 8,30,180 people died worldwide in 2020 due to liver cancer [8]. About 85% of liver cancers are hepatocellular carcinoma (HCC) and are frequently observed in people with chronic liver diseases. HCC development is a multiplex process that includes inflammatory damage that leads to hepatocyte necrosis, regeneration, and fibrotic deposition [9, 10]. As many signaling pathways are involved in HCC development and progression, it is better to target these pathways by therapeutic molecules. These days, various efforts including chemotherapeutic approaches, immunotherapy, transplantation, anticancer therapies, and so on have been utilized to manage HCC [11]. But chemoresistance, side effects of drugs, and recurrence of disease in the case of surgery are the major limiting factors for the successful treatment of HCC. Exploring promising and cost-effective natural products for HCC management is a sensible approach [4, 6, 12, 13]. Hepatocarcinoma is predominant among various cancers that persists as a major cause of death having limited treatment possibilities globally. There is a need to discover innovative preventive and therapeutic approaches to effectively eliminate this disease. In this scenario, the relevance of potential in several naturally occurring dietary as well as non-dietary phytochemicals has to be validated. A plethora of preclinical studies demonstrated the anti-hepatocarcinoma activity of many phytoactive constituents. Chemopreventive agents work by inhibiting liver enzymes that activate carcinogens, preventing carcinogen interaction with cellular DNA, altering intracellular signaling pathways, halting the progression of malignant cells, inhibiting angiogenesis, arresting cell cycle, and triggering apoptosis [14]. This chapter focuses on HCC, chemoprevention, phytochemicals used in HCC, their mechanism of action, and their clinical trial.

2. Hepatocellular Carcinoma

Liver diseases are very harmful to life and are categorized into four major types: cirrhosis, fatty liver, hepatitis, and HCC. Among these, hepatitis and HCC are the most life-threatening diseases that affect public health globally. **Cirrhosis** emerges following prolonged liver inflammation over a period of years, especially in men. According to MacDonald 2001, 75% of HCC develop in cirrhotic livers [15]. **Fibrosis** is the abnormal accumulation of extracellular matrix proteins, which results in cirrhosis, liver failure, and so on. It is a condition preceding cirrhosis. The main reasons for liver fibrosis in developed countries are chronic hepatitis C virus (HCV) infection, alcohol abuse, and non-alcoholic steatohepatitis [16, 17]. Although **fatty liver** is a non-threatening condition, it has the potential for progress to severe liver scarring and cirrhosis. Oxidative stress, excessive production, and release of toxic inflammatory proteins and necrosis are the various causes of fatty liver [18]. **Hepatitis** is caused by one of five hepatitis viruses: hepatitis A, B, C, D, and E, cytomegalovirus, Epstein-Barr virus, yellow fever, parasites, drugs and toxins. However, hepatitis B and C viruses can establish persistent infections and thereby cause chronic hepatitis, which may lead to cirrhosis and liver cancer [19]. HCC, most common liver cancer, is a deadly disease in both developed and developing countries.

HCC is a unique cancer, and its survival rate is very less after diagnosis [20]. Globally, HCC ranked as the fifth most prevalent form of cancer and stands as the third highest contributor to cancer-related deaths [21]. Liver cancer incidence, mainly HCC cases, are steadily increasing worldwide, and around 7,00,000 people are diagnosed with HCC per annum [21–24]. In the United States, because of growing number of people diagnosed with advanced HCV or non-alcoholic steatohepatitis (NASH), HCC incidences will continue to increase over the next 20 years. At its present rate, HCC over lead breast and colorectal cancers in the United States by 2030 [25]. This high HCC mortality rate is due to many reasons: (a) the diagnosis of HCC often occurs late in its progression due to the absence of specific symptoms during its early stages. (b) The liver's detoxification role makes it highly resilient against many therapies, resulting in insufficient treatment options for liver cancer [20, 26].

3. Risk Factors

HCC development is a complex and multifactorial process, associated with chronic and persistent infection. This multistep process may include the alteration in host gene expression, DNA methylation, loss of heterozygosity, and point mutation, but still the rate-limiting step for initiation and progression of HCC is not determined [27]. Infection by HCV and cirrhosis are widely recognized etiological agents in HCC. Usually, HCC develops in patients with chronic liver disease, and it is estimated that 66% are due to hepatitis B virus (HBV) and 42% are attributable to HCV [28].

Exposure to various environmental chemicals such as aflatoxin, vinyl chloride (occupational exposure), arsenic compounds, polychlorinated biphenyls, and radioactive compounds has also been implicated in HCC carcinogenesis [29, 30]. Studies revealed that aflatoxin B1 causes cancer development in humans and animals [31]. Regions with significant aflatoxin exposure showed a 70-fold high risk of HCC development [32]. Non-alcoholic fatty liver disease (NAFLD) or non-alcoholic steatohepatitis (NASH) becomes a prominent cause of HCC. The mechanism of HCC carcinogenesis due to NAFLD is not completely known. Smoking is a major lifestyle factor that increases the chance of HCC development. Tobacco contains many carcinogens, including aromatic hydrocarbons [33], diethyl nitrosamine [34], and 4-aminobiphenyl [35], and about 13% of all HCC cases worldwide are attributed to this factor [36]. Glycogen storage disease I, or Von Gierke's disease [37], hemochromatosis [38], alpha 1-antitrypsin (AAT) deficiency [39], and hereditary tyrosinemia type 1 [40] can lead to hepatocellular adenomas and HCC [37].

Some endocrine risk factors are also seen in HCC. Hypothyroidism is more prevalent among individuals diagnosed with HCV. Research indicates that patients with hypothyroidism face twice the risk of HCC compared to those without any history of thyroid issues [41–43]. Compared to females, HCC predominantly occurs in males, with the male-to-female ratio for this condition ranging from 15:1 to 11:1. Females demonstrate notably better HCC prognosis, survival rates, and disease-free survival after surgery than males [44]. This difference is mainly due to hormonal differences between males and females. In males, androgen/androgen receptors (ARs) promote HBV viral replication and contribute to HBV-induced HCC [45]. In females, estrogen/estrogen receptors (ERs) exhibit protective qualities against HCC, while postmenopausal females experience higher incidences of HCC [46, 47]. Long-term use of contraceptives, duration of infection, viral load, family history, co-infections with hepatitis D virus (HDV), human immunodeficiency virus (HIV), and angiogenic therapy are some other factors contribute to HCC development [29]. The two major secondary factors associated with increased risk of liver carcinogenesis are obesity and diabetes [48]. Various factors linked with an increased risk of HCC are shown in Figure 1.

4. Histopathology of HCC

Various factors such as aflatoxins, viral infections, and alcoholism result in liver cell regeneration, proliferation, cell cycle activation and uncontrolled cell growth associated with hyperplasia, dedifferentiation, and development of HCC. So, HCC often develops as a result of continuum of pathological changes in the liver tissues [49–51]. Understanding this histological progression from regeneration to malignant transformation is essential for understanding the stages of HCC, which helps in the development of appropriate treatment methods.

5. Molecular Pathology of HCC

The molecular aspect of HCC development is reported by Ozturk [52]. The process of transformation of normal liver cells to malignant cells requires more than 20 genes and involves four genetic pathways: (1) p53 pathway (in DNA damage and response), (2) pRB/p16INK4A

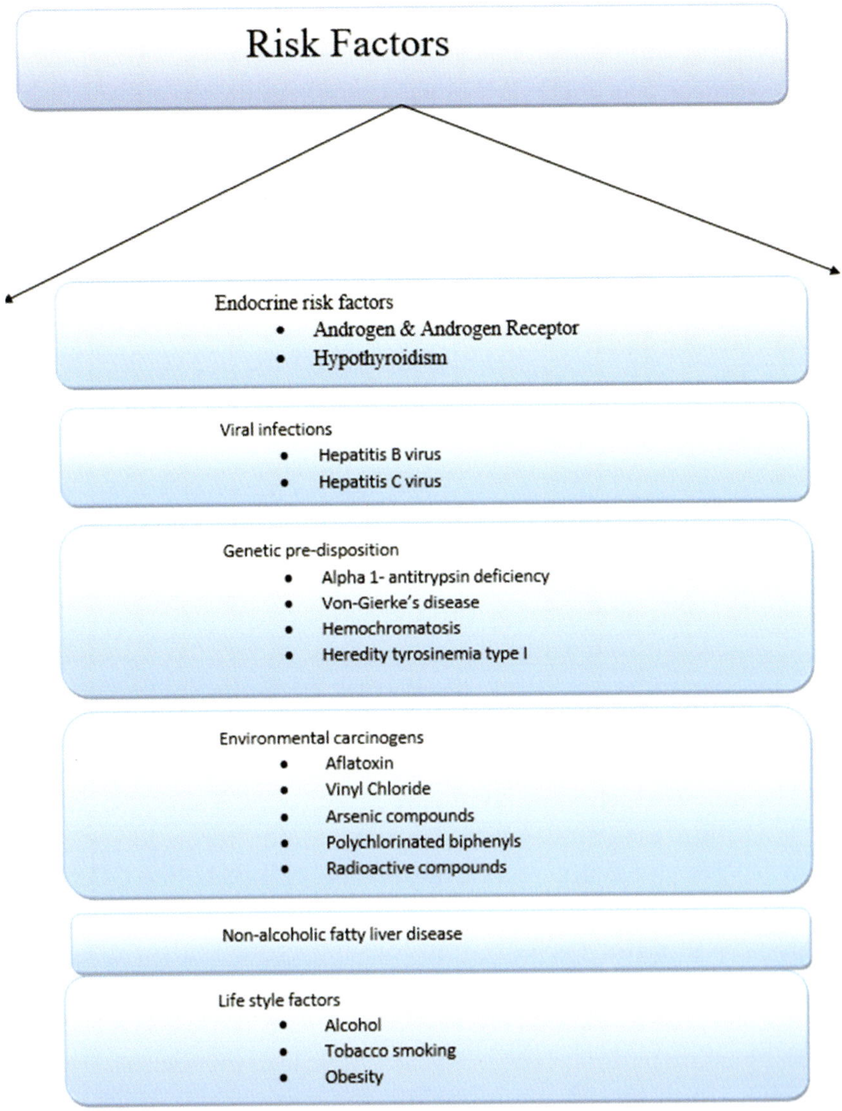

Figure 1: Various factors linked with an increased risk of hepatocellular carcinoma

pathway (in cell cycle control), (3) TGF-β1 pathway (in growth inhibition), and (4) apoptosis and β-catenin/Axin1 pathway (in morphogenesis and signal transduction). Some *in vitro* studies revealed that viral infections upregulate hexosamine and membrane lipid biosynthesis by modulating glutamine-fructose-6-phosphate transaminase 1 (GFAT) and cholinekinase A expression [53–55]. Human hepatocytes infected with the hepatitis virus alter glycolysis and gluconeogenesis with the activation of transcription factor, PPARγ, related to lipid-metabolism [56].

HBV-induced HCC carcinogenesis operates through two mechanisms. First, active HBV-specific T cells, chemokine-mediated neutrophils, macrophages, and natural killers in chronic HBV patients foster cancer development by stimulating hepatocyte regeneration, producing reactive oxygen species, and causing DNA damage [57, 58]. Second, integration of HBV DNA into the host genome can activate proto-oncogenes [59], induce chromosomal instability [60], and prompt the transcription of pro-carcinogenic HBV genes [61]. Hepatitis B viral proteins induce lipid accumulation by upregulating sterol regulatory element-binding protein (SREBP)1, peroxisome proliferator-activated receptor γ(PPAR), and various lipogenic and adipogenic enzymes [62, 63].

The excessive action of HCV core proteins, NS3 and NS5, causes the inhibition of genes, which suppress tumor formation such as TP53, TP73, and factors which impede the cell cycle like CDKN1A [64, 65]. Crucial signaling pathways of HCC involve vascular endothelial growth factor (VEGF), transforming growth factor (TGF)-β, Wnt/B-catenin, hedgehog, notch, epidermal growth factor (EGF), hepatocyte growth factor (HGF), Janus kinase (JAK)/STAT3, and hippo signaling pathways [66]. The alcoholic liver disease (ALD) triggers HCC through changes in the metabolic pathways, which causes excessive buildup of acetaldehyde. This causes cancer through the creation of DNA — protein adducts [67].

Various molecular pathways involved in HCC are shown in Figure 2.

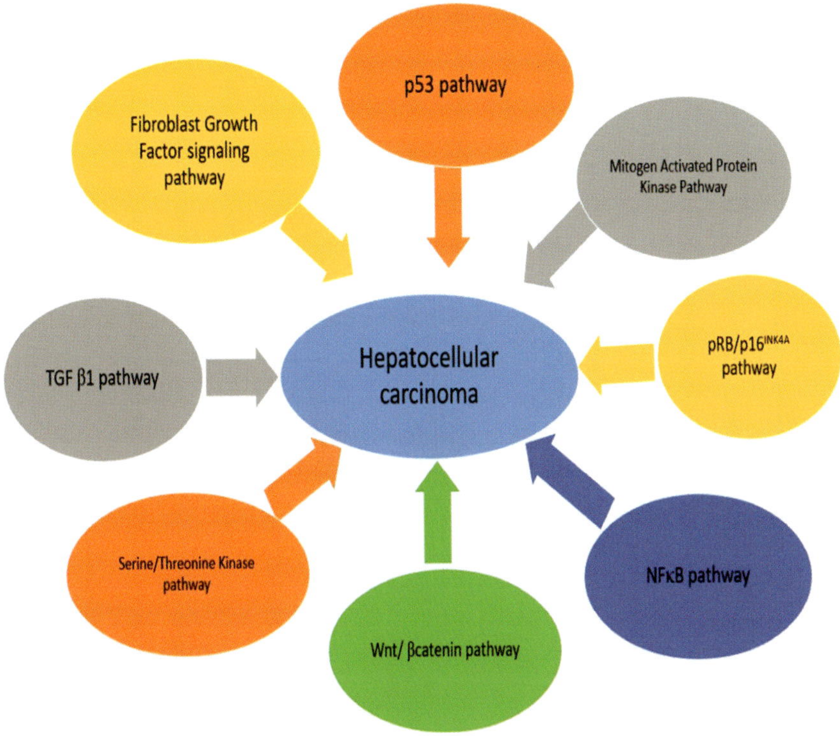

Figure 2: Signaling pathways associated with hepatocellular carcinoma

6. Available Medications and Challenges

As the liver is detoxifying the body, it exhibits high resistance to available chemotherapeutic agents, and early-stage liver cancer often lacks specific symptoms [20, 68]. Late diagnosis of the disease, poor prognosis, recurrent disease occurrence, and insufficient treatment modalities lead to high prevalence and increased death rates of liver cancer. Advanced cancer therapies including surgery and transplantation are exist in the majority of tumor cases, but treatments for HCC are restricted to patients with small nodules and optimal liver function [29, 48]. High recurrence rates in surgery, organ shortage, and high cost of transplantation are the three significant challenging points in this field [69, 70]. Highly complex and heterogenous genetic aberrations in HCC tumors is another major obstacle in the identification of therapeutic strategies [71]. Various combinations of chemotherapeutic agents have shown increase response against HCC, but most of the combinations are not clinically proved yet [72, 73]. Other treatment options include liver resection, radiofrequency ablation (RFA), percutaneous ethanol injection (PEIT), transarterial chemoembolization (TACE), and molecular targeted therapy (MTT) such as sorafenib [74]. Until recently, FDA has only clinically approved "Sorafenib" as the drug for advanced HCC, but it has several adverse effects [75]. For second-line treatments, additional multikinase inhibitors such as Cabozantinib and Ramucirumab [76–78] and Checkpoint inhibitors such as Nivolumab [79] and Pembrolizumab [80] have been endorsed from 2017 onwards. Managing the adverse side effects of systemic therapies is a very difficult task in patients with cirrhosis [81], and there is no established treatment regimen achieves complete remission in HCC patients. Consequently, preventing and treating HCC pose a considerable challenge in medical and research fields, and there is a pressing need for identifying new agents and discovering novel strategies against HCC.

Because of high cost of approved therapies, addressing the prevention of HCC emerges as an important concern within highly populated, low-income nations. A successful and alternative approach for HCC management in high-risk groups is prevention. Various prevention strategies [82] include primary prevention, secondary prevention and tertiary prevention.

7. Prevention Strategies

7.1. *Primary prevention*

Primary prevention of HCC aimed to eradicate the factors that increase the development of cancer through early vaccination, changes in lifestyle and interventions in environment. It mainly focuses to reduce the risk factors such as infections caused by HBV and HCV, exposure to aflatoxin B1, diabetes, obesity, excessive use of tobacco and alcohol before the onset of cirrhosis [83]. Oncogenic hepatitis viruses are responsible for 80 percent of HCC cases, prompting 181 countries to initiate "Expanded Program of Immunization" (EPI) against HBV, which results 10-fold decrease in HCC incidence in vaccinated chronic HBV carriers [84–86]. But due to the hypervariable genomic structure of HCV and several mutated strains in the patients, it is a challenging task to synthesize universally efficient vaccine against HCV. To reduces the risk of viral HCC development, we need to take precautions to prevent the spreading of these viruses through intravenous injection, avoid contaminated blood transfusion and treating infected individuals with antiviral drugs [75, 82].

Exposure to Aflatoxin B1 (AFB1) in crops increases the risk of HCC development in low-income nations, because food lacks screening for this particular toxin in these countries. Providing necessary crop storage facilities and replacing them with low-risk crops like rice are the two major solutions of this problem. *Aspergillus*-resistant crop lines formed by genetic recombination and application of non-aflatoxigenic strains of *Aspergillus* for crop inoculation are other cost-effective alternative solutions for low-income countries [75, 82].

Raising awareness for healthy food consumption, regulating obesity and diabetes, and limiting alcohol intake are valid approaches for prevention of HCC [48].

7.2. *Secondary prevention/chemoprevention*

Secondary prevention or chemoprevention aims to reduce HCC or delay the progression of chronic liver diseases. It mainly depends on the daily consumption of fruits and vegetables through our diet. Natural constituents present in fruits, vegetables, nuts, and spices have demonstrated the ability to inhibit or potentially reverse the cancer development in liver cells and even eliminate the neoplastic cells [75, 82, 83, 87]. Generally, chemopreventive agents are reasonable, suitable for prolonged treatment without any adverse effects, and accessible to the general public.

7.3. *Tertiary prevention*

Tertiary prevention is aimed at the recurrence of cancer, that is, preventing the formation of new HCC lesions following successful surgery or curative treatment [88]. Therefore, immunosuppressive drugs such as interferons and glucocorticoids have been employed to reducing inflammation, thus halting the advancement of HCC [87, 89, 90].

Among the three prevention approaches, chemoprevention is the most comprehensive approach to HCC prevention.

8. Chemoprevention

Cancer chemoprevention means the application of particular natural or man-made chemical agents to counteract or inhibit the process of carcinogenesis and prevent the onset of invasive cancer by altering physiological pathways [91]. Interferon (IFN) is able to inhibit the reoccurrence of HCC after successful therapy [92–94], but its use is often impeded due to adverse side effects such as general tiredness, depression, and pancytopenia. As chemopreventive agents can be administered for an extended period of time without any adverse effects and even elderly patients exhibit good tolerance toward this medication, it is worth to develop an efficient chemopreventive compound offering both effectiveness and less toxicity. So dietary agents from every day food and compounds in medicinal plants are more preferable and acceptable than pharmaceutical agents [95].

Many plants possess anticancer activity, reducing the risk of developing chronic diseases [96, 97]. Phytochemicals are also acted as adjuvants of chemotherapeutic drugs to improve their potency and alleviate their side effects [98]. Chlorophyllin is a chemopreventive agent, which binds with chemical carcinogens like aflatoxins and forms molecular complexes that lower their bioavailability and carcinogenicity [99, 100]. As a secondary prevention of HCC, oltipraz (*4-methyl-5-(2-pyrazinyl)-3-dithiolethione*) is used because it induces phase II detoxifying and anti-oxidative enzymes and blocks AFB1-induced HCC [101]. Using polyprenoic acid might help to restore retinoid levels during hepatic damage induced by alcohol [102].

Some other compounds that show promise in the chemoprevention of HCC are isothiocyanates, glycosinolates, and terpenoids. Consumption of vegetables correlates with low risk of HCC as it contains many biologically active phytochemicals [23]. Different strategies of chemoprevention are following.

8.1. *Etiology-specific chemoprevention*

Hepatitis B vaccination: More than 175 countries worldwide implemented HBV vaccination, which significantly reduced the risk of HCC related with HBV.

Antiviral therapy against HBV and HCV: Managing viral replication in patients with chronic hepatitis B and C viral infection by antiviral therapy plays an important role in reducing the risk of HBV- and HCV-associated liver carcinogenesis [103].

8.2. *Generic chemoprevention strategies*

Statins: 3-hydroxy-3-methylglutaryl coenzyme A (HMG-CoA) reductase inhibitors or statins are among the most globally accepted medications. It prevents cardiovascular diseases and has antineoplastic properties through antiproliferative, proapoptotic, antiangiogenic, immunomodulatory, and anti-infective effects [104]. Earlier studies revealed that statins might be protective against inflammation-driven cancers such as esophageal adenocarcinoma [105], *Helicobacter pylori*-associated gastric cancer [106], and colitis-associated colorectal cancer [107]. Studies also showed a positive correlation between statin use and low risk of HCC incidence [108–110].

Antidiabetic medications: Research proved that traditional medicines used for diabetes might influence the risk of carcinogenesis in diabetic patients: metformin and thiazolidinediones help to decrease the possibility of cancer [111], and insulin and insulin secretagogues increase the chance of cancer development [112]. Several population-based studies have proved the association between metformin and low risk of HCC in diabetic patients [113, 114].

Aspirin: In addition to anti-inflammatory effects, an antiplatelet agent, aspirin showed antineoplastic effects against inflammation-mediated cancers like esophageal adenocarcinoma [115]. A comparison study proved that aspirin use causes 41% reduction in the risk of developing liver cancer [116].

8.3. *Dietary agents for prevention of HCC*

Coffee: Previous studies reported that consumption of coffee lowers the risk of HCC [117, 118]. There is a 23% reduction in the risk of HCC for each cup of coffee consumption per day [119]. Diterpenes, cafestol, and kahweol present in coffee show antineoplastic effects by modulating various enzymes involved in carcinogen detoxification, and caffeine shows antioxidant properties [120]. Coffee's ability to lower the chances of advanced fibrosis and cirrhosis indirectly impacts the risk of developing HCC as well [121].

Vitamin D and Vitamin E: The protective association of intake of vitamin D and vitamin E and risk of HCC is due to their potent antioxidant effect [122, 123]. These vitamins prevent damage of DNA, enhance repair of DNA, and promote inactivation of cancer-causing agents [124].

Fish consumption: There is a dose-dependent protective association between fish consumption and risk of HCC. Earlier studies observed that daily intake of fishes rich in *n*-3 polyunsaturated fatty acids causes 36% reduction in risk of developing HCC [125].

8.4. *Phytochemicals*

Based on some preclinical studies, several plant-based chemicals in our diet that possess potent antioxidant, anti-inflammatory and antineoplastic properties have a major role in chemoprevention of HCC [126]. Glucosinolates and metabolites in broccoli sprouts exert antineoplastic effects by modulating Keap1/Nrf2 signaling and activate cytoprotective responses against oxidants [127]. Curcumin in turmeric showed a protective effect in mouse models of aflatoxin-induced hepatocarcinogenesis [128] and other cancers such as oral, breast, prostate, pancreatic, and colorectal cancers [129]. Resveratrol is a dietary polyphenol seen in grapes, berries, and peanuts which suppresses hepatic-carcinogen-activating enzymes like cytochrome P450, oxidoreductases, and glutathione S-transferase and thus inhibits carcinogenesis [130].

9. Role of Plants in Chemoprevention

Herbs have been used as a healing agent since ancient times, and its customary action has been coevolved with mankind. The pharmacological efficiency of plants was recognized through trial and failure technique and conveyed the expertise to successors verbally or through practice. A single plant or its parts as such had been used for the cure of various pharmacological conditions before sixteenth century and in between sixteenth and eighteenth century combination of plants or its parts were used. Since the onset of the eighteenth century, active phytoconstituents have been separated from herbs and applied as drugs. Till date, about 6 lakh phytochemicals have been isolated from different plants and identified their therapeutic potential. Out of the total basic and essential 252 drugs considered by the WHO, 11% are solely of herbal origin, and a notable number are designer drugs developed from natural compounds [131].

Phytochemicals can stop or impede the alteration of precancerous cells into the malignant ones. Nonetheless, reviews proclaimed that the positive health advantages of phytomolecules in fresh or uncooked plant-based foods would be even greater than its current value, regarding the involvement of free radical-induced oxidative stress in various chronic diseases. Hepatocarcinoma is predominant among various cancers that persist as a major cause of death having limited treatment possibilities globally. Advanced preventive measures and effective treatment modalities need to be discovered to eradicate this disease. In this scenario, the relevance of potential in various naturally available dietary as well as non-dietary phytochemicals has to be validated. A plethora of preclinical studies demonstrated the antihepatocarcinoma of many phytoactive constituents (Table 1) as depicted in Figure 3–8.

Table 1: Plants, phytoactive constituents, and their mechanism of action against hepatocarcinoma. ↑ indicate upregulation and ↓ indicate downregulation of various genes or proteins

Phytochemicals	Plant Name	Mechanism of Action	References
Quercetin	*Foeniculum vulgare* and *Capsicum fruitescens*	HepG2 — ↓ Cell proliferation, ↑ Apoptosis ↑ Bad and Bax ↓ Bcl-2	[132]
Resveratrol	*Polygonum cuspidatum*	Rat hepatic lesions — DENA induced — ↓ COX2; ↓ hepatic HSP70 protein expression CCL 4-induced HCC rat model — ↓ lipid peroxidation; ↑ GSH and GST serum levels HepG2 — ↑ Apoptosis; ↓ HIF-1a; VEGF, PI3K and TNF; ↑ p53, p21 TRAIL-based TNF-α NDEA-induced HCC rats — ↓ neoplastic lesions, AST, ALT, ALP, and GGT	[133–138]
Peonidin-3-glucoside Delphinidin-3-glucoside Cyanidin-3-glucoside Quercetin-3-glucoside Tricin Kaempferol Isorhamnetin-3-glucoside Catechin Protocatechuic acid	*Oryza sativa*	Synergetic effect: DEN-induced hepatic preneoplastic lesions in rats. ⊥ glutathione *S*-transferase ↑ nitric oxide synthase, interleukin-6, interleukin-1 beta, apoptotic gene and Bcl2 associated X ↓ cyclin E, COX 2	[139]

Vanillic acid			
β-Sitosteryl ferulate			
Campesteryl ferulate (Cycloartenyl ferulate)			
24-methylene cycloartanyl ferulate			
Epigallocatechin gallate	*Pinus densiflora* and *Cammellia sinensis*	SK-Hep-1 cells — ↑ MMPs HLE, HepG2, HuH-7, PLC/PRF/5, HCC-LM3, HepG2, SMMC-7721, LO2, Hep3B, HCCLM6, MHCC-97H, MHCC-97L, MHCC-97H, and L02 — ↓ oxidative stress, hepatitis virus infection, angiogenesis, proliferation, invasion, migration, autophagy, apoptosis, and tumor metabolism	[140–142]
Epigallocatechin	*Pinus densiflora;* Walnuts, pomegranates, strawberries, blackberries, cloudberries, and raspberries		
Catechin gallate	*Pinus densiflora*		
Ellagitannins	*Rubusidaeus*	Synergism: HepG2 and Huh7 — ↑ PTEN; ↓P-AKT(Ser473)	[143]
Cyanidin-3-O-sophoroside			
Campothecin	*Ophirrhiza mungos*	Topoisomerase inhibition	[144]
Uttroside B	*Solanum nigrum*	HepG2 and Hep3B — ⊥mTOR signaling; ↑ autophagy markers, that is, LC3 II, Beclin 1, ATG5, and ATG7 ↑ AMPK signaling; ↑ ATG protein; modulates autophagy; regulates AMPK-mTOR signaling axis	[145]

(*Continued*)

Table 1: (*Continued*)

Phytochemicals	Plant Name	Mechanism of Action	References
6,8-diprenylorobol	*Glycyrrhiza uralensis*	HuH-7 and HepG2 — ↑ apoptosis; ↑ cleaved caspase-3, Bax, Bim, PARP1, FOXO3, p21, and p27; ↓ cell viability and proliferation; ↓ Bcl2, BclXLebastine hydroxylase and CYP2J2-mediated astemizole O-demethylation	[146]
α-Mangosteen	*Garcinia mangostana*	HepG2 — cytotoxicity ↓ ROS, MDA, and PC	[147]
Ellagic acid	Berries, black currents, grapes, pomegranates, walnuts, and dried fruits	NDEA-induced hepatocarcinogenesis in rats — tumor markers — ↓ AST, ALT, ALP, and G6PD; serum protein ↓GSH, GPX, and c-GT	[148]
Sesamol	*Sesamum indicum*	HepG2 — autophagy and mitophagy ↓ upstream signal of AMPK/PGC1α and mitochondrial complex I subunit ND1 HepG2 injected mice — ↓ tumor volume	[149]
Hesperidin Sesamin	*Sesamum indicum*	Synergetic effect with orange seed extract: rat hepatic lesions — DENA induced — ↓ ALT and PI3K/Akt pathway	[150]
Hesperidin	Citrus seed	HepG2 — ↑ Caspase-9, -8, and -3	[151]
Silymarin	Milk thistle plant	HepG2 — ↑ apoptosis	[152]
Silybin (Silibinin)		Genotoxic effects in HepG2; ↓ cell viability	

		H4IIE cell proliferation, cytochrome P450 2E1 (CYP2E1) induction, metabolism of ethanol, Hep-55.1C — ROS generation ↑ apoptosis TRAIL	
Dehydrosilybin		HepG2 — ↓ viability of cells	
Geraniol		HepG2 — ↓ HMG-CoA reductase	[153]
Excisanin A	*Isodon macrocalyxin* and *Rabdosia excise*	Heo3B cells — ↑ apoptosis; ↓ p-AKT; BALB/c nude mice (implanted with Hep3B cells) — ↓ p-AKT; ↓ apoptosis	[154]
Gnidimacrin	*Gnidia subcordata*	HLE — ⊥ G2; ↓ cdc2; ↑ p21WAF1/CIP1	[155]
Oridonin	*Isodon* sp., and *Rabdosia rubescens*	HepG2 cells — ↑ apoptosis; ↑ ROS; ↑ p53; ↑ p38	[156]
Actein	*Actaea racemose* and *Cimidifuga racemosa*	Growth inhibition of p53 — positive HepG2 cells	[157]
Ardisiacrispin (A+B)	*Ardisia crenata*	BEL-7402 cells — ↑ apoptosis; ↓ proliferation; microtubule disassembly	[158]
Astragaloside IV	*Astragalus* sp. and *Radix Astragali*	HepG2 — ↓ Vav3.1; ↑ HSP70; ↑ HSPA1A; ↑ HSPA8; ↑ BiP/GRP78; ⊥ anchorage-independent growth and colonogenic survival	[159]
Asiatic acid	*Centella asiatica*	HepG2 — ↑ apoptosis; ↑ Ca^{2+}; ↑ p53	[160]
Betulinic acid	*Betula pendula*	HepT1, HepT3, and HUH6 cells — ↑ caspase 3; ↑ apoptosis; ↓ GLI1; ↓ PI3K/AKT; ↓ IGF2; ↓ PTCH1	[161]

(*Continued*)

Table 1: (*Continued*)

Phytochemicals	Plant Name	Mechanism of Action	References
Cucurbitacin B	*Cucurbitaceae* members	HepG2 cells — ↑ apoptosis; ↓ Bcl-2; ↓ pSTAT3 HepG2 xenograft mouse model — ↓ tumor growth and volume BEL-7402 xenograft mouse model — ↓ tumor growth	[162, 163]
Cucurbitacin D		Hep3b — ↑ apoptosis; ↑ caspase-3; ↑ pJNK	[164]
Cucurbitacin D, I		BEL-7402 Cells — ⊥ G1/S	[165]
Echinocystic acid	*Gleditsia sinensis*	HepG2 — ↓ Bcl-2; ↓ ΔΨm; ↑ apoptosis; ↑ caspase-3, -9, -8;↑ PARP cleavage; ↓ cyt. *c*; ↑ p38; ↑ JNK	[166]
Escin	*Aesculus hippocastanum*	HepG2 — ↑ apoptosis; ⊥ G1/S; ↑ bax; ↑ AIF; ↑ cyt. *c*; ↓ Bcl-2; ↓ E2F; ↓ pRb; ↓ cyclin E/cdk2 H22 tumor-bearing female Kunming mice	[167, 168]
Ganoderic acid	*Ganoderma lucidum*	BEL-7402 cells — ⊥ G1/S	[169]
Ganoderiol F	*Ganoderma* sp.	HepG2, Hep3B, and HuH7 cells ⊥G1; ↑pERK2; ↓ p21; ↓ DNA synthesis; ↓ topo I and II; ↑ p16	[170]
Ginsenoside-Rg1	*Panax ginseng*	SK-Hep-1 cells — ↑ cdk2; ↑ cyclin E	[171]
Ginsenoside-Rg5		SK-Hep-1 cells — ⊥ G1/S; ↑ p21WAF1/CIP1; ↓ cdc25A; ↓ cyclin E; ↓ cdk2;	[172]
Ginsenoside Rh2		SK-Hep-1 cells — ⊥G1/S; ↑ p27kip1; ↓ cdc25A; ↓ cyclin E SK-Hep-2 — ↑ apoptosis; ↑ PARP; ↑ caspase-3	[173]
Ginsenoside Rk1		HepG2 cells — ↑ apoptosis; ↑ caspase-3, -8; ↓ telomerase activity; ↓FADD	[174]

Ginsenoside-Rs3		SK-Hep-1 cells — ↑ apoptosis; ↓ cyclin E, A; ↑ p53; ↑ p21WAF1/CIP1; ↓ cdk2	[175]
Ginsenosides		HuH7, HA22T, and Hep3B — ↑ apoptosis; ↑ Bak; ↑ Bax; ↑ Bcl-XL; ↑ caspase-3, -9,-8; ↑ cyt. *c*; ↓ Bcl-2; ↓ Bad	[176]
IH-901		HepG2 cells — ↑ apoptosis; ↑ PARP; ↑ caspase-3, -8, -9; ↑ cyt. *C* SMMC7721 cells — ↑ apoptosis; ⊥ G0/G1; ↑ p53; ↑ Bax; ↑ cyt. *c*; ↓ pro-caspase-3, -9	[177, 178]
Kalopanax saponins A, I	*Kalopanax septemlobus*	HepG2 and R-HepG2 cells — ↑ apoptosis	[179]
Keto- and acetyl-keto-boswellic acids	*Boswellia serrata*	HepG2 cells — ⊥ G1; ↑ caspase-3, -8, -9; ↑ apoptosis	[180]
Lucidenic acid A, B, C, N	*Ganoderma lucidum*	HepG2 cells — ↓ MMP-9; ↓NF-κB; ↓ ERK1/2; ↓ c-Jun; ↓AP-1; ↓ c-Fos	[181]
Lupeol	Mango, grapes, strawberry, olive, and white cabbage	SMMC7721 cells — ↑ FADD ↑ apoptosis; ↓ DR3; ↑ caspase-3, -8;	[182]
25-Methoxyhispidol A	*Poncirus trifoliata*	SK-Hep1 cells — ↑ apoptosis; ↓ cyclin D1; ↓ CDK4; ⊥ G0/G1; ↓ pRb; ↓ c-myc; ↑ p21	[183]
Oleanolic acid	*Olea europaea*	HepG2, Hep3B HA22T, and HuH7cells — ↑ apoptosis; ↑ caspase-3, -8; ↓ ΔΨm; ↓ VEGF; ↓ ICAM-1; ↓ Na^+-K^+- ATPase	[184]

(*Continued*)

Table 1: (*Continued*)

Phytochemicals	Plant Name	Mechanism of Action	References
Ursolic acid	Apples and berries; *Salvia nementosa*	HepG2 and R-HepG2 cells — ⊥ G1/G0; ↑ apoptosis; ↑ HSP105 ; ↓ COX-2 HepG2 — ↑ apoptosis; ↑ caspase-3; ↑ p53; ↓ Bcl-2; ↓ PI3K/Akt ↓ survivin; HepG2, HuH7, Hep3B, and HA22T cells — ↑ apoptosis; ↑ caspase-3, -8; ↓ Na^+-K^+-ATPase; ↓ ΔΨm; ↓ VEGF; ↓ ICAM-1 Huh7 cells — ↑ apoptosis; ↑ Bax; ↑ caspase-3, -9; ↑ cyt. *c*; ↓ Bcl2; ↓ NF-κB; ↓ ΔΨm; ↓ XIAP Male CD-1 mice (H22 hepatoma implanted)— ↓ growth DENA + PB caused hepatocarcinogenesis in male Wistar rats — ↓ Tumor; ↓ PC; ↓ MDA; ↓membrane damage; ↑ Mg^{2+} ATPase; ↑ Na^+K^+ ATPase; ↑ Ca^{2+} ATPase	[185, 186, 187]
Waltonitone	Gentianaceae members; *Gentiana waltonii*	BEL-7402 cells — ↑ apaf-1; ↑ apoptosis; ↑ cyt. *c*; ↑ caspase-3, -8, -9; ↑ Bax; ↑ FasL; ↑ Fas BALB/c nu/nu mice (BEL-7402 cells implanted) — ↓ pro-caspase-9; ↑cleaved caspase-3, -9	[162, 188]
Astaxanthin (Tetraterpene)	Freshwater microalgae	AH109A cells — Antioxidant mechanisms SK-Hep-1 cells — ↑ albumin; ↑ fibrinogen; ↑ Hapatoglobin HepG2 cells — ↑ apoptosis; ↑ necrosis; ↑ TBARS	[189]

Fucoxanthin	Sea weeds	SK-Hep-1 cells — ⊥G0-G1; ↑ apoptosis; ↑ Cx43; ↑ GJIC ↑ Cx32; ↑ [Ca]++; ↓ pJNK; ↓ pERK	[190, 191]
Lycopene	*Lycopersicon esculentum*	AH109A cells and Hep3b cells — ⊥ G0/G1; DNA damage SK-Hep-1 cells — ↑ nm23-H1; ↓ MMP-9, -2; ↓ Sp1; ↓ NF-κB; ↓ IGF-1R; ↑ IκBα; ↓ ROS	[189, 192–194]
α-Bisabolbol	*Matricaria recutita*	HepG2 cells — ↑ apoptosis; ↑ cyt. *c*; ↑ caspase-8, -9; ↑ Fas; ↑ NF-κB; ↑ Bax; ↑ Bak; ↑p53; ↓ Bcl-2	[195]
Dehydrocostus lactone	*Compositae* members	HepG2, PLC/PRF/5 cells — ↑ apoptosis; ↑ AIF; ↑ caspase-4, -9; ↑ ER stress; ↑ Bak, Bax, Endo G, Bcl-XL, Bcl-2, and CHOP/GADD153; ↑ BiP, pJNK, ERK1/2, MAPK, and p38	[196]
Furanodiene	*Rhizoma curcumae*	HepG2 cells — ⊥ G2/M; altered ΔΨm; ↑ apoptosis; ↑ cyt. *c*; ↑ caspase-3; ↑ pp38, pERK1/2	[197]
Zerumbone	*Zingiber zerumbet*	HepG2 cells — ↑ apoptosis; ↑ Bax; ↓ Bcl-2 Sprague-Dawley rats (DENA/2-AAF induced) — ↑ Apoptosis; ↓ ALP, AST, AFP, ALT; ↓ lipid peroxidation; ↓ GSH, PCNA, Bcl-2; ↑ Bax	[198, 199]
Auraptene (Monoterpene)	*Citrus* sp.	DENA-induced carcinoma and TGF-α foci in male F344 rats — ↓ cell proliferation ↑ apoptosis	[200]

(*Continued*)

Table 1: (*Continued*)

Phytochemicals	Plant Name	Mechanism of Action	References
Geraniol	Carrot. Grape and berries	DENA + 2-AAF-promoted hepatocarcinogenesis in male Wistar rats — ↓ cell proliferation; ↑ apoptosis	[201, 202]
d-Limonene		DENA/PB in male AKR mice — ↓ c-jun; ↓ c-myc; Reduced the frequency, number, and dimensions of neoplastic nodules and GSTpfoci caused by NNM in male Sprague-Dawley rats — ↓ cell proliferation; ↑ apoptosis; DENA-induced hepatocellular carcinoma in male WR rats — ↓ hepatic tumor growth and preneoplasia; ↑ GJIC	[203–206]
Perillyl alcohol	Lavender, peppermint, and Cherries	DENA in male F344 rats — ↑ apoptosis; ↑ TGFβ type I, II, III R; ↑ M6P/IGF II R; ↑ TGFβ	[207]
Andrographolide (Diterpenoid)	*Andrographis* sp.	Nodules (BHC induced) in Swiss male albino mice — ↑ GSH; ↑ GPX; ↑ GR; ↑ SOD; ↓ GGT; ↑ CAT; ↓ GST BHC-induced hepatocarcinogenesis male Swiss mice — ↑ SDH; ↑ G-6-Pase; ↑ ATPase; ↓ SGPT; ↓ SGOT; ↓ OCT; ↓ ACP; ↓ALP Hep3B cells — ↑ apoptosis; ↑ MAPKs; ↑ pJNK; ↑ ERK1/2	[208–210]
Epoxy clerodane	*Tinospora cordifolia*	Nodules (DENA induced) in male Wistar rats — ↓ LDH; ↓ SGOT; ↓ SGPT; ↓ GST; ↓ GGT; ↑ SOD; ↑ GSH; ↑ GPX; ↑ CAT	[211]

Geranyl geraniol	*Citrus* sp.	DENA/2-AAF — ↓ occurrence, number, and size of visible nodules and GSTp foci; ↓ cell proliferation; ↓ NF-κB p65; ↓ plasma cholesterol; ↓ DNA strand break	[212]
Bacoside A (Triterpenoid)	*Bacopa monnieri*	Neoplastic nodules (DENA induced) in male Wistar albino rats — ↓ lipid peroxidation; ↓ AFP; ↓ ROS; ↑ Vit A; ↑ Vit E; ↓ CEA; ↑ GSH; ↓ 5′-nucleotidase; ↓ ALT; ↓ LDH; ↓ AST; ↓ ALP; ↑ SOD; ↓ GGT ↑CAT; ↑ GR; ↓ MMP-2; ↓ MMP-9; ↑ GPX;	[213, 214]
Glycyrrhizin	*Glycyrrhiza glabra*	↓ Nodules aHCC induced by DENA in BALB/c mice — ↑ albumin; ↑ AST reduced the size, volume number of preneoplastic liver lesions	[215, 216]
α-Carotene	Carrot and sweet potatoes	Male C3H/He mice — ↓ hepatomas number Multiorgan carcinogenesis in male and female B6C3F1 mice — ↓ tumors	[217, 218]
β-Carotene		Male Wistar rats (DENA + 2-AAF induced) — ↓ growth of nodules GGT foci (DENA/2-AAFinduced) in male Wistar rats — ↓ tumor induction; number of GGT foci and nodules HepG2 cells — ↓ pRb; ↓ cyclin D1, D3; ↓ cdk4; ⊥ G0/G1	[219–235]

(*Continued*)

Table 1: (*Continued*)

Phytochemicals	Plant Name	Mechanism of Action	References
β-Ionone	*Osmanthus fragrans* and *Thymus vulgaris*	↓ incidence, number and size of GSTp foci Male Wistar rats (DENA/2-AAF induced) — ↓ DNA damage; ↓ plasma cholesterol; ↓ cell proliferation	[202, 212]
Dehydrocostus lactone	*Costus* sp.	Mouse (PLC/PRF/5 cells implanted) — ↑ apoptosis; ↓ tumor growth; ↑ IRE-1; ↑ pPERK	[196]
Farnesol	Peaches, apricots, plums, and tomatoes	Male Wistar rats (DENA + 2-AAF induced)-↓ growth of GSTp foci and nodules; ↓ cell proliferation; ↓ DNA damage; ↓ HMG-CoA reductase; ↓ plasma cholesterol	[201]
Xanthohumol	*Humulus lupulus*	HepG2 cells — the induction of GSTs and HO-1, ↑ NQO1 expression	[236]
18b-Glycyrrhetinic acid	*Glycyrrhiza glabra*	HepG2 — ↑ apoptosis (caspase-3, caspase-9, Bax:Bcl-2 ratio, and cleaved PARP)	[237]
Rutin	*Cammellia sinensis*	HepG2 — ↓ Cell proliferation	[238–241]
Myricetin		HepG2 — ↑ apoptosis	
Naringenin	Citrus sp.	Antioxidant activity — ↓ oxidative stress	[240–244]
Naringin		Cell growth inhibition	
Daidzein	Soya and other legumes	HuH-7, HepG2, BEL-7402 — ↑ apoptosis	[240, 244–246]
Genistein		HuH-7, HepG2, BEL-7402 — ↑ apoptosis	
Glycitein		HuH-7, HepG2, B7402 — ↑ apoptosis	

Apigenin	Capsicum, celery, broccoli, and parsley	HepG2 — ⊥ G2/M phase cell cycle arrest; ↓ cell Proliferation; ↑ apoptosis	[241, 244, 247–249]
Luteolin			
Tangeritin			
Catechins	*Malus pumila*, *Camellina sinensis*, and *Theobroma cacao*	LM6 — ↑ apoptosis	[238, 241, 244]
Malvidin		HepG2 — ↑ apoptosis	[240, 241, 244, 250]
Peonidin		HepG2 — ↑ apoptosis	
Petunidin		HepG2 — ↓ cell proliferation	
Cyanidin-3-O-rutinoside	*Ribes nigrum*	NPC1L1 in Caco-2 — ↓ mRNA expression	[251]
Polyphenon-B	*Camellina sinensis*	DAB-induced hepatomas — ↑ markers of invasion, angiogenesis and epigenetic histone deacetylation	[252]
Curcumin	*Curcuma longa*	DEN-induced hepatocarcinogenic rat — ↓ tumor growth; ↓ $p21^{ras}$, PCNA, CDC2	[253–255]
Caffeine	*Coffea arabica*, *Theobroma cacao*, and *Camellina sinensis*	DEN-induced hepatocarcinogenesis — ↓ glutathione S-transferase-P antibodies and proliferating cell nuclear antigen	
Capsaicin	*Capsicum* sp.	SK-Hep-1 — ↓ Bcl2; ↑ caspase-3	[256]
1,8-cineole	Eucalyptus, rosemary, cardamom, and sweet basil	Rats (DEN/2-AAF induced) — ↓TGF-β1; ↓ FSCN1; ↑ MiR-122; ↓ VEGF; ↓ Vimentin; ↓ MMP-9	[257]

(*Continued*)

Table 1: (*Continued*)

Phytochemicals	Plant Name	Mechanism of Action	References
Caffeic acid, Chlorogenic acid, Gentisic acid, Ferulic acid, Iso-chlorogenic acid, Sinapic acid, p-Coumaric acid, and Robinin	*Brssica oleracea* var. *italica*	Synergetic effect — HepG2 and SW480 — ↑ Apoptosis and necrosis	[258]
Dieckol	*Ecklonia cava*	NDEA rats — tumor markers — ↑ p450, TBARS, HP, PCC, and CD; ↓AST, ALT, ALP, GGT, LDH, AFP SOD, CAT, GPx, GST, GR, and G6PD; ↓ lipid peroxidative markers, ↑ antioxidant cascade and ↓NDEA concentration	[259]
Galangin	*Alpinia officinarum*, *Alnus pendula*, *Plantago major*, and *Scutellaria galericulata*	HepG2, Hep3B, and PLC/PRF/5 — ↓ Cell proliferation, mitochondrial membrane potential; ↑ Apoptosis	[260]
γ-mangostin	*Garcinia mangostana*	HepG2 — ↓ Cell proliferation; ↑ Apoptosis; inhibit LPO and scavenge DPPH	[261]
Corosolic acid	*Camptotheca acuminata*, *Ugni molinae*, *Crataegus pinnatifida*, *Psidium guajava*, *Tiarella polyphylla*,	HepG2-enhanced ROS level; ↑ Apoptosis: ↓ NF-κB; ↑ fragmentation PARP protein expression and Bax expression	[262]

	Eriobotrya japonica, and *Lagerstroemia speciosa*		
Delphinidin	*Vaccinium myrtillus*	SMMC7721, HCCLM3, and MHCC-97L — Macroautophagy	[263]
Nobiletin	*Garcinia indica*	HepG2 and MH1C1 — ↓ HGF-induced cell invasion; ↑ Apoptosis	[264]
		DEN-induced HCC in rats — ↓ tumor growth	
Garcinol		HepG2 and MH1C1 — ↓ HGF-induced cell invasion; ↑ Apoptosis	
Auraptene			
β-Cryptoxanthin			
Hesperidine			
1′-acetoxychavicol acetate	*Languas galangal*		
Guggulsterone	*Commiphora mukul*	HepG2 — ↓ Cell proliferation; ↑ Apoptosis	[265]
Indole-3-carbinol	*Cruciferae members*	SK-Hep-1 and SNU-449 — ↓ PTEN/AKT pathway	[266, 267]
		SK-Hep-1 xenograft tumors in mice — ↓ tumor growth	
		HepG2 — ↓ EMT; ↑ NOX-1	
Glucomoringin-isothiocyanate	*Mangifera indica*	DEN-induced HCC in rats — ↓ AST and ALT; ↑ antioxidant capacity	[268]

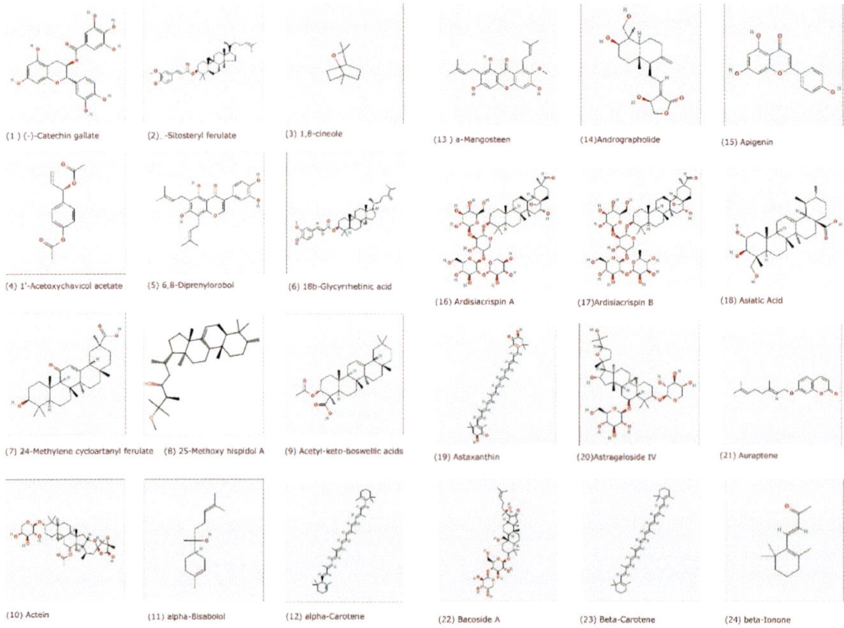

Figure 3: Phytoactive molecules

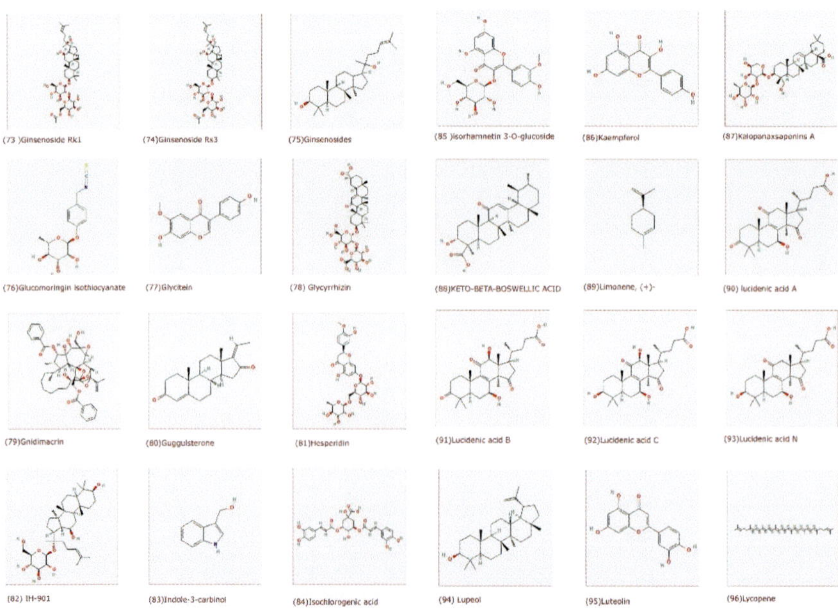

Figure 4: Phytoactive molecules

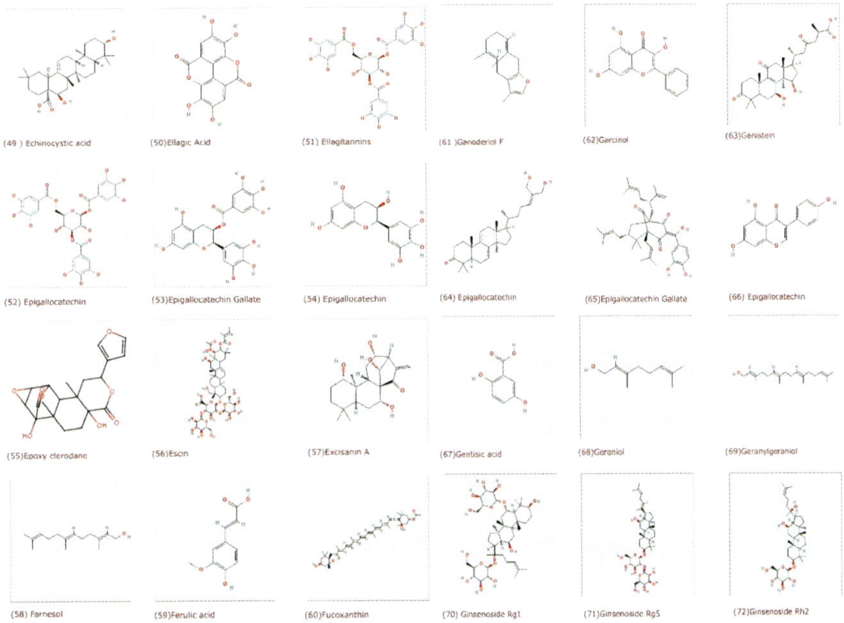

Figure 5: Phytoactive molecules

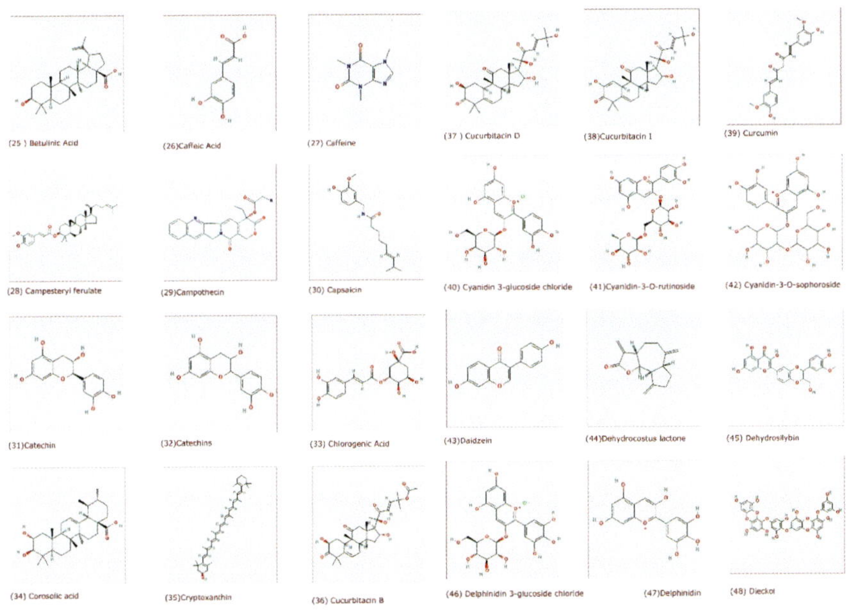

Figure 6: Phytoactive molecules

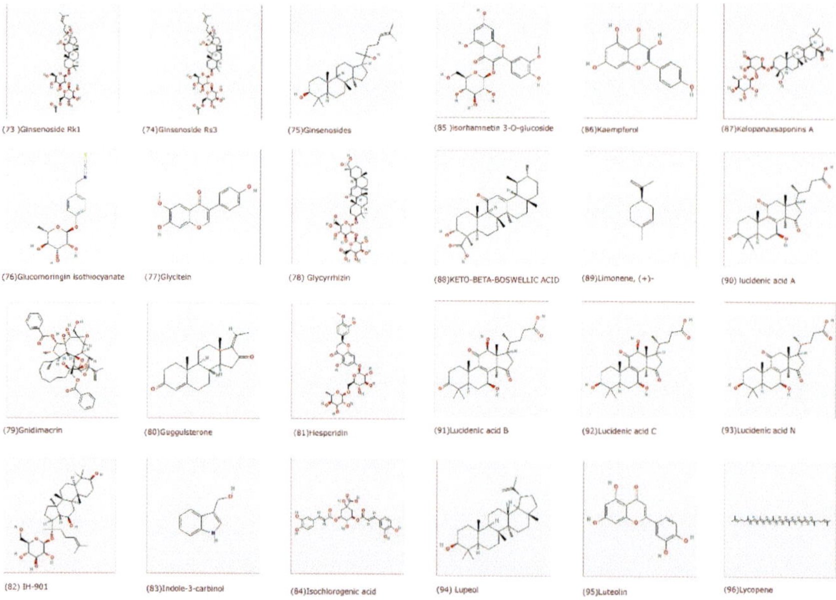

Figure 7: Phytoactive molecules

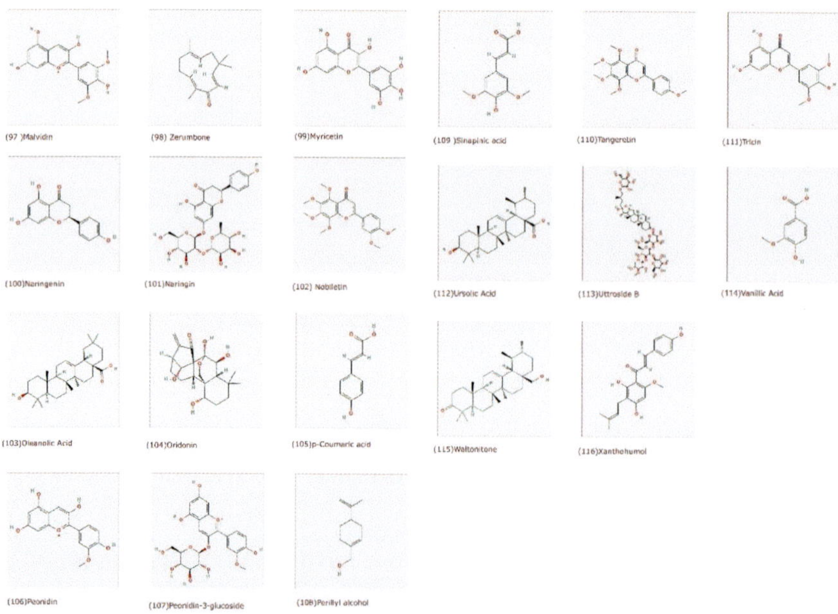

Figure 8: Phytoactive molecules

10. Role of Major Classes of Phytochemicals in Liver Cancer

10.1. *Phenolics*

Naturally occurring phenolic compounds are considered as one of the most relevant chemopreventive and chemotherapeutic phytochemicals against different types of cancers. Culinary spices are rich in polyphenols and flavonoids that are responsible for their antioxidant activity. Phenolics including flavonoids usually scavenge the free radicals and have a pivotal role in therapy as well as prevention of cancer. Fruit juice of pomegranate and peel extracts is a very good repository of polyphenols; thus, it has antioxidant potentials [269, 270]. The HPLC analysis of *Acacia nilotica* bark extract affirmed the occurrence of various polyphenol constituents, namely protocatechuic, gallic, ellagic, caffeic acids, and quercetin. Antihepatocarcinogenic efficacy of orally administered *A. nilotica* bark extract reduced NDEA (*N*-nitrosodiethylamine) induced liver injury and elevated amounts of liver cancer markers, namely alanine transaminase (ALT), α-feto protein (AFP), alkaline phosphatase (ALP), γ-glutamyl transferase (γ-GT), aspartate transaminase (AST), carcinoembryonic antigen (CEA), and total bilirubin level (TBL). The plant extract accelerated the antioxidant enzymes such as catalase (CAT), superoxide dismutase (SOD), glutathione-*S*-transferase (GST), and glutathione peroxidase (GPx) and thereby reduced hepatic injury and reinstated liver cancer markers [271]. Shen *et al.* [272] studied the anticancerous potential of polyphenols present in green tea and found that lipid-soluble polyphenols impeded the advancement of liver carcinogenesis and arrested DBN/PB-induced hepatotoxicity in Sprague-Dawley rats. The administration of Polyphenon-B remarkably lowered the occurrence of DAB-induced hepatomas as proved by regulation of invasion markers, namely matrix metalloproteinase, MMP-9, MMP-2, TIMP-2, tissue inhibitor of matrix metalloproteinase, and reversion-induction cysteine-rich protein with Kazal motifs (RECK). Similarly, the compound declined angiogenic effects such as HIF1α, VEGF, and VEGF receptor, hypoxia-inducible factor 1α, VEGF, VEGFR1, and histone deacetylase HDAC-1 activity [252].

Rezq (2017) reported [273] that the quantity of sinapic, chlorogenic, *P*-coumaric and ferulic acids, and total phenolics in red cabbage was greater than those present in white cabbage. However, white cabbage exceeded the content of caffeic and gallic acids as that of red cabbage. Total flavonoids (lutein, quercetin, kaempferol, and rutin) content was higher in white cabbage than red cabbage. Oral administration of ethanolic extract of red and white cabbage to NDEA and CCl_4 injected rats lessened serum TNF-α AFP, and NF-κβ levels and reduced the highest serum activities of ALT, AST, and ALP enzymes as that of the drug-administered positive control group in dose-dependent manner. Furthermore, administrations of the extracts to drug-administered rats, the activity of inhibited SOD, CAT enzymes and hepatic GPx, increased significantly. Histological analysis pointed out that white cabbage extract increased mild kupffer cells activation.

Quercetin exhibits various antitumor effects such as apoptosis and autophagy stimulation, cell cycle cessation at S and G2/M phases, cell viability reduction, cell motility, and invasion suppression by JAK2/STAT3 signaling pathway inhibition in HCC [274]. *Prunus avium* is a good source of polyphenols that exhibits anticancerous potential. Saeed *et al.* [275] reported that the *P. avium* extract revealed antimutagenic and anticancerous activity through reduction of elevated tumor markers and hepatic transaminases. The extract reduced oxidative stress, tumor growth and proliferation as well as enhanced hepatic function, namely improved expression of cellular checkpoint kinases and P21.

Resveratrol is one among the prominent phytophenol which is abundant in grapes and peanuts can be used for the protection of liver from development of early-stage HCC [134, 276]. Fresh grape skins possess resveratrol ranges from 50 to 100 mg per gram and in wine it ranges from 0.2 to 7.7 mg/liter. Hence, the historical evidence of resveratrol started from the use of grape wine and a renowned ayurvedic formulation Draksharistam [277]. Resveratrol of 50/100/300 mg/kg body weight/day was supplemented with food 4 weeks prior to initiation of hepatocarcinoma followed by histopathological analysis of liver substantiated the safeguarding effect of the compound [278]. The investigations done by Yeh *et al.* (2013) [279] in HuH7 cells through modified Boyden chamber assays showed that resveratrol remarkably hindered cell motility and invasion. Resveratrol inhibited the cell functions and levels of urokinase-type plasminogen activator in casein zymography and western blotting studies. Likewise, chromatin immunoprecipitation assay revealed that resveratrol suppressed the nuclear factor SP-1 transcription protein to the u-PA promoters in Huh7 cells. In another *in vitro* and *in vivo* investigation, resveratrol-coated liposomes showed improved anticancer activity in HepG2 cell line in comparison with free resveratrol [135]. Parekh *et al.* [136] reported that flow cytometry and PCNA western blot analysis of resveratrol-treated HepG2 cells displayed diminution in the cell proliferation. In addition to this, they found that resveratrol treatment downregulated the activity of cyclin D1 and expression of Pak1, p38 MAP kinase and Akt in HepG2 cells. Bishayee *et al.* [137, 138] showed that resveratrol substantially inhibited the expression of HIF-1 α, indicating that this transcription factor is a possible target of resveratrol in the anticipation of VEGF-mediated angiogenesis of hepatic neoplasia. Another *in vivo* study revealed that the compound can reduce oxidative stress and anti-inflammatory response facilitated by Nrf2 and thus validated the chemoprotective potential of this nutritional compound against chemically triggered hepatocarcinoma in rats. Resveratrol administration in the initial or advanced phases of hepatocarcinogenesis remarkably minimized the level of α-fetoprotein, the serum marker of HCC in DEN-induced male Wistar rats [280].

Sesamol, another phenolic constituent found in sesame, has antagonistic effect on hepatic carcinoma [281]. Silymarin extracted from *Silybum marianum*, "milk thistle" seeds, has been prescribed for liver ailments. Silymarin, a mixture of polyphenols of flavonolignans, namely silybin A, silybin B, silychristin, isosilychristin, isosilybin A, isosilybin B, and silydianin and a flavonoid, namely taxifolin [152, 282]. Silymarin has hepatoprotective activity [283, 284] and anti-hepato tumorogenesis [285–287]. The antihepatocarcinogenic potential made by silymarin lowers the cell proliferation and stimulates apoptosis in hepatic carcinoma cells [288]. The anticancerous potential of silymarin is due to the interruption of cell proliferation and apoptosis initiation through cell cycle arrest and interference of both extrinsic and intrinsic mitochondrial pathways. Silymarin constituents can affect several signaling pathways such as ERK, PTEN/Akt, Wnt/β-catenin, mTOR, and Notch in HCC [152].

10.1.1. *Flavonoids*

Flavonoids are one among the class of polyphenolic compounds seen in plants that exhibits anticancerous property. Anticarcinogenic mechanism exhibited by flavonoids (natural polyphenols) through upregulation of tumor inhibitors and autophagy by regulating signaling pathways such as canonical (Beclin-1-dependent) and non-canonical (Beclin-1-independent) pathways. In addition to this, the phytopolyphenols inhibit angiogenesis and metastasis through cross-talk with multiple intracellular signals and decline the risk of HCC [289]. Phytophenols, namely epigallocatechin, epigallocatechin gallate and catechin gallate present in red pine, restrict the invasion and motility of SK-Hep-1 (human HCC cells) by suppressing the activity of matrix metalloproteinases, especially gelatinase-A and -B. In addition to this, they found that epigallocatechin gallate imparts a major effect of red pine extract against hepatic carcinoma cells [290]. Xanthohumol, a prenylflavonoid chalcone, is the main constituent in female flowers of *Humulus lupulus* L., or "hop." This active molecule can enhance Nrf2 pathway in HCC in immortalized human liver THLE-2 and HepG2 cells [236].

10.1.2. *Anthocyanins*

As other naturally existing phenolic compounds, anthocyanins possess antioxidant activity against various induced reactive oxygen species and the potential to hinder lipid oxidation. Longo *et al.* [291, 292] explored anthocyanin present in *Rubia peregrina* L., *Philly realatifolia* L., and *Pistacia lentiscus* L., and their free radical scavenging efficacy. The principal anthocyanin compound of *P. lentiscus* berries was cyanidin 3-O-glucoside; however cyanidin 3-O-arabinoside and delphinidin 3-O-glucoside were also seen in trivial quantities. Alternatively, major anthocyanin found in the berry extracts of *R. peregrina* and *P. latifolia* was cyanidin 3-O-rutinoside and a small proportion of cyanidin 3-O-glucoside. The effectiveness of these anthocyanins to scavenge H_2O_2 was compared with standard reference antioxidant compound Troloxand BHA. The results endorsed that the H_2O_2 scavenging effect was declined in the order of Trolox > *P. lentiscus* > BHA > *R. peregrina* > *P. latifolia* at a concentration of 0.05 mg/mL. On the other hand, DPPH antioxidant activity was reduced in the order of a-tocopherol >*P. lentiscus* > *R. peregrina* > BHA >*P. latifolia*.

Ribes nigrum L., or black currant, is known as "superfruit," possessing different pharmacological properties together with mitigation of persisting oxidative stress and inflammatory conditions. The fruit is a very rich source of anthocyanins and thus has potent anticarcinogenic properties. In order to substantiate the chemopreventive efficacy, the skin extract of the fruit was used in rat liver carcinoma induced by intraperitoneal administration of diethylnitrosamine (DENA). The histopathological examinations revealed that the fruit skin extract successfully decreased tumor incidence, multiplicity, size, number, and volume of precancerous liver nodules dose-dependently. Immunohistochemical analysis and mechanistic studies substantiated inhibitory activity on abnormal cell proliferation and proapoptotic signal through the increase of Bax and decrease of Bcl-2 expression at the level of translation, respectively [293]. Delphinidin, another anthocyanidin compound, accelerated cellular vacuolization in different HCC cell lines [263].

10.2. *Terpenoids*

Terpenoids, another class of secondary metabolites present in plants, are constituted of isoprenoid units. Depending upon the number of these isoprenoid units, terpenoids are categorized into mono, di, tri, and tetra terpenes. Terpenoids have been administered in India to cure various diseases. Terpenoids showed cytotoxicity against different tumor cells including hepatic carcinoma cells and cancer prevention in preclinical *in vitro* and *in vivo* studies [23]. The major phytoactive compound astragaloside IV in *Radix astragali* reduced the efficiency of cell foci development and growth of anchorage-independent manner in HepG2. In order to analyze the protein expression activity of astragaloside IV in HepG2 cells, astragaloside IV affected stress response proteins, biosynthesis of proteins, and cell signaling cascade that were detected by MALDI/MS technology, proposing a novel triterpenoid mediated anticancer mechanism [159].

10.3. *Carotenoids*

Lycopene is a non-provitamin A and a natural carotenoid with high nutraceutical value, possesses the utmost antioxidant activity among the group of carotenoids, and present in limited number of fruits. Gupta *et al.* [294] studied the regulatory effectiveness of lycopene from tomato extracts towards N-diethylnitrosamine (NDEA)-induced liver cancer. The evaluation on the parameters such as survival rate, tumor burden, multiplicity, and incident rate along with histopathological analysis proclaimed ameliorating the deleterious effects by lycopene extract of N-diethylnitrosamine-induced liver carcinoma.

10.4. *Alkaloids*

Chuang *et al.* [253] studied the antagonistic effect of curcumin, a major alkaloid reported in *Curcuma longa* L., on murine hepatocarcinogenesis. Curcumin-containing diet was given to C3H/HeN mice for 4 days before N-diethylnitrosamine (DEN) injection and observed for 42 weeks. The results showed that curcumin-given animals had 81% reduction in tumor multiplicity and 62% reduction in tumor incidence. The hepatic tissue of curcumin-administered animals exposed a remarkable decrease in p21, PCNA, and CDC2 proteins than DEN-treated control group. Chemopreventive effects of two alkaloids, namely curcumin and caffeine, were compared in the diethylnitrosamine-treated hepatocarcinogenic rat model. The macroscopic and microscopic features of hepatic cells in the G2 stage, following a 10-week treatment with curcumin and caffeine (G3-10w,

G4-10w), as well as a 14-week treatment (G3-14w, G4-14w) recommended that treatment with caffeine could effectively attenuate hepatocarcinogenesis than curcumin. Moreover, the assessment through western blot and immunohistochemical analyses of glutathione S-transferase-P antibodies and proliferating cell nuclear antigen confirmed that the reduction in expression levels of these hepatocarcinogenic markers was more effectively achieved through administration of caffeine compared to curcumin [254].

Curcumin (diferuloylmethane) possesses potent antioxidant and anti-inflammatory activities and can inhibit chemical carcinogenesis in liver. However, poor bioavailability and hydrophobicity of curcumin obstruct to use it as a strong anticancer drug. To evade this, Farazuddin *et al.* [255] formulated a dual-core microcell of curcumin by the encapsulation of curcumin in microcells. It enhances the solubility and bioavailability of curcumin and enables gradual release kinetics over prolonged time periods. The *in vitro* and *in vivo* assays ratified improved ADMET properties of this formulation as well. Histopathological examinations substantiated that microcells that contain curcumin facilitated reduction of HCC and sustainment of cell architecture in hepatic cells. Jung *et al.* [256] reported that Capsaicin, an alkaloid found in red pepper and its derivative 4-methoxy capsaicin or met-capsaicin repressed SK-Hep-1 hepatocarcinoma cell growth through initiation of apoptosis and capsaicin depleted the proportion of Bax to Bcl-2 and accordingly accelerated the activity of caspase-3.

11. Combinatorial Activity of Phytoactive Constituents Against Hepatocarcinoma

Profusion of diversity of phytochemicals in phytoextracts synergizes its pharmacological potential and mitigates the adverse reactions of the active principle present in it. Phytoactive compounds function as a competent immunotherapeutic agent in single or in combination effectuate synergistic pharmacological activity. The combinatorial effects of different phytochemical, including polyphenols, carotenoids, and terpenoids as anticancer drugs, are either on the epigenetics mechanisms by furnishing insights into their precise epigenetics targets or mechanisms involved in prevention and therapy of cancer.

Synergistic, antagonistic activity of the following phytochemicals, namely phenethyl isothiocyanate, indole-3-carbinol reported from cruciferous plants; xanthohumol, from *Humulus lupulus* L., (hop plant) and resveratrol, active component of grape skin and seeds on liver carcinoma was investigated. In HepG2 HCC cells, synergism was shown by phenethyl isothiocyanate and indole-3-carbinol, indole-3-carbinol and xanthohumol, phenethyl isothiocyanate and resveratrol, phenethyl isothiocyanate and xanthohumol, indole-3-carbinol and resveratrol and xanthohumol and resveratrol combinations. However, mixtures of indole-3-carbinol and resveratrol and phenethyl isothiocyanate and resveratrol seem to act mostly antagonistically. All tested phytochemicals, except phenethyl isothiocyanate, increased the number of apoptotic cells, but phenethyl isothiocyanate and xanthohumol were the most potential apoptosis inducers and exhibited an increase of approximate 55% apoptotic cells [295]. Similarly, the combinatorial treatment of Thymoquinone from *Nigella sativa* and resveratrol from *Polygonum cuspidatum* in HCC cells (HepG2) revealed potent cell inhibition and acceleration of cell apoptosis. The molecules elevated ROS leading to depletion of glutathione and negligible activity on lipid peroxidation. These findings enlighten the novel promising combination against hepatic carcinoma [133]. The cotreatment of ethanolic extracts of *Punica granatum* and *Silybum marianum* exhibited remarkable decrease in HepG2 cell viability in albino rats [296]. Nath *et al.* [145] reported that Uttroside B, a saponin from *Solanum nigrum* L., in combination with the malaria drug, Cqn applied on HepG2 demonstrated induced autophagy. The cytotoxic assay conducted on HepG2 treated with methanolic extract of *Cousinia davisiana,* Cass confirmed the synergetic cytotoxic potential of its flavonoids, terpenes, and sterols compared to other *Cousinia* sp [297].

Oleo-gum-resin contained in *Boswellia Serrata* was separated with methanol and petroleum ether. GC/MS data of methanol extract fractions I, II, and III uncovered seven active principles such as 2-methyl-levulinicacid methyl ester; pent-2-ene-1,4-dione;

3,5-dimethyl-1-hexane and methyl,1-methylpentadecanoate in fraction I. Nevertheless, fractions II and III showed the presence of 17a-hydroxy-17a-cyano, preg-4-en-3-one; 1-methoxy- 4-(1-propenyl) benzene and 1,1-dimethoxy cyclohexane. The competent cytotoxicity of *B. serrata* methanolic chromatographic fractions I, II, III, and IV was validated in HepG2 cell lines [298].

Radiation resistance is a major issue during radiotherapy, and the possible efficacious alternative therapy is the use of naturally occurring phytochemicals. A commercial product, Breast Safeguard (BSG) is a combination of seven proven anticancerous plant-derived bioactive compounds, namely indol-3-carbinol, curcumin, quercetin, resveratrol, genistein, gallic acid, and C-Phycocyanine. Abdraboh *et al.* [298] validated the radio-sensitizing and anticancer potential of BSG in HepG2 cells treated with ionizing radiations. Application of ionizing radiations and/or BSG in HepG2 cells resulted in remarkable downregulation at cell growth as observed through the reduction of proliferation marker (Ki67) expression, ratio of formation of colony as well as G2/M cell cycle arrest. The concurrent intervention triggered apoptosis through a P53-dependent pathway, as evidenced by a notable rise in the expression of early apoptosis marker (Annexin V), DNA fragmentation, P53, and Bax, along with a reduction in Bcl2 expression. Synergetic treatment remarkably reduced motility of HepG2 cells which was confirmed through wound healing migration assay and observed the remarkable decrease at CD95 expression. Hence, the results demonstrated the synergetic effect of combined phytochemicals as effective radiosensitizer that accelerated the response of cell to IR to subsequently weaken the growth of HepG2 cells, its survival, and motility.

Administration of aqueous extract of *Curcuma longa* L., to HBx transgenic mice reactivated p53, suppressed HBx and elevated its downstream genes cyclin D1 and p21, thereby regulating the anomalous cell cycle. The reduced HBx expression by enhancing its breaking down is due to the synergetic chemopreventive activity of phytochemicals present in *C. longa* [299]. The *in vitro* and *in vivo* experiments on Curcuma oil revealed hepatoprotective and anti-HCC effects [300]. The probable inhibitory activity of a standardized ginger rhizome extract against liver cancer in Wistar rats treated with diethylnitrosamine (DEN) was studied. The ginger extract neutralized DEN-influenced oxidative stress and reduced protein carbonyl concentrations, malondialdehyde, and myeloperoxidase in the liver tissue. In addition to these, the reinstatement of catalase, GST, superoxide dismutase, and glutathione was observed. Rat liver immunohistochemical bleaching revealed that ginger extract restricted the rise in cyclooxygenase-2, Ki-67, and nuclear factor-kappa B p65 cell-positive numbers. In addition to these, the extract declined the quantity of positive cells in DEN/2-AAF-administered rats [301].

Potential antitumor activity of plant-derived antioxidant molecules has been recognized as alternate means of cancer prevention and treatment. Combinatorial therapeutic approaches have advantages like synergistic effect, reduce side effects, and decrease drug resistance [302]. Sorafenib is an FDA-approved multikinase inhibitor drug that causes side effects such as neurological disorders, hypertension, hematological disorders, and renal toxicity attributed to its prolonged use [303, 304]. *In vitro* application of sorafenib in combination with trans-charcone, vitamin K1 (plant derived) in HepG2 cell line accelerated the resistance against H_2O_2 induced oxidative stress [305].

Fumaria indica extract showed chemopreventive effect on DEN and CCl_4-mediated hepatocarcinogenesis by reducing the tumor and reinstating the functions of marker enzymes of hepatocarcinoma in Wistar rats [306]. Jin *et al.* [307] reported that ethanolic extract of *Osmanthus matsumuranus* successfully inhibited the growth of HepG2 cells by causing both apoptosis and G2/M arrest by extrinsic and intrinsic pathways. The *in vitro* and *in vivo* studies of *Piper betle* leaf extract proved its potential chemopreventive effect through activated cAbl, ATM and p73 expressions, p38 and JNK pathways that result in the arrest of cell cycle and apotopsis [308].

Phytochemicals in pomegranate fruit have strong anti-inflammatory and antioxidant effects, and it can prevent DENA-initiated hepatocarcinogenesis in rats by Nrf2-mediated antioxidant activities [309]. Bhatiya *et al.* [310] reported that pomegranate extract prevented diethylnitrosamine-mediated rat hepatocarcinogenesis through suppression of nuclear factor-kappaB (NF-κB). The polyphenolic antioxidant property of this superfruit is attributed to the compounds such as condensed tannins (proanthocyanidins), hydrolyzable tannins (gallotannins and ellagitannins), and anthocyanins. Bishayee *et al.* [311] reported pomegranate-mediated chemopreventive action against experimental hepatocarcinogenesis. Celery (*Apium graveolens* L.) seed oil is a repository of various classes of phytoactive molecules endowed with potential anti-inflammatory and antioxidant effects. Immunohistochemical analyses of DENA-induced HCC rats treated with celery seed oil confirmed remarkable raise in upregulation of PCNA, COX-2, NF-kB serum, liver nitric oxide content and TNF-α level. As the celery seed oil extract elevated caspase-3 expression and declined the PCNA expression, implying apoptotic and antiproliferative properties, respectively [312]. Maideen *et al.* [313] corroborated the hepatoprotective and antioxidant activity of *Phyllanthus polyphyllus* methanol extract on liver tumor in DEN-induced male Wistar rats through decline of increased mitochondrial lipid peroxidation, RNA, DNA, and weight of liver. Likewise, the extract elevated non-enzymatic antioxidants and mitochondrial antioxidants, namely SOD, glutathione peroxidase, and catalase.

Pulsatilla koreana extract inhibited hepatic carcinoma by decreasing the activity of VEGF and hypoxia-inducible factor (HIF-1α) [314]. Four varieties of raspberry extract noticeably affected the growth of HepG2 cells. Similarly, the dose-dependent application of raspberry extract on DEN-induced hepatic nodule formation revealed that the HCC masses decreased in accordance with increasing doses of the extract [315]. Various analyses revealed that red raspberry extract can potentially inhibit S phase cell growth and cell cycle advancement in HepG2 cells. Also, raspberry extract accelerated the activity of tensin homolog deleted on chromosome 10 (PTEN) and phosphatase through depleting the PTEN gene promoter methylation and DNMT1 expression and modulated signaling pathway of AKT [143].

A comparative investigation on the anticancerous activity of free C6, a coumarin derivative, and C6 entrapped liposome was tested preclinically, and the result showed that free C6 possessed reduced cell internalization [135, 316]. *Trigonella foenum-graecum* L., or "fenugreek" contains diverse phytoactive constituents that impart various pharmacological activities, especially anticancerous effect. Fenugreek seed extract treated HepG2 cell line exhibited cytotoxicity through apoptosis induction. The HepG2 cells, 48 hours after the treatment, expressed cytotoxic features such as shrinkage, condensation of DNA, development of apoptotic bodies and enucleation [317]. Subfractions of methanolic extract of *Amorphophallus companulatus* showed antiproliferative and apoptotic effect in PLC/PRF/5 liver cancer cell line [318]. Likewise, methanolic extract of *Annona muricata* fruit [319], chlorofom extract of Fig latex [320], and ethanolic extract of *Ficus odorata* [321] exhibited apoptotic potency in HepG2 cell lines. *Costus speciosus*is is a prominent herb that has been administered for the cure of different diseases in Ayurveda. The apoptosis induced by the methanolic extract of *C. speciosus* is investigated in HepG2 through caspase-3 simulation and assay of annexin V/7-AAD. The declined membrane potential of mitochondria verified the occurrence of mitochondrial apoptotic pathway *via* opening of mitochondrial permeability transition pore. Apoptosis was in accordance with the breakdown of the transmembrane potential that leads to the eviction of cytochrome C, key apoptogenic molecule from mitochondria. The investigation ensured significant cell growth arrest by the methanolic extract with apoptotic-inducing activities associated with cell cycle inhibition at S and G2/M phases [322]. Desert plants such as *Achillea fragrantissima* (Compositae), *Varthemia iphionoides* Boiss (Compositae), *Phlomis platystegia* Post, *Origanum dayi* Post(Lamiaceae), and *Ochradenus baccatus* Delile (Resedaceae), against HepG2 cell line study [323] affirmed their anticancerous potential.

Crocus sativus, the golden spice "saffron" contains phytochemicals, namely crocin, crocetin, carotene, and safranal, which have proven antioxidant and anticancerous properties [324–330]. The *in vivo* studies of this plant in DEN-treated animals showed antiproliferative activity through cell cycle inhibition and decrease in the quantity of Ki-67-positive cells, phosphorylated tumor necrosis factor receptor, inducible nitric oxide synthase, nuclear factor-kappa B p-65, and cyclooxygenase 2. In addition to this, by reinstatement of superoxide dismutase, glutathione-S-transferase and catalase levels and reduction of protein carbonyl formation, malondialdehyde and myeloperoxidase activity in liver, saffron inhibited oxidative stress caused by DEN in rats [257, 326].

Studies on HepG2 cells treated with sesamol in a dose response revealed reduction in cell viability. Further, colony formation assay confirmed the triggered apoptotic potential and S phase cell cycle arrest. The analysis of both intrinsic and extrinsic pathways revealed that the sesamol impaired the expression of Bcl-2 (anti-apoptotic protein) and enhanced the release of cytochrome c from mitochondria, poly-ADP-ribose polymerase, activity of Fas/FasL and stimulated caspase-8 and tBid. Meanwhile, mitochondrial membrane potential loss, a characteristic of cell apoptosis, was also observed [281]. Administration of a mixture of sesame and orange seed extract that contains hesperidin and sesaminin in rats with diethylnitrosamine (DEN)-induced hepatocarcinogenesis showed enhanced chemopreventive effect against an early stage of hepatocarcinogenesis [150].

The prophylactic effect of *Averrhoa carambola* "star fruit" on DENA-treated and CCl4-enhanced Swiss albino mice hepatocarcinoma was studied. Oral administration of star fruit extract at a dose of 25 mg/kg b.wt/day was done only for five successive days before the 48 hours of first administration of DENA. CCl_4 was administered after two weeks of DENA treatment and found that a considerable reduction in hepatic carcinoma [331]. Sulforaphane ([1-isothioyanato-4-(methyl-sulfinyl) butane], SFN) is the major phytoactive constituent seen in broccoli and cauliflower, the vegetables belonging to Cruciferae [332], and has potent antioxidant, anti-inflammatory, cytotoxicity and cytoprotection effects. Liu *et al.* [149] validated the *in vitro* anticancerous potential of sulphoraphane in HepG2 cell and human umbilical vein endothelial (HUVEC) cell lines. They reported that SFN hindered HepG2-induced angiogenesis through the hindrance of STAT3/HIF-1α/VEGF signaling.

Phytochemical screening of *Tephrosia purpurea* unveiled the occurrence of flavonoids (quercetin, rutin, lanceolatin A, B, C, purpuritenin, purpurenone, osyritin, and purpurin) and carotenoids (elliptone, deguelin, rotenone and tephrosin, and β-sitosterol) [333].

Meanwhile an isoflavone, 7,4′- dihydroxy-3′,5′-dimethoxyisoflavone, and a chalcone (+)-tephropurpurin was also explored in *T. Purpurea* [334]. Antitumerigenesis study of *T. purpurea* was performed in Wistar rats; interestingly, the analysis of status of serum marker enzymes, nodule incidence, liver tumor markers and antioxidant enzymes indicated the counteraction of *T. purpurea* extract toward HCC [335].

Histopathology, immunohistochemical analysis (cell proliferation) and DNA fragmentation assay (apoptosis) of DENA-initiated liver tumors in Sprague-Dawley rats undoubtedly substantiated that sulfated polysaccharides of *Ulva lactuca* showed a remarkable chemoprevention, namely abnormal cell growth arrest and apoptosis induction [336]. *Ribes nigrum* L., berries (black currant) are also recognized to possess various other antioxidant constituents such as anthocyanins and phenolics, including flavonoids and phenolic acids [337]. Aqueous extract of the black currant berries to be an efficient chemoprotective agent against hepatocarcinogenesis (DENA-induced) through its antioxidant (Nrf2-mediated) mechanisms. Moreover, the extract was able to conquer NF-kB-mediated inflammatory pathways together with the inflammation-driven activity of HSP70, HSP90, and COX-2 during an initial stage of liver carcinogenesis in rats [338]. Abdellah *et al.* [339] studied the potential of two herbal components, ellagic acid (phytophenol) and 1,8-cineole (a monoterpenoid) against DEN/2-AAF-induced HCC in rats. DEN/2-AAF administration caused degradation of hepatic cells with a weakened liver functional capacity, and tumor markers increase such as alpha-L-fucosidase, alpha-fetoprotein, arginase-1, and ferritin. The treatment with EA (60 mg/kg) and Cin (100 mg/kg) strongly reinstated these biochemical modifications. Likewise, Cin and EA administration resulted in the decrease in VEGF, Fascin-1 (FSCN1), transforming growth factor beta-1 (TGF-β1), matrix metalloproteinase-9 (MMP-9), and epithelial-mesenchymal transition (EMT) key marker, vimentin, in association with a revival of anatomical features related to HCC cell lines.

The research conducted by Bharathi *et al.* [340] in leaf extract of *Azadiracta indica* indicated its efficacy as chemoprotective agent on

NDEA-mediated hepatocarcinogenesis. Administration of extract showed remarkable decrease in multiplicity (42%), tumor occurrence (33%), and increase in survival (34%). Further, scanning and transmission electron microscopic studies revealed acute variations in organization of organelles, morphology, metabolism, cellular arrangement, and degree of differentiation. Chemopreventive effects of hydrophilic polysaccharides from *Ganoderma resinaceum* against HCC were studied by Sipping *et al.* [341]. *In vitro* antiproliferative effect of polysaccharide-rich fractions of *G. resinaceum*(GRP I and GRP II) was tested in HeLa, MDA-MB 231 and HepG2 using the MTT assay followed by animal model studies. Hepatocarcinoma initiation and development was analyzed through histopathology of liver, hematology, cytokines/chemokines levels, hepatic injury markers and stress oxidative markers. Furthermore, GRP I and GRP II inhibited the changes of the histoarchitecture in DEN-induced lever cells. Aspartate aminotransferase (AST), alanine aminotransferase (ALT), proinflammatory cytokines (G-CSF, IFN*c*, and TNFα), alpha-fetoprotein (AFP) and chemokines (fractalkine and eotaxin) levels were remarkable reduced in groups treated with GRP I and GRP II, although anti-inflammatory cytokines (IL-12p70 and IL-10) levels were amplified. The antioxidant activity was enhanced by decreasing nitric oxide (NO_2) and malondialdehyde (MDA) levels, increasing superoxide dismutase (SOD) and catalase (CAT) activities, and decreasing glutathione (GSH) levels. The overall outcomes implicated that GRP I has chemoprotective activity through preventing cell growth and reinstating antioxidant enzymes, liver architecture and chemokine/cytokine balance.

Chang *et al.* [261] isolated γ-Mangostin from *Garcinia mangostana* fruit and demonstrated its free radical scavenging, antiproliferative, and apoptotic activities in HepG2 cells. Qualitative phytochemical analysis of epicarp and endocarp of the extracts of *G. mangostana* fruit affirmed the presence of phenols and flavonoids. However, HPLC and GC phytochemical profiling verified that phenolic constituents were greater in chloroform extract of epicarp than in hexane extract of endocarp, and flavonoids and triterpenoid content were greater in hexane extract of endocarp. Quantifiable HPLC and GC-MS studies also substantiated that the chloroform epicarp extract possessed 166 compounds, and hexane endocarp extract contained 105 compounds. The extracts treated HCC (HeP-G2) cells revealed the best antiproliferative activity. The cell proliferation inhibition of Hep-G2 cells might be attributed to the occurrence of flavonoids, phenols, and triterpenoids in mangosteen fruit wall [342]. The groups with HCC exposed to either high or low dose of extract prompted remarkable reduction of serum hepatic hydroxy proline, CEA, AFP, and increase in total serum proteins related to the untreated HCC rats [343]. The inhibitory activity of *Garcinia mangostana* fruit extract (GME) against overexpressed enzymes and apoptotic proteins in DEN-mediated HCC rats was studied. They observed that the GME-treated groups of rats showed remarkable decrease in lysosomal enzymes, ornithine decarboxylase and decreased cell growth with elevated apoptosis. The evaluation on the level of beta-D-glucosidase (lysosomal enzyme) showed that it was increased due to DEN induction, and after GME treatment, the level was declined; thus, the experiment substantiated the chemoprotective action of GME on liver cancer [344].

12. Clinical Trials

The preclinical efficacy and safety of promising chemical compounds derived from plants have been assessed in suitable clinical trials. Most of these clinical trials were conducted in patients or high-risk individuals, and only 20% of the studies have reported their results due to various factors such as problems of bioavailability, toxicity, and other unidentified reasons. Among the various compounds used in clinical trials, only retinoids have been tested against liver cancer along with cancer of several other origins [345–347].

13. Conclusion and Remarks

HCC is the third deadliest and fifth common malignancy worldwide, having high morbidity and mortality. Among the various treatment strategies reported against HCC, chemoprevention using phytochemicals is found to be the most efficient one. A significant quantity of phytochemicals demonstrated high efficacy in treating HCC, either individually or in combination with others, both *in vitro* or in animal models; none of them have been entered in clinical trials till date except retinoids to finally prove their efficacy, bioavailability and toxicity if any during treatment in patients. More clinical studies should be conducted using the preclinically effective phytochemicals to bring all of them to market for therapeutic use.

Conflict of Interest

The authors declare no conflict of interest.

References

1. Von Meyenfeldt, M. Cancer-associated malnutrition: an introduction. *European Journal of Oncology Nursing*, 2005. **9**: p. S35–S38.
2. Van Zandwijk, H., Reid, G., and Frank, A.L. Asbestos-related cancers: the 'Hidden Killer' remains a global threat. *Expert Review of Anticancer Therapy*, 2020. **20** (4): p. 271–278.
3. Kanwal, F., *et al.* Risk factors for HCC in contemporary cohorts of patients with cirrhosis. *Hepatology*, 2022.
4. Ganguly, R., Gupta, A., and Pandey, A.K. Role of baicalin as a potential therapeutic agent in hepatobiliary and gastrointestinal disorders: A review. *World Journal of Gastroenterology*, 2022. **28**: p. 3047–3062.
5. Jeng, K.S., *et al.* Upper gastrointestinal cancer and liver cirrhosis. *Cancers (Basel)*, 2022. **14**: p. 2269.
6. Singh, A.K., Kumar, R., and Pandey A.K. Hepatocellular carcinoma: causes, mechanism of progression and biomarkers. *Current Chemical Genomics and Translational Medicine*, 2018. **12**: p. 9–26.
7. Kim, J.Y., *et al.* HBx-induced hepatic steatosis and apoptosis are regulated by TNFR1- and NF-kappaB-dependent pathways. *Journal of Molecular Biology*, 2010. **397**: p. 917–931.
8. Flores, J.E., *et al.* The global impact of hepatitis B vaccination on hepatocellular carcinoma. *Vaccines (Basel)*, 2022. **10**: p. 793.
9. Rodina, A.S., *et al.* Hepatocellular damage and inflammation in various forms of alcoholic liver disease. *Ter Arkh*, 2021. **93**: p. 15–19.

10. Yasmin, A., *et al.* Transcriptional regulation of alcohol induced liver fibrosis in a translational porcine hepatocellular carcinoma model. *Biochimie*, 2021. **182**: p. 73–84.
11. Liu, B.J., *et al.* Real-world study of hepatic artery infusion chemotherapy combined with anti-PD-1 immunotherapy and tyrosine kinase inhibitors for advanced hepatocellular carcinoma. *Immunotherapy*, 2021. **13**: p. 1395–1405.
12. Xiang, M., *et al.* Chemical composition of total flavonoids from Polygonum amplexicaule and their pro-apoptotic effect on hepatocellular carcinoma cells: potential roles of suppressing STAT3 signaling. *Food and Chemical Toxicology*, 2015. **80**: p. 62–71.
13. Sreekumar, S., and Nisha, N.C. Plants are renewable source of medicine and nanoparticles: a review in current aspects in pharmaceutical research and development. *BP International, UK*, 2021. p. 44–56.
14. Christopher, D., *et al.* Phytochemicals as potential chemopreventive and chemotherapeutic agents in hepatocarcinogenesis. *European Journal of Cancer Prevention*, 2009. **18**: p. 13–25.
15. Macdonald, G.A. Pathogenesis of hepatocellular carcinoma. *Clinical Liver Disease*, 2001. **5** (1): p. 69–85.
16. Bataller, R. and Brenner, D.A., Liver fibrosis. *Journal of Clinical Investigation*, 2005. **115** (2): p. 209–218.
17. Koike, K. Steatosis, liver injury, and hepatocarcinogenesis in hepatitis C viral infection. *Journal of Gastroenterology*, 2009. **44** (19): p. 82–88.
18. Schütte, K., Bornschein, J., and Malfertheiner, P. Hepatocellular carcinoma-epidemiological trends and risk factors. *Journal of Digestive Diseases*, 2009. **27** (2): p. 80–92.
19. Farinati, F., *et al.* Hepatitis C virus: from oxygen free radicals to hepatocellular carcinoma. *Journal of Viral Hepatitis,* 2007. **14** (12): p. 821–9.
20. El-Serag, H.B. Hepatocellular carcinoma. *New England Journal of Medicine*, 2011. **365** (12): p. 1118–1127.
21. Forner, A., Llovet, J.M., and Bruix, J. Hepatocellular carcinoma. *Lancet*, 2012. **379** (9822): p. 1245–1255.
22. Forner, A., *et al.* Treatment of intermediate-stage hepatocellular carcinoma. *Nature Reviews Clinical Oncology*, 2014. **11** (9): p. 525–535.

23. Thoppil, R.J., and Bishayee, A. Terpenoids as potential chemopreventive and therapeutic agents in liver cancer. *World Journal of Hepatology*, 2011. **3** (9): p. 228–249.
24. Villanueva, A., and Llovet, J.M. Impact of intra-individual molecular heterogeneity in personalized treatment of hepatocellular carcinoma. *Hepatology*, 2012. **56** (6): p. 2416–2419.
25. Njei, B., Rotman, Y., and Ditah, I. Emerging trends in hepatocellular carcinoma incidence and mortality. *Hepatology*, 2015. **61**: p. 191–199.
26. Thun, M.J., *et al.* The global burden of cancer: priorities for prevention. *Carcinogenesis*, 2010. **31** (1): p. 100–110.
27. Parkin, D.M. *et al.* Estimating the world cancer burden: Globocan. *International Journal of Cancer*, 2000. **94** (2): p. 153–156.
28. EL-Kenawy, A.E.-M., and El-Bendary, A.H. Hepatocellular carcinoma: an update. *International Journal of Cancer Research and Prevention*, **6** (1): p. 1554–1134.
29. Kumar, V. *Herbs and bioactive compounds in prevention and treatment of hepatocellular carcinoma*. ResearchGate, 2012.
30. Shen, Li., *et al.* Risk factors, pathogenesis, and strategies for hepatocellular carcinoma prevention: emphasis on secondary prevention and its translational challenges. *Journal of Clinical Medicine*, 2020. **9**: p. 3817.
31. Yu, M.-W., *et al.* Effect of aflatoxin metabolism and DNA adduct formation on hepatocellular carcinoma among chronic hepatitis B carriers in Taiwan. *Journal of Hepatology*, 1997. **27**: p. 320–330.
32. Yang, J.D., *et al.* Characteristics, management, and outcomes of patients with hepatocellular carcinoma in Africa: A multicounty observational study from the Africa Liver Cancer Consortium. *Lancet Gastroenterology and Hepatology*, 2017. **2**: 103–111.
33. Staretz, M.E., *et al.* Comparative metabolism of the tobacco-related carcinogens benzo[a]pyrene, 4-(methylnitrosamino)-1-(3-pyridyl)-1-butanone, 4-(methylnitrosamino)-1-(3-pyridyl)-1-butanol, and N′-nitrosonornicotine in human hepatic microsomes. *Drug Metabolism and Disposition*, 1997. **25**: p. 154–162.
34. Barbieri, S.S., *et al.* Cytokines present in smokers' serum interact with smoke components to enhance endothelial dysfunction. *Cardiovascular Research*, 2011. **90**: p. 475–483.

35. Piña, J.M.D., *et al.* Tumor necrosis factor as an early marker of inflammation in healthy smokers. *Journal of Clinical Medicine*, 2012. **139**: p. 47–53.
36. Baecker, A., *et al.* Worldwide incidence of hepatocellular carcinoma cases attributable to major risk factors. *European Journal of Cancer Prevention*, 2018. **27**: p. 205–212.
37. Bianchi, L. Glycogen storage disease I and hepatocellular tumours. *European Journal of Nuclear Medicine and Molecular Imaging*, 1993. **152**: p. 63–70.
38. Elmberg, M., *et al.* Cancer risk in patients with hereditary hemochromatosis and in their first-degree relatives. *Gastroenterology*, 2003. **125**: p. 1733–1741.
39. Eriksson, S.G. Liver disease in α1-antitrypsin deficiency: aspects of incidence and prognosis. *Scandinavian Journal of Gastroenterology*, 1985. **20**: p. 907–911.
40. Scott, C.R. The genetic tyrosinemias. *American Journal of Medical Genetics Part C: Seminars in Medical Genetics*, 2006. **142**: p. 121–126.
41. Antonelli, A., *et al.* Thyroid disorders in chronic hepatitis C. *American Journal of Medicine*, 2004. **117**: p. 10–13.
42. Hassan, M.M., *et al.* Association between hypothyroidism and hepatocellular carcinoma: a case-control study in the United States. *Hepatology*, 2009. **49**: p. 1563–1570.
43. Lonardo, A., *et al.* Pathogenesis of hypothyroidism-induced NAFLD: evidence for a distinct disease entity? *Digestive and Liver Disease*, 2019. **51**: p. 462–470.
44. Yeh, S.H., and Chen, P.J. Gender disparity of hepatocellular carcinoma: the roles of sex hormones. *Oncology*, 2010. **78**: p. 172–179.
45. Wu, M.H., *et al.* Androgen receptor promotes hepatitis B virus-induced hepatocarcinogenesis through modulation of hepatitis B virus RNA transcription. *Science Translational Medicine*, 2010. **2**: p. 32ra35.
46. Shimizu, I. Impact of oestrogens on the progression of liver disease. *Liver International*, 2003. **23**: p. 63–69.
47. McGlynn, K.A., *et al.* Reproductive factors, exogenous hormone use and risk of hepatocellular carcinoma among US women: results from the Liver Cancer Pooling Project. *British Journal of Cancer*, 2015. **112**: p. 1266–1272.

48. Ozen, C. ***Current prevention approaches for hepatocellular carcinoma.*** Research Gate, 2016.
49. Feitelson, M.A., ***et al.*** Genetic mechanisms of hepatocarcinogenesis. *Oncogene*, 2002. **21** (16): p. 2593–2604.
50. Osawa, M., ***et al.*** Prognosis and predictors of hepatocellular carcinoma in elderly patients infected with hepatitis B virus. *Journal of Medical Virology*, 2017. **89**: p. 2144–2148.
51. El-Serag, H.B. Epidemiology of viral hepatitis and hepatocellular carcinoma. *Gastroenterology*, 2012. **142**: p. 1264–1273.
52. Ozturk, M. Genetic aspects of hepatocellular carcinogenesis. *Seminars in Liver Disease*, 1999. **19** (3): p. 235–242.
53. Farcas, M., ***et al.*** SIRT1 in the development and treatment of hepatocellular carcinoma. *Frontiers in Nutrition*, 2019. **6**: p. 148.
54. Tommasi, S., ***et al.*** Molecular pathways and related target therapies in liver carcinoma. *International Journal of Current Pharmaceutical Research*, 2007. **13**: p. 3279–3287.
55. Yang, C., ***et al.*** High expression of GFAT1 predicts poor prognosis in patients with pancreatic cancer. *Scientific Reports*, 2016. **6**: p. 39044.
56. Nath, A., ***et al.*** Elevated free fatty acid uptake via CD36 promotes epithelial-mesenchymal transition in hepatocellular carcinoma. *Scientific Reports*, 2015. **5**: p. 14752.
57. Soussan, P., ***et al.*** ***In vivo*** expression of a new hepatitis B virus protein encoded by a spliced RNA. *The Journal of Clinical Investigation*, 2000. **105**: p. 55–60.
58. Edmunds, W.J., ***et al.*** The influence of age on the development of the hepatitis B carrier state. *Proceedings of the Royal Society B: Biological Sciences*, 1993. **253**: p. 197–201.
59. Sung, W.K., ***et al.*** Genome-wide survey of recurrent HBV integration in hepatocellular carcinoma. *Nature Genetics*, 2012. **44**: p. 765–769.
60. Yan, H., ***et al.*** Characterization of the genotype and integration patterns of hepatitis B virus in early- and late-onset hepatocellular carcinoma. *Hepatology*, 2015. **61**: p. 1821–1831.
61. Chemin, I., and Zoulim, F. Hepatitis B virus induced hepatocellular carcinoma. *Cancer Letters*, 2009. **286**: p. 52–59.
62. Sundaram, V., ***et al.*** Acute on chronic liver failure from nonalcoholic fatty liver disease: a growing and aging cohort with rising mortality. *Hepatology*, 2021. **73**: p. 1932–1944.

63. Yuan, R.H., *et al.* Tumor-matrix interaction induces phenotypic switching in liver cancer cells. *Hepatology International*, 2022. **16**: p. 562–576.
64. Vescovo, T., *et al.* Molecular mechanisms of hepatitis C virus–induced hepatocellular carcinoma. *Clinical Microbiology and Infection*, 2016. **22**: p. 853–861.
65. Street, A., *et al.* Hepatitis C virus NS5A-mediated activation of phosphoinositide 3-Kinase results in stabilization of cellular β-catenin and stimulation of β-catenin-responsive transcription. *Journal of Virology*, 2005. **79**: p. 5006–5016.
66. Farzaneh, Z., *et al.* Critical signaling pathways governing hepatocellular carcinoma behavior; small molecule-based approaches. *Cancer Cell International*, 2021. **21**: p. 208.
67. Setshedi, M., Wands, J.R., and De La Monte, S.M. Acetaldehyde adducts in alcoholic liver disease. *Oxidative Medicine and Cellular Longevity*, 2010. **3**: p. 178–185.
68. Thun, M.J., *et al.* The global burden of cancer: priorities for prevention. *Carcinogenesis*, 2010. **31** (1): p. 100–110.
69. Nakagawa, S., *et al.* Molecular liver cancer prevention in cirrhosis by organ transcriptome analysis and lysophosphatidic acid pathway inhibition. *Cancer Cell*, 2016. **30**: p. 879–890.
70. Parikh, N.D., Singal, A.G., and Hutton, D.W. Cost effectiveness of regorafenib as second-line therapy for patients with advanced hepatocellular carcinoma. *Cancer*, 2017. **123**: p. 3725–3731.
71. Cancer Genome Atlas Research Network Electronic address: wheeler@bcm.edu Cancer Genome Atlas Research Network. Comprehensive and integrative genomic characterization of hepatocellular carcinoma. *Cell*, 2017. **169**: p. 1327–1341.
72. Wörns, M.I., and Galle, P.R. Novel inhibitors in development for hepatocellular carcinoma. *Expert Opinion on Investigational Drugs*, 2010. **19** (5): p. 615–629.
73. Zhu, A.X. Molecularly targeted therapy for advanced hepatocellular carcinoma in 2012: current status and future perspectives. *Seminars in Oncology Nursing*, 2012. **39** (4): p. 493–502.
74. Shen, Y.C., Hsu, C., and Cheng, A.L. Molecular targeted therapy for advanced hepatocellular carcinoma: current status and future perspectives. *Journal of Gastroenterology*, 2010. **45**: p. 794–807.

75. Bishayee, A., *et al.* Dietary phytochemicals in the chemoprevention and treatment of hepatocellular carcinoma: *in vivo* evidence, molecular targets, and clinical relevance. *Current Cancer Drug Targets*, 2012. **12** (9): p. 1191–1232.
76. Llovet, J.M., *et al.* Sorafenib in advanced hepatocellular carcinoma. *The New England Journal of Medicine*, 2008. **359**: p. 378–390.
77. Merle, P., *et al.* Cabozantinib in patients with advanced and progressing hepatocellular carcinoma. *The New England Journal of Medicine*, 2018. **379**: p. 54–63.
78. Zhu, A.X., *et al.* A study of ramucirumab (LY3009806) versus placebo in patients with hepatocellular carcinoma and elevated baseline alpha-fetoprotein (REACH-2). *Journal of Clinical Oncology*, 2018. **36**: p. TPS538.
79. El-Khoueiry, A.B., *et al.* Nivolumab in patients with advanced hepatocellular carcinoma (CheckMate 040): An open-label, non-comparative, phase 1/2 dose escalation and expansion trial. *Lancet*, 2017. **389**: p. 2492–2502.
80. Finn, R.S., *et al.* Results of KEYNOTE-240: Phase 3 study of pembrolizumab (Pembro) vs. best supportive care (BSC) for second line therapy in advanced hepatocellular carcinoma (HCC). *Journal of Clinical Oncology*, 2019. **37**: p. 4004.
81. Pinter, M., Jain, R.K., and Duda, D.G. The current landscape of immune checkpoint blockade in hepatocellular carcinoma. *JAMA Oncology*, 2020. 22.
82. Kew, M.C. Prevention of hepatocellular carcinoma. *HPB (Oxford)*, 2005. 7 (1): p. 16–25.
83. Colombo, M. Prevention of hepatocellular carcinoma and recommendations for surveillance in adults with chronic liver disease. *UptoDate*, 2015.
84. Zanetti, A.R., Van Damme, P., and Shouval, D. The global impact of vaccination against hepatitis B: a historical overview. *Vaccine*, 2008. **26**: p. 6266–6273.
85. Ni, Y.H., *et al.* Hepatitis B virus infection in children and adolescents in a hyperendemic area: 15 years after mass hepatitis B vaccination. *Annals of Internal Medicine*, 2001. **135**: p. 796–800.
86. Chen, C.-H., *et al.* Estimation of seroprevalence of hepatitis B virus and hepatitis C virus in Taiwan from a large-scale survey of free hepatitis

screening participants. *Journal of the Formosan Medical Association*, 2007. **106**: p. 148–155.

87. Singh, S., *et al.* Chemo preventive strategies in hepatocellular carcinoma. *Nature Reviews Gastroenterology and Hepatology*, 2014. **11** (1): p. 45–54.
88. Luedde, T., and Schwabe, R.F. NF-κB in the liver — linking injury, fibrosis and hepatocellular carcinoma. *Nature Reviews Gastroenterology and Hepatology*, 2011. **8**: p. 108–118.
89. Ikeda, K., *et al.* Interferon beta prevents recurrence of hepatocellular carcinoma after complete resection or ablation of the primary tumor—a prospective randomized study of hepatitis C virus–related liver cancer. *Hepatology*, 2000. **32**: p. 228–232.
90. Mazzaferro, V., *et al.* Prevention of hepatocellular carcinoma recurrence with alpha-interferon after liver resection in HCV cirrhosis. *Hepatology*, 2006. **44**: p. 1543–1554.
91. Hong, W.K., and Lippman, S.M. Cancer chemoprevention. *Journal of the National Cancer Institute Monographs*, 1995. p. 49–53.
92. Suou, T., *et al.* Interferon alpha inhibits intrahepatic recurrence in hepatocellular carcinoma with chronic hepatitis C: a pilot study. *Hepatology Research*, 2001. **20**: p. 301–311.
93. Uenishi, T., *et al.* Influence of interferon therapy on outcome after surgery for hepatitis C virus-related hepatocellular carcinoma. *Hepatology Research*, 2006. **36**: p. 195–200.
94. Ishikawa, T. Secondary prevention of recurrence by interferon therapy after ablation therapy for hepatocellular carcinoma in chronic hepatitis C patients. *World Journal of Gastroenterology*, 2008. **14**: p. 6140–6144.
95. Okano, J.-I. Chemoprevention against hepatocellular carcinoma. *Journal of Clinical Gastroenterology*, 2011. **4**: p. 185–197.
96. Liu, R.H. Potential synergy of phytochemicals in cancer prevention: mechanism of action. *Journal of Nutrition*, 2004. **134**: p. 3479S–3485S.
97. Zhang, Y., and Tang, L. Discovery and development of sulforaphane as a cancer chemopreventive phytochemical. *Acta Pharmacologica Sinica*, 2007. **28**: p. 1343–1354.
98. Shu, L., *et al.* Phytochemicals: cancer chemoprevention and suppression of tumor onset and metastasis. *Cancer Metastasis Reviews*, 2010. **29**: p. 483–502.

99. Dashwood, R.H. The importance of using pure chemicals in (anti) mutagenicity studies: chlorophyllin as a case in point. *Mutation Research*, 1997. **381** (2): p. 283–286.
100. Breinholt, V., *et al.* Mechanisms of chlorophyllin anticarcinogenesis against aflatoxin B1: complex formation with the carcinogen. *Chemical Research in Toxicology*, 1995. **8** (4): p. 506–514.
101. Morel, F., *et al.* Preferential increase of glutathione S-transferase class alpha transcripts in cultured human hepatocytes by phenobarbital, 3-methylcholanthrene, and dithiolethiones. *Cancer Research*, 1993. **53** (2): p. 231–234.
102. Okuno, M., Kojima, S., and Moriwaki, H. Chemoprevention of hepatocellular carcinoma: concept, progress and perspectives. *Journal of Gastroenterology and Hepatology*, 2001. **16** (12): p. 1329–1335.
103. Singh, S. Chemo preventive strategies in hepatocellular carcinoma. *Nature Reviews Gastroenterology and Hepatology*, 2014. **11** (1): p. 45–54.
104. Demierre, M.F., *et al.* Statins and cancer prevention. *Nature Reviews Cancer*, 2005. **5**: p. 930–942.
105. Singh, S., *et al.* Statins are associated with reduced risk of esophageal cancer, particularly in patients with Barrett's esophagus: a systematic review and meta-analysis. *Clinical Gastroenterology and Hepatology*, 2013. **11**: p. 620–629.
106. Singh, P.P., and Singh, S. Statins are associated with reduced risk of gastric cancer: a systematic review and meta-analysis. *Annals of Oncology*, 2013. **24**: p. 1721–1730.
107. Samadder, N.J., *et al.* Risk of colorectal cancer in self-reported inflammatory bowel disease and modification of risk by statin and NSAID use. *Cancer*, 2011. **117**: p. 1640–1648.
108. El-Serag, H.B., *et al.* Statins are associated with a reduced risk of hepatocellular carcinoma in a large cohort of patients with diabetes. *Gastroenterology*, 2009. **136**: p. 1601–1608.
109. Tsan, Y.T. Statins and the risk of hepatocellular carcinoma in patients with hepatitis B virus infection. *Journal of Clinical Oncology*, 2012. **30**: p. 623–630.
110. Chiu, H.F. Statin use and the risk of liver cancer: a population-based case-control study. *American Journal of Gastroenterology Supplements*, 2011. **106**: p. 894–898.

111. Decensi, A., *et al.* Metformin and cancer risk in diabetic patients: A systematic review and meta-analysis. *Cancer Prevention Research (Phila)*, 2010. **3**: p. 1451–1461.
112. Chang, C.H., *et al.* Oral insulin secretagogues, insulin, and cancer risk in type 2 diabetes mellitus. *The Journal of Clinical Endocrinology and Metabolism*, 2012. **97**: p. E1170–E1175.
113. Chen, H.P., *et al.* Metformin decreases hepatocellular carcinoma risk in a dose-dependent manner: population-based and *in vitro* studies. *Gastroenterology and Hepatology*, 2012. **62**: p. 606–615.
114. Ruiter, R., *et al.* Lower risk of cancer in patients on metformin in comparison with those on sulfonylurea derivatives: results from a large population-based follow-up study. *Diabetes Care*, 2012. **35**: p. 119–124.
115. Falk, G.W., *et al.* A combination of esomeprazole and aspirin reduces tissue concentrations of prostaglandin E(2) in patients with Barrett's esophagus. *Gastroenterology*, 2012. **143**: p. 917–926. e911.
116. Sahasrabuddhe, V.V., *et al.* Nonsteroidal anti-inflammatory drug use, chronic liver disease, and hepatocellular carcinoma. *Journal of the National Cancer Institute*, 2012. **104**: p. 1808–1814.
117. Gelatti, U., *et al.* Coffee consumption reduces the risk of hepatocellular carcinoma independently of its aetiology: a case–control study. *Journal of Hepatology*, 2005. **42**: p. 528–534.
118. Inoue, M., *et al.* Influence of coffee drinking on subsequent risk of hepatocellular carcinoma: a prospective study in Japan. *Journal of National Cancer Institute*, 2005. **97**: p. 293–300.
119. Bravi, F., *et al.* Coffee drinking and hepatocellular carcinoma risk: a meta-analysis. *Hepatology*, 2007. **46**: p. 430–435.
120. Tao, K.S., *et al.* The multifaceted mechanisms for coffee's anti-tumorigenic effect on liver. *Medical Hypotheses*, 2008. **71**: p. 730–736.
121. Torres, D.M., and Harrison, S.A. Is it time to write a prescription for coffee? Coffee and liver disease. *Gastroenterology*, 2013. **144**: p. 670–672.
122. Wong, G.L.H., *et al.* Adverse effects of vitamin D deficiency on outcomes of patients with chronic hepatitis B. *Clinical Gastroenterology and Hepatology*, 2015. **13**: p. 783–790. e1.

123. Fedirko, V., *et al.* Prediagnostic circulating vitamin D levels and risk of hepatocellular carcinoma in European populations: A nested case-control study. *Hepatology*, 2014. **60**: p. 1222–1230.
124. Zhang, W., *et al.* Vitamin intake and liver cancer risk: a report from two cohort studies in China. *Journal of National Cancer Institute*, 2012. **104**: p. 1173–1181.
125. Sawada, N., *et al.* Consumption of n-3 fatty acids and fish reduces risk of hepatocellular carcinoma. *Gastroenterology*, 2012. **142**: p. 1468–1475.
126. Bishayee, A., *et al.* Dietary phytochemicals in the chemoprevention and treatment of hepatocellular carcinoma: *in vivo* evidence, molecular targets, and clinical relevance. *Current Cancer Drug Targets*. 2012. **12**: p. 1191–1232.
127. Kensler, T.W., *et al.* Keap1-nrf2 signaling: a target for cancer prevention by sulforaphane. *Topics in Current Chemistry*, 2013. **329**: p. 163–177.
128. Soni, K.B., *et al.* Protective effect of food additives on aflatoxin-induced mutagenicity and hepatocarcinogenicity. *Cancer Letters*, 1997. **115**: p. 129–133.
129. Anand, P., *et al.* Curcumin and cancer: an "old-age" disease with an "age-old" solution. *Cancer Letters*, 2008. **267**: p. 133–164.
130. Bishayee, A., Politis, T. and Darvesh, A.S. Resveratrol in the chemoprevention and treatment of hepatocellular carcinoma. *Cancer Treatment Reviews*, 2010. **36**: p. 43–53.
131. Sreekumar, S., and Nisha, N.C. Plants are renewable source of medicine and nanoparticles: a review in current aspects in pharmaceutical research and development. *BP International, UK*, 2021. p. 44–56.
132. Dai, W., *et al.* Quercetin induces apoptosis and enhances 5-FU therapeutic efficacy in hepatocellular carcinoma. *Tumor Biology*, 2016. **37** (5): p. 6307–6313.
133. Ismail, N., *et al.* Novel combination of thymoquinone and resveratrol enhances anticancer effect on hepatocellular carcinoma cell line. *Future Journal of Pharmaceutical Sciences*, 2018. **4**: p. 41–46.
134. Bhattacharya, S., *et al.* Therapeutic role of resveratrol against hepatocellular carcinoma: a review on its molecular mechanisms

of action. *Pharmacological Research — Modern Chinese Medicine*, 2023. **6**: p. 1–11.

135. Jagwani, S., *et al.* Pharmacokinetic and pharmacodynamic evaluation of resveratrol loaded cationic liposomes for targeting hepatocellular Carcinoma. *ACS Biomaterial Science & Engineering*, 2020. **6**: p. 4969–4984.
136. Parekh, P., *et al.* Downregulation of cyclin D1 is associated with decreased levels of p38 MAP kinases, Akt/PKB and Pak1 during chemopreventive effects of resveratrol in liver cancer cells. *Experimental and Toxicologic Pathology*, 2011. **63**: p. 167–173.
137. Bishayee, A., *et al.* Angioprevention implicated in resveratrol chemoprevention of experimental hepatocarcinogenesis. *Journal of Carcinogenesis & Mutagenesis*, 2010. **1** (1): p. 1–8.
138. Bishayee, A., *et al.* Resveratrol suppresses oxidative stress and inflammatory response in diethylnitrosamine-initiated rat hepatocarcinogenesis. *Cancer Prevention Research*, 2010. **3** (6): p. 753–763.
139. Guo, H., *et al.* Cancer chemopreventive potential of cooked glutinous purple rice on the early stages of hepatocarcinogenesis in rats. *Frontiers in Nutrition*, 2022. **9**: p. 1032771.
140. Lee, S.J., *et al.* Phenolic phytochemicals derived from Red Pine (*Pinus densiflora*) inhibit the invasion and migration of SK-Hep-1 human hepatocellular carcinoma cells. *Annals of the New York Academy of Sciences,* 2007. **1095**: p. 536–544.
141. Li, D., *et al.* The potential of epigallocatechin gallate in the chemoprevention and therapy of hepatocellular carcinoma. *Frontiers in Pharmacology*, 2023. **14**: p. 1–21.
142. Liao, S., *et al.* Chemoprevention of elite tea variety CFT-1 rich in EGCG against chemically induced liver cancer in rats. *Food Science & Nutrition*, 2019. 7: p. 2647–2665.
143. Zhang, H., *et al.* Fresh red raspberry phytochemicals suppress the growth of hepatocellular carcinoma cells by PTEN/AKT pathway. *International Journal of Biochemistry and Cell Biology*. 2018. **104**: p. 55–65.
144. Li, F., *et al.* Camptothecin (CPT) and its derivatives are known to target topoisomerase I (Top1) as their mechanism of action: did we miss something in CPT analogue molecular targets for treating human

disease such as cancer? *American Journal of Cancer Research*, 2017. 7 (12): p. 2350–2394.

145. Nath, L.R., *et al.* Blockade of Uttroside B-induced autophagic pro-survival signals augments its chemotherapeutic efficacy against hepato-cellular carcinoma. *Frontiers in Oncology*, 2022. **12**: p. 812598.
146. Lee, C.M., *et al.* 6,8-diprenylorobol induces apoptosis in human hepatocellular carcinoma cells via activation of FOXO3 and inhibition of CYP2J2. *Oxidative Medicine and Cellular Longevity*, 2020: p. 8887251.
147. Harliansya, *et al.* α-Mangosteen as an oxidative inhibitor in hepatocellular carcinoma. *Indonesian Journal of Cancer Chemoprevention*, 2021. **12** (2): p. 106–113.
148. Hussein, R.H., and Khalifa, F.K. The protective role of ellagitannins flavonoids pretreatment against N-nitrosodiethylamine induced-hepatocellular carcinoma. *Saudi Journal of Biological Sciences*, 2014. **21**: p. 589–596.
149. Liu, Z., *et al.* Sesamol induces human hepatocellular carcinoma cells apoptosis by impairing mitochondrial function and suppressing autophagy. *Scientific Reports*, 2017. 7: p. 45728.
150. Khuanphram, N., *et al.* Sesame extract promotes chemopreventive effect of hesperidin on early phase of Diethylnitrosamine-initiated hepatocarcinogenesis in rats. *Pharmaceutics*, 2021. **13**: p. 1687.
151. Banjerdpongchai, R., *et al.* Hesperidin from Citrus seed induces human hepatocellular carcinoma HepG2 cell apoptosis via both mitochondrial and death. *Tumor Biology*. 2016. **37**: p. 227–237.
152. Mastron, J.K., *et al.* Silymarin and hepatocellular carcinoma: a systematic, comprehensive, and critical review. *Anti-Cancer Drugs*, 2015. **26** (5): p. 475–486.
153. Polo, M.P., and M.G. de Bravo. Effect of geraniol on fatty-acid and mevalonate metabolism in the human hepatoma cell line Hep G2. *Biochemistry and Cell Biology*, 2006. **84**: p. 102–111.
154. Deng, R., *et al.* Excisanin A, a diterpenoid compound purified from Isodon Macrocalyxin D, induces tumor cells apoptosis and suppresses tumor growth through inhibition of PKB/AKT kinase activity and blockade of its signal pathway. *Molecular Cancer Therapeutics*, 2009. **8**: p. 873–882.

155. Yoshida, M., *et al.* G2-phase arrest through p21(WAF1/Cip1) induction and cdc2 repression by gnidimacrin in human hepatoma HLE cells. *Anticancer Research*, 2009. **29**: p. 1349–1354.
156. Huang, J., *et al.* Reactive oxygen species mediate oridonin-induced HepG2 apoptosis through p53, MAPK, and mitochondrial signaling pathways. *Journal of Pharmacological Sciences*, 2008. **107**: p. 370–379.
157. Einbond, L.S., *et al.* Actein activates stress- and statin-associated responses and is bioavailable in Sprague-Dawley rats. *Fundamental & Clinical Pharmacology*, 2009. **23**: p. 311–321.
158. Li, M., *et al.* Proapoptotic and microtubule-disassembly effects of ardisiacrispin(A+B), triterpenoid saponins from Ardisia crenata on human hepatoma Bel-7402 cells. *Journal of Asian Natural Products Research,* 2008. **10**: p. 739–746.
159. Qi, H., *et al.* Proteomic characterization of the cellular response to chemopreventive triterpenoid astragaloside IV in human hepatocellular carcinoma cell line HepG2. *International Journal of Oncolology*, 2010. **36**: p. 725–735.
160. Lee, Y.S., *et al.* Asiatic acid, a triterpene, induces apoptosis through intracellular Ca^{2+} release and enhanced expression of p53 in HepG2 human hepatoma cells. *Cancer Letters*, 2002. **186**: p. 83–91.
161. Eichenmüller, M., *et al.* Betulinic acid treatment promotes apoptosis in hepatoblastoma cells. *International Journal of Oncology*, 2009. **35**: p. 873–879.
162. Zhang, M., *et al.* Targeted constitutive activation of signal transducer and activator of transcription 3 in human hepatocellular carcinoma cells by cucurbitacin B. *Cancer Chemotherapy and Pharmacology*, 2009. **63**: p. 635–642.
163. Chan, K.T., *et al.* Cucurbitacin B induces apoptosis and S phase cell cycle arrest in BEL-7402 human hepatocellular carcinoma cells and is effective via oral administration. *Cancer Letters*, 2010. **294**: p. 118–124.
164. Takahashi, N., *et al.* Cucurbitacin D isolated from *Trichosanthes kirilowii* induces apoptosis in human hepatocellular carcinoma cells *in vitro. International Immunopharmacology*, 2009. **9**: p. 508–513.
165. Meng, D., *et al.* Cytotoxic cucurbitane-type triterpenoids from *Elaeocarpus hainanensis. Planta Medica*, 2008. **74**: p. 1741–1744.

166. Tong, X., *et al.* Molecular mechanisms of echinocystic acid-induced apoptosis in HepG2 cells. *Biochemical and Biophysical Research Communications*, 2004. **321**: p. 539–546.
167. Zhou, X.Y., *et al.* Escin, a natural mixture of triterpene saponins, exhibits antitumor activity against hepatocellular carcinoma. *Planta Medica*, 2009. **75**: p. 1580–1585.
168. Zhou, X.Y., *et al.* Escin, a natural mixture of triterpene saponins, exhibits antitumor activity against hepatocellular carcinoma. *Planta Medica*, 2009. **75**: p. 1580–1585.
169. Yang, H.L. Ganoderic acid produced from submerged culture of Ganoderma lucidum induces cell cycle arrest and cytotoxicity in human hepatoma cell line BEL7402. *Biotechnology Letters*, 2005. **27**: p. 835–838.
170. Chang, U.M., *et al.* Ganoderiol F, a ganoderma triterpene, induces senescence in hepatoma HepG2 cells. *Life Sciences*, 2006. **79**: p. 1129–1139.
171. Lee, K.Y., and Lee, S.K. Ginsenoside-Rg1 positively regulates cyclin E-dependent kinase activity in human hepatoma SK-HEP-1 cells. *Biochemistry and Molecular Biology International*, 1996. **39**: p. 539–546.
172. Lee, K.Y., *et al.* Ginsenoside-Rg5 suppresses cyclin E-dependent protein kinase activity via up-regulating p21Cip/WAF1 and down-regulating cyclin E in SK-HEP-1 cells. *Anticancer Research*, 1997. **17**: p. 1067–1072.
173. Lee, K.Y., *et al.* Ginsenoside-Rh2 blocks the cell cycle of SK-HEP-1 cells at the G1/S boundary by selectively inducing the protein expression of p27kip1. *Cancer Letters*, 1996. **110**: p. 193–200.
174. Park, J.A., *et al.* Activation of caspase-3 protease via a Bcl-2-insensitive pathway during the process of ginsenoside Rh2-induced apoptosis. *Cancer Letters*, 1997. **121**: p. 73–81.
175. Kim, Y.J., *et al.* Anti-tumor activity of the ginsenoside Rk1 in human hepatocellular carcinoma cells through inhibition of telomerase activity and induction of apoptosis. *Biological and Pharmaceutical Bulletin*, 2008. **31**: p. 826–830.
176. Wang, Q.F., *et al.* Regulation of Bcl-2 family molecules and activation of caspase cascade involved in gypenosides-induced apoptosis in human hepatoma cells. *Cancer Letters*, 2002. **183**: p. 169–178.

177. Oh, S.H., and Lee, B.H. A ginseng saponin metabolite-induced apoptosis in HepG2 cells involves a mitochondria-mediated pathway and its downstream caspase-8 activation and bid cleavage. *Toxicology and Applied Pharmacology*, 2004. **194**: p. 221–229.
178. Ming, Y.L., *et al.* Anti-proliferation and apoptosis induced by a novel intestinal metabolite of ginseng saponin in human hepatocellular carcinoma cells. *Cell Biology International*, 2007. **31**: p. 1265–1273.
179. Tian, Z., *et al.* Cytotoxicity of two triterpenoids from *Nigella glandulifera*. *Molecules*, 2006. **11**: p. 693–699.
180. Liu, J.J., *et al.* Keto and acetyl-keto-boswellic acids inhibit proliferation and induce apoptosis in Hep G2 cells via a caspase-8 dependent pathway. *International Journal of Molecular Medicine*, 2002. **10**: p. 501–505.
181. Weng, C.J., *et al.* Lucidenic acid inhibits PMA-induced invasion of human hepatoma cells through inactivating MAPK/ERK signal transduction pathway and reducing binding activities of NF-κB and AP-1. *Carcinogenesis*, 2008. **29**: p. 147–156.
182. Zhang, L., *et al.* Lupeol, a dietary triterpene, inhibited growth, and induced apoptosis through down-regulation of DR3 in SMMC7721 cells. *Cancer Investigations*, 2009. **27**: p. 163–170.
183. Hong, J., *et al.* Growth inhibition and G1 cell cycle arrest mediated by 25-methoxyhispidol A, a novel triterpenoid, isolated from the fruit of *Poncirus trifoliata* in human hepatocellular carcinoma cells. *Planta Medica*, 2008. **74**: p. 151–155.
184. Shyu, M.H., *et al.* Oleanolic acid and ursolic acid induce apoptosis in HuH7 human hepatocellular carcinoma cells through a mitochondrial-dependent pathway and downregulation of XIAP. *Journal of Agricultural and Food Chemistry*, 2010. **58**: p. 6110–6118.
185. Tian, Z., *et al.* Antihepatoma activity and mechanism of ursolic acid and its derivatives isolated from *Aralia decaisneana*. *World Journal of Gastroenterology*, 2006. **12**: p. 874–879.
186. Tang, C., *et al.* Downregulation of survivin and activation of caspase-3 through the PI3K/Akt pathway in ursolic acid-induced HepG2 cell apoptosis. *Anticancer Drugs*, 2009. **20**: p. 249–258.
187. Gayathri, R., *et al.* Ursolic acid attenuates oxidative stress-mediated hepatocellular carcinoma induction by diethylnitrosamine in male

Wistar rats. *Asian Pacific Journal Cancer Prevention*, 2009. **10**: p. 933–938.

188. Zhang, Z., *et al.* Waltonitone induces human hepatocellular carcinoma cells apoptosis *in vitro* and *in vivo*. *Cancer Letters*, 2009. **286**: p. 223–231.
189. Kozuki, Y., *et al.* Inhibitory effects of carotenoids on the invasion of rat ascites hepatoma cells in culture. *Cancer Letters*, 2000. **151**: p. 111–115.
190. Das, S.K., *et al.* Growth inhibition of human hepatic carcinoma HepG2 cells by fucoxanthin is associated with down-regulation of cyclin D. *Biochimica et Biophysica Acta*, 2008. **1780**: p. 743–749.
191. Liu, C.L., *et al.* Inhibition of proliferation of a hepatoma cell line by fucoxanthin in relation to cell cycle arrest and enhanced gap junctional intercellular communication. *Chemico-Biological Interactions*, 2009. **182**: p. 165–172.
192. Park, Y.O., *et al.* The effect of lycopene on cell growth and oxidative DNA damage of Hep3B human hepatoma cells. *Biofactors.* 2005. **23**: p. 129–139.
193. Huang, C.S. Lycopene inhibits matrix metalloproteinase-9 expression and down-regulates the binding activity of nuclear factor-kappa B and stimulatory protein-1. *Journal of Nutritional Biochemistry*, 2007. **18**: p. 449–456.
194. Hwang, E.S., and Lee, H.J. Inhibitory effects of lycopene on the adhesion, invasion, and migration of SK-Hep1 human hepatoma cells. *Experimental Biology and Medicine*, 2006. **231**: p. 322–327.
195. Chen, W., *et al.* Alpha-Bisabolol induces dose- and time-dependent apoptosis in HepG2 cells via a Fas- and mitochondrial-related pathway, involves p53 and NF-κB. *Biochemical Pharmacology*, 2010. **80**: p. 247–254.
196. Hsu, Y.L., *et al.* Dehydrocostus lactone, a medicinal plant-derived sesquiterpene lactone, induces apoptosis coupled to endoplasmic reticulum stress in liver cancer cells. *Journal of Pharmacology and Experimental Therapeutics,* 2009. **329**: p. 808–819.
197. Xiao, Y., *et al.* Furanodiene induces G2/M cell cycle arrest and apoptosis through MAPK signalling and mitochondria-caspase pathway in

human hepatocellular carcinoma cells. *Cancer Biology and Therapy,* 2007. **6**: p. 1044–1050.

198. Sakinah, S.A., *et al.* Zerumbone induced apoptosis in liver cancer cells via modulation of Bax/Bcl-2 ratio. *Cancer Cell International,* 2007. **7**: p. 4.
199. Taha, M.M.E., *et al.* Potential chemoprevention of diethylnitrosamine-initiated and 2-acetylaminofluorene-promoted hepatocarcinogenesis by zerumbone from the rhizomes of the subtropical ginger (*Zingiber zerumbet*). *Chemico-Biological Interactions,* 2010. **186**: p. 295–305.
200. Sakata, K., *et al.* Dietary supplementation of the citrus antioxidant auraptene inhibits N,N-diethylnitrosamine-induced rat hepatocarcinogenesis. *Oncology,* 2004. **66**: p. 244–252.
201. Ong, T.P., *et al.* Farnesol and geraniol chemopreventive activities during the initial phases of hepatocarcinogenesis involve similar actions on cell proliferation and DNA damage, but distinct actions on apoptosis, plasma cholesterol and HMGCoA reductase. *Carcinogenesis,* 2006. **27**: p. 1194–1203.
202. Cardozo, M.T., *et al.* Chemopreventive effects of β-ionone and geraniol during rat hepatocarcinogenesis promotion: distinct actions on cell proliferation, apoptosis, HMGCoA reductase, and RhoA. *Journal of Nutritional Biochemistry,* 2011. **22**: p. 130–135.
203. Hirose, M., *et al.* Inhibitory effects of 1-O-hexyl-2,3,5-trimethylhydroquinone (HTHQ), green tea catechins and other antioxidants on 2-amino-6-methyldipyrido[1,2-a: 3′,2′-d]imidazole (Glu-P-1)-induced rat hepatocarcinogenesis and dose-dependent inhibition by HTHQ of lesion induction by Glu-P-1 or 2-amino-3,8-dimethylimidazo[4,5-f]quinoxaline (MeIQx). *Carcinogenesis,* 1995. **16**: p. 3049–3055.
204. Parija, T., and Das, B.R. Involvement of YY1 and its correlation with c-Myc in NDEA induced hepatocarcinogenesis, its prevention by d-limonene. *Molecular Biology Reports,* 2003. **30**: p. 41–46.
205. Kaji, I., *et al.* Inhibition by d-limonene of experimental hepatocarcinogenesis in Sprague-Dawley rats does not involve p21(ras) plasma membrane association. *International Journal of Cancer,* 2001. **93**: p. 441–444.
206. Bodake, H.B. Chemopreventive effect of orange oil on the development of hepatic preneoplastic lesions induced by N-nitrosodiethylamine

in rats: an ultrastructural study. *Indian Journal of Experimental Biology*, 2002. **40**: p. 245–251.

207. Mills, J.J., *et al.* Induction of apoptosis in liver tumors by the monoterpene perillyl alcohol. *Cancer Research,* 1995. **55**: p. 979–983.
208. Ji, L., *et al.* Andrographolide inhibits human hepatoma-derived Hep3B cell growth through the activation of c-Jun N-terminal kinase. *Planta Medica*, 2007. **73**: p. 1397–1401.
209. Trivedi, N.P., *et al.* Hepatoprotective effect of andrographolide against hexachlorocyclohexane-induced oxidative injury. *Integrative Cancer Therapies,* 2007. **6**: p. 271–280.
210. Trivedi, N.P., *et al.* Potency of andrographolide as an antitumor compound in BHC-induced liver damage. *Integrative Cancer Therapies,* 2009. **8**: p. 177–189.
211. Dhanasekaran, M., *et al.* Chemopreventive potential of epoxy clerodane diterpene from *Tinospora cordifolia* against diethylnitrosamine-induced hepatocellular carcinoma. *Investigational New Drugs*, 2009. **27**: p. 347–355.
212. De Moura Espíndola R., *et al.* Geranylgeraniol and beta-ionone inhibit hepatic preneoplastic lesions, cell proliferation, total plasma cholesterol and DNA damage during the initial phases of hepatocarcinogenesis, but only the former inhibits NF-κB activation. *Carcinogenesis*, 2005. **26**: p. 1091–1099.
213. Janani, P., *et al.* Chemopreventive effect of bacoside A on N-nitrosodiethylamine-induced hepatocarcinogenesis in rats. *Journal of Cancer Research Clinical Oncology*, 2010. **136**: p. 759–770.
214. Janani, P., *et al.* Bacoside A downregulates matrix metalloproteinases 2 and 9 in DEN-induced hepatocellular carcinoma. *Cell Biochemistry & Function*, 2010. **28**: 164–169.
215. Shiota, G., *et al.* Inhibition of hepatocellular carcinoma by glycyrrhizin in diethylnitrosamine-treated mice. *Carcinogenesis,* 1999. **20**: p. 59–63.
216. Wan, X.Y., *et al.* Hepatoprotective and antihepatocarcinogenic effects of glycyrrhizin and matrine. *Chemico-Biological Interactions*, 2009. **181**: p. 15–19.
217. Murakoshi, M., *et al.* Potent preventive action of alpha-carotene against carcinogenesis: spontaneous liver carcinogenesis and promoting stage

of lung and skin carcinogenesis in mice are suppressed more effectively by alpha-carotene than by beta-carotene. *Cancer Research*, 1992. **52**: p. 6583–6587.

218. Tsuda, H., *et al.* Demonstration of organotropic effects of chemopreventive agents in multiorgan carcinogenesis models. *IARC Scientific Publications*, 1996. **139**: p. 143–150.
219. Moreno, F.S., *et al.* Inhibitory effects of beta-carotene on preneoplastic lesions induced in Wistar rats by the resistant hepatocyte model. *Carcinogenesis*, 1991. **12**: p. 1817–1822.
220. Rizzi, M.B., *et al.* beta-carotene inhibits persistent and stimulates remodelling gamma GT-positive preneoplastic lesions during early promotion of hepatocarcinogenesis. *International Journal for Vitamin and Nutritional Research*, 1997. **67**: p. 415–422.
221. Dagli, M.L., *et al.* Beta-carotene reduces the ductular (oval) cell reaction in the liver of Wistar rats submitted to the resistant hepatocyte model of carcinogenesis. *Pathology*, 1998. **30**: p. 259–266.
222. Ambrogi, F., *et al.* Multiple correspondence analysis in S-PLUS. *Computational Methods and Programs in Biomedicine*, 2005. **79**: p. 161–167.
223. Sampaio, A.R., *et al.* Vitamin A and beta-carotene inhibitory effect during 1,2-dimethylhydrazine induced hepatocarcinogenesis potentiated by 5-azacytidine. *Food and Chemical Toxicology*, 2007. **45**: p. 563–567.
224. Sarkar, A., *et al.* Inhibition of 3′-methyl-4-dimethylaminoazobenzene-induced hepatocarcinogenesis in rat by dietary beta-carotene: changes in hepatic antioxidant defense enzyme levels. *International Journal of Cancer*, 1995. **61**: p. 799–805.
225. Sarkar, A., *et al.* Beta-carotene prevents lipid peroxidation and red blood cell membrane protein damage in experimental hepatocarcinogenesis. *Cancer Biochemistry Biophysics*, 1995. **15**: p. 111–125.
226. Sarkar, A., *et al.* Beta-carotene inhibits rat liver chromosomal aberrations and DNA chain break after a single injection of diethylnitrosamine. *British Journal of Cancer*, 1997. **76**: p. 855–861.
227. Bishayee, A., *et al.* Further evidence for chemopreventive potential of beta-carotene against experimental carcinogenesis: diethylnitrosamine-initiated and phenobarbital-promoted hepatocarcinogenesis is

prevented more effectively by beta-carotene than by retinoic acid. *Nutrition and Cancer*, 2000. **37**: p. 89–98.

228. Tsuda, H., *et al.* Chemopreventive effects of beta-carotene, alpha-tocopherol and five naturally occurring antioxidants on initiation of hepatocarcinogenesis by 2-amino-3-methylimidazo[4,5-f]quinoline in the rat. *Japanese Journal of Cancer Research*, 1994. **85**: p. 1214–1219.
229. Ogawa, T., *et al.* Role of reactive oxygen in synthetic estrogen induction of hepatocellular carcinomas in rats and preventive effect of vitamins. *Carcinogenesis*, 1995. **16**: p. 831–836.
230. Uehara, N., *et al.* Decreased levels of 2-amino-3-methylimidazo[4,5-f]quinoline-DNA adducts in rats treated with beta-carotene, alpha-tocopherol and freeze dried aloe. *Japanese Journal of Cancer Research*, 1996. **87**: p. 342–348.
231. Gradelet, S., *et al.* Modulation of aflatoxin B1 carcinogenicity, genotoxicity and metabolism in rat liver by dietary carotenoids: evidence for a protective effect of CYP1A inducers. *Cancer Letters*, 1997. **114**: p. 221–223.
232. Gradelet, S., *et al.* Dietary carotenoids inhibit aflatoxin B1-induced liver preneoplastic foci and DNA damage in the rat: role of the modulation of aflatoxin B1 metabolism. *Carcinogenesis*, 1998. **19**: p. 403–411.
233. Sadek, I.A., and Hayat, L.G. Initiation and post-initiation chemopreventive effects of beta-carotene in toad liver carcinogenesis. *Histology and Histopathololy*, 1996. **11**: p. 357–360.
234. Chattopadhyay, M.B., *et al.* Combined supplementation of vanadium and beta-carotene suppresses placental glutathione S-transferase positive foci and enhances antioxidant functions during the inhibition of diethylnitrosamine-induced rat liver carcinogenesis. *Journal of Gastroenterology and Hepatology*, 2004. **19**: p. 683–693.
235. Chattopadhyay, M.B., *et al.* Proton-induced X-ray emission (PIXE) analysis and DNA-chain break study in rat hepatocarcinogenesis: a possible chemopreventive role by combined supplementation of vanadium and beta-carotene. *Cancer Cell International*, 2005. **5**: p. 16.
236. Krajka-Kuźniak, V., *et al.* Xanthohumol induces phase II enzymes via Nrf2 in human hepatocytes *in vitro*. *Toxicology in vitro*, 2013. **27**: p. 149156.

237. Hasan, S.K., ***et al.*** Chemopreventive effect of 18b-glycyrrhetinic acid via modulation of inflammatory markers and induction of apoptosis in human hepatoma cell line (HepG2). ***Molecular and Cell Biochemistry***, 2016. **416**: p. 169–177.
238. Xia, J. Flavonoids as potential anti-hepatocellular carcinoma agents: recent approaches using HepG2 cell line. ***Drug Discoveries & Therapeutics***, 2013. 7 (1): p. 1–8.
239. Zhao, P. Quercetin induces HepG2 cell apoptosis by inhibiting fatty acid biosynthesis. ***Oncology Letters***, 2014. **8** (2): p. 765–769.
240. Panche, A.N., ***et al.*** Flavonoids: an overview. ***Journal of Nutritional Science***, 2016. **5**: p. 41.
241. Manach, C., ***et al.*** Polyphenols: food sources and bioavailability. ***American Journal of Clinical Nutrition***, 2004. **79** (5): p. 727–747.
242. Arul, D., and Subramanian, P. Inhibitory effect of naringenin (citrus flavanone) on N-nitrosodiethylamine induced hepatocarcinogenesis in rats. ***Biochemical and Biophysical Research Communications***, 2013. **434** (2): p. 203–209.
243. Hernández-Aquino, E., and Muriel, P. Beneficial effects of naringenin in liver diseases: molecular mechanisms. ***World Journal of Gastroenterology***, 2018. **24** (16): p. 1679–1707.
244. Yao, L.H., ***et al.*** Flavonoids in food and their health benefits. ***Plant Foods for Human Nutrition***, 2004. **59** (3): p. 113–122.
245. Gu, Y., ***et al.*** Inhibitory effects of genistein on metastasis of human hepatocellular carcinoma. ***Journal of Gastroenterology***, 2009. **15** (39): p. 4952–4957.
246. Lee, S.R., ***et al.*** Dietary intake of genistein suppresses hepatocellular carcinoma through AMPK-mediated apoptosis and anti-inflammation. ***BMC Cancer***, 2019. **19** (1): p. 6.
247. Chiang, L.-C., ***et al.*** Anti-proliferative effect of apigenin and its apoptotic induction in human Hep G2 cells. ***Cancer Letters***, 2006. **237** (2): p. 207–214.
248. Balamurugan, K., and Karthikeyan, J. Evaluation of luteolin in the prevention of N-nitrosodiethylamine-induced hepatocellular carcinoma using animal model system. ***Indian Journal of Clinical Biochemistry***, 2012. **27** (2): p. 157–163.

249. Cao, Z., *et al.* Luteolin promotes cell apoptosis by inducing autophagy in hepatocellular carcinoma. *Cellular Physiology and Biochemistry*, 2017. **43** (5): p. 1803–1812.
250. Martinez, M.J., *et al.* Plant polyphenolic extracts as potential anti-human hepatocarcinoma agents. *Plant Science Today*, 2014. **1** (4): p. 213–218.
251. Thilavech, T., and Adisakwattana, S. Cyanidin-3-rutinoside acts as a natural inhibitor of intestinal lipid digestion and absorption. *BMC Complementary and Alternative Medicine*, 2019. **19** (1): p. 242.
252. Murugan, R.S., *et al.* Black tea polyphenols target matrix metalloproteinases, RECK, proangiogenic molecules and histone deacetylase in a rat hepatocarcinogenesis model. *Anticancer Research*, 2009. **29**: p. 2301–2306.
253. Chuang, S.E., *et al.* Curcumin-containing diethylnitosamine-induced murine hepatocarcinogenesis. *Carcinogenesis*. 2000. **21** (2): p. 331–335.
254. Fujise, Y., *et al.* Preventive effect of caffeine and curcumin on hepatocarcinogenesis in diethylnitrosamine-induced rats. *International Journal of Oncology*, 2012. **40**: p. 1779–1788.
255. Farazuddin, M., *et al.* Chemotherapeutic potential of curcumin-bearing microcells against hepatocellular carcinoma in model animals. *International Journal of Nanomedicine*, 2014. **9**: p. 1139–1152.
256. Jung, M.-Y., *et al.* Capsaicin-induced apoptosis in SK-Hep-1 hepatocarcinoma cells involves Bcl-2 downregulation and caspase-3 activation. *Cancer Letters*, 2001. **165**: p. 139–145.
257. Abdalla, Y., *et al.* Safranal prevents liver cancer through inhibiting oxidative stress and alleviating inflammation. *Frontiers in Pharmacology*, 2022. **12**: p. 1–13.
258. Paśko, P., *et al.* Comparative study of predominant phytochemical compounds and proapoptotic potential of broccoli sprouts and florets. *Plant Foods for Human Nutrition*, 2018. **73**: p. 95–100.
259. Sadeeshkumar, V., *et al.* Protective effects of dieckol on N-nitrosodiethylamine induced hepatocarcinogenesis in rats. *Biomedicine & Pharmacotherapy*, 2016. **84**: p. 1810–1819.

260. Zhang, H.T., *et al.* Galangin induces apoptosis of hepatocellular carcinoma cells via the mitochondrial pathway. *World Journal of Gastroenterology,* 2010. **16** (27): p. 3377–3384.
261. Chang, H.-F., *et al.* Antitumour and free radical scavenging effects of γ-mangostin isolated from *Garcinia mangostana* pericarps against hepatocellular carcinoma cell. *Journal of Pharmacy and Pharmacology.* 2013. **65**: p. 1419–1428.
262. Al-Assaf, A.H. Chemopreventive effect of corosolic acid in human hepatocellular carcinoma cells. *African Journal of Biotechnology,* 2013. **12** (19): p. 2733–2742.
263. Feng, R., *et al.* Delphinidin induces necrosis in hepatocellular carcinoma cells in the presence of 3-methyladenine, an autophagy inhibitor. *Journal of Agricultural and Food Chemistry,* 2010. **58**: p. 3957–3964.
264. Ohnishi, H., *et al.* Inhibition of cell proliferation by nobiletin, a dietary phytochemical, associated with apoptosis and characteristic gene expression, but lack of effect on early rat hepatocarcinogenesis *in vivo. Cancer Science,* 2004. **95** (12): p. 936–942.
265. Shi, J.-J., *et al.* Guggulsterone induces apoptosis of human hepatocellular carcinoma cells through intrinsic mitochondrial pathway. *World Journal of Gastroenterology.* 2015. **21** (47): p. 13277–13287.
266. Wang, X., *et al.* Indole-3-carbinol inhibits tumorigenicity of hepatocellular arcinoma cells via suppression of microRNA-21 and upregulation of phosphatase and tensin homolog. *Biochimica et Biophysica Acta,* 2015. **1853**: p. 244–253.
267. Abdelmageed, M.M., *et al.* Indole-3-carbinol enhances sorafenib cytotoxicity in hepatocellular carcinoma cells: A mechanistic study. *Scientific Reports,* 2016. **6**: p. 32733.
268. Zhang, Y., *et al.* Anticarcinogenic effects of isothiocynates on hepatocellular carcinoma. *International Journal of Molecular Sciences,* 2022. **23**: p. 13834.
269. Gil, M.I., *et al.* Antioxidant activity of pomegranate juice and its relationship with phenolic composition and processing. *Journal of Agriculture Food Chemistry,* 2000. **48** (10): p. 4581–4589.
270. Li, Y., *et al.* Evaluation of antioxidant properties of pomegranate peel extract in comparison with pomegranate pulp extract. *Food Chemistry,* 2006. **96** (2): p. 254–260.

271. Singh, B.N., *et al.* Potential chemoprevention of N-nitrosodiethylamine-induced hepatocarcinogenesis by polyphenolics from Acacianilotica bark. *Chemico-Biological Interactions*, 2009. **181**: p. 20–28.
272. Shen, T., *et al.* Chemoprevention by lipid-soluble tea polyphenols in diethylnitrosamaine/phenobarbital-induced hepatic pre-cancerous lesions. *Anticancer Research*, 2014. **34**: p. 683–694.
273. Rezq AA. Antioxidant role of cabbage (*Brassica oleracea*) ethanolic extract in hepatoprotective of N-nitrosodiethylamine induced initiation of hepatocellular carcinoma in rat liver. *Egyptian Journal of Nutrition*, 2017. **32** (2): p. 1–53.
274. Basu A. Effect of flavonoid quercetin in MicroRNA and transcription factor regulatory network in hepatocellular carcinoma. *International Journal of Advanced Life Science Research*, 2020. **3** (1): p. 16–23.
275. Saeed, R.A., *et al.* Phytochemical screening of *Prunus avium* for its anti-oxidative and anti-mutagenic potential against DMBA-induced hepato-carcinogenesis. *Frontiers in Nutrition*, 2023. **12** (10): p. 1132356.
276. Bishayee, A., *et al.* Resveratrol in the chemoprevention and treatment of hepatocellular carcinoma. *Cancer Treatment Reviews*, 2020. **36**: p. 43–53.
277. Paul, B., *et al.* Occurrence of resveratrol and pterostilbene in age-old darakchasava, an ayurvedic medicine from India. *Journal of Ethnopharmacology*, 1999. **68**: p. 71–76.
278. Bishayee, A., and Dhir, N. Resveratrol-mediated chemoprevention of diethylnitrosamine-initiated hepatocarcinogenesis: inhibition of cell proliferation and induction of apoptosis. *Chemico-Biological Interactions*, 2009. **179**: p. 131–144.
279. Yeh, C.B., *et al.* The antimetastatic effects of resveratrol on hepatocellular carcinoma through the downregulation of a metastasis-associated protease by SP-1 modulation. *PLoS One*, 2013. **8** (2): p. 1–10.
280. Rajasekaran, D., *et al.* Resveratrol interferes with N-nitrosodiethylamine-induced hepatocellular carcinoma at early and advanced stages in male Wistar rats. *Molecular Medicine Reports*, 2011. **4**: p. 1211–1217.
281. Liu, P., *et al.* Sulforaphane exerts antiangiogenesis effects against hepatocellular carcinoma through inhibition of STAT3/HIF-1α/VEGF signalling. *Scientific Reports*, 2017. **7**: p. 12651.
282. Luper, S. A review of plants used in the treatment of liver disease: part 1. *Alternative Medicine Review*, 1998. **3**: p. 410–421.

283. Polyak, S.J., *et al.* Identification of hepatoprotective flavonolignans from silymarin. *Proceedings of the National Academy of Sciences USA*, 2010. **107**: p. 5995–5999.
284. Freedman, N.D., *et al.* HALT-C trial group: silymarin use and liver disease progression in the hepatitis C antiviral long-term treatment against cirrhosis trial. *Aliment Pharmacology & Therapeutics*, 2011. **33**: p. 127–137.
285. Varghese, L., *et al.* Silibinin efficacy against human hepatocellular carcinoma. *Clinical Cancer Research*, 2005. **11**: p. 8441–8448.
286. Féher, J., and Lengyel, G. Silymarin in the prevention and treatment of liver diseases and primary liver cancer. *Current Pharmaceutical Biotechnology*, 2012. **13**: p. 210–217.
287. Bousserouel, S., *et al.* Silibinin inhibits tumor growth in a murine orthotopic hepatocarcinoma model and activates the TRAIL apoptotic signaling pathway. *Anticancer Research*, 2012. **32**: p. 2455–2462.
288. Gopalakrishnan, R., *et al.* Dietary supplementation of silymarin is associated with decreased cell proliferation, increased apoptosis, and activation of detoxification system in hepatocellular carcinoma. *Molecular Cell Biochemistry*, 2013. **377**: p. 163–176.
289. Kiruthiga, C., *et al.* Autophagy: A potential therapeutic target of plyphenol in hepatocellular carcinoma. *Cancers*, 2020. **12** (562): p. 1–31.
290. Lee, S.J., *et al.* Phenolic phytochemicals derived from Red Pine (*Pinus densiflora*) inhibit the invasion and migration of SK-Hep-1 human hepatocellular carcinoma cells. *Annals of the New York Academy of Sciences*, 2007. **1095**: p. 536–544.
291. Longo, L., *et al.* Identification an quantification of antocyanins in the berries of *Pistacia lentiscus* L., *Phillyrea latifolia* L., and *Rubia peregrina* L. *Innovative Food Science & Emerging Technology*, 2007. **8**: p. 360–364.
292. Longo, L., *et al.* Autophagy inhibition enhances anthocyanin-induced apoptosis in hepatocellular carcinoma. *Molecular Cancer Therapy*, 2008. 7 (8): p. 2476–2485.
293. Bishayee, A., *et al.* Anthocyanin-rich black currant (*Ribes nigrum* L.) extract affords chemoprevention against diethylnitrosamine-induced hepatocellular carcinogenesis in rats. *Journal of Nutritional Biochemistry*, 2011. **22**: p. 1035–1046.

294. Gupta, P., *et al.* Spectroscopic characterization of lycopene extract from *Lycopersicum esculentum* (tomato) and its evaluation as a chemopreventive agent against experimental hepatocarcinogenesis in mice. *Phytotherapy Research*, 2013. **27**: p. 448–456.
295. Cykowiak, M., *et al.* Comparison of the impact of xanthohumol and phenethyl isothiocyanate and their combination on Nrf2 and NF-κB pathways in HepG2 cells *in vitro* and tumor burden *in vivo*. *Nutrients*, 2021. **13**: p. 3000.
296. Tag, H.M., *et al.* Chemopreventive efficacy of *Punica granatum* and *Silybum marianum* extracts on chemically-induced hepatocellular carcinomain rats. *Asian Journal of Applied Sciences*, 2019. 7 (2): p. 229–249.
297. Paşayeva, L., *et al.* Phytochemical composition and cytotoxic activity of four Cousinia Species against human hepatocellular carcinoma (HepG2) cell line. *Phytomedicine Plus*, 2021. **1**: p. 100068.
298. Abdraboh, M.E., *et al.* Radio-sensitizing effect of a cocktail of phytochemicals on HepG2 cell proliferation, motility and survival. *Biomedicine & Pharmacotherapy*, 2020. **131**: p. 110620.
299. Kim, J., *et al.* Chemopreventive effect of *Curcuma longa* Linn on liver pathology in HBx transgenic mice. *Intergrative Cancer Therapies*, 2011. **10** (2): p. 168–177.
300. Li, Y., *et al.* Hepatic protection and anticancer activity of Curcuma: a potential chemopreventive strategy against hepatocellular carcinoma. *International Journal of Oncology*, 2014. **44**: p. 505–513.
301. Hamsa, A.A., *et al.* Standardized extract of ginger ameliorates liver cancer by reducing proliferation and inducing apoptosis through inhibition oxidative stress/inflammation pathway. *Biomedicine & Pharmacotherapy*, 2021. **134**: p. 111102.
302. Chou, T.-C. Drug combination studies and their synergy quantification using the Chou-Talalay method. *Cancer Research*, 2010. **70**: p. 440–446.
303. Takimoto, C.H., and Awada, A. Safety and anti-tumor activity of sorafenib (Nexavar) in combination with other anti-cancer agents: a review of clinical trials. *Cancer Chemotherapy Pharmacology*, 2008. **61**: p. 535–548.
304. Kim, A. Sorafenib and sunitinib. *Oncologist*, 2009. **14**: p. 800–805.

305. Mishra, S., and Katare, P. Synergistic combination for chemoprevention of hepatocellular carcinoma: an *in silico* and *in vitro* approach. *Basic & Clinical Pharmacology & Toxicology*, 2017. **120**: p. 532–540.
306. Hussain, T., *et al.* Evaluation of chemopreventive effect of *Fumaria indica* against N-nitrosodiethylamine and CCl4-induced hepatocellular carcinoma in Wistar rats. *Asian Pacific Journal Tropical Medicine*, 2012. **5**: p. 623–629.
307. Jin, S., *et al.* Anti-cancer activity of *Osmanthus matsumuranus* extract by inducing G2/M arrest and apoptosis in human hepatocellular carcinoma Hep G2 cells. *Journal Cancer Prevention*. 2015. **20** (4): p. 241–249.
308. Wu, P.F., *et al.* Piper betle leaf extracts induced human hepatocellular carcinoma Hep3B cell death via MAPKs regulating the p73 pathway *in vitro* and *in vivo*. *Food & Function*, 2014. **5** (12): p. 3320–3328.
309. Bishayee, A., *et al.* Pomegranate phytoconstituents blunt the inflammatory cascade in a chemically induced rodent model of hepatocellular carcinogenesis. *Journal of Nutritional Biochemistry*, 2013. **24** (2013): p. 178–187.
310. Bhatia, D., *et al.* Pomegranate bioactive constituents suppress cell proliferation and induce apoptosis in an experimental model of hepatocellular carcinoma: role of Wnt/β-catenin signalling pathway. *Evidence-Based Complementary and Alternative Medicine*, 2013. **2013**: p. 1–11.
311. Bishayee, A., *et al.* Pomgranate-mediated chemoprevention of experimental hepatocarcinogenesis involves Nrf2-reulated antioxidant mechanisms. *Carcinogenesis*, 2011. **32** (6): p. 888–896.
312. Ahmedy, *et al.* Study of the anticancer potential of celery seed oil against chemically induced hepatocellular carcinoma in rats: a mechanistic approach. *Al Azhar Journal of Pharmaceutical Sciences*, 2016. **53**: p. 14–28.
313. Maideen, N.M.P. Chemopreventive effect of *Phyllanthus polyphyllus* against N-nitrosodiethylamine induced liver tumors by regulating liver enzymes, lipid peroxidation and antioxidants. *Middle-East Journal of Scientific Research*, 2011. **9** (6): p. 696–703.
314. Hong, S., *et al.* Apoptotic and anti-angiogenic effects of *Pulsatilla koreana* extract on hepatocellular carcinoma. *International Journal of Oncology*, 2012. **40**: p. 452–460.

315. Liu, Y., *et al.* Fresh raspberry phytochemical extract inhibits hepatic lesion in a Wistar rat model. *Nutrition & Metabolism*, 2010. **25** (7): p. 84.
316. Parvathaneni, V. Systematic development and optimization of inhalable pirfenidone liposomes for non-small cell lung cancer treatment. *Pharmaceutics*, 2020. **12** (3): p. 206.
317. Khalil, M.I.M., *et al. Trigonella foenum* (Fenugreek) induced apoptosis in hepatocellular carcinoma cell line, HepG2, mediated by upregulation of p53 and proliferating cell nuclear antigen. *BioMed Research International*, 2015. **2015**: p. 1–11.
318. Ansil, P.N., *et al.* Cytotoxic and apoptotic activities *Amorphophallus campanulatus* tuber extracts against human hepatoma cell line. *Research in Pharmaceutical Sciences*, 2014. **9** (4): p. 269–277.
319. Hemalatha, G., *et al.* Phytochemical profiling, anticancer and apoptotic activity of Graviola (*Annona muricata*) fruit extract against human hepatocellular carcinoma (HepG-2) cells. *International Journal of Zoology and Applied Biosciences*, 2020. **5** (1): p. 32–47.
320. Jeivad, F., *et al. Ficus carica* L. Latex: possible chemo-preventive, apoptotic activity and safety assessment. *Iranian Journal of Pharmaceutical Research*, 2020. **19** (3): p. 231–240.
321. Santiago, L.A., *et al.* Cytotoxic and genotoxic activities of the crude ethanolic leaf extract of *Ficus odorata* (Blco). Merr. Against human hepatocellular carcinoma. *Journal of Pharmacognosy and Phytochemistry*, 2014. **3** (3): p. 33–38.
322. Nair, S.V.G., *et al.* Apoptotic and inhibitory effects on cell proliferation of hepatocellular carcinoma HepG2 cells by methanol leaf extract of *Costus speciosus. BioMed Research International*, 2014. **2014**: p. 637098.
323. Thoppil, R.J., *et al.* Antitumor activities of extracts from selected desert plants against HepG2 human hepatocellular carcinoma cells. *Pharmamaceutical Biology*, 2013. **51** (5): p. 668–674.
324. Abdullaev, F.I., and Espinosa-Aguirre, J.J. Biomedical properties of saffron and its potential use in cancer therapy and chemoprevention trials. *Cancer Detection Prevention*, 2004. **28**: p. 426–432.
325. Hodek P., *et al.* Chemopreventive compounds view from the other side. *Chemico-Biological Interaction*, 2009. **180**: p. 1–9.

326. Amin, A., *et al.* Saffron: A potential candidate for a novel anticancer drug against hepatocellular carcinoma. *Hepatology*, 2011. **2011**: p. 857–867.
327. Amin, A., *et al.* Saffron-based crocin prevents early lesions of liver cancer: *in vivo*, *in vitro* and network analyses. *Recent Patents on Anticancer Drug Discovery*, 2016. **11** (1): p. 121–133.
328. Milajerdi, A. The toxicity of saffron (*Crocus sativus* L.) and its constituents against normal and cancer cells. *Journal of Nutrition & Intermediary Metabolism*, 2016. **3**: p. 23–32.
329. Mollaei, H., *et al.* The anti-proliferative and apoptotic effects of crocin on chemosensitive and chemoresistant cervical cancer cells. *Biomedicine & Pharmacotherapy*. 2017. **94**: p. 307–316.
330. Khorasanchi, Z., *et al. Crocus sativus* a natural food coloring and flavoring has potent anti-tumor properties. *Phytomedicine*, 2018. **43**: p. 21–27.
331. Singh, R., *et al.* Prophylactic role of *Averrhoa carambola* (star fruit) extract against chemically induced hepatocellular carcinoma in Swiss albino mice. *Advances in Pharmacological Sciences*, 2014. **2014**: p. 158936.
332. Nakagawa, K., *et al.* Evaporative light-scattering analysis of sulforaphane in broccoli samples: quality of broccoli products regarding sulforaphane contents. *Journal of Agricultural Food Chemistry*, 2006. **54**: p. 2479–2483.
333. Khatria, A., *et al.* Evaluation of hepatoprotective activity of aerial parts of *Tephrosia purpurea* L. and stem bark of *Tecomella undulata*. *Journal of Ethnopharmacology*, 2009. **122**: p. 1–5.
334. Chang, L.C., *et al.* Activity-guided isolation of constituents of *Tephrosia purpurea* with the potential to induce the phase II enzyme, quinone reductase. *Journal of Natural Products*, 1997. **60**: p. 869–873.
335. Hussain, T., *et al.* Chemopreventive evaluation of *Tephrosia purpurea* against N-nitrosodiethylamine-induced hepatocarcinogenesis in Wistar rats. *Journal of Pharmacy and Pharmacology*, 2012. **64**: p. 1195–1205.
336. Hussein, U.K., *et al.* Chemoprevention of diethylnitrosamine-initiated and phenobarbital-promoted hepatocarcinogenesis in rats by sulfated polysaccharides and aqueous extract of *Ulva lactuca*. *Integrative Cancer Therapies*, 2015. **14** (6): p. 525–545.

337. Wu, X., *et al.* Characterization of anthocyanins and proanthocyanins in some cultivars of Ribes, Aronia, and Sambucus and their antioxidant capacity. *Journal of Agricultural Food Chemistry*, 2004. **52**: p. 7846–7856.
338. Bishayee, A., *et al.* Black Currant phytoconstituents exert chemoprevention of diethylnitrosamine-initiated hepatocarcinogenesis by suppression of the inflammatory response. *Molecular Carcinogenesis*, 2013. **52**: p. 304–317.
339. Abdallah, H.M.I., *et al.* 1,8 Cineole and Ellagic acid inhibit hepatocarcinogenesis via upregulation of MiR-122 and suppression of TGF-β1, FSCN1, Vimentin, VEGF, and MMP-9. *PLoS One*, 2022. **17** (1): e0258998.
340. Bharati, S., *et al. Azadirachta indica* exhibits chemopreventive action against haptic cancer: studies on associated histopathological and ultrastructural changes. *Microscopy Research and Technique*, 2012. **75**: p. 586–595.
341. Sipping, M.T.K., *et al.* Polysaccharide-rich fractions from *Ganoderma resinaceum* (Ganodermataceae) as chemopreventive agents in N-Diethylnitrosamine-induced hepatocellular carcinoma in Wistar rats. *Evidence-Based Complementary and Alternative Medicine*, 2022. **2022**: p. 8198859.
342. Manimekalai, I., *et al.* Phytochemical profiling of mangosteen fruit, *Garcinia mangostana. World Journal of Pharmacy and Pharmaceutical Sciences*, 2016. **5** (2): p. 221–252.
343. Priya, V.V., *et al.* Biochemical evidence for the antitumor potential of *Garcinia mangostana* Linn. on diethylnitrosamine-induced hepatic carcinoma. *Pharmacognosy Magazine*, 2018. **14**: p. 186–190.
344. Veeraraghavan, V.P., *et al.* Chemopreventive action of *Garcinia mangostana* Linn. On hepatic carcinoma by modulating ornithine decarboxylase activity. *Pharmacognosy Journal*, 2020. **12** (6): p. 1383–1388.
345. Maru G.B., *et al.* Understanding the molecular mechanisms of cancer prevention by dietary phytochemicals: from experimental models to clinical trials. *World Journal of Biological Chemistry*, 2016. 7 (1): p. 88–99.
346. Ryningen A., *et al. In vivo* biological effects of ATRA in the treatment of AML. *Expert Opin Investig Drugs*, 2008. **17**: p. 1623–1633.

347. Blot W.J., *et al.* Nutrition intervention trials in Linxian, China: supplementation with specific vitamin/mineral combinations, cancer incidence, and disease-specific mortality in the general population. *Journal of National Cancer Institute*, 1993. **85**: p. 1483–1492.
348. Lee, Y., and Kwon, Y.H. Regulation of apoptosis and autophagy by luteolin in human hepatocellular cancer Hep3B cells. *Biochemical and Biophysical Research Communications*, 2019. **517** (4): p. 617–622.
349. Jung, M.-Y., *et al.* Capsaicin-induced apoptosis in SK-Hep-1 hepatocarcinoma cells involves Bcl-2 downregulation and caspase-3 activation. *Cancer Letters*, 2001. **165**: p. 139–145.
350. Ahmed, H.H., *et al.* Phytochemical analysis and anti-cancer investigation of *Boswellia serrata* bioactive constituents *In Vitro*. *Asian Pacific Journal of Cancer Prevention*, 2015. **16**: p. 7179–7188.

https://doi.org/10.1142/9789811293320_0003

Chapter 3

Role of Dietary Supplementation in the Management of Liver Disease

KL Ajee[1*] and KT Moly[2]

[1]*Foundations of Nursing, Amrita College of Nursing, AMRITA Vishwa Vidhyapeetham, Kochi, Kerala, India*
[2]*Amrita College of Nursing, AMRITA Vishwa Vidhyapeetham, Kochi, Kerala, India*

Table of Contents:

*Corresponding author: E-mail address: capt.ajee@gmail.com

Abbreviations:

CLD — Chronic liver disease
HCC — Hepatocellular carcinoma
BCAA — Branched-chain amino acid
EASL — European Association for the Study of the Liver
ESPEN — European Society for Parenteral and Enteral Nutrition
ESLD — End-stage liver disease
REE — Resting energy expenditure
TEE — Total energy expenditure
CTP Score — Child-Turcotte-Pugh score
ESRD — End-stage renal disease
BEE — Basal energy expenditure
IBD — Inflammatory bowel disease
IGF — Insulin growth factor
IL-6 — Interleukin-6
GI — Gastro intestinal
NS — Nervous system
GH — Growth hormone
TNF — Tumor necrosis factors
EN — Enteral nutrition
PN — Parenteral nutrition
ERAS — Enhanced recovery after surgery
HE — Hepatic encephalopathy
MELD — Model for end-stage liver disease
DNA — Deoxyribonucleic acid
PAHs — Polycyclic aromatic hydrocarbons
HCA — Heterocyclic amines
NAFLD — Non-alcoholic fatty liver disease
NASH — Non-alcoholic steatohepatitis
BMI — Body mass index
PCM — Protein calorie malnutrition
RQ — Respiratory quotient
MAC — Mid-arm circumference
SGA — Subjective global assessment
PEG — Percutaneous endoscopic gastrostomy
BIA — Bioelectric impedance analysis

Abstract

Dietary supplementation is often required in liver disease because the liver has a role in nutrient metabolism, and liver dysfunction can pose several potential challenges. Impaired protein synthesis, malnutrition from hypercatabolic status, decreased nutrient absorption, decreased caloric intake, vitamin and mineral deficiencies, and so on are some of the reasons for malnutrition. Hence, detailed nutrition assessments are crucial in all types of liver diseases. This chapter discusses the dietary requirements of patients with cirrhosis of the liver, end-stage liver disease (ESLD), liver transplant, hepatocellular carcinoma (HCC), and alcoholic steatohepatitis. A stage-dependent gradual impairment of lipid, protein, and carbohydrate metabolism accompanied by a deficit of trace elements, protein, and hepatic glycogen is anticipated in these patients. Patients on oral nutrition may have protein and micronutrient deficiencies and need a low-sodium diet. Severe cases need enteral or parenteral nutrition. Probiotics and synbiotics are advantageous in managing the recurrent septic episodes that coincide with liver decompensation. The customized diets for various HCC stages are also specified. Treating the side effects of cancer treatment with diet and the vital role of antioxidants and phytochemicals in HCC prevention give the readers quite new information.

1. Introduction

Liver disorders have grown into a significant threat to global health beyond doubt. Chronic liver disease (CLD) is one of the most prevalent and harmful forms of liver disease. It is marked by a more than six-month period of increasing hepatic parenchymal deterioration and ultimately results in liver cirrhosis, fibrosis, and possibly hepatocellular carcinoma (HCC). The three main interrelated events during the course are inflammation, dysregulated angiogenesis, and fibrosis.

Protein-energy malnutrition is linked to all stages of CLD, and patients with these conditions need to follow a regular diet and take supplements as needed [1]. Treating malnutrition is challenging for these patients since the issues they face concerning their nutrition are complex. Enhancing individuals' nutritional status has the potential to improve their overall quality of life and mitigate the occurrence of medical issues associated with dietary factors [2].

Dietary supplementation is often required in liver disease for several reasons because the liver has a role in nutrient metabolism, and liver dysfunction can pose several potential challenges. A review of the functions of the liver and the changes that occur in liver dysfunctions would help the reader better comprehend the need for dietary supplements in liver disease.

2. Role of the Liver in Nutrient Metabolism — Review

The liver performs many critical tasks central to metabolism and vital for maintaining the body's overall homeostasis. Here are some essential aspects of the role of the liver in metabolism:

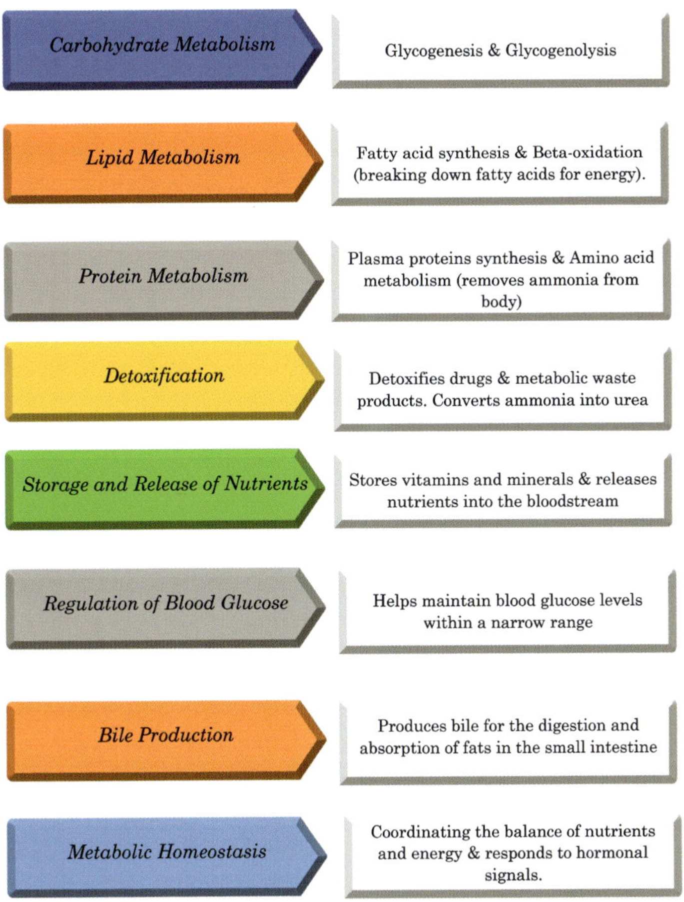

Figure 1: Role of the liver in nutrient metabolism

3. Reasons for Dietary Supplementation in Liver Disease in General

Compared to the worldwide population, Indians have a higher prevalence of malnutrition in cirrhosis. The severity of liver illness is correlated with an increase in malnutrition, and sarcopenia is more common in men [3].

1. Malabsorption of nutrients: Bile, an emulsifier the liver produces, is essential for absorbing lipids and fat-soluble vitamins. Cirrhosis can impair absorption of fat-soluble vitamins, including A, D, E, and K.
2. Impaired protein synthesis: Albumin, a protein produced by the liver, is needed for blood volume maintenance and clotting factors. Protein supplements may be necessary in cases of liver illness since synthesizing these proteins may be hampered.
3. Malnutrition and energy balance: Malnutrition is a frequent concern, and liver illness can increase the body's energy needs. Supplements are required to supply extra calories and minerals, mainly if there is unintentional weight loss.
4. Vitamin and mineral deficiencies: Impaired conversion or storage of vitamins and minerals can result from liver disorders. For instance, a vitamin K shortage may cause issues with liver disease since it is necessary for blood clotting.
5. Branched-chain amino acids (BCAAs): Supplementing with valine, leucine, and isoleucine (BCAAs) may be advised in certain situations. Essential amino acids, known as BCAAs, are involved in synthesizing proteins and generating energy. Supplementing with them can aid in the management of liver disease consequences.
6. Antioxidant support: Increased oxidative stress is a potential side effect of liver illnesses. Vitamins C and E, two antioxidant supplements, may help lessen oxidative damage to liver cells.
7. Preventing the build-up of Hazardous Compounds: Dietary restrictions or supplements may be required in cases of certain liver disorders, such as hemochromatosis or Wilson's disease, to prevent the accumulation of hazardous compounds like copper or iron.

Prominent organizations, such as the European Association for the Study of the Liver (EASL) and the European Society for Parenteral and Enteral Nutrition (ESPEN), have recently published guidelines that emphasize the significance of nutrition in the context of liver diseases and individuals awaiting liver transplantation [4, 5]. However, it is essential to note that these suggestions may not universally apply to the Indian population, as specific considerations must be made while addressing malnutrition and assessing nutritional status within the Indian context.

The authors of this chapter aim to provide dietary guidelines on the four central diseases closely related to diet: liver cirrhosis, ESLD, liver transplantation, and HCC.

4. Dietary Management in Liver Cirrhosis

4.1. *Malnutrition in liver cirrhosis and end-stage liver disease (ESLD)*

People with liver cirrhosis have an incidence of 50% to 90% malnutrition [6]. This condition is associated with an increased risk of infections, hepatic encephalopathy, and ascites, in addition to the advancement of liver failure. Malnutrition, obesity, and sarcopenic obesity may worsen a patient's prognosis and decrease their likelihood of survival. Therefore, in cases of CLD or ESLD, nutrition assessment and management are crucial [7].

Rapid post-absorptive cirrhosis is distinguished by an elevation in appetite and a decrease in the respiratory quotient (RQ) [8, 9]. Due to the metabolic transition from glucose to fatty acids as the principal fuel, the RQ decreases. As a consequence of this state of heightened hunger, protein synthesis is diminished, and gluconeogenesis from amino acids is increased; this ultimately results in sarcopenia. An additional escalation in these patients' resting energy expenditure (REE) may be attributed to gluconeogenesis, an energy-intensive process. Reduced nutritional intake due to many factors — including dysgeusia, anorexia caused by a chronic disease, unappealing, salt-restricted food, and portal hypertension, which impairs gastrointestinal motility and nutrient absorption — accelerates the onset of hunger [10].

Reduced nutritional intake can also result from encephalopathy, gastrointestinal bleeding, hospitalization with fasting periods for diagnostic and therapeutic procedures, and inappropriate dietary protein restriction. The energy supply must balance total energy expenditure (TEE), which includes food-associated thermogenesis, REE, and energy expenditure from physical activity. Individuals suffering from decompensated cirrhosis have reduced or virtually non-existent levels of physical activity. In persons with cirrhosis, TEE varies from 28 to 37.5 kcal/kg/body weight/day [11]. Inadequate dietary protein limitation, hospitalization accompanied by intermittent fasting for diagnostic and therapeutic interventions, encephalopathy, and gastrointestinal bleeding are among the supplementary factors contributing to diminished nutritional consumption.

The balance between energy supply and TEE is crucial, as TEE encompasses REE, thermogenesis linked with meals, and energy expenditure resulting from physical activity. The most effective methods for assessing TEE are often conducted within a controlled respiratory chamber or using doubly-labeled water. Nevertheless, these approaches are neither feasible nor applicable within a clinical setting. Physical activity is significantly reduced and virtually absent in individuals diagnosed with decompensated cirrhosis. The TEE in persons with cirrhosis often falls between the range of 28 to 37.5 kcal/kg/body weight/day.

A condition known as hypermetabolism occurs when the measured REE is higher than usual. Ascites development, liver cirrhosis severity, etiology, or laboratory or clinical criteria cannot be used to diagnose hypermetabolism [12]. The bedside hand-held calorimeter can calculate a patient's daily calorie requirements [9].

The malnutrition associated with more excellent rates of morbidity and death gets worse with increasing Child-Turcotte-Pugh (CTP) scores. One method for predicting death in people with cirrhosis is the Child-Pugh score system. It categorizes patients into three groups based on clinical nutrition status: ascites, neurological disorders, blood bilirubin, and albumin levels. Group A represents a good liver function, B represents moderately impaired hepatic function, and C represents advanced hepatic dysfunction. Malnutrition frequently needs to be noticed. Because of this, malnutrition screening should be performed on all patients with cirrhosis, irrespective of etiology or severity [6, 13].

4.2. *End-stage liver disease*

ESLD, or chronic liver failure, advances gradually over a period of months, years, or even decades. Chronic liver failure is frequently caused by cirrhosis, a pathological condition characterized by the progressive fibrosis of healthy liver tissue to the point where its functionality is compromised. ESLD is characterized by the presence of variceal hemorrhage, hepatic encephalopathy, ascites, or renal impairment in patients with aberrant liver function. Although liver transplantation is a viable treatment option for end-stage renal disease (ESRD), nearly 17% of patients on the transplant waiting list pass away annually due to the lengthening process [14].

The impaired functionality of the liver results in the inability to effectively eliminate toxins from the bloodstream, leading to their gradual accumulation inside the brain. The collection of toxins in the brain, known as hepatic encephalopathy, can lead to a decline in cognitive function and even result in a state of coma. Indications of diminished cognitive function include symptoms such as mental disorientation, alterations in personality, reduction in memory capacity, difficulties sustaining focus, and modifications in sleep patterns. This intricate neurological illness manifests due to hepatic failure and the presence of portosystemic shunting. Liver cirrhosis is frequently linked with this condition.

5. Myths on Malnutrition in Liver Cirrhosis and End-Stage Liver Disease

There are several myths regarding the etiology and management of malnutrition in cirrhosis.

Protein restriction has been one of the principal treatments for hepatic encephalopathy for more than 50 years [15, 16]. It has been well accepted that individuals with cirrhosis should follow a low-protein

Table 1: Etiology of malnutrition

Hypercatabolic Status		**Decreased Nutrient Absorption**		**Decreased Caloric Intake**	
↑BEE	↑Sympathetic NS Inflammation Fever Peritonitis Bacterial translocation	Drug-induced diarrhea	Antibiotics← Lactulose Diuretics Antimetabolites Cholestyramine	Anorexia	Zinc deficiency Hyperglycemia ↑TNF-α, leptin, IL6 *H. pylori* infection
				Unpalatable diets	Low salt Low protein
Insulin resistance	↓Glycogen Stores ↓Glycogenolysis ↑Gluconeogenesis ↑Lipid peroxidation ↑AA mobilization	Fat malabsorption	Alcoholic LD Cholestatic LD IBD Pancreatic insufficiency	Altered gustatory sensation	Hypomagnesemia Autonomic neuropathy
				Early satiety	Tense ascites ↓GI Peristalsis Organomegaly
↓IGFI	↑GH resistance	Delayed bowel function recovery	Surgery GI reperfusion injury Immunosuppressors Corticosteroids	↑Protein losses	GI bleeding Portal hypertensive gastro enteropathy Paracentesis

Source: Etiology of malnutrition in end-stage liver disease. Bunchorntavakul and Reddy [6]. BEE: basal energy expenditure; IBD: inflammatory bowel disease; IGF1: insulin growth factor 1; IL6: interleukin-6; GI: gastrointestinal tract; GH: growth hormone; LD: liver disease; NS: the nervous system; TNF-α: tumor necrosis factor-alpha.

diet due to earlier clinical studies suggesting that a high-protein diet may exacerbate encephalopathy [17]. However, more recent research has demonstrated that protein restriction does not significantly aid in managing or avoiding hepatic encephalopathy. On the other hand, muscles, which play a crucial role in buffering ammonia and supplying amino acids for gluconeogenesis, are negatively impacted by protein restriction or hunger [18].

The second misconception is that those who have cirrhosis should not eat fat. Due to their low glycogen stores, patients with cirrhosis frequently switch to fatty acid oxidation for energy extraction [19]. To some extent, the easy access to fatty acids may prevent muscle breakdown. Additionally, Indian patients think that taking herbal products will not hurt them and that they are safe. These traditional medicines should not be used by people who have liver illness because there have been multiple reports of hepatotoxicity from them [20].

6. Nutritional Assessment

6.1. *Goal of nutritional assessment*

A nutritional assessment aims to identify morbidity and mortality-influencing health risks that may be modifiable through targeted dietary therapy. A nutritional assessment enables the evaluation of an individual's micro and macronutrient status. Examinations of muscle function and body composition provide additional information. Regarding the nutritional assessment of patients with cirrhosis, no gold standard exists.

The dietary requirements of individuals with liver illnesses are contingent upon the liver's capacity to carry out its physiological tasks within the human body. A comprehensive nutritional evaluation will facilitate the formulation of personalized dietary and physical activity regimens. The dietary intervention should establish daily caloric goals emphasizing consuming high-quality protein and addressing deficits in vitamins and micronutrients. This can only be achieved after a comprehensive nutritional evaluation conducted by a multidisciplinary team, as outlined in the following manner.

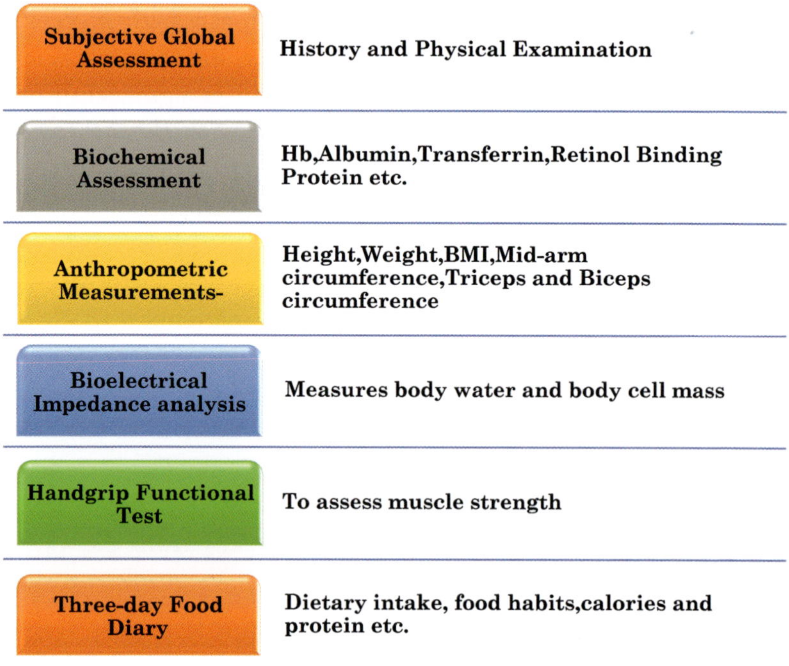

Figure 2: Nutritional assessment [21]

7. Dietary Management in Liver Cirrhosis and HCC

The dietary management in patients with liver cirrhosis depends on the category the patient may belong to after the nutritional assessment. Accordingly, the classes are

- patients at risk for malnutrition,
- patients on oral nutrition, and
- patients on medical nutrition.

7.1. *Patients at risk for malnutrition*

A stage-dependent gradual impairment of lipid, protein, and carbohydrate metabolism accompanied by a deficit of trace elements, protein, and hepatic glycogen is anticipated in these patients. Therefore, after assessing the nutritional status, specialized nutrition counseling is needed [22].

Eating three to five meals per day, in addition to a late-evening snack, effectively reduces the duration of fasting periods. In contrast to individuals who are overweight or obese, it is recommended to increase energy intake in situations characterized by heightened energy expenditure, such as acute complications and refractory ascites, as well as cases of malnutrition. It is recommended that individuals consider making lifestyle modifications.

7.2. *Patients on oral nutrition*

Protein requirement: Individuals suffering from malnourishment and compensated cirrhosis should take 1.2 gm/kg daily. It is recommended that individuals who exhibit signs of malnutrition and sarcopenia have a daily dietary intake of 30 to 35 kcal/kg body weight, along with 1.5 gm of protein per kg body weight. Given that protein enhances protein catabolism, it is advisable to refrain from imposing restrictions on protein intake in individuals with cirrhosis and hepatic encephalopathy.

BCAA requirement: To enable sufficient protein intake, oral BCAA 0.25/kg/day is advised for cirrhotic individuals intolerant to

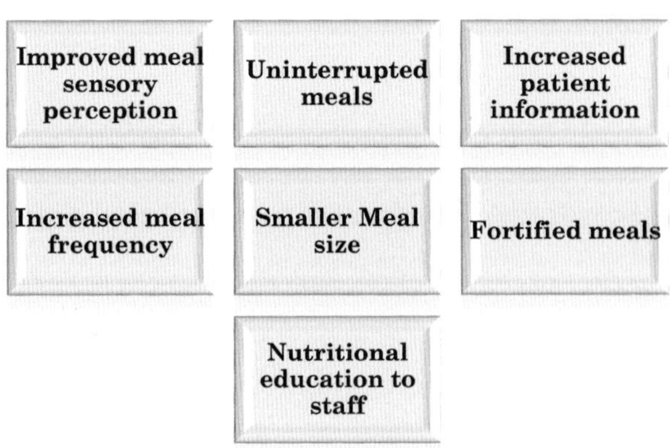

Figure 3: Methods to improve oral intake

protein. To enhance event-free survival in individuals diagnosed with advanced cirrhosis, it is imperative to implement long-term supplementation of BCAAs.

7.2.1. *Micronutrient deficiencies*

7.2.1.1. Deficiency of fat-soluble vitamins

Severe cirrhosis patients sometimes have deficiencies in fat-soluble vitamins [23]. Elevations of serum retinol can be used to diagnose vitamin A deficiency, resulting in night blindness. (32.5–78.0 g/dL is typical). Therefore, taking 25,000 units of vitamin A daily for four to eight weeks is recommended.

Deficiency of vitamin D may result in osteopenia, osteoporosis, and osteomalacia. One should take 2000 IU of vitamin D2 or D3 and 1200–150 mg of calcium daily. Patients with vitamin D deficiency (25-hydroxyvitamin D level below 20 ng/mL) are advised to consume 50,000 IU of vitamin D.

An insufficient amount of vitamin K raises the chance of bleeding. The choice of treatments for vitamin K deficiency depends on whether individuals require intramuscular or intravenous assistance [4].

7.2.1.2. Deficiency of water-soluble vitamins

A thiamine [vitamin B1] deficiency can cause high-output heart failure, also known as "wet beriberi," and brain dysfunction, including Wernicke encephalopathy and Korsakoff psychosis. Vitamin B12, cobalamin, and folate deficits are less common. Pyridoxine is a vitamin B6). Alternatively, inactive cobalamin mimics in cirrhotic people seep into the circulation, leading to elevated blood vitamin B12 levels despite lower tissue levels [4].

Deficits in zinc have been associated with dysgeusia, which can worsen food aversion and are common in cirrhotic patients. Other symptoms include hypogonadism, glossitis, acrodermatitis, and impaired wound healing. The measurement of serum zinc levels may provide limitations since it may not provide a comprehensive representation of the overall zinc storage throughout the body. If a deficiency is present, it is recommended to administer a daily dose of 50 mg of elemental zinc (equivalent to 220 mg of zinc sulfate). This dosage has been found to have no negative impact on the absorption of copper [24]. There exists a correlation between muscle cramps and magnesium deficiency. In clinical practice, it is customary to administer a standard dosage of 400 mg of magnesium oxide as a supplement [13].

Low-sodium diet: When considering the recommended use of a low-sodium diet, it is essential to carefully weigh the potential decrease in food consumption against the mild benefits it offers in treating ascites. Compromising the palatability of the diet should be prevented.

7.3. *Patients on medical nutrition*

7.3.1. *Enteral nutrition and parenteral nutrition (EN and PN)*

The initiation of enteral nutrition is indicated for cirrhotic patients who cannot achieve their dietary goals by oral feeding. Parenteral nutrition is required in whom oral or EN are ineffective or not feasible. No absolute contraindication exists, including esophageal varices for positioning a nasogastric tube.

For malnourished sarcopenics suffering from severe liver disease, getting enough calories and protein to eat might be difficult. With varying degrees of effectiveness, clinical studies have addressed this issue with BCAA and oral nutritional supplements [25]. While establishing a substantial survival benefit remains uncertain, it is recommended that individuals with malnutrition and cirrhosis who cannot adequately address underfeeding through oral intake, including oral supplements, should be administered short-term enteral or parenteral nutrition [26].

When gastrointestinal bleeding, encephalopathy, reduced gut motility, or ileus impede oral intake for an extended period, parenteral nutritional supplementation may benefit cirrhotic patients. When individuals have encephalopathy, gastrointestinal hemorrhage, or reduced gut motility or ileus for an extended duration, relying on oral information may be advantageous [27].

7.3.2. *Use of probiotics and synbiotics*

Probiotics and synbiotics are advantageous in managing the recurrent septic episodes that coincide with liver decompensation [28]. Probiotics refer to living microorganisms, while prebiotics are indigestible carbohydrates that promote the growth and functionality of advantageous bacteria within the intestinal flora. Synbiotics, conversely, encompass a combination of both probiotics and prebiotics [29].

A growing body of evidence suggests that the transfer of intestinal flora bacteria, in conjunction with the compromised antibacterial defense mechanisms, plays a crucial role in the pathogenesis of sepsis. According to the study conducted by Wiest in 2005, probiotic or prebiotic treatment aims to increase the presence of lactic acid-producing bacteria in the intestines while decreasing the prevalence of other species that have a higher likelihood of causing disease. This approach is intended to reduce the occurrence of sepsis.

A randomized study assessed the incidence of postoperative infections in a cohort of 95 liver transplant recipients. The recipients were divided into two groups: one group had an early supply of conventional enteral feed supplemented with a synbiotic regimen, while the other group underwent intestinal cleaning. The results showed that the group receiving the synbiotic regimen had a much lower rate of bacterial infections (13%) than those with intestinal decontamination (48%) [30].

Moreover, data supports the notion that administering synbiotic or probiotic supplements enhances liver function. The administration of synbiotic medication resulted in an enhancement in the Child score among a cohort of 55 individuals diagnosed with cirrhosis and exhibiting little hepatic encephalopathy. This intervention led to noteworthy improvements in bilirubin levels, albumin levels, and prothrombin time [31].

7.4. *Diet in liver transplantation*

Even now, nutritional therapy presents difficulties for liver transplant recipients. Malnutrition is frequently observed in severe liver illnesses, such as cirrhosis, as a result of reduced calorie intake, hypercatabolic state, and impaired nutrient absorption. Malnutrition is a common condition among liver transplant candidates.

One of the most influential determinants of survival and malnutrition after liver transplantation is nutritional status before the procedure. Anorexia, ascites, dietary restrictions, metabolic and inflammatory derangements, polypharmacy, multiple paracenteses, bleeding varices, and prolonged fasting periods for lab and diagnostic procedures can be summed up as the factors linked to malnutrition in patients waiting for liver transplantation [32].

Early retrospective studies found that malnutrition harms liver transplantation [15, 33]. The success of transplantation was predicted by preoperative hypermetabolism and body cell mass reduction [34, 35]. It has been suggested that glycogen depletion intensifies the pro-inflammatory cytokine response, which leads to postoperative systemic inflammatory response syndrome and multi-organ failure in these individuals [35]. Proper diet and repairing vitamin and mineral shortages are essential to preserve residual hepatic function, enhance the patient's metabolic reserves, and improve liver transplant results. As a result, prompt nutrition assessments and interventions are crucial. Every single liver transplant candidate waiting for transplantation should undergo the subjective global assessment (SGA) for patients described early in this chapter [36].

7.4.1. *Diet in pre-liver transplant*

Emphasis should be placed on the fact that most patients do not need or should not be advised to fast from midnight before surgery, nor should they stop eating after that [33]. The ERAS technique is recommended during the initial preoperative phase to avoid needless hunger. The multimodal, evidence-based enhanced recovery after surgery (ERAS) program of treatment was created to lessen the body's reaction to surgical stress and is linked to a lower rate of perioperative morbidity and brief hospital stays. The ERAS protocol encompasses several fundamental principles, including preoperative counseling, preoperative nutrition, early mobilization, standardized anesthetic and analgesic regimens (including epidural and non-opioid

Table 2: Nutritional recommendations in pre-liver transplant

Diet	Recommendations	Observations
Calories	35–40 kcal/kg	No fasting for more than 3–6 hours during daytime; Small, frequent meals daily
Protein	1.2–1.5 g/kg	A diet rich in vegetables and dairy protein
Carbohydrates	50%–70%	A late-evening snack (50 g) of carbohydrates
Fat	30%	There is no fat restriction unless fat malabsorption or slower gastric emptying
Fiber	25–45 g/d	Beneficial on neuropsychiatric performance
Vitamin and minerals	Dietary reference intakes	Therapeutic doses in case of deficiency

Source: Hammad et al. [15].

analgesic analgesics), and avoidance of perioperative fasting and carbohydrate loading for a maximum of two hours before surgery. Before surgery, 1.2–1.5 kg of protein should be consumed daily, and a total calorie intake of 30–35 kcal/kg should be the goal.

7.4.2. *Diet in post-liver transplant*

Within 12 to 24 hours after surgery, regular diet and enteral nourishment should be started to lower the infection rate. Aim for a daily total calorie intake of 30–35 kcal/kg after the acute phase and a daily protein consumption of 1.2–1.5 kg. Early enteral feeding should be administered using nasogastric or naso-jejunal tubes. Enteral formula and specific probiotics should be taken post-surgery to lower the infection rate. When patients with HE require enteral nutrition, a BCAA-enriched recipe is typically given.

Parenteral nutrition should be utilized instead of oral food or EN to reduce the length of mechanical ventilation, the time spent in the intensive care unit, and the incidence of complications. When respiration and swallow reflexes are affected, PN is indicated for patients with unprotected airways and HE, as opposed to EN, which is contraindicated.

Regarding deceased donor transplants, the exact timing of a patient's transplant cannot be predicted. Patients who achieve the highest MELD scores should receive prompt postoperative nutrition support, preferably through enteral feeding, mainly if they are malnourished, unable to consume, or unable to sustain oral intake exceeding 60% of the recommended amount for a duration exceeding ten days. Scores for the Model for End-Stage Liver Disease (MELD) vary from 6 to 40. Your odds of passing away from liver failure within the following 3 months increase with your score.) Nutrition therapy can be better organized around the transplant procedure timeline for patients receiving transplants from living donors.

Weeks after the liver transplant procedure, there is still an increase in energy and protein needs. Liver transplant recipients' metabolism gets better 4 weeks later. Protein catabolism is significantly elevated in the postoperative period, and patients should consume 1.5–2.0 g/kg of protein. Because of the frequent use of diuretics, abdominal drains, and fluid overload, electrolyte abnormalities such as serum potassium, phosphorus, and magnesium levels should be evaluated [37].

In conclusion, early ordinary food or enteral nutrition is recommended 12 hours after liver transplantation, provided the patient is

Table 3: post-liver transplant diet

Nutrients/Diet	Recommendations	Observations
	Post-transplant	
Calories	25–30 kcal/kg	Use indirect calorimetry when possible
Proteins	1.5–2.0 g/kg	In the immediate postoperative phase, protein catabolism is markedly increased
Food/enteral nutrition		Post-transplant, if the patient is hemodynamically stable and has no nausea or vomiting, Early average food or enteral nutrition (12 h) after liver transplant is advisable

hemodynamically stable and does not experience nausea or vomiting [38]. Patients undergoing liver transplantation will be required to take immunosuppressant drugs such as cyclosporine, tacrolimus, and corticosteroids lifelong. These also may lead to nutrition-associated implications. New-onset diabetes is common initially [39] diabetic dietary advice is usually required.

Hyperkalemia may present in some patients shortly after the operation, ordinarily due to the nephrotoxicity of the prescribed immunosuppressant medication. Then, control of potassium food sources may be essential [40]. The condition mostly disappears in the long term. Hypomagnesemia arising from immunosuppression requires magnesium supplementation through dark cocoa, whole grains, nuts, legumes, fruits, and green vegetables.

In the post-transplant period, transplant, weight gain becomes an issue over time. As these individuals lose an average of 9.1 kg over the duration of liver illness, it is fine at first [41]. Significant relative weight gain occurs most frequently within the initial half-year following the transplant procedure, with complete restoration of weight loss arising within the initial year following the operation [41]. Nevertheless, regrettably, patients continue to accumulate weight in the years that follow, culminating in the development of overweight and obesity [42]. Despite this, the high incidence of sarcopenia persists even after transplantation. Efforts should be made to prevent metabolic complications associated with weight gain and immunosuppression through counseling, exercise, and other means. Lastly, malnutrition is a potentially treatable condition that, when appropriately identified and managed, can yield favorable outcomes for individuals afflicted with chronic liver dysfunctions.

7.5. *Diet in hepatocellular carcinoma*

HCC, or hepatoma, is one of the most common forms of primary liver cancer. It ranks as the sixth most prevalent form of cancer worldwide and is the third leading cause of death due to cancer. HCC exhibits a higher prevalence in Asia and Africa, although its occurrence is progressively rising in developed countries. It originates from hepatocytes, the functional units of the liver. The process of HCC is facilitated by the persistent presence of liver inflammation and subsequent cellular injury, leading to the malignant transformation of hepatocytes. The primary risk factors associated with HCC encompass chronic viral hepatitis, excessive alcohol intake, non-alcoholic fatty liver disease (NAFLD), exposure to certain toxins formed by specific fungi, and inherited liver disorders [43–45].

Early detection of HCC is difficult since symptoms may be quiet or misinterpreted as liver diseases. Later symptoms include stomach pain, weight loss, jaundice, and a palpable lump. HCC has a dismal prognosis due to its aggressiveness and late diagnosis. Prevention and early intervention are vital in fighting HCC. Hepatitis B vaccination, viral hepatitis treatment, and lifestyle changes can lower cancer risk. Patients at risk need screening programs such as liver function testing and imaging early detection. Depending on stage and health, HCC treatments include surgical excision, liver transplantation, locoregional therapy, systemic therapies, and palliative care [46].

8. Nutrition and Diet Are Essential for Cancer Prevention, Treatment, and Recovery

8.1. *Cancer prevention*

Cancer risk can be reduced by eating well. Eat plenty of fruits, veggies, and whole grains, and minimize processed meats, red meat, and sugary drinks.

8.2. *Specific dietary components associated with lower cancer risk*

- Fiber: Fiber aids digestion and lowers colon cancer risk.
- Folate is a B vitamin needed for cell growth and repair. A folate-rich diet may lower breast cancer and other cancer risks.
- Antioxidants protect cells. Carotenoids, vitamin C, and vitamin E are antioxidants in fruits and vegetables [47].

8.3. *Cancer treatment*

Cancer therapy can also affect diet and nutrition. Side effects of cancer and cancer therapies include fatigue, nausea, vomiting, and diarrhea. Side effects can make it hard to eat enough or absorb nutrition. Malnutrition can weaken the body and make cancer and treatment harder.

8.3.1. *Role of nutrition in cancer care*

Healthy eating during cancer treatment helps to

- Reduce side effects
- Maintain weight
- Boost energy
- Boost Immune system
- Help the body heal and recover from cancer.

Healthy eating is essential after cancer therapy. This may prevent cancer recurrence and improve quality of life [48].

9. Dietary Recommendations for Patients with Cancer

There is no optimal dietary approach that is universally acceptable for cancer patients. The optimal nutritional regimen for each individual depends on their specific cancer type, stage, and concurrent medical issues. Nevertheless, it is worth noting that specific fundamental dietary guidelines may benefit individuals diagnosed with cancer. It is recommended to consume an ample amount of fruits and vegetables. As fruits and vegetables are rich in vitamins, minerals, and antioxidants that promote optimal health, eating at least five servings of fruits and vegetables daily is recommended.

It is advised to eat whole grains rather than refined grains. Whole grains are considered a favorable dietary component due to their high fiber content, which is associated with promoting optimal digestive system functioning and potentially mitigating the likelihood of developing cancer. It is advisable to restrict the consumption of processed meats and red meat. Evidence suggests a positive association between consuming processed meats and red meat and an elevated susceptibility to cancer. The recommended dietary guideline is to consume 500 gm of red meat per week while completely abstaining from consuming processed meats.

Select protein sources that are low in fat. Consuming lean protein sources, such as fish, chicken, beans, and paneer, is crucial in preserving muscle mass and facilitating the body's healing processes. It is recommended to restrict the consumption of beverages high in added sugars. Drinks with high sugar content possess a significant caloric load and have the potential to contribute to the accumulation of body weight. Consuming water, unsweetened tea, or coffee as an alternative is advisable.

It is essential to work with a dietician for a personalized diet plan [49, 50].

10. Role of Nutrition in Cancer Development

10.1. *The Connection between diet and development of hepatocellular carcinoma*

An increasing body of empirical research indicates a correlation between dietary patterns and HCC, which is recognized as the prevailing form of liver cancer [51].

a. Alcohol: Excessive alcohol consumption significantly contributes to the development of HCC. Alcohol consumption has been found to adversely affect hepatocytes, resulting in hepatocellular injury and triggering an inflammatory response that leads to fibrosis and carcinogenesis [52].
b. Obesity: It represents an additional risk factor for HCC. Adipocytes secrete hormones and inflammatory mediators that can potentially facilitate cancer cell proliferation [53].
c. Aflatoxins: These are a class of toxins synthesized by specific fungal species and potentially contaminate several food crops,

including peanuts, maize, and soybeans. Aflatoxins are recognized for their carcinogenic properties and are associated with an elevated susceptibility to HCC [54].

d. Red meat: The consumption of red meat has been associated with an elevated risk of HCC. Red meat is known to possess high levels of iron, a mineral related to potential adverse effects on liver health and the facilitation of cancer progression [55, 56].
e. Processed meats, bacon, sausage, and hot dogs are correlated with a heightened likelihood of developing HCC. Nitrates and nitrites, present in processed meats, can potentially convert within the human body, resulting in the formation of chemicals that possess carcinogenic properties [57].

10.1.1. *Protective dietary factors include*

- Fruits and vegetables are abundant sources of antioxidants and various nutrients that can safeguard the liver against potential harm.
- Whole grains are considered a valuable dietary component due to their high fiber content, associated with potential benefits such as inflammation reduction and a decreased likelihood of developing cancer.
- Coffee is known to possess bioactive chemicals that have anti-inflammatory and antioxidant properties. Drinking coffee has decreased the likelihood of developing HCC [58].
- The Mediterranean diet is a nutritionally beneficial eating regimen distinguished by its emphasis on abundant intake of fruits, vegetables, whole grains, and olive oil. Several studies have established a correlation between adherence to the Mediterranean diet and a decreased likelihood of developing HCC [58, 59].

10.2. *Dietary sources of carcinogenic substances*

Carcinogens are defined as compounds that have the potential to induce the development of cancer. These entities can be observed within the natural surroundings, occupational settings, and dietary sources. Several dietary carcinogens are commonly found in various food sources.

a. Processed meats refer to meats that have undergone preservation techniques such as smoking, curing, or salting. This process has the potential to generate deleterious substances known as N-nitroso compounds, which have been associated with the development of colorectal cancer. Processed meats encompass a variety of food products, such as bacon, sausage, and hot dogs.
b. Red meat refers to the flesh of mammals, including beef, pork, and lamb. Red meat contains heme iron, a compound associated with potential DNA damage and an elevated susceptibility to cancer.
c. Alcohol is a known carcinogen, and it can cause DNA damage and increase susceptibility to different types of cancer, such as carcinoma of the oral cavity, pharynx, esophagus, liver, and colon.
d. Aflatoxins are toxins produced by particular fungi and can potentially infect various food sources such as peanuts, cereals, and

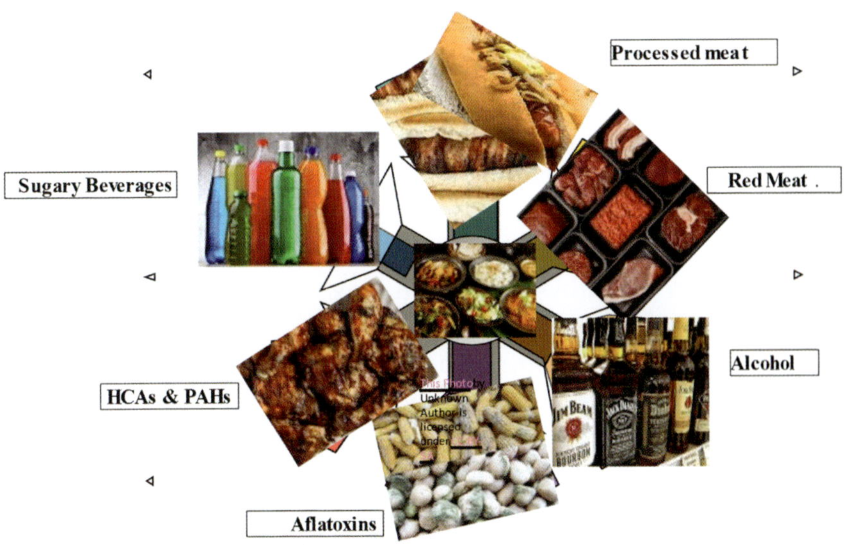

Figure 4: Dietary sources of carcinogens

legumes. Aflatoxins are highly carcinogenic and have been linked to the development of liver cancer.

e. Chemical molecules known as polycyclic aromatic hydrocarbons (PAHs) and heterocyclic amines (HCAs) are created when meat is prepared using high-temperature cooking techniques, including grilling, frying, or barbecuing. There is a connection between HCAs and PAHs with breast, stomach, and colon cancer.

Apart from the carcinogens mentioned above, a dietary pattern characterized by a high consumption of processed foods, sugary beverages, and unhealthy fats has been associated with an increased susceptibility to cancer. This phenomenon can be attributed to the development of obesity and inflammation, both of which have been identified as significant risk factors for the onset of cancer [52, 60].

10.3. *The role of diet and lifestyle in liver diseases*

Diet significantly affects liver health because the liver is essential for metabolizing nutrients and detoxifying the body. A nutritious diet can aid in the maintenance of optimal liver function and the prevention of liver-related diseases. Diet influences liver health as follows [61].

i) Weight maintenance: Maintaining a healthy body weight is crucial in preventing the development and progression of NAFLD, a condition closely associated with obesity. NAFLD has the potential to advance into more severe illnesses such as non-alcoholic steatohepatitis (NASH) and cirrhosis. It is vital to maintain a healthy weight by having a well-balanced diet.
ii) Consumption of essential macronutrients: A healthy diet depends on adhering to a balanced macronutrient regimen, encompassing suitable portions of proteins, carbohydrates, and lipids. Fat accumulation in the liver may result from consuming excessive foods with higher calories, sugar, and fat content.
iii) Restrict sugar intake: Excessive dietary intake of sugar, particularly fructose, may play a role in the pathogenesis of NAFLD.

Restricting processed food, sugary beverages, and dessert intake is crucial to maintain optimal liver health.

iv) Restriction of saturated fat: Limiting saturated fat intake is recommended. Increased cholesterol levels and a higher chance of developing fatty liver disease are consequences of consuming saturated and trans fats. It is suggested that prioritization be given to consuming unsaturated fats, like olive oil, avocados, or seafood rich in fat. It is advisable to restrict the intake of saturated fats and refrain from trans fats, as the former may likely contribute to inflammation of liver cells.

v) Sufficient protein intake: Protein is essential for optimal liver function. The diet should contain poultry, fish, paneer, and lentils that are low in fat and calories. Limiting the intake of red and processed meats is advisable due to their potential to exert pressure on the liver.

vi) Fiber-rich food: Dietary sources rich in dietary fiber, such as fruits, vegetables, and whole grains, have a crucial role in the regulation of digestion and the promotion of a healthy gut microbiome. This, in turn, has indirect positive effects on liver function.

vii) Adequate hydration: Sufficient hydration facilitates the liver's detoxifying mechanisms. Water plays a crucial role in eliminating toxins and waste products from the body.

viii) Micronutrients: It is essential to take food rich in vitamin E, vitamin C, and selenium as they support liver functions.

ix) Limiting processed meat, red meat, and food rich in HCA and PAHs is essential for liver health.

x) Avoid excessive salt intake: Excess salt intake leads to fluid retention and adversely affects liver health [62, 63].

11. Role of Antioxidants and Phytochemicals in HCC Prevention

- Vitamin C, known as ascorbic acid, possesses potent antioxidant properties that contribute to cellular protection against oxidative stress-induced damage.

- Vitamin E can safeguard cells against potential injury.
- Beta-carotene is classified as a carotenoid compound, which can convert into vitamin A within the human body. Carotenoids have potent antioxidant properties, exhibiting the capacity to safeguard cells against oxidative harm.
- Selenium is a trace mineral known for its potential to mitigate cellular damage.
- Sulforaphane, a phytochemical, is abundantly present in cruciferous vegetables such as broccoli, cauliflower, and Brussels sprouts. Research has demonstrated that sulforaphane possesses anticancer properties [64, 65].

12. Nutrition During Cancer Treatment

12.1. *Significance of proper nutrition during cancer treatment*

Ensuring adequate nutrition throughout cancer therapy is crucial for many reasons. It is essential to consistently manage one's weight and body mass index (BMI) to promote optimal health and well-being. This aspect has significance as individuals with a low body weight may encounter challenges in tolerating medical interventions and recuperating from surgical procedures [66].

It is imperative to provide an adequate intake of protein. Protein plays a crucial role in tissue repair and regeneration, particularly in the context of cancer and its associated treatments.

Ensure an adequate caloric intake. Caloric intake is essential for sustaining energy levels, a critical factor in maintaining physical activity and bolstering the body's ability to combat cancer [67].

Ensure enough intake of vitamins and minerals. Vitamins and minerals play an essential role in various physiological processes in the human body, encompassing cellular proliferation and restoration, immune system functionality, as well as the facilitation of wound healing.

Minimize the adverse consequences associated with therapeutic interventions. Specific cancer treatments have the potential to induce adverse effects, including but not limited to nausea, vomiting, diarrhea, and alterations in taste perception. Sufficient nutritional intake can ameliorate these negative consequences and augment the ability to ingest food and withstand medical procedures [58].

The consumption of a nutritionally balanced diet has the potential to positively impact an individual's overall well-being and augment their levels of energy. It can also improve an individual's emotional well-being and regulate sleep patterns.

12.2. *Treating the side effects of cancer treatment with diet*

The relevance of diet in the management of side effects associated with cancer therapy is substantial. By consuming suitable beverages and selecting diets, individuals may experience relief from symptoms, increase their energy levels, and maintain an ideal body weight. With a healthy diet, the following adverse effects may be mitigated.

1) Severe nausea and vomiting: Eat smaller, more frequent meals daily. Choose light, easily digested foods such as bread, crackers, plain yogurt, and clear soup. It is best to avoid eating anything fried, spicy, or heavy in fat. It is recommended to drink enough fluids, focusing primarily on clear liquids such as broth, sports drinks, and water. Drinking ginger ale, ginger tea, or sucking on ginger candies may alleviate nausea.
2) Loose stools or diarrhea: Adopt a bland, low-fiber diet consisting primarily of potatoes, white bread, and rice. It is recommended to abstain from consuming uncooked fruits and vegetables and fiber-rich foods, including cereals made with bran, whole grains, and legumes. Adequate fluid consumption is recommended to ensure proper hydration. It is advisable to avoid the consumption of caffeine and alcohol, as it may cause dehydration and worsen diarrhea symptoms.
3) Constipation: It is advised to have a diet high in fiber-containing foods, such as fruits, vegetables, and whole grains. It is essential to have adequate fluid intake, especially water and prune juice (dry plum), to maintain proper hydration. Regular exercise promotes the best possible motility of the colon.

4) Loss of appetite: Eat small, frequent meals throughout the day. Make sure the foods chosen are tasty and high in calories. Eat high-calorie snacks such as nuts, seeds, avocados, and yogurt as part of the diet. Add various herbs and spices to the diet to improve the flavor.
5) Oral ulcers: Soft, flavorless dishes that are freely masticated and swallowed should be followed. Avoiding acidic foods and beverages, such as pineapple, citrus fruits, and tomatoes, is recommended. Engaging in regular oral cavity rinsing using either saltwater or baking soda solution is recommended.
6) Fatigue: Consuming a balanced diet with ample protein, carbs, and nutritious fats is recommended. It is advisable to refrain from drinking beverages and snacks high in sugar, as such dietary choices can induce a subsequent decline in energy levels. Consume smaller, regular meals throughout the course of the day.

It is essential to have adequate sleep. It is imperative to consult a medical professional, such as a doctor or a qualified dietitian, to address and discuss one's individualized dietary requirements. Professionals in the field can assist individuals in formulating a customized dietary regimen tailored to mitigate the adverse effects of cancer treatment and maintain overall well-being [68, 69].

13. Customized Diets for Various Stages of Hepatocellular Carcinoma (HCC)

13.1. *Early stage of Hepatocellular carcinoma (HCC)*

A standard dietary regimen is required for individuals with early-stage HCC. All food items that can irritate hepatocytes, such as alcohol, spicy foods, and food rich in fat, must be restricted. Refraining from processed foods and beverages with high sugar content is highly recommended to avoid weight gain and inflammation of the liver [70].

13.2. *Late or advanced stage of hepatocellular carcinoma (HCC)*

As the patient's taste alters and the general condition does not permit a regular, well-balanced diet, a special diet is prepared per the individual's need.

Modified diet may be as follows:

a. Restriction in protein intake: In the advanced stage of HCC or portal hypertension, there is a need to restrict protein intake. This phenomenon can be attributed to the liver's possible incapacity to metabolize an excessive quantity of protein efficiently.
b. Sodium restriction: In patients with fluid retention and ascites, sodium must be restricted.
c. Restrict fat intake: In the case of patients with hyperlipidemia, cholesterolemia, and elevated triglycerides, fat intake needs to be restricted.
d. Adequate micronutrients: Ensure adequate intake of vitamins, minerals, and other micronutrients [71].

Collaborating with a certified nutritionist:

The assistance of a qualified dietician can be sought to develop a customized meal plan that aligns with one's specific requirements and dietary limitations. Additionally, they can offer recommendations about maintaining a balanced diet throughout cancer treatment and the subsequent recovery period.

14. Nutritional Assessment in Liver Diseases

Protein calorie malnutrition (PCM) affects 50%–100% of decompensated cirrhosis patients and at least 20% of compensated patients. PCM can lead to consequences such as variceal bleeding, ascites, increased surgical mortality, lower survival, and worsened hepatic

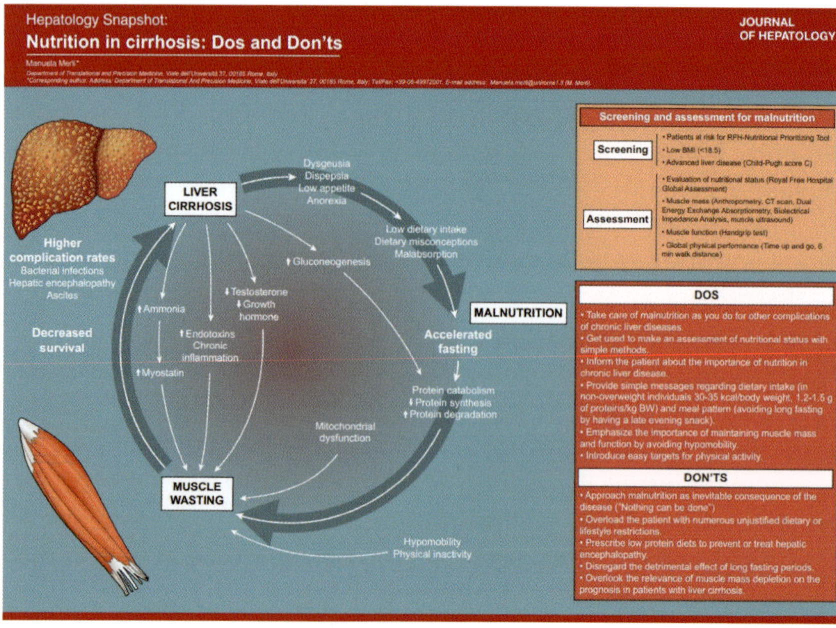

Figure 5: Nutrition in cirrhosis: dos and dont's

Source: Merli [72].

function (in some trials). Cirrhosis patients, especially those with severe disease, may have vitamin deficits.

Since supplemental nutrition reduces infection and in-hospital mortality and improves liver function, macro- and micronutrient deficiencies must be identified [73–75].

Malnutrition in liver cirrhosis has a complex etiology. Liver diseases alter lipid, carbohydrate, and protein metabolism. Undernutrition, poor digestion, and altered metabolism contribute to it. The causes are:

- Nutritional intake may be affected by anorexia, nausea, encephalopathy, gastritis, ascites, sodium-restricted diet, and alcohol consumption.
- Reasons for nutritional malabsorption include lack of bile salt, bacterial overgrowth, altered intestinal motility, portal hypertension, damage to intestinal mucosal, and increased intestinal permeability.

- Due to cirrhosis and increased hunger, protein and lipids are used as fuels instead of glucose. The loss of total protein occurs due to reduced urea and hepatic protein synthesis, malabsorption of intestinal protein, and decreased excretion of nitrogen in urine. A correlation exists between liver disease and a reduced ratio of BCAAs to aromatic amino acids.
- When carbohydrate metabolism is abnormal, it leads to insulin resistance, gluconeogenesis impairment, and decreased glycogen reserves. Lipids are oxidized for energy, resulting in a lower RQ than those without CLD [76, 77].

14.1. *Tool for nutritional assessment*

A nutritional assessment aims to identify morbidity and mortality-influencing health risks that may be modifiable through targeted dietary therapy. A nutritional assessment enables the evaluation of an individual's micro and macronutrient status. Examinations of muscle function and body composition provide additional information. Regarding the nutritional assessment of patients with cirrhosis, no gold standard exists.

There needs to be a standard nutritional assessment tool. However, the nutritional assessment includes:

A) History Taking:
   1. Weight and BMI: It includes the history of their usual weight or loss of weight over the past two weeks and the past 6 months. Any weight loss (unintentional) of more than 10% is considered severe.
   2. Dietary history: 3 days from a food diary or 24-hour dietary recall will help assess dietary intake, which can be compared with the recommended diet.
   3. Smoking and alcohol history: This must be quantified as it can alter the dietary intake.
   4. History of gastrointestinal symptoms: History of anorexia, nausea, vomiting, early satiety, and its onset and frequency need to be obtained. Symptoms that endure beyond two weeks and are accompanied by a constraint in consuming essential nutrients give rise to concern.

5. History of Liver Disease: a detailed history of the onset and duration of the disease will help understand the course of malnutrition. The disease severity can be assessed with the help of the Child-Pugh Score and MELD Score.
6. Micronutrient deficiency: Micronutrients such as vitamins A, B, C, and K and trace elements like niacin Zink can cause dermatitis, night blindness, mouth ulcers, easy bruising, and paresthesia. A detailed history of these symptoms needs to be obtained.
7. Medication history: Certain medications can alter the taste and lead to appetite loss.
8. History of allergies and intolerance: Food allergies and discrimination can affect dietary choices.
9. Social and lifestyle factors: Dietary changes are influenced by sociocultural factors, living conditions, and availability of support systems.
10. Functional capacity and metabolic demand: It is essential to obtain a history of the patient's daily activities, including occupational activities, social activities, and history of comorbidities, to understand nutritional needs and metabolic demand.

B) Physical Examination:

Conduct a comprehensive physical examination, with particular attention to identifying biological indicators that suggest the presence of deficiencies in macronutrients or micronutrients.

1. General appearance: Look for body-built (thin, emaciated patients with sarcopenia), icteric, and edematous bodies.
2. Height, weight, and body mass index: A body mass less than 18.5 kg/m^2 suggests underweight status and malnutrition in individuals diagnosed with liver disease.
3. Anthropometric measures: Additional information such as mid-arm circumference (MAC) and triceps skinfold thickness will give an idea about body composition and muscle wastage.
4. Assessment of ascites and edema: The ascites and edema indicate salt and fluid deficiency and body albumin loss.

5. Loss of subcutaneous fat: The depletion of subcutaneous adipose tissue is an additional malnutrition marker. To evaluate subcutaneous fat storage, it is necessary to do palpation on specific locations such as the chest wall, eye sockets, and triceps region.
6. Look for pallor, keratitis, dermatitis, bruising, glossitis, and angular stomatitis for micronutrient deficiencies such as iron, vitamin A, Vitamin C, K, B12, Folate, and niacin.
7. Dynamometry: A mechanical handgrip dynamometer is used to assess the hand grip strength [8, 78].
8. Subjective Global Assessment: A clinical instrument extensively employed to assess the nutritional status of various patient populations is the SGA. This assessment is performed uncomplicated at the patient's bedside, eliminating the requirement for specialized apparatus or laboratory methodologies. The SGA employs a holistic method integrating functional appraisals, somatic assessments, and historical data. The historical analysis focuses on the recent occurrence of weight loss, changes in dietary patterns, and the presentation of symptoms indicative of malnutrition. Subcutaneous adipose tissue, muscular atrophy, fluid retention, and abdominal cavity fluid accumulation (ascites) are assessed during the physical examination. The functional assessment evaluates the individual's ability to perform activities that are essential for the performance of daily tasks [79].

The patient classification system employed by the SGA consists of three discrete groups: group A comprises individuals who are sufficiently nourished; Group B includes patients who are experiencing mild to moderate malnourishment; and Group C contains patients who are severely malnourished. Individuals classified as B or C are more prone to complications related to malnutrition, such as increased rates of illness and death. The SGA is a valuable tool for identifying patients who demonstrate indicators of malnutrition susceptibility; this underscores the potential benefits of incorporating nutrition intervention strategies [80].

C) Laboratory Evaluation.
   1. Blood tests:
      a. Total blood count
      b. Total protein and serum albumin
      c. Retinol binding protein
      d. Transferrin
      e. Water and fat-soluble vitamin levels in plasma.

In malnutrition, the value of all the above-said tests will be less than usual.

   2. Tests used to assess body composition.
      a. CT and MRI-based muscle mass assessment
      b. DEXA scan
      c. Deuterium oxide dilution *in vivo* neutron activation analysis
      d. Bioelectrical impedance
   3. A 6-minute walk and physical frailty tests are done to assess the nutritional status.

15. Nutrition Guidelines

Patients who are identified as malnourished necessitate the implementation of nutritional intervention. In such instances, seeking guidance from a certified dietician is imperative. General guidelines have been established to guide diet treatment in individuals suffering from CLD. The procedures commonly employed in clinical practice are those set by the European Society for Clinical Nutrition and Metabolism (ESPEN) in 2006 [81, 82].

15.1. *For alcoholic steatohepatitis*

- Apply simple techniques, like SGA or anthropometry, to discern individuals susceptible to undernutrition.
- The recommended energy intake for individuals is 35 to 40 kcal/kg/day (147–168 kJ/kg/day).
- The recommended daily protein consumption ranges from 1.2 to 1.5 gm/kg/day.

- The use of additional enteral nutrition, particularly oral supplements, is recommended for patients who cannot fulfill their caloric needs through regular food consumption.
  - ✓ It is often advised to use whole protein formulas in clinical practice.
  - ✓ It is worth considering the utilization of more concentrated high-energy formulas in patients presenting with ascites.
  - ✓ It is recommended to incorporate BCAAs in treating hepatic encephalopathy in patients receiving enteral nutrition.
- Tube feeding should be employed in cases where patients cannot sustain sufficient oral intake.
- It is not recommended to put a percutaneous endoscopic gastrostomy (PEG) tube as it is associated with many problems.
- The installation of PEG tubes is correlated with an elevated incidence of problems, thereby rendering it not advised [23].

15.2. *Patients with cirrhosis of the liver*

- Utilize basic bedside techniques, such as the SGA or anthropometry, to ascertain individuals susceptible to undernutrition.
- Bioelectric impedance analysis (BIA) can be employed to quantify undernutrition, although its application may be limited in individuals presenting with ascites.
- The recommended energy intake for individuals is between 35 to 40 kcal/kg/day (147–168 kJ/kg/day).
- The recommended protein intake ranges from 1.2 to 1.5 gm/kg/day.
- The utilization of additional enteral nutrition is employed in cases where patients cannot fulfill their caloric needs through regular dietary intake.
  - ➢ It is usually advised to consume whole protein formulations.
  - ➢ It is advisable to contemplate the utilization of more potent high-energy formulations in individuals presenting with ascites.
  - ➢ It is recommended to employ formulas enhanced with BCAAs in individuals diagnosed with hepatic encephalopathy that

occurs during enteral nutritional assessment in cases of chronic liver illness.

- Tube feeding should be employed in cases where patients cannot sustain sufficient oral intake.
- The installation of PEG tubes is correlated with an elevated incidence of problems, thereby rendering it not advised [83–85].

16. Conclusion

Nutrition is of utmost importance in managing liver diseases. Consuming a nutritionally balanced diet can enhance hepatic function, mitigate inflammatory responses, and decelerate the advancement of hepatic impairment. In certain instances, modifications to one's food habits may suffice as the sole intervention required.

Individuals diagnosed with liver disease should collaborate with a registered dietitian to establish a personalized nutrition regimen. The dietician possesses the expertise to ascertain individualized nutrient requirements and guide dietary choices, including recommended and discouraged food items.

Several overarching nutritional guidelines are recommended for individuals with liver disease.

It is advisable to

- have a well-rounded combination of protein, carbs, and fats to maintain a balanced diet.
- choose whole grains instead of refined grains.
- consume a substantial amount of fruits and vegetables.
- restrict the consumption of saturated and trans fats.
- restrict the consumption of cholesterol.
- restrict the consumption of salt.
- abstain from using alcohol.

References

1. Silva M, Gomes S, Peixoto A, Torres-Ramalho P, Cardoso H, Azevedo R, Cunha C, Macedo G. Nutrition in chronic liver disease. *GE Port J Gastroenterol.* 2015;22:268–276.

2. Mandato C, Di Nuzzi A, Vajro P. Nutrition and liver disease. *Nutrients.* 2017;10:9.
3. Puri P, Dhiman RK, Taneja S, Tandon P, Merli M, Anand AC, et al. Nutrition in chronic liver disease: consensus statement of the Indian National Association for Study of the Liver. *J Clin Exp Hepatol.* 2021 Jan 1;11(1):97–143.
4. European Association for the Study of the Liver. EASL clinical practice guidelines on nutrition in chronic liver disease. *J Hepatol.* 2019;70: 172–193.
5. Plauth M, Bernal W, Dasarathy S. ESPEN guideline on clinical nutrition in liver disease. *Clin Nutr.* 2019;38:485–521. Mazurak VC, Tandon P, Montano-Loza AJ. Nutrition and the transplant candidate. *Liver Transpl.* 2017;23:1451–1464.
6. Bunchorntavakul C, Reddy KR. Malnutrition/sarcopenia and frailty in patients with cirrhosis. *Aliment Pharmacol Ther.* 2020;51:64–77.
7. Merli M, Berzigotti A, Zelber-Sagi S, Dasarathy S, Montagnese S, Genton L, Parés A. EASL Clinical practice guidelines on nutrition in chronic liver disease. *J Hepatol.* 2019;70:172–193.
8. Glass C, Hipskind P, Tsien C, Malin S, Kasumov T, Shah SN, Kirwan JP, Dasarathy S. Sarcopenia and a physiologically low respiratory quotient in patients with cirrhosis: a prospective controlled study. *J Appl Physiol.* 2013;114:559–565.
9. Glass C, Hipskind P, Cole D, Lopez R, Dasarathy S. Handheld calorimeter is a valid instrument to quantify resting energy expenditure in hospitalized cirrhotic patients: a prospective study. *Nutr Clin Pract.* 2012;27:677–688.
10. Dasarathy S, Merli M. Sarcopenia from mechanism to diagnosis and treatment in liver disease. *J Hepatol.* 2016;65:1232–1244.
11. Dasarathy J, McCullough AJ, Dasarathy S. Sarcopenia in alcoholic liver disease: clinical and molecular advances. *Alcohol Clin Exp Res.* 2017;41:1419–1431.
12. Peng S, Plank LD, McCall JL, Gillanders LK, McIlroy K, Gane EJ. Body composition, muscle function, and energy expenditure in patients with liver cirrhosis: a comprehensive study. *Am J Clin Nutr.* 2007;85: 1257–1266.
13. Calmet F, Martin P, Pearlman M. Nutrition in patients with cirrhosis. *Gastroenterol Hepatol.* 2019;15:248–254.

14. https://surgery.ucsf.edu/conditions--procedures/end-stage-liver-disease-(esld).aspx
15. Hammad A, Kaido T, Aliyev V, Mandato C, Uemoto S. Nutritional therapy in liver transplantation. *Nutrients.* 2017 Oct 16;9(10):1126.
16. Phillips GB, Schwartz R, Gabuzda GJ, Davidson CS. The syndrome of impending hepatic coma in patients with cirrhosis of the liver given certain nitrogenous substances. *N Engl J Med.* 1952;247:239–246.
17. Riordan SM, Williams R. Treatment of hepatic encephalopathy. *N Engl J Med.* 1997;337:413–419.
18. Seymour CA, Whelan K. Dietary management of hepatic encephalopathy. *BMJ.* 1999;318:1364–1365.
19. Les I, Planas M, Cardenas G. Effects of the proteins of the diet in patients with cirrhosis and a prior episode of hepatic encephalopathy. A long-term randomized study. *Hepatology.* 2009;50:313A.
20. Merli M, Eriksson LS, Hagenfeldt L, Wahren J. Splanchnic and leg exchange of free fatty acids in patients with liver cirrhosis. *J Hepatol.* 1986;3:348–355.
21. The Lancet Gastroenterology. Hepatology herbal assault: liver toxicity of herbal and dietary supplements. *Lancet Gastroenterol Hepatol.* 2018;3:141.
22. Perumpail BJ, Li AA, Cholankeril G, Kumari R, Ahmed A. Optimizing the nutritional support of adult patients in the setting of cirrhosis. *Nutrients.* 2017 Oct 13;9(10):1114.
23. Bischoff SC, Bernal W, Dasarathy S, Merli M, Plank LD, Schütz T, Plauth M. ESPEN practical guideline: clinical nutrition in liver disease. *Clin Nutr.* 2020 Dec 1;39(12):3533–3562.
24. Young S, Kwarta E, Azzam R, Sentongo T. Nutrition assessment and support in children with end-stage liver disease. *Nutr Clin Prac.* 2013; 28:317–329.
25. Vidot H, Carey S, Allman-Farinelli M, Shackel N. Systematic review: the treatment of muscle cramps in patients with cirrhosis. *Aliment Pharmacol Ther.* 2014;40:221–232.
26. Nakaya Y, Harada N, Kakui S, Okada K, Takahashi A, Inoi J, Ito S. Severe catabolic state after prolonged fasting in cirrhotic patients: effect of oral branched-chain amino-acid-enriched nutrient mixture. *J Gastroenterol.* 2002;37:531–536.

27. Fialla AD, Israelsen M, Hamberg O, Krag A, Gluud, LL. Nutritional therapy in cirrhosis or alcoholic hepatitis: a systematic review and meta-analysis. *Liver Int.* 2015;35:2072–2078.
28. Ayers P, Adams S, Boullata J, Gervasio J, Holcombe B, Kraft MD, American Society for Parenteral and Enteral Nutrition. ASPEN parenteral nutrition safety consensus recommendations. *J Parenteral Enteral Nutr.* 2014;38:296–333.
29. O'Brien A, Williams R. Nutrition in end-stage liver disease: principles and practice. *Gastroenterology.* 2008 May 1;134(6):1729–1740.
30. Rayes N, Seehofer D, Theruvath T, Mogl M, Langrehr JM, Nüssler NC, Bengmark S, Neuhaus P. Effect of enteral nutrition and synbiotics on bacterial infection rates after pylorus-preserving pancreatoduodenectomy: a randomized, double-blind trial. *Ann Surg.* 2007;246(1):36–41. DOI: 10.1097/01.sla.0000259442.78947.19
31. Ferolla SM, Couto CA, Costa-Silva L, Armiliato GN, Pereira CA, Martins FS, Ferrari MdeL, Vilela EG, Torres HO, Cunha AS, Ferrari TC. Beneficial effect of Synbiotic supplementation on hepatic steatosis and anthropometric parameters, but not on gut permeability in a population with nonalcoholic steatohepatitis. *Nutrients.* 2016;8(7):397. DOI: 10.3390/nu8070397
32. Riordan SM. Williams R. The intestinal flora and bacterial infection in cirrhosis. *J Hepatol.* 2006;45:744–757.
33. Selberg O, Böttcher J, Tusch G, Pichlmayr R, Henkel E, Müller MJ. Identification of high- and low risk patients before liver transplantation: a prospective cohort study of nutritional and metabolic parameters in 150 patients. *Hepatology.* 1997;25:652–657.
34. Chen L, Deng H, Cui H, Fang J, Zuo Z, Deng J, Li Y, Wang X, Zhao L. Inflammatory responses and inflammation-associated diseases in organs. *Oncotarget.* 2017;9(6):7204–7218. DOI: 10.18632/oncotarget.23208
35. Shaw B, Wood R, Gordon R, Iwatsuki S, Gillquist W, Starzl, T. Influence of selected patient variables and operative blood loss on six-month survival following liver transplantation. *Semin Liver Dis.* 1985;5:385–393.
36. Hasse J, Strong S, Gorman MA, Liepa G. Subjective global assessment: alternative nutrition-assessment technique for liver-transplant candidates. *Nutrition.* 1993;9:339–343.

37. Ney M, Abraldes JG, Ma M, Belland D, Harvey A, Robbins S, Den Heyer V, Tandon P. Insufficient protein intake is associated with increased mortality in 630 patients with cirrhosis awaiting liver transplantation. *Nutr Clin Pract.* 2015;30:530–536.
38. Montejo González JC, Mesejo A, Bonet Saris A. Guidelines for specialized nutritional and metabolic support in the critically-ill patient: Update. Consensus SEMICYUC-SENPE: liver failure and liver transplantation. *Nutr Hosp.* 2011;26 Suppl 2:27–31.
39. Bodziak KA, Hricik DE. New-onset diabetes mellitus after solid organ transplantation. *Transpl Int.* 2009;22:519–530.
40. Bethke PC, Jansky SH. The effects of boiling and leaching on the content of potassium and other minerals in potatoes. *J Food Sci.* 2008;73:H80–H85.
41. DiMartini A, Cruz RJ, Dew MA, Myaskovsky L, Goodpaster B, Fox K, Kim KH, Fontes P. Muscle mass predicts outcomes following liver transplantation. *Liver Transpl.* 2013;19:1172–1180.
42. Richards J, Gunson B, Johnson J, Neuberger J. Weight gain and obesity after liver transplantation. *Transpl Int.* 2005;18:461–466.
43. Kouz J, Vincent C, Leong A, Dorais M, Räkel A. Weight gain after orthotopic liver transplantation: is non-alcoholic fatty liver disease cirrhosis a risk factor for greater weight gain? *Liver Transpl.* 2014; 20:1266–1274.
44. Ioannou GN, Splan MF, Weiss NS, McDonald GB, Beretta L, Lee SP. Incidence and predictors of hepatocellular carcinoma in patients with cirrhosis. *Clin Gastroenterol Hepatol.* 2007 Aug;5(8):938–45;945: e1–e4.
45. Ferlay J, Soerjomataram I, Dikshit R, Eser S, Mathers C, Rebelo M, Parkin DM, Forman D, Bray F. Cancer incidence and mortality worldwide: sources, methods and major patterns in GLOBOCAN 2012. *Int J Cancer.* 2015 Mar 01;136(5):E359–E386.
46. Mann J, Truswell S, Hodson L. Essentials of Human Nutrition 6e. 2023.
47. Beudeker BJB, Boonstra A. Circulating biomarkers for early detection of hepatocellular carcinoma. *Ther Adv Gastroenterol.* 2020;13: 1756284820931734. DOI: 10.1177/1756284820931734.

48. Donaldson MS. Nutrition and cancer: a review of the evidence for an anti-cancer diet. *Nutr J.* 2004;3:19. DOI: 10.1186/1475-2891-3-19.
49. Milliron BJ, Packel L, Dychtwald D, Klobodu C, Pontiggia L, Ogbogu O, Barksdale B, Deutsch J. When eating becomes torturous: understanding nutrition-related cancer treatment side effects among individuals with cancer and their caregivers. *Nutrients.* 2022;14(2):356. DOI: 10.3390/nu14020356.
50. Bazzan AJ, Newberg AB, Cho WC, Monti DA. Diet and nutrition in cancer survivorship and palliative care. Evid based complement *Alternat Med.* 2013;2013:917647. DOI: 10.1155/2013/917647.
51. Champ CE, Mishra MV, Showalter TN, Ohri N, Dicker AP, Simone NL. Dietary recommendations during and after cancer treatment: consistently inconsistent? *Nutr Cancer.* 2013;65(3):430–439. DOI: 10.1080/01635581.2013.757629.
52. George ES, Sood S, Broughton A, Cogan G, Hickey M, Chan WS, Sudan S, Nicoll AJ. The association between diet and hepatocellular carcinoma: a systematic review. *Nutrients.* 2021;13(1):172. DOI: 10.3390/nu13010172.
53. Ramadori P, Cubero FJ, Liedtke C, Trautwein C, Nevzorova YA. Alcohol and hepatocellular carcinoma: adding fuel to the flame. *Cancers.* 2017;9(10):130. DOI: 10.3390/cancers9100130.
54. Yang J, He J, Feng Y, Xiang M. Obesity contributes to hepatocellular carcinoma development via immunosuppressive microenvironment remodeling. *Front Immunol.* 2023;14:1166440. DOI: 10.3389/fimmu.2023.1166440.
55. Wenndt A, Mutua F, Grace D, Thomas LF, Lambertini E. Quantitative assessment of aflatoxin exposure and hepatocellular carcinoma (HCC) risk associated with consumption of select Nigerian staple foods. *Front Sustain Food Syst.* 2023;7:1128540. DOI: 10.3389/fsufs.2023.1128540.
56. Ma Y, Yang W, Li T, Liu Y, Simon TG, Sui J, Wu K, Giovannucci EL, Chan AT, Zhang X. Meat intake and risk of hepatocellular carcinoma in two large US prospective cohorts of women and men. *Int J Epidemiol.* 2019;48(6):1863–1871. DOI: 10.1093/ije/dyz146.
57. Bouvard V, Loomis D, Guyton KZ, Grosse Y, Ghissassi FE, Benbrahim-Tallaa L, Guha N, Mattock H, Straif K. International agency for research on cancer monograph working group. Carcinogenicity of

consumption of red and processed meat. *Lancet Oncol.* 2015; 16(16):1599–1600. DOI: 10.1016/S1470-2045(15)00444-1.
58. Petrick JL, Freedman ND, Graubard BI, Sahasrabuddhe VV, Lai GY, Alavanja MC, et al. Coffee consumption and risk of hepatocellular carcinoma and intrahepatic cholangiocarcinoma by sex: the Liver Cancer Pooling Project. *Cancer Epidemiol Biomarkers Prev.* 2015 Sep 1;24(9):1398–1406.
59. Turati F, Trichopoulos D, Polesel J, Bravi F, Rossi M, Talamini R, Franceschi S, Montella M, Trichopoulou A, La Vecchia C, Lagiou P. Mediterranean diet and hepatocellular carcinoma. *J Hepatol.* 2014; 60(3):606–611. doi:10.1016/j.jhep.2013.10.034
60. Abnet CC. Carcinogenic food contaminants. *Cancer Invest.* 2007; 25(3):189–196. doi:10.1080/07357900701208733
61. National Research Council (US) Committee on Diet, Nutrition, and Cancer. Washington (DC): national Academies Press (US);1982.
62. Aller de la Fuente R. Nutrition and chronic liver disease. *Clin Drug Invest.* 2022;42(Suppl 1):55–61. doi:10.1007/s40261-022-01141-x
63. Storck LJ, Imoberdorf R, Ballmer PE. Nutrition in gastrointestinal disease: liver, pancreatic, and inflammatory bowel disease. *J Clin Med.* 2019;8(8):1098. doi:10.3390/jcm80810
64. European Association for the Study of the Liver. EASL clinical practice guidelines on nutrition in chronic liver disease. *J Hepatol.* 2018;69(2): 508–531. doi:10.1016/j.jhep.2018.06.024
65. Zhang YJ, Gan RY, Li S, Zhou Y, Li AN, Xu DP, Li HB. Antioxidant phytochemicals for the prevention and treatment of chronic diseases. *Molecules.* 2015;20(12):21138–21156. doi:10.3390/molecules201219753
66. Rodriguez S, Skeet K, Mehmetoglu-Gurbuz T, Goldfarb M, Karri S, Rocha J, Shahinian M, Yazadi A, Poudel S, Subramani R. Phytochemicals as an alternative or integrative option, in conjunction with conventional treatments for hepatocellular carcinoma. *Cancers.* 2021;13(22):5753. doi:10.3390/cancers13225753
67. Ravasco P. Nutrition in cancer patients. *J Clin Med.* 2019;8(8):1211. doi:10.3390/jcm8081211
68. Fagbohun OF, Gillies CR, Murphy KPJ, Rupasinghe HPV. Role of antioxidant vitamins and other micronutrients on regulations of specific

genes and signaling pathways in the prevention and treatment of cancer. *Int J Mol Sci.* 2023;24(7):6092. doi:10.3390/ijms24076092

69. Barrera S, Demark-Wahnefried W. Nutrition during and after cancer therapy. *Oncology (Williston Park, NY.).* 2009;23(2 Suppl Nurse Ed):15–21.
70. Conigliaro T, Boyce LM, Lopez CA, Tonorezos ES. Food intake during cancer therapy: a systematic review. *Am J Clin Oncol.* 2020;43(11): 813–819. doi:10.1097/COC.0000000000000749
71. Ruiz-Margáin A, Román-Calleja BM, Moreno-Guillén P, González-Regueiro JA, Kúsulas-Delint D, Campos-Murguía A, Flores-García NC, Macías-Rodríguez RU. Nutritional therapy for hepatocellular carcinoma. *World J Gastrointest Oncol.* 2021;13(10):1440–1452. doi:10.4251/wjgo.v13.i10.1440
72. Merli M. Nutrition in cirrhosis: dos & dont's. *J Hepatol.* 2020 Dec;73(6):1563–1565. doi: 10.1016/j.jhep.2020.07.019
73. Kumar M, Panda D. Role of supportive care for terminal stage hepatocellular carcinoma. *J Clin Exp Hepatol.* 2014;4(Suppl 3):S130–S139. doi:10.1016/j.jceh.2014.03.049
74. Haj Ali S, Abu Sneineh A, Hasweh R. Nutritional assessment in patients with liver cirrhosis. *World J Hepatol.* 2022;14(9):1694–1703. doi:10.4254/wjh.v14.i9.1694
75. Tandon P, Raman M, Mourtzakis M, Merli M. A practical approach to nutritional screening and assessment in cirrhosis. *Hepatology (Baltimore, Md.).* 2017;65(3):1044–1057. doi:10.1002/hep.29003
76. Wang T, Shen J. Usefulness of simplified nutritional appetite questionnaire (SNAQ) in appetite assessment in elder patients with liver cirrhosis. *J Nutr Health Aging.* 2018;22(10):1273–1278.
77. Teiusanu A, Andrei M, Arbanas T, Nicolaie T, Diculescu M. Nutritional status in cirrhotic patients. *Maedica.* 2012;7(4):284–289.
78. Johnson TM, Overgard EB, Cohen AE, DiBaise JK. Nutrition assessment and management in advanced liver disease. *Nutr Clin Pract.* 2013;28(1):15–29. DOI: 10.1177/0884533612469027
79. Parkash O, Jafri W, Munir SM, Iqbal, R. Assessment of malnutrition in patients with liver cirrhosis using protein calorie malnutrition (PCM) score versus bio-electrical impedance analysis (BIA). *BMC Res Notes.* 2018;11:545. DOI: 10.1186/s13104-018-3640-y

80. Detsky AS, McLaughlin JR, Baker JP, Johnston N, Whittaker S, Mendelson RA, et al. What is subjective global assessment of nutritional status? *JPEN J Parenter Enteral Nutr.* 1987;11(1):8–13. DOI: 10.1177/014860718701100108
81. Perumal N, Pike V, Ho C, Bradley B, Wong J, Zlotkin S. Global nutrition. *Curr Dev Nutr.* 2018;2(11):nzy039. DOI: 10.1093/cdn/nzy039
82. Cook F, Rodriguez JM, & McCaul, LK. Malnutrition, nutrition support and dietary intervention: the role of the dietitian supporting patients with head and neck cancer. *Br Dent J.* 2022;233(9):757–764. DOI: 10.1038/s41415-022-5107-8
83. Plauth M, Bernal W, Dasarathy S, Merli M, Plank LD, Schütz T, Bischoff SC. ESPEN guideline on clinical nutrition in liver disease. *Clin Nutr (Edinburgh, Scotland).* 2019;38(2):485–521. DOI: 10.1016/j.clnu.2018.12.022
84. Elsebaie EM, Abdel-Fattah AN, Bakr NA, Attalah KM, Aweas A-HA. Principles of nutritional management in patients with liver dysfunction — A narrative review. *Liver.* 2023;3(2):190–218. DOI: 10.3390/livers3020013
85. "Nutrition Counseling and Nutrition Tidbits." Nutritional Care of the Patient with Gastrointestinal Disease, 2015.

https://doi.org/10.1142/9789811293320_0004

Chapter 4

Therapeutic Potential of Phytochemicals: Preclinical Insights in Hepatocellular Carcinoma

Anisha Vadakkepatt[1,*] and Rafia Islam[2]

[1]*Assistant Professor, Amrita College of Nursing, AMRITA Vishwa Vidyapeetham, Health Sciences Campus, Kochi 41, Kerala, India*
[2]*Associate Professor, New Royal College of Nursing, East Point group of Institutions, RGUHS, Bangalore-49, India*

Table of Contents:

*Corresponding author: Tel.: 9061559280; E-mail address: anisha56433@gmail.com

Abbreviations:

HCC — Hepatocellular carcinoma; the most common type of liver cancer.
EGCG — Epigallocatechin gallate; a polyphenol and catechin found in green tea.
CDKs — Cyclin-dependent kinases; a group of protein kinases that regulate the cell cycle and its progression.
CKIs — Cyclin-dependent kinase inhibitors; proteins that stop the cell cycle when conditions are unfavorable.
UV — Ultraviolet
ROS — Reactive oxygen species; molecules capable of independent existence, containing at least one oxygen atom and one or more unpaired electrons.
COX — Cyclooxygenase; officially known as prostaglandin-endoperoxide synthase (PTGS), is an enzyme that is responsible for biosynthesis of prostanoids, including thromboxane and prostaglandins such as prostacyclin, from arachidonic acid.
LOX — Lipoxygenase; dioxygenases that catalyze the formation of corresponding hydroperoxides from polyunsaturated fatty acids such as linoleic acid and arachidonic acid.
NSAID — Nonsteroidal anti-inflammatory drugs.

AA — Achyranthes aspera.
APG — Apigenin.
Nrf2 — Nuclear factor erythroid 2–related factor 2.
CYP450 — Cytochrome P450; a group of enzymes encoded by P450 genes and expressed as membrane-bound proteins mostly found in the endoplasmic reticulum of the liver.
MAPK — Mitogen-activated protein kinases; a family of protein kinases that are specific to the amino acids, serine and threonine.
Akt — Protein kinase B; a collective name for three serine/threonine-specific protein kinases.
JAK/STAT — Janus kinase/signal transducers and activators of transcription.
Wnt/-catenin — Wingless-related integration site; a cell-cell communication system that is important for stem cell renewal, cell proliferation, and cell differentiation.
p53 — A tumor suppressor protein that regulates cell division by preventing cells from growing and dividing too quickly or in an uncontrolled manner.
NF-B — Nuclear factor kappa-light-chain-enhancer of activated B cells; comprises a family of five transcription factors that form distinct protein complexes, which bind to consensus DNA sequences at promoter regions of responsive genes regulating cellular processes.
miRNAs — MicroRNAs; a class of non-coding RNAs that play important roles in regulating gene expression.
MAPK/ERK — Microtubule-associated protein kinases/extracellular signal-regulated kinases.
NF-κB — Nuclear factor kappa B.
PI3K/Akt — Phosphoinositide-3-kinase–protein kinase.

Abstract

Phytochemicals, such as curcumin, resveratrol, epigallocatechin-3-gallate (EGCG), silibinin, and quercetin, have gained significant attention for their potential anticancer properties, including antioxidant, anti-inflammatory, and antitumor effects. These compounds have demonstrated promising capabilities, such as inhibiting cancer cell growth, inducing apoptosis, promoting cell cycle arrest, and reducing angiogenesis in preclinical studies. Although phytochemicals cannot replace conventional therapies, they may serve as complementary or alternative approaches to enhance treatment efficacy and reduce adverse effects. However, the translation of these findings into clinical practice remains challenging due to limited human studies. Further research is essential to validate the safety, efficacy, and mechanisms of phytochemicals in liver cancer therapy. Healthcare professionals must be consulted before incorporating phytochemicals into treatment plans to prevent potential interactions with existing therapies. This chapter explores the therapeutic potential, mechanisms of action, and current research status of phytochemicals in liver cancer therapy, emphasizing their role as adjunctive agents in integrated oncology care.

1. Introduction

In the United States, 41,210 people (27,980 men and 13,230 women) are estimated to have primary liver cancer in 2023. Since 1980, the incidence of liver cancer has more than tripled. However, between 2014 and 2015, the incidence rates for women decreased while they remained constant for men. A diagnosis is roughly three times more likely to be given to men than to women. There were approximately 905,677 new liver cancer cases reported globally in 2020. According to unpublished data from multiple tertiary care institutes in India, the incidence of Hepatocellular carcinoma (HCC) is rising [6]. The age-incidence rate of HCC in India for men ranges from 4 to 7.5 and for women from 1.2 to 2.2 per 100,000 population each year, according to the currently available data [1].

The seventh most common cause of cancer-related death in men is liver cancer. It comes in at number eight on the list of causes of cancer-related deaths in women. Despite more than doubling since 1980, the mortality rate from liver cancer stabilized between 2016 and 2020 for both men and women.

The third most frequent cancer that causes death globally is liver cancer [2]. In 2020, the sickness is predicted to claim the lives of 830,180 persons worldwide. When compared to the United States, sub-Saharan Africa and Southeast Asia have significantly higher rates of liver cancer. It is the most prevalent type of cancer in many different countries [3].

HCC typically manifests between the ages of 40 and 70, with a 4:1 male-to-female ratio. East Asia and Africa continue to have the highest rates of HCC incidence and mortality, even though these rates are increasing in some regions of Europe and the USA. HCC has, in fact, had the highest rate of deaths from cancer-related causes in the USA since the early 2000s. By 2030, HCC is anticipated to rank third among causes of death from cancer if current trends continue [4].

Phytochemical liver cancer therapy uses phytochemicals, or natural plant substances, to prevent and treat liver cancer. The nonnutritive bioactive substances known as phytochemicals can be found in various fruits, vegetables, herbs, and other plant-based meals. Due to their assumed anticancer characteristics, they have drawn interest in cancer research. The use of phytochemicals in treating liver cancer is the subject of continuing research. They may support standard cancer treatments such as surgery, chemotherapy, radiation therapy, and targeted therapy, even though they are not a stand-alone treatment for liver cancer [5].

2. Phytochemicals

Phytochemicals, often known as "phytonutrients," are organic substances found in plants. Fruits, vegetables, grains, legumes, nuts, seeds, and herbs have a variety of colors, flavors, and disease-preventing qualities because of these substances. Like vitamins and minerals, phytochemicals are not regarded as essential nutrients, but when included in a balanced diet, they have many positive health effects. Their ability to improve health and prevent chronic illnesses such as cancer, heart disease, and other conditions has been thoroughly researched. Numerous phytochemicals exist, each with unique qualities and possible health advantages [6]. The following is the ***pictorial representation of phytochemicals used in liver cancer therapy***: Figure 1

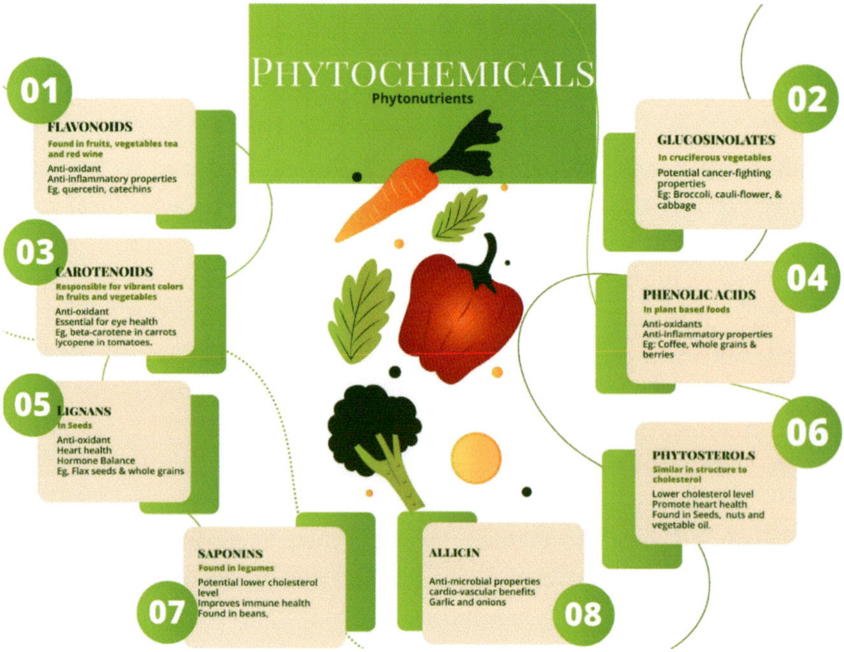

Figure 1: Phytochemicals

It is important to note that the specific health benefits of phytochemicals can vary depending on the type of phytochemical and the foods they are found in. Eating diverse fruits, vegetables, and plant-based foods can provide a broad spectrum of phytochemicals contributing to overall health and well-being. Including various colorful foods in your diet is an excellent way to ensure you benefit from the vast array of natural phytochemicals. Additionally, phytochemicals are often best consumed in whole foods rather than supplement forms, as the overall food matrix may enhance their effectiveness.

3. Mechanism of Action of Phytochemicals in Cancer Prevention

Phytochemicals are plant-derived compounds such as flavonoids, alkaloids, and carotenoids. They have been used to treat and prevent diseases alone or with other medications [7].

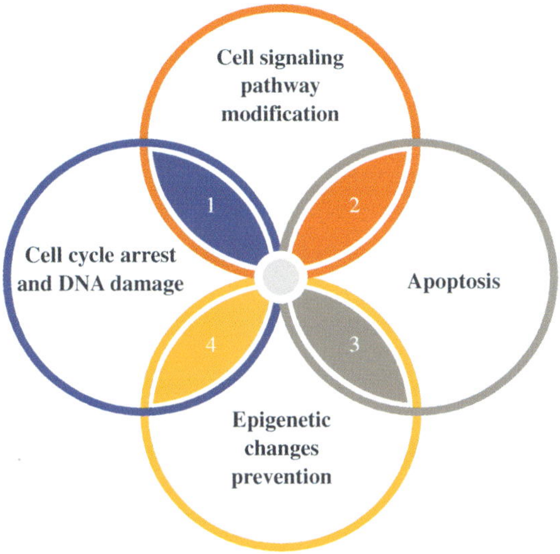

Figure 2: Mechanism of action of phytochemicals

It exerts anticancer activity via a variety of pathways, including Figure 2:

1. Cell signaling pathway modification.
2. Apoptosis.
3. Prevention of epigenetic changes.
4. Cell cycle arrest and DNA damage.

3.1. *Cell signaling pathway modification*

Phytochemicals impact the cell cycle by modulating crucial cell division and growth proteins. They target various cell signaling pathways at different levels, including protein activation, intercellular communication, and transcriptional and post-transcriptional control, to demonstrate anticancer characteristics. These substances regulate the cell signaling transduction of important players such as Nrf2, CYP450, MAPK, Akt, JAK/STAT, Wnt/-catenin, p53, NF-B, and cancer-related miRNAs to prevent carcinogenesis.

- Dysregulated pathways such as microtubule-associated protein kinases/extracellular signal-regulated kinases (MAPK/ERK), NF-κB, and JAK/STAT drive cancer progression, promoting angiogenesis, proliferation, dedifferentiation, and metastasis.
- Modulating these pathways with drugs is a rational approach to preventing and treating cancer. For example, phytochemicals such as apigenin, crocetin, quercetin, and rhein inhibit overactive MAPK/ERK signaling in tumors like melanoma.
- Quercetin inhibits ERK and PI3K/Akt pathways, reducing proliferation in human hepatoma HepG2 cells. Gallic acid from *Bergenia ciliata* downregulates Ras/MAPK and PI3K/Akt pathways, reducing invasiveness in brain endothelial and glioblastoma cells.
- The NF-κB pathway plays a crucial role in cancer progression, with phytochemicals such as anethole, capsaicin, eugenol, sedanolide, genistein, gingerol, ursolic acid, and 3,3′-diindolylmethane inhibiting it.

3.2. *Apoptosis*

Necrosis and apoptosis are the two main types of cell death. Given that apoptosis is the most prevalent type of programed cell death, it is an essential therapeutic target in the fight against cancer. Resveratrol, quercetin, EGCG, curcumin, apigenin, chrysin, silymarin, and ellagic acid are a few dietary chemopreventive substances that have shown they can reduce carcinogenesis by triggering apoptosis, which kills tumor cells by programed cell death.

- Epigallocatechin gallate (EGCG) can promote apoptosis and cell cycle arrest in specific cancer cells. It exhibits effects on cell lines at both millimolar and micromolar doses.
- Quercetin inhibits cellular proliferation in various cancers by triggering the intrinsic apoptotic pathway. It enhances the activity of pro-apoptotic protein family members and activates caspase-9 and caspase-3.

- Resveratrol, found in red wine, is an antioxidant that reduces the activity of the antiapoptotic protein Bcl-2 while enhancing the activity of pro-apoptotic Bcl-2 family members.
- Colorectal and small-cell lung carcinomas undergo apoptosis when phytochemicals increase caspase-3 and -9 activity. Esculetin increases oxidative stress and inhibits protein to cause apoptosis in a mouse lung cancer model. In colon cancer cells, diosgenin induces apoptosis by upregulating caspase-3 activity and downregulating Bcl-2. Glioma cells undergo apoptosis when artabotryside A arrests the cell cycle at the G2/M phase. In breast cancer cells that are hormone-sensitive, caffeine causes apoptosis.

3.3. *Prevention of epigenetic changes*

Cancer occurs when genetic and epigenetic changes lead to an abnormal behavior of certain genes. These changes can be influenced by chemicals affecting gene activity. Some phytochemicals, such as resveratrol and curcumin, can block enzymes that silence genes by adding methyl groups to DNA. By doing so, they prevent harmful DNA changes, helping maintain normal gene behavior and reducing the risk of cancer.

3.4. *Cell cycle arrest and DNA damage*

Activating cyclin-dependent kinases (CDKs) is necessary for cell cycle advancement, and cyclin-dependent kinase inhibitors (CKIs) control cell cycle arrest. Both processes require synchronized breakdown. Numerous phytochemicals, including alkaloids, flavonoids, phenolic acids, coumarins, and steroidal derivatives, have been shown to obstruct cell cycle advancement.

For instance, it has been revealed that ferulic acid stops the cell cycle at the S phase and increases the production of genes necessary for centrosome assembly. Inhibiting colon cancer Caco-2 cell multiplication as a result.

4. Properties of Phytochemicals

4.1. *Antioxidant effects*

Phytochemicals frequently include antioxidant qualities that safeguard cells from oxidative damage, a condition associated with cancer development. Antioxidants are molecules that aid in shielding the body from the damaging effects of free radicals and oxidative stress, which can contribute to several health issues, including chronic illnesses and aging. The following are some salient points regarding phytochemicals' antioxidant properties:

- ✓ Free radicals and oxidative stress: Oxidative stress is a condition where unstable chemicals, such as free radicals, cause harm to DNA, proteins, and cells. Numerous illnesses such as cancer, heart disease, and neurological disorders are linked to this damage.
- ✓ Many free radicals can overpower the body's natural antioxidant defense mechanism. By scavenging free radicals and halting oxidative damage, phytochemicals from plants can support this defense system.
- ✓ Rich food sources: Phytochemicals having antioxidant properties are abundant in fruits, vegetables, whole grains, nuts, seeds, and spices. A wide variety of antioxidants can be obtained by consuming these foods.

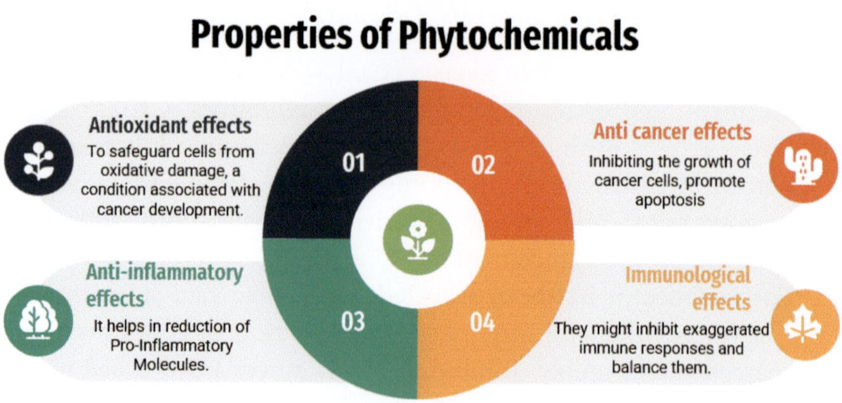

Figure 3: Properties of phytochemicals

✓ Benefits to health: Antioxidants may also help to maintain healthy skin and delay the effects of aging.
✓ Protection against ultraviolet (UV) damage: Some phytochemicals, such as the carotenoids present in fruits and vegetables, can defend against the harmful effects of sun UV radiation.
✓ Individual variability: Depending on things such as heredity, food, and general health, the efficiency of phytochemical antioxidants can differ from person to person.
✓ Supplements versus whole foods: Although antioxidant supplements are offered, it is typically advised to receive antioxidants from whole foods since they contain a complex mixture of phytochemicals that collaborate to protect against damage. Supplements might not offer the same health advantages, and taking too much of them in certain situations can be detrimental.
✓ Dietary balance: One of the most excellent methods to guarantee you acquire a variety of phytochemical antioxidants is to eat a balanced and mixed diet that contains a wide range of colorful fruits and vegetables.

4.2. *Anti-inflammatory effects*

Chronic inflammation can contribute to the development and progression of liver cancer. Some phytochemicals have anti-inflammatory properties that may help reduce this risk. Although inflammation is a normal immune system reaction to damage or infection, chronic inflammation has been related to several chronic disorders. Through various processes, phytochemicals can aid in reducing inflammatory responses in the body. The following are some essential details regarding phytochemicals' anti-inflammatory properties:

✓ Reduction of pro-inflammatory molecules: Pro-inflammatory molecules, such as cytokines and prostaglandins, are essential to the inflammatory process and can be reduced by various phytochemicals.
✓ Some phytochemicals have antioxidant properties, scavenging reactive oxygen species (ROS), and free radicals that can cause

inflammation. They indirectly lessen inflammation by lowering oxidative stress.

- ✓ Enzyme inhibition: Some phytochemicals can block certain inflammatory enzymes, including cyclooxygenase (COX) and lipoxygenase (LOX), which produce inflammatory mediators.
- ✓ Foods that reduce inflammation: Foods high in phytochemicals, such as fruits, vegetables, teas, herbs, and spices, are frequently regarded as reducing inflammation and are advised as a component of an anti-inflammatory diet.

4.3. *Specific illustrations*

Some phytochemicals with well-established anti-inflammatory effects include:

- ✓ Turmeric contains a powerful anti-inflammatory chemical called curcumin, which has various possible health advantages.
- ✓ Tea, apples, and onions contain the antioxidant and anti-inflammatory compound quercetin.
- ✓ Red wine and red grapes contain resveratrol, which is thought to have anti-inflammatory and heart-protective properties.
- ✓ Gingerol: Found in ginger, gingerol has both analgesic (pain-relieving) and anti-inflammatory effects.
- ✓ Omega-3 fatty acids: Omega-3 fatty acids present in foods such as fatty fish, flaxseed, and walnuts have anti-inflammatory solid properties despite not being phytochemicals.
- ✓ Individual variability: Depending on elements including heredity, diet, and general health, phytochemicals' capacity to reduce inflammation may differ from person to person.
- ✓ Phytochemicals can work with other anti-inflammatory measures such as regular exercise, stress reduction, and a healthy diet.

While phytochemicals might support an anti-inflammatory diet, it is critical to remember that no one food or substance is a miracle cure for inflammation. Together with a healthy lifestyle, a well-balanced, varied diet high in phytochemicals and other nutrients can help reduce chronic inflammation and promote general well-being. People with chronic inflammatory problems should consult a medical expert or a qualified nutritionist.

4.4. *Anticancer effects*

Certain phytochemicals have demonstrated direct anticancer effects by inhibiting the growth of cancer cells, promoting apoptosis (programed cell death), or interfering with cancer-promoting pathways. The following are the critical points on the anticancer effects of phytochemicals.

✓ Anti-proliferative properties: Several phytochemicals have been demonstrated to prevent cancer cells from proliferating and multiplying. They can interfere with the signaling pathways that support cancer's unchecked cell proliferation.
✓ Apoptosis induction: Programed cell death, also known as apoptosis, is a natural mechanism that aids in the elimination of damaged or abnormal cells from the body. Some phytochemicals can cause cancer cells to undergo apoptosis, which kills the cells.
✓ Angiogenesis Inhibition: Phytochemicals can prevent the growth of new blood vessels (angiogenesis), which feed tumors with nutrients. They can restrict the tumor's capacity to develop and spread.
✓ Support for the immune system: Some phytochemicals may improve the immune system's capacity to identify and destroy cancer cells. This may strengthen the body's inherent anticancer defenses.
✓ Metastasis, or the spread of cancer cells to other parts of the body, is what is meant by anti-metastatic properties. Some phytochemicals can stop cancer cells from spreading to distant organs and invading neighboring tissues.
✓ Enhancement of DNA repair mechanisms: Some phytochemicals may aid DNA repair processes in cells, maintaining the integrity of the genetic code and preventing cancer-causing mutations.
✓ Chemopreventive Effects: Phytochemicals are being investigated for their ability to shield those at high risk from developing cancer.

They could function as chemopreventive drugs by preventing cancer development or halting its spread.

4.5. *Immunological modulation*

Phytochemicals can alter immunological function, balancing the immune response. They might inhibit exaggerated immune responses that cause persistent inflammation [8].

5. Evidence Acquisition in Phytochemical in Cancer Prevention

Curcumin: Found in turmeric, curcumin has antioxidant and anti-inflammatory properties and has shown the potential to inhibit the growth of liver cancer cells.

Resveratrol: In grapes and red wine, resveratrol has antioxidant properties and may have anticancer effects.

Epigallocatechin-3-gallate (EGCG): Found in green tea, EGCG has been studied for its potential in preventing and treating various cancers, including liver cancer.

Quercetin: In various fruits and vegetables, quercetin has antioxidant and anti-inflammatory properties and may help inhibit the growth of liver cancer cells [9].

It is essential to note that while these phytochemicals show promise in laboratory and animal studies, more research is needed to determine their effectiveness in humans. Additionally, phytochemicals should not be used as a sole or primary treatment for liver cancer. Instead, they may be considered part of a comprehensive treatment plan alongside conventional therapies under the guidance of a healthcare professional.

Patients interested in incorporating phytochemicals into their diet or treatment plan should consult with their healthcare team to ensure that it is safe and appropriate for their situation. Liver cancer treatment decisions should always be made in consultation with medical professionals who can provide personalized guidance based on the individual's condition and needs.

6. Potential Risks of Using Phytochemicals

1. **Interactions with medications**: Phytochemicals can interact with medications, either enhancing or inhibiting their effects. Individuals taking specific medications should consult a healthcare professional to avoid adverse interactions.
2. **Excessive consumption:** Excessive intake of certain phytochemicals may have adverse effects. For instance, excessive beta-carotene intake from supplements has been associated with increased lung cancer risk in smokers.
3. **Individual variability:** People respond differently to phytochemicals. What works as a protective agent for one person may affect another differently.
4. **Allergic reactions**: Some individuals may be allergic to specific phytochemicals or plant-based foods rich in these compounds.
5. **Incomplete understanding:** The mechanisms by which phytochemicals affect cancer prevention are not fully understood. This makes it essential to exercise caution and not rely solely on phytochemical-rich foods or supplements for cancer prevention.

It is essential to note that while phytochemicals show promise in cancer prevention, a balanced and varied diet, and a healthy lifestyle are still the most reliable approaches to reducing cancer risk. Consult with a healthcare provider or registered dietitian for personalized advice and recommendations related to cancer prevention.

7. New Insights into the Role of Phytochemicals in Preventing Cancer

Genetic disorders frequently cause cancer, which is characterized as aberrant cell proliferation that can spread to other parts of the body. Interest in cancer prevention measures has increased due to difficulties with treatment resistance and rising cancer rates worldwide. Chemoprevention is the use of organic, synthetic, or biological substances to slow down or stop cancer development and prevent the spread of precancerous cells. It is a risk-free and economical strategy that

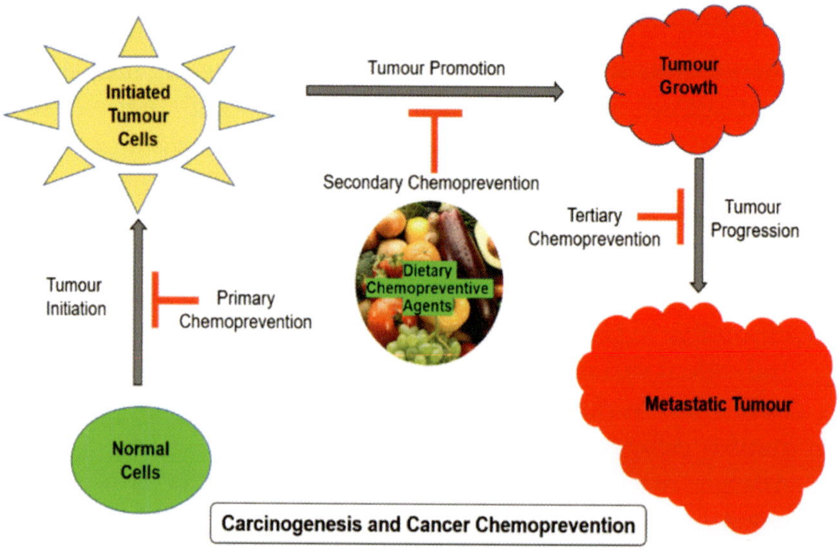

Figure 4: Cancer chemoprevention

Sources: George BP, Chandran R, Abrahamse H. Role of phytochemicals in cancer chemoprevention: Insights. Antioxidants. 2021 Sep 14;10(9):1455.

focuses mostly on dietary adjustments. Extensive epidemiological and preclinical studies support the effectiveness of dietary elements in preventing and treating cancer [9]. The chemopreventive abilities of these natural substances have also been studied in clinical trials (Figure 4).

Chemoprevention involves using natural, synthetic, or biological agents to prevent, suppress, or reverse the early stages of cancer development and inhibit the invasion of precancerous cells. Interest in this field has grown significantly due to advances in cancer biology, the identification of molecular targets, and the successful prevention of cancer cases. Cancer chemoprevention influences various pathways crucial in the three fundamental stages of carcinogenesis: initiation, promotion, and progression [10].

Chemoprevention has been classified clinically as primary, secondary, and tertiary.

- Primary chemoprevention is appropriate for people without cancer in general and for those who have a high lifetime risk of getting cancer.

- Aiming at those with pre-malignant lesions that may develop into invasive cancer, secondary chemoprevention is directed at these individuals.
- Tertiary chemotherapy is used to stop the spread of cancer. For instance, breast cancer patients may take tamoxifen.
- Common chemopreventive therapies include dietary phytochemicals and nonsteroidal anti-inflammatory drugs (NSAID) [11].

7.1. *Exploring the Evidence: Phytochemicals in Cancer Prevention*

In multistep carcinogenesis, phytochemicals can impede or reverse the promotion step. Additionally, they can stop or delay the development of malignant cells from precancerous ones. However, considering the importance of oxidative stress-induced free radicals in several chronic diseases, the study revealed that the health benefits of phytochemicals in fruits and vegetables might be significantly more significant than previously believed [12].

7.2. *Phenolics*

Fruits contain many phenolics. These substances contain hydroxyl groups in one or more aromatic rings. the most prevalent phenolic substances found in the diet. They serve as defense mechanisms against diseases, parasites, and predators and are essential for plant growth and reproduction.

7.3. *Alkaloids*

A class of chemical substances known as alkaloids has anticancer properties. These medications help prevent cancer by reducing the activity of the DNA replication enzyme topoisomerase, which results in apoptosis and boosts gene expression.

8. Cancer Therapy with Phytochemicals: Evidence from Clinical Studies

The increasing worldwide prevalence and often fatal nature of cancer underscore the urgency of discovering new remedies. Medicinal plants have long been valuable sources for exploring novel therapies for human diseases. Traditional recommendations and experimental research have identified numerous medicinal plants with potential anticancer effects, making them promising candidates for developing new anticancer agents. Of the many plants studied for their anticancer properties, only a select few have passed in vitro experiments and animal studies and are currently undergoing clinical trials.

One study has indicated that a water-soluble compound from *Coriandrum sativum* (coriander) possesses neuroprotective properties. Certain plant constituents may act as cytotoxic agents under stressful conditions such as hypoglycemia and serum limitations.

Another study reveals that an extract of *Allium sativum* (garlic) exerts an anti-proliferative effect on both Hep2 and L929 cell lines.

Notably, recent research has demonstrated that garlic consumption can inhibit the progression of colorectal adenomas in humans, as reported in a study by Tanaka et al. in 2006. These findings highlight the efficacy of medicinal plants in cancer treatment and point to their potential in the creation of novel therapeutic strategies [13].

- ***Achyranthes aspera* (AA):** This plant has been used for a long time to treat various illnesses. When you use the roots of this plant, it can work like medicine to fight cancer, especially in colon cancer. It stops cancer cells from growing and can even kill them. The effect depends on how much you use and for how long. Using extracts from this plant in water could be a good way to treat cancer [14].
- **Garlic (*A. sativum*):** Garlic is good for your health because it helps your immune system and fights harmful things in your body. They tested a special garlic extract on people with a certain kind of cancer, but it did not make them feel better, even though it improved their immune system in some ways. A part of garlic called allicin can stop tumors from growing. In some types of cancer, such as cholangiocarcinoma and lung adenocarcinoma, allicin was studied as a treatment and showed promise.
- **Apigenin (APG):** Apigenin is a natural substance in fruits and vegetables that fights cancer.

- **Curcumin:** Curcumin comes from a plant called Curcuma longa. It can stop melanoma cells from growing differently, which is important for treating cancer.
- **Green Tea:** Green tea is a healthy drink. It has something called epigallocatechin (EGCG) that can slow down tumor growth and make cancer cells die in breast cancer. In one study, green tea helped treat prostate cancer.

  In summary, these natural substances from plants and food such as *A. aspera*, garlic, apigenin, curcumin, and green tea have shown potential in fighting cancer or helping cancer patients differently. However, more research is needed to confirm their effectiveness in various types of cancer.
- ***Rhus Verniciflua***: This is a plant from Asia. It is being used in traditional Korean medicine because it is good for many things, including being an antioxidant, stopping inflammation, and maybe fighting cancer. Tests showed that things from this plant can slow down the growth of different cancer cells such as lymphoma, breast cancer, and more. It might also help people with pancreatic, colorectal, and lung cancer. It could be a valuable part of cancer treatment [15].
- ***Viscum album***
  - ➢ European mistletoe (*V. album*): People in Europe often use European mistletoe as an extra treatment for cancer [16].
  - ➢ Clinical trials: Before 2003, there were 23 scientific tests done on this mistletoe, and 19 showed it helped cancer patients live longer, have a better life, or make their tumors get smaller [17].
  - ➢ Reducing side effects: New research shows that a unique water-based mistletoe extract can help cancer patients by reducing chemotherapy's harmful effects and improving their lives.
  - ➢ Iscador: There is a particular mistletoe product called Iscador, made from fresh mistletoe sap, that has been seen to help people with cancers in the colon, rectum, stomach, breast, and bronchial area. But it did not work for high-risk melanoma patients.
  - ➢ Aviscumine: Another substance called aviscumine can boost the immune system to control tumors in lab tests. We are unsure if

it works for cancer patients, especially those with diabetes, so more tests are needed.

- **Panax ginseng**

Ginseng is a plant with different types such as American, Japanese, and Korean/Chinese ginseng. People in Asia have used ginseng to treat illnesses for a very long time. Studies have found that ginseng might help prevent cancer and make cancer patients feel better. Different forms of ginseng, such as slices, juice, or tea, can lower the chances of cancer, including those in the throat, stomach, and liver. A study also shows Korean ginseng can make people with certain cancers feel mentally and physically better.

9. Conclusion

Finally, there is significant potential for employing phytochemicals to treat liver cancer. This chapter has examined numerous organic substances that can be obtained from plants and other sources and have been shown to have anti-liver cancer properties. Curcumin, resveratrol, and silymarin can inhibit the growth of cancer cells, increase cell death, and even improve the efficacy of chemotherapy [18].

Additionally, research has shown that phytochemicals can lessen the adverse side effects of conventional therapies, enhance the general quality of life for people with liver cancer, and, in some cases, raise their chances of survival. These chemicals' low toxicity and advantageous effects on the liver make them very appealing for treating this complex condition [19].

Although the results are encouraging, it is essential to recognize that more study, including clinical trials, is required to determine the safety and effectiveness of these phytochemical substances in treating liver cancer. Not all patients will benefit similarly from phytochemical therapy, and individual reactions may differ [20].

However, using phytochemicals to treat liver cancer is still a promising research topic. These natural substances may be valuable complements or alternatives to currently available liver cancer treatments as science continues to delve deeper into their therapeutic properties,

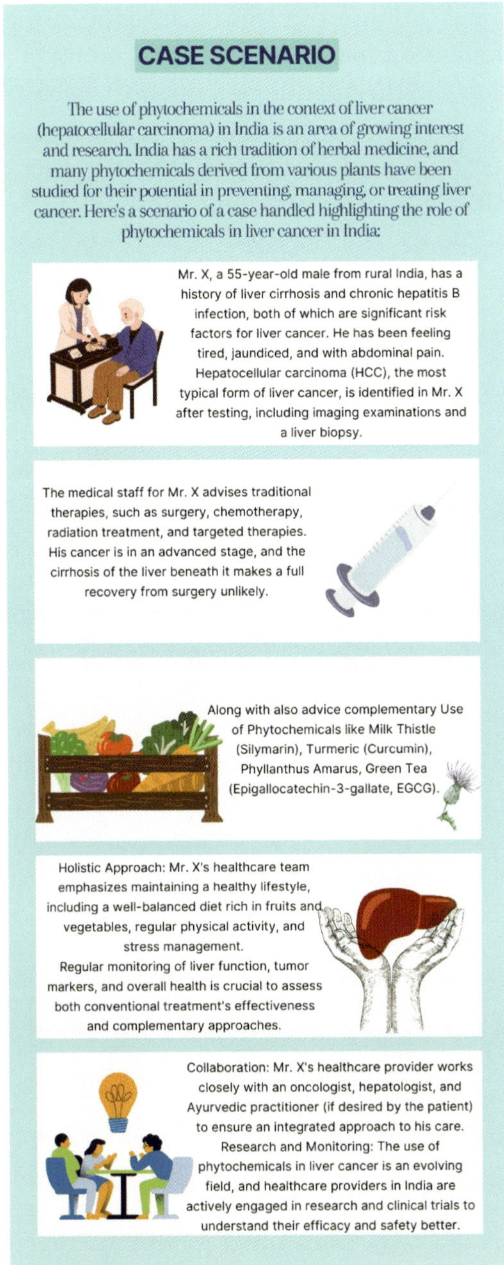
CASE SCENARIO
The use of phytochemicals in the context of liver cancer (hepatocellular carcinoma) in India is an area of growing interest and research. India has a rich tradition of herbal medicine, and many phytochemicals derived from various plants have been studied for their potential in preventing, managing, or treating liver cancer. Here's a scenario of a case handled highlighting the role of phytochemicals in liver cancer in India:
Mr. X, a 55-year-old male from rural India, has a history of liver cirrhosis and chronic hepatitis B infection, both of which are significant risk factors for liver cancer. He has been feeling tired, jaundiced, and with abdominal pain. Hepatocellular carcinoma (HCC), the most typical form of liver cancer, is identified in Mr. X after testing, including imaging examinations and a liver biopsy.
The medical staff for Mr. X advises traditional therapies, such as surgery, chemotherapy, radiation treatment, and targeted therapies. His cancer is in an advanced stage, and the cirrhosis of the liver beneath it makes a full recovery from surgery unlikely.
Along with also advice complementary Use of Phytochemicals like Milk Thistle (Silymarin), Turmeric (Curcumin), Phyllanthus Amarus, Green Tea (Epigallocatechin-3-gallate, EGCG).
Holistic Approach: Mr. X's healthcare team emphasizes maintaining a healthy lifestyle, including a well-balanced diet rich in fruits and vegetables, regular physical activity, and stress management.
Regular monitoring of liver function, tumor markers, and overall health is crucial to assess both conventional treatment's effectiveness and complementary approaches.
Collaboration: Mr. X's healthcare provider works closely with an oncologist, hepatologist, and Ayurvedic practitioner (if desired by the patient) to ensure an integrated approach to his care.
Research and Monitoring: The use of phytochemicals in liver cancer is an evolving field, and healthcare providers in India are actively engaged in research and clinical trials to understand their efficacy and safety better.

Figure 5: Case scenario

giving patients and healthcare professionals hope in the ongoing fight against this complicated and life-threatening condition [21, 22].

By leveraging the therapeutic potential of phytochemicals in preclinical studies and integrating them into clinical practice, advanced personalized and multidisciplinary approaches to liver cancer therapy, to improve patient outcomes and quality of life can be used, illustrations shown as case scenario in Figure 5.

References

1. Siddiqui MA, Siddiqui HH, Mishra A, Usmani A. Epidemiology of hepatocellular carcinoma. *Virus.* 2018;18:19.
2. International Journal of Pharmaceutical Sciences and Research. *Int J Pharm Sci Res.* 2018;9.
3. Cancer facts & figures 2023 [Internet]. Cancer.org. [cited 2024 Feb 16]. Available from: https://www.cancer.org/research/cancer-facts-statistics/all-cancer-facts-figures/2023-cancer-facts-figures.html.
4. Bray F, Ferlay J, Soerjomataram I, Siegel RL, Torre LA, Jemal A. Global cancer statistics 2018: GLOBOCAN estimates of incidence and mortality worldwide for 36 cancers in 185 countries. *CA Cancer J Clin.* 2018 Nov;68(6):394–424. doi: 10.3322/caac.21492. Epub 2018 Sep 12. Erratum in: *CA Cancer J Clin.* 2020 Jul;70(4):313. PMID: 30207593.
5. Rudzińska A, Juchaniuk P, Oberda J, Wiśniewska J, Wojdan W, Szklener K, Mańdziuk S. Phytochemicals in cancer treatment and cancer prevention-review on epidemiological data and clinical trials. *Nutrients.* 2023 Apr 14;15(8):1896. doi: 10.3390/nu15081896. PMID: 37111115; PMCID: PMC10144429.
6. What are phytochemicals? (And why should you eat more of them?) [Internet]. Uclahealth.org. [cited 2024 Feb 16]. Available from: https://www.uclahealth.org/news/what-are-phytochemicals-and-why-should-you-eat-more-them
7. George BP, Chandran R, Abrahamse H. Role of phytochemicals in cancer chemoprevention: Insights. *Antioxidants (Basel).* 2021 Sep 14; 10(9):1455. doi: 10.3390/antiox10091455. PMID: 34573087; PMCID: PMC8466984.

8. Huang W, He J, Nisar MF, Li H, Wan C. Phytochemical and pharmacological properties of *Chaenomeles speciosa*: An edible medicinal Chinese Mugua. *Evid Based Complement Alternat Med*. 2018 Dec 9;2018:9591845. doi: 10.1155/2018/9591845. PMID: 30622618; PMCID: PMC6304597.
9. George BP, Chandran R, Abrahamse H. Role of phytochemicals in cancer chemoprevention: Insights. *Antioxidants*. 2021 Sep 14;10(9):1455.
10. Pratheeshkumar P, Son YO, Korangath P, Manu KA, Siveen KS. Phytochemicals in cancer prevention and therapy. *BioMed Res Int*. 2015 Jan 1;2015:324021.
11. Ayaz M, Nawaz A, Ahmad S, Mosa OF, Eisa Hamdoon AA, Khalifa MA, Sadiq A, Ullah F, Wadood A, Kabra A, Ananda Murthy HC. Underlying anticancer mechanisms and synergistic combinations of phytochemicals with cancer chemotherapeutics: Potential benefits and risks. *J Food Qual*. 2022 Jun 15;2022:1–5.
12. Newman DJ, Cragg GM. Natural products as sources of new drugs from 1981 to 2014. *J Nat Prod*. 2016 Mar 25;79(3):629–661.
13. Ashraf MA. Phytochemicals as potential anticancer drugs: Time to ponder nature's bounty. *BioMed Res Int*. 2020 Jan 31;2020:1–7.
14. Hosseini A, Ghorbani A. Cancer therapy with phytochemicals: Evidence from clinical studies. *Avicenna J Phytomed*. 2015;5(2):84–97.
15. Choudhari AS, Mandave PC, Deshpande M, Ranjekar P, Prakash O. Phytochemicals in cancer treatment: From preclinical studies to clinical practice. *Front Pharmacol*. 2020 Jan 28;10:1614.
16. Choudhari AS, Mandave PC, Deshpande M, Ranjekar P, Prakash O. Phytochemicals in cancer treatment: From preclinical studies to clinical practice. *Front Pharmacol*. 2020 Jan 28;10:1614.
17. Meybodi NM, Mortazavian AM, Monfared AB, Sohrabvandi S, Meybodi FA. Phytochemicals in cancer prevention: A review of the evidence. *Iran J Cancer Prev*. 2017 Jan 31;10(1):e7219.
18. Dimri M, Satyanarayana A. Molecular signaling pathways and therapeutic targets in hepatocellular carcinoma. *Cancers*. 2020 Feb 20;12(2):491.
19. Rodriguez S, Skeet K, Mehmetoglu-Gurbuz T, Goldfarb M, Karri S, Rocha J, Shahinian M, Yazadi A, Poudel S, Subramani R. Phytochemicals as an alternative or integrative option, in conjunction with conventional

treatments for hepatocellular carcinoma. *Cancers.* 2021 Nov 17; 13(22):5753.

20. Wang Y, Li J, Xia L. Plant-derived natural products and combination therapy in liver cancer. *Front Oncol.* 2023 Feb 14;13:1116532.
21. Batta A. A review on phytochemicals and their activities. *Int J Res Med Sci.* 2016;2(1):20–28.
22. Arora S, Ranvir S. Phytochemicals: Benefits, concerns and challenges. In *Advancement in Functional Food Ingredients.* 2019:225.

https://doi.org/10.1142/9789811293320_0005

Chapter 5

Phytochemicals to Target Sorafenib Resistance Pathways in Liver Cancer

Shreyas Hulusemane Karunakara[1], Varsha Dilip Shiragannavar[1], Nirmala Gollarahalli Sannappagowda[1], Shama Prasada Kabekkodu[2], Divya Prasanna Kumar[1], and Prasanna Kumar Santhekadur[1,*]

[1]*Centre of Excellence in Molecular Biology and Regenerative Medicine, Department of Biochemistry, JSS Medical College, Mysuru, India*
[2]*Department of Cell and Molecular Biology, Manipal School of Life Sciences, Manipal Academy of Higher Education, Manipal, India*

Table of Contents

*Corresponding author: E-mail address: prasannakumars@jssuni.edu.in

Abbreviations:

HCC — Hepatocellular carcinoma
FDA — Food and Drug Administration
MEK — Mitogen-activated protein kinase
VEGFR — Vascular endothelial growth factor receptor
PDGFR — Platelet-derived growth factor receptor
PI3K/AKT pathway — Phosphoinositide-3-kinase–protein kinase B/AKT pathway
Mcl1 — Myeloid cell leukemia sequence 1
FOXO3 — Forkhead box O-3
CDKN1A — Cyclin-dependent kinase 1A
JAK/STAT — Janus kinase/statin
VEGF-A — Vascular endothelial growth factor-A
bHLH — Basic helix-loop-helix
p70S6K — p70 ribosomal S6 kinase
RP-S6 — Ribosomal protein S6
4E-BP1 — Eukaryotic translation initiation factor 4E-binding protein 1
eIF4E — Eukaryotic initiation factor 4E
CD4/8/25$^+$ — Cluster of differentiation 4/8/25$^+$
NK cells — Natural killer cells
iAST — Inducible albumin-specific SV40 T antigen
IL — Interleukins
IFNG — Interferon gamma
CSF2 — Colony stimulating factor 2
mTORC1 — mammalian target of rapamycin (mTOR) complex 1
ER — Endoplasmic reticulum
Ca^{2+} — Calcium ions
pERK — Extracellular signal-regulated kinase (phosphorylated)
IFNα — Interferon-alpha
pMAPK — Phosphorylated mitogen-activated protein kinase (active)

TGF-α/β — Transforming growth factor-alpha/beta
COX2/PGE2 — Cycloxygenase-2/prostaglandin E2
RTK — Receptor tyrosine kinase
ERK — Extracellular signal-regulated kinase
ETS1 — ETS proto-oncogene-1
PXR — Pregnane X receptor
CCL2 — CC motif chemokine ligand 2
CCL17 — CC motif chemokine ligand 17
CCR4 — CC motif chemokine receptor 4
DNMT1 — DNA methyl transferase 1
SREBP1 — Sterol regulatory element-binding protein 1
c-MET — Mesenchymal epithelial transition
DNMT3a/3b — DNA methyl transferase 3a/3b
OCT4 — Octamer-binding transcription factor 4
METTL3 — RNA modification enzyme methyltransferase-like 3
PFKFB3 — 6-phosphofructo-2-kinase/fructose-2,6-biphosphatase 3
HK2 — Hexokinase-2
PKM2 — Pyruvate kinase M2
AMPK — Adenosine monophosphate kinase
ETC — Electron transport chain
NRF2 — Nuclear factor erythroid 2-related factor 2
TXNRD1L — Thioredoxin reductase 1
MT1G — Metallothionein 1 G
MTHFD1L — Monofunctional C1-tetrahydrofolate synthase
NADPH — Nucleotide adenine di-nucleotide phosphate hydrogenase
ROS — Reactive oxygen species
EZH2 — Enhancer of zeste homolog 2
DNA — Deoxyribonucleic acid
MORC2 — Microrchidia 2
NF2 — Neurofibromatosis type 2
KIBRA — KIdney/BRAin protein
FOXO1 — Forkhead box O 1
PPARγ — Peroxisome proliferator-activator receptor gamma
PTEN — Phosphatase and tensin homolog
Zbtb7a — Zinc finger and BTB domain-containing protein 7A

RASSF1 — Ras association domain family member 1
ANT2 — Adenine nucleotide translocase 2
FBP2 — Fructose-1,6-bisphosphatase-2
KRAS — Kirsten rat sarcoma virus
TYRO3 — TYRO3 protein tyrosine kinase-3
MDR — Multidrug resistance mutation
MRP1 — Multidrug resistance protein 1
AEG-1 — Astrocyte elevated gene-1
IGF-1R — Insulin-like growth factor-1 receptor
TNF-α — Tumor necrosis factor-alpha
NF-κB — Nuclear factor-kappa B

Abstract

Hepatocellular carcinoma (HCC) is the primary form of liver cancer. With more than 70% of liver cancer cases identified as HCC, it is ranked second in terms of cancer-related mortality across the world. Viral infections such as hepatitis B and C, cirrhosis, are the dominant factors for the causation of this deadly disease. With the etiology of the disease changing every year due to factors like lifestyle changes and increased exposure to factors like alcohol, the epidemiology of HCC is morphing continuously limiting the available diagnosis and treatment options. Sorafenib is a multi-kinase inhibitor approved for HCC treatment by the FDA since 2007. Also used as a first-line treatment for renal cell carcinoma, this chemotherapeutic agent has previously been shown to increase the median survival expectancy in patients with advanced HCC. However, the increase in the side effects and resistance against the drug has pivoted researchers from across the globe to find alternatives from natural sources such as phytochemicals. This interactive book chapter discusses the details of sorafenib as a therapeutic target to treat HCC, its mode of action, modes and mechanisms of sorafenib resistance in HCC patients, and the advances in the field of phytochemical research to overcome sorafenib resistance in liver cancer.

1. Introduction

Sorafenib is a class of tyrosine-kinase inhibitors approved for treating several advanced forms of cancers such as renal cell carcinoma [1] and thyroid cancer [2]. This antineoplastic chemotherapeutic drug was first commercially sold as Nexavar by Bayer as a treatment for advanced renal cell carcinoma and has been subjected to rigorous clinical trials to treat primary liver cancer or hepatocellular carcinoma (HCC) [3]. The physicochemical and pharmaco-toxicological properties of sorafenib are described in Table 1.

Table 1: Physicochemical properties of sorafenib

Property	Details
Chemical structure	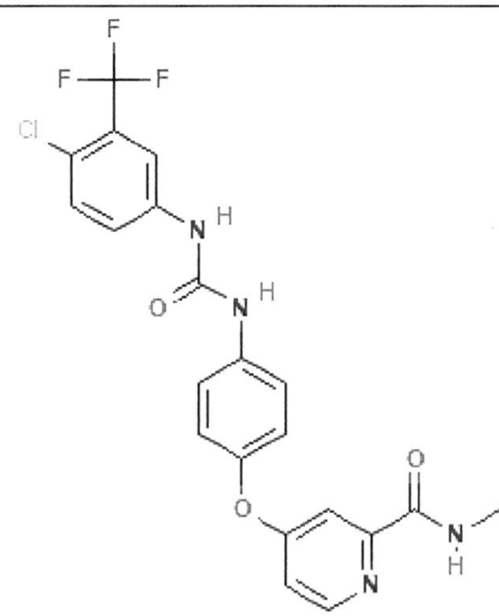 https://pubchem.ncbi.nlm.nih.gov/image/imgsrv.fcgi?cid=216239&t=l
Molecular formula	$C_{21}H_{16}ClF_3N_4O_3$
IUPAC nomenclature	4-[4-[[4-chloro-3-(trifluoromethyl)phenyl]carbamoylamino] phenoxy]-*N*-methylpyridine-2-carboxamide
Molecular weight	464.8 g/mol
Melting point	205.6°C

(*Continued*)

Table 1: (*Continued*)

Property	Details
Color	White solid
Solubility	Insoluble in aqueous solutions, partially soluble in ethanol
Pharmacological class	Protein kinase inhibitor
Biological half-life	25–48 hours
Mean bioavailability	38%–49% when administered during fasting orally as tablets

2. Mechanisms of Action

Sorafenib acts as a serine/threonine kinase inhibitor and can target multiple signaling pathways such as the Raf-MEK-ERK signaling to abrogate tumor growth, and other receptor-mediated signaling pathways involving vascular endothelial growth factor receptors (VEGFRs-VEGFR1, VEGFR2, and VEGFR3) and platelet-derived growth factor receptor-mediated signaling (PGDFR) which mediate neo-angiogenesis in HCC [4]. Various studies have shown the molecular mechanisms underlining the modes of action of sorafenib on HCC in various *in-vitro* as well as *in-vivo* models. The current section of the chapter explains the mechanisms through which sorafenib acts on tumor cells in HCC in detail.

2.1. *Sorafenib induces cell death in HCC through various mechanisms*

Evasion of apoptosis is a major cancer hallmark and various studies have shown that sorafenib induces apoptosis in HCC. Cell line studies involving HepG2, PLC/PRF/5 treated with sorafenib showed induction of apoptosis [5]. It was observed that both the cell lines and xenograft models displayed nuclear condensation, DNA fragmentation upon treatment, and an increase in cell populations in the sub-G_0 phase indicative of cells in the late-apoptotic stage. These cellular changes were attributed to the inhibition of phosphorylation of key proteins such as the MEK and ERK involved in the RAF/MEK/ERK signaling cascade. Also, cyclin D1, a well-known downstream target of MEK/ERK activation and PI3/AKT signaling, was found to be significantly reduced upon sorafenib treatment. Further, it is shown that sorafenib inhibits the phosphorylation of eIF4e, resulting in the downregulation of antiapoptotic proteins like Mcl-1 [5, 6] through MEK/ERK-independent mechanism and survivin [6] to induce apoptosis.

Sorafenib is shown to induce apoptosis by regulating the DNA methylome of apoptotic genes, suggesting the possible role of epigenetic effects induced by the multi-kinase inhibitor drug. Abeni et al. have determined the differential methylated regions (DMRs) in various pro-apoptotic and anti-apoptotic genes in sorafenib-treated HA22T/VGH cell lines and have reported that pro-apoptotic genes like FOXO3 as hypomethylated in treated cells as compared to the control cells [7]. Additionally, sorafenib-treated cells showed hypermethylation of a prominent antiapoptotic gene, p21 or CDKN1A, which is generally upregulated in HCC, suggesting that hypermethylation of CDKN1A upon sorafenib treatment at the gene level might be involved in decreased transcription of its mRNA and the subsequent protein [7].

JAK/STAT pathway is a critical pathway regulating key cellular processes such as cellular proliferation, differentiation, and apoptosis. Cyclin D3 (CCND3) is an important target of this pathway. Both STAT3 and STAT5 act as transcription factors and are known to activate CCND3 and aid in the G_0/S transition during the cell cycle. Interestingly, Cervello et al. have shown that sorafenib treatment downregulated CCND3 [6], which is further demonstrated to be regulated by DNA methylation epigenetically by Abeni et al. where several upstream regulators of this gene such as JAK1, STAT3, STAT5A, STAT5B, and CCND3 itself were hypermethylated upon sorafenib treatment [7].

Tumor hypoxia is a well-known driving factor for the progression of HCC [8–10]. It is described that sorafenib-induces apoptosis by inhibiting HIF-1α/VEGF-A activation in hepatoma cells with cobalt-induced hypoxia [11]. Hypoxia is mediated by a broad family of transcription factors called hypoxia-inducible factors (HIFs).

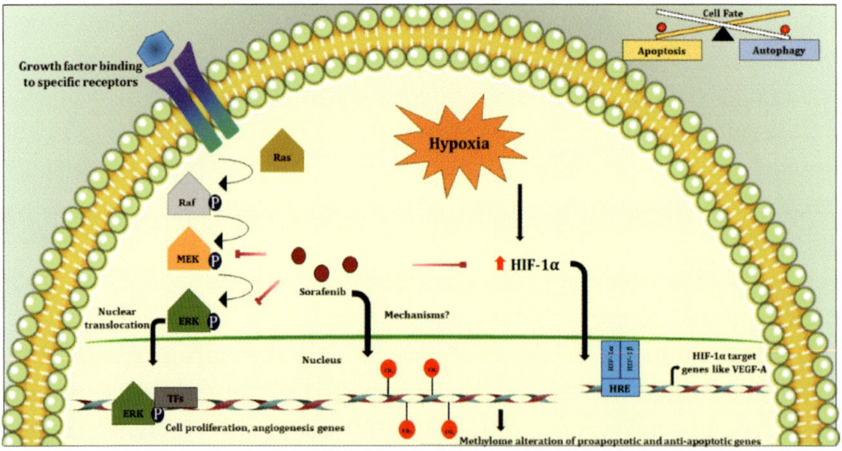

Figure 1: An overview of apoptotic mechanisms mediated by sorafenib treatment

Hypoxia-inducible transcription factor-1 (HIF-1) contains two bHLH proteins, namely HIF-1α and HIF-1β [12, 13]. Liu et al. showed that sorafenib inhibited angiogenesis through suppression of HIF-1α and its downstream targets such as ERK, p70S6K, RP-S6, 4E-BP1, and eIF4E [14]. It is noteworthy to mention that an elegant study by Horwitz et al. reported that murine models and human HCC tumors carrying amplifications in VEGF-A were found to be more sensitive to sorafenib than those without any amplification in the VEGF-A gene [15]. Figure 1 summarizes the mechanisms of sorafenib-induced apoptosis in HCC.

2.2. *Sorafenib mediates immunomodulation in HCC tumor microenvironment (TME)*

Besides regulating these conventional apoptotic mediators, sorafenib is also said to induce immune-mediated cell death or pyroptosis, where the effect of sorafenib on key immune cellular players such as macrophages, $CD4^+$ and $CD8^+$ T-cell populations, dendritic cell (DC), monocytes, and granulocytic myeloid-derived suppressor cell

(MDSC), NK cells and pro-inflammatory markers such as cytokines are already extensively investigated. Tumor induction and immune cell depletion studies using xenograft and iAST (inducible albumin-specific SV40 T antigen) models treated with sorafenib by Hage et al. showed an increase in pyroptosis of MΦ (M phi-lineage of macrophages) and subsequent NK cell activation, but there was no effect of sorafenib on T-cell mediated tumor reduction in both these models [16]. Further, several pro-inflammatory cytokines such as IL1A, IL1B, IL6, IL12, IL15, IL18, IFNG, and CSF2 were upregulated upon sorafenib treatment. Among these, MΦ-derived IL1B and IL18 secreted as a result of caspase-1 mediated pyropotosis of macrophages was shown to accelerate the degranulation of NK cells which resulted in enhanced perforin activity which ultimately targeted HCC cells and resulted in their programmed cell death [16].

Effector T-cells such as $CD8^+$ cytotoxic T cells and regulatory T-cells (Tregs) constitute a critical niche of the TME and mediate crucial hallmarks such as immunosuppression critical to the proliferation and growth of tumors including HCC. Programmed cell death ligand-1 (PD-1) is usually highly expressed in tumor-associated cytotoxic T-cells, suggesting its role in immune evasion [17–19]. Additionally, specific gene signatures like transcription factor forkhead box P3 (Foxp3) expression in $CD4^+CD25^+$ Tregs are also commonly associated with immune suppression mechanisms [20]. Interestingly, studies involving murine models have elaboratively demonstrated the possible immunomodulatory functions of sorafenib treatment on effector T-cell populations in HCC. Chen et al. have shown a strong correlation between HCC amelioration through sorafenib-mediated alterations in cell populations and expression signatures of specific gene signatures in these immune cells [21]. Sorafenib treatment is shown to decrease the PD-1 expressing $CD8^+$ T cells and $CD4^+CD25^+Foxp3^+$Treg subsets which subsequently results in the active release of cytokines by other effector T cells which can act on tumor cells and eliminate them [21]. Figure 2 summarizes different modes of immunomodulation mechanisms mediated by sorafenib treatment.

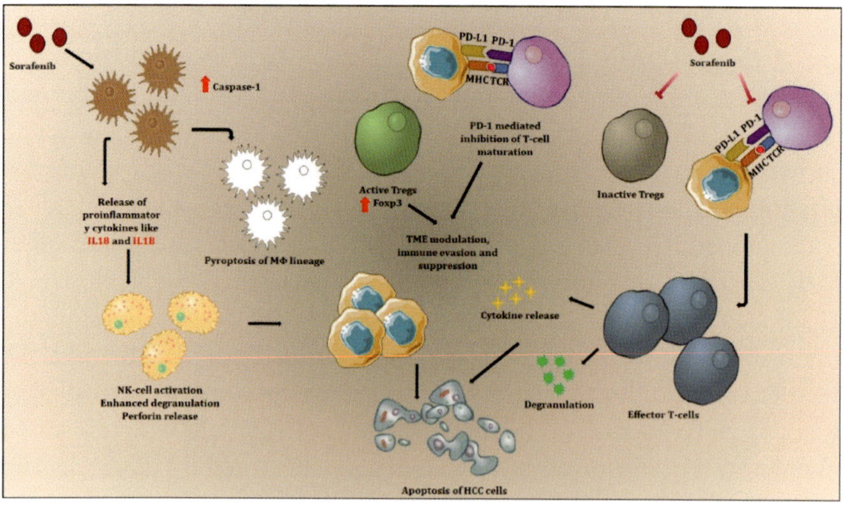

Figure 2: An overview of immunomodulation mechanisms mediated by sorafenib treatment in HCC

2.3. *Sorafenib-mediated autophagy mechanisms*

Autophagy or macro-autophagy is a mass-degradation process where damaged cellular components, organelles, and misfolded proteins are broken down through a self-engulfing body referred to as the autophagolysosome resulting from the fusion of a double-membraned vesicle called autophagosome and lysosome. The role of autophagic processes in balancing cellular homeostasis is well appreciated [22]. It is also reported that excessive stimulation of autophagic processes can result in cell death [23], suggesting the existence of a fine balance between autophagy-mediated cell survival and autophagy-mediated cell death. In mammals, the formation of autophagosomes is initiated by various stress mechanisms including nutrient deprivation and hypoxic stress which targets the formation of ULK1 (unc-51-like kinase) complex, which recruits various autophagy-related proteins (Atgs) [24]. Next, the phagosome nucleation is initiated at the endoplasmic reticulum as omegasome through phosphorylation of the Beclin1-Vps34 (vacuolar protein sorting 34) complex, which activates local production of phosphatidyl-inositol-3-phosphate (PIP3) [25].

Subsequently, the elongation of the phagosome occurs through the incorporation of certain lipids and proteins through Atg9 and WIPI (WD-repeat protein interacting with phosphoinositides) system [26]. Finally, the cargo-sequestration to the omegasome occurs through WIPI2-recruitment of ATG12~ATG5–ATG16L1 complex and conjugation of microtubule-associated protein light chain 3 (LC3) proteins and γ-aminobutyric acid receptor-associated proteins (GABARAPs) to phosphatidylethanolamine (LC3-II) [18], resulting in an autophagosome. This is followed by the subsequent fusion with lysosomes and maturation into an auto-phagolysosome [23, 27].

Sorafenib treatment in *in-vitro* cell line models such as HepG2, MHCC97-L, Huh7, HLF, and PLC/PRF/5 has been shown to promote LC3-II formation in a dose-dependent manner [28, 29]. Other autophagy markers such as Beclin1, Atg5, and Atg12 expression are also shown to be induced by this drug in HCC cells *in vitro* [29, 30].

mTOR-pathway is a commonly upregulated pathway in HCC as a response to oxidative stress, hypoxia, and misfolding of proteins [31–33]. Sorafenib has been shown to repress the phosphorylation of mTORC1 in both HCC *in-vitro* as well as xenograft models [9]. Further other studies by Liu et al. and Zhai et al. have demonstrated that the subsequent phosphorylation of mTORC1 downstream targets such as p70S6K, 4E-BP1, and eIF-4E was also dampened as a result of the treatment in *in-vivo* models [14, 34]. Concerning the fact that PI3/AKT is the upstream regulator of mTOR activity and that the pathway is upregulated in HCC, studies have a positive view that a combination of PI3/AKT inhibitors coupled with sorafenib can provide better treatment for HCC [35].

The critical cellular organelle for protein synthesis, folding, and modifications is the endoplasmic reticulum. ER stress can result in the accumulation of misfolded proteins that can give rise to unfolded protein response (UPR) [36] as a counterbalance mechanism which is mediated by macromolecules such as inositol requiring enzyme 1α (IRE1α), protein kinase R-like ER kinase (PERK) and activating transcription factor (ATF6) [37]. UPR can ultimately result in the degradation of parts of ER through autophagy, reduction in protein translation, alleviation of chaperones, or stimulation of

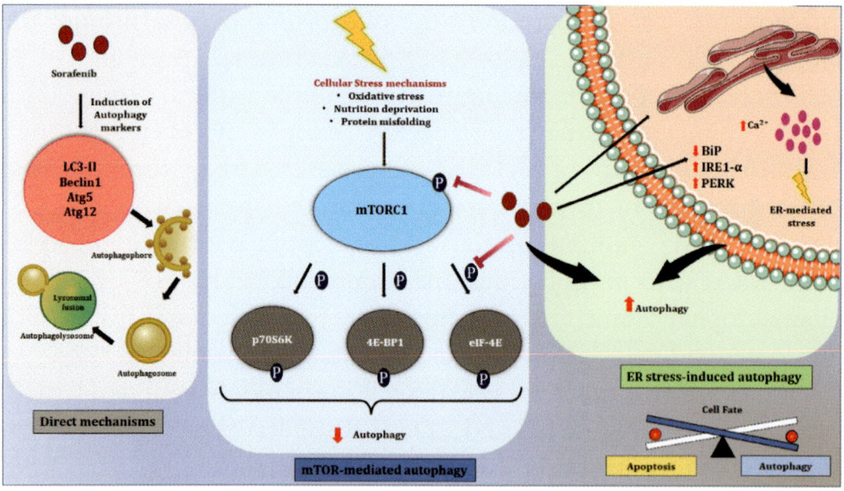

Figure 3: Sorafenib-mediated extracellular and intracellular stress mechanisms and activation of downstream autophagy mechanisms in HCC

ubiquitin-proteasome machinery. Sorafenib is shown to inhibit the expression of chaperone BiP located on the basal ER membrane, thereby alleviating the expressions of IRE1α, and PERK [38, 39]. Additionally, sorafenib is also shown to disrupt Ca^{2+} homeostasis within the ER resulting in the accumulation of calcium in the cytosol, in turn inducing oxidative stress and subsequent activation of cell death mechanisms [39, 40]. An overwhelmed UPR can result in the activation of programmed cell death mediated through C/EBP homologous protein (CHOP) transcription factor [41]. Sorafenib is shown to induce CHOP expression in MHCC97-L, HepG2, and PLC/PRF/5 HCC cells [29]. Figure 3 summarizes sorafenib-mediated extracellular and intracellular stress and downstream activation of autophagy mechanisms in HCC cells.

3. Modes and Mechanisms of Sorafenib Resistance

Tumor heterogeneity is a critical driving factor in HCC resistance. Recently, a large cohort involving 1114 HCC subjects from a random phase-III clinical (STORM) trial who had already undergone surgical resection and ablation, were reclassified into two groups receiving placebo and sorafenib (400 mg) as an adjuvant therapy, twice a day for a total period of 4 years [3]. Surprisingly, it was observed that there were no improvements in terms of both overall survival (OS) and recurrence-free survival (RFS) among the sorafenib group in comparison with the group that received the placebo. Other studies such as the SHARP and the Asian-pacific trials targeted advanced HCC without any systemic treatment of sorafenib making it difficult to conclude the efficiency of sorafenib treatment in HCC treatment and management, and restricting the study's power to test the efficiency of sorafenib only as an adjuvant therapy [42]. This further suggests that larger cohorts involving much larger sample sizes, and diverse subpopulations are essential to explore the practicality of sorafenib in the treatment of HCC. The current section elaboratively explains the know-how of different modes and mechanisms involved in sorafenib resistance (summarized in Figure 4).

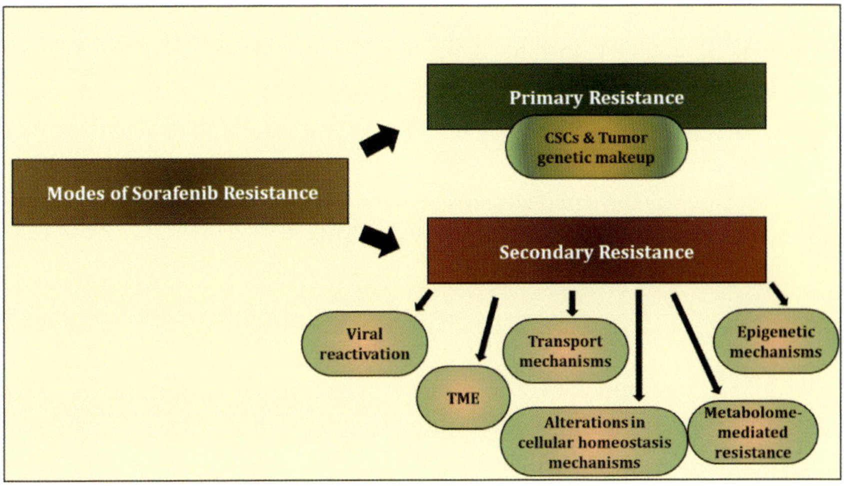

Figure 4: Figure summarizing the various modes of sorafenib resistance in HCC

3.1. *Primary sorafenib resistance*

Primary resistance refers to the resistance of HCC cells during the initial stages of tumor development [43]. While the mechanisms of primary sorafenib resistance remain undefined, studies have pointed toward epithelial-to-mesenchymal transition (EMT) and cellular stemness driven by Cancer Stem Cells (CSCs) as the driving factors of phenotypic diversity and tumor heterogeneity resulting in the primary resistance to drugs like sorafenib [44]. It is commonly observed that HCC tumors display certain anomalies in terms of genotypic aberrations. For example, a commonly encountered proto-oncogene ce-rbB1 and its product EGFR is abnormally activated in more than 50% of all HCCs [45]. Another study demonstrated that EGFR overexpression or its ligand or the activation of downstream targets of EGFR-signaling such as Ras/Raf/MEK//ERK signaling and pERK might be the driving factors for primary resistance and reduced sensitivity to sorafenib exposure [46].

3.2. *Secondary or acquired sorafenib resistance*

3.2.1. *Sorafenib resistance is mediated by viral reactivation*

Hepatitis B (HBV) and hepatitis C (HCV) infections are the two prominent viral infections responsible for HCC [47]. Viral reactivation upon the onset of chemotherapy remains a controversial link in the failure of therapy [48, 49]. A summary of the contradictory findings associated with the mechanisms associated with sorafenib resistance and viral reactivations can be found in Table 2.

3.2.2. *Tumor microenvironment (TME)*

The TME encompasses the unique internal environment present within the tumor comprising various cellular and extracellular players, their secretions, and their interactions. The common cellular players apart from the tumor mass include various immune cells like NK cells, and $CD8^+$ cytotoxic T-cells (CTLs) which are usually in a dampened or inactive state prominently in the periphery of the tumor [55].

Table 2: Table summarizing various viral-mediated sorafenib resistance in HCC

Publications	Major findings	Reference
Descamps et al.	Sorafenib imparts an anti-viral effect on HCV in *in-vitro* models by modulation of the viral entry through modulation of Claudin-1 expression and localization.	[50]
Cabrera et al.	Sorafenib has no significant effect on HCV expression.	[51]
Himmelsbach et al.	Sorafenib is shown to inhibit c-Raf-independent phosphorylation of STAT1 and subsequent impaired IFNα expression, promoting immune suppression and subsequent progression of HCV replication.	[52]
Zhang et al.	Sorafenib suppresses NK cell populations, creating a pro-tumorigenic environment for HCC progression and metastasis.	[53]
Witt-Kehati et al.	• HBV induces sorafenib resistance in HCC. • HBV X protein expression is associated with pMAPK14-mediated sorafenib resistance. • Combinatorial treatment of pMAPK14 inhibitors and sorafenib might be beneficial in HBV-associated HCC.	[54]

TME also has other activated immune cells such as MDSCs and Tregs which inhibit the activity of effector T-cells and create a pro-tumorigenic condition, favoring proliferation and spread of cancers [55].

The extracellular matrix (ECM) is a critical factor in TME. Interestingly it was shown that ECM deposition promoted the formation of "fibrotic nests" which prevented CTLs from infiltrating the tumor core and restricting it to the periphery [55]. ECM components such as hyaluronic acid and collagen are known to affect critical processes such as angiogenesis, tumor growth, immunosuppression, and resistance [56].

Cancer-associated fibroblasts (CAFs) form an abundant niche of TME, and along with its several secretions such as chemokines, angiogenic factors, exosome secretions, growth factors, and metabolites, these cells are known to modulate the reconstitution and reshaping of the ECM [57, 58]. The current subsection explains the different relations between sorafenib resistance and TME.

3.2.2.1. Hypoxia

Several studies have pointed toward an increasing role of hypoxic environments and its possible links to sorafenib resistance in several cancers including HCC [59]. It is shown that sorafenib-resistant HCCs favor an increasingly higher state of intra-tumoral hypoxic condition than HCCs that are sensitive to sorafenib [60, 61]. Prolonged sorafenib treatment is shown to increase the tumor hypoxia stabilizing HIF-1α and HIF-2α [62, 63] or promoting HIF-1α-to-HIF-2α switching [64] resulting in the activation of downstream target oncogenes involved in processes like angiogenesis. Sorafenib is shown to induce HIF-2α and the subsequent activation of genes such as VEGF and cyclin D1 [14, 62]. Zhao et al. demonstrated that sorafenib treatment upregulated HIF-2α by a positive feedback mechanism and activated the TGF-α/EGFR through the COX2/PGE2 axis, promoting HCC tumorigenesis and reduced sorafenib sensitivity [62]. Liu et al. noted that another downstream pathway of HIF-2α activation, the β-catenin/c-Myc pathway enhances tumor metabolism and promotes hepatocarcinogenesis, and drug resistance. Further, it was also demonstrated that targeted downregulation of HIF-2α improved the antitumor effect of sorafenib by targeting the β-catenin/c-Myc-dependent pathway which was reportedly upregulated in resistant cancer cells under hypoxic condition [65]. Figure 5 summarizes sorafenib-induced resistance through hypoxia-activated downstream mechanisms.

3.2.2.2. Tumor-associated immune and stromal cells (TAISCs)

a. Tumor-associated macrophages

Polarization of tumor-associated macrophages (TAM) from classically activated macrophages (M1) to alternatively activated macrophages (M2) is a critical step associated with tumor progression and metastasis [66]. The link between sorafenib resistance and TAMs was

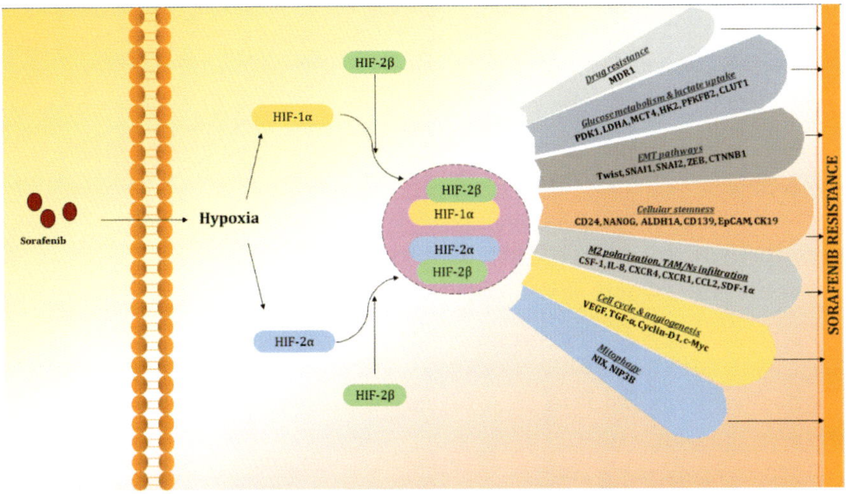

Figure 5: Sorafenib-induced resistance through hypoxia-activated mechanisms

demonstrated by Wei et al. [67]. It was shown that M2-TAMs enhanced the proliferative, migratory behavior and invasiveness of sorafenib-resistant HCC cells. It is increasingly evident from different studies that the M2 lineage of activated macrophages can cause sorafenib resistance in HCC [30, 68]. Notably, it is also reported that TAMs enhance the EMT state and the stemness of cancerous cells treated with sorafenib [69].

b. Cancer-associated fibroblasts (CAFs)

CAFs along with their secretions are known to influence tumor growth, metastasis, immune evasion, and drug resistance [70, 71]. Co-culturing studies involving the culture of liver organoids alongside CAFs has showed compromised efficiency of drugs such as sorafenib, 5-fluoro uracil (5-FU), and regorafenib [72]. Several molecular pathways are attributed to CAF-mediated sorafenib resistance in HCC. Gao et al. reported that CAFs activated NF-κB signaling which promoted sorafenib resistance in liver cancer [73]. Peng et al. reported that the secretions of CAFs, particularly hepatocyte-growth-factor (HGF) secretion, imparted sorafenib resistance through Met/ERK1/2 activation [74].

c. Tumor-associated neutrophils (TANs)

Similar to TAMs, TANs also undergo polarization, and two phenotypes of TANs exist: the pro-tumorigenic "N2" and anti-tumorigenic "N1" phenotypes. TANs undergo N1-switching as a response to interferons while N2-switching is driven by TGF-β [75]. Immune enrichment in terms of N2 phenotype was associated not only with poor prognostic markers but also as an indicator of low efficacy of sorafenib in treated HCC patients [76, 77]. Also, N2-TANs promoted sorafenib resistance by enhancing the stemness as well as by recruiting other key immune suppressor cells like the Tregs and macrophages which can lead to subsequent progression of HCC [78].

d. Other immune players

Multiple immunosuppressive cells that constitute the heterogenous population of TME can regulate sorafenib resistance. Deng et al. identified that MDSCs were associated with poor prognosis and early recurrence in patients who had undergone interventions such as curative resection, chemotherapy, and radiotherapy [79]. The same study also deciphered that MDSCs supplemented CAF-activation and subsequent sorafenib resistance through fibroblast-growth factor 1 (FGF1) expression. Other studies have pointed toward immune cell cross-talks wherein MDSCs were shown to inhibit $CD8^+$ T cell, induce Treg, and impair NK cell functions adding to HCC progression. Additionally, CCR4-Treg cells, another intra-tumoral form of Tregs, were shown to be associated with sorafenib resistance, particularly in HBV-associated HCC [80]. Figure 6 summarizes the sorafenib-resistant mechanisms mediated through different tumor-associated immune cells and their secretions in HCC.

3.2.2.3. Immunosuppressive molecules and factors

The secretions from immune cells or stromal cells also play an important role in creating an immunosuppressive environment favorable for tumor development and progression. Table 3 summarizes the role of different immune factors and secretions that are known to promote resistance toward sorafenib in HCC.

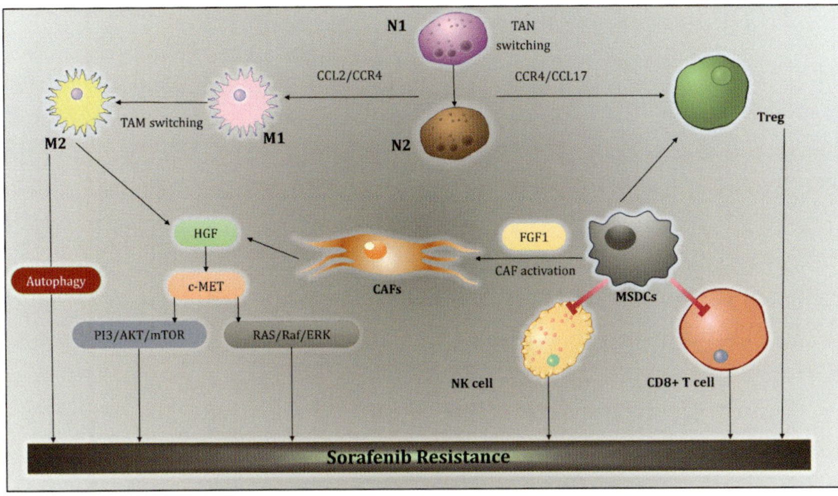

Figure 6: Mechanisms of sorafenib resistance mediated through different tumor-associated immune cells and their secretions in HCC

Table 3: Immune secretions or factors and their subsequent pathways active in sorafenib-resistant HCC

Immune secretion/factor	Pathways activated	References
TGF-β	• TGF-β/EMT/PD-L1 • TGF-β/RTK • ERK/ETS1/PXR	[81] [82] [83]
CCL-2	• CCL2/CCR4/TAM	[78]
PD-L1	• PD-L1/STAT3/DNMT1 • PI3K/AKT/SREBP-1 • c-MET/PD-L1/RAS/RAF/ MEK/ERK1/2	[84] [85] [86]
IL-6	• IL6/STAT3 • IL-6/STAT3/DNMT3b/OCT4	 [87]
CCL17	• CCL17/CCR4/Treg	[78]
CXCR3	• MAPK pathway/adipocytokine signaling	[88]

3.2.3. *Transport mechanisms and sorafenib resistance*

The existing literature points toward two prominent mechanisms responsible for the efflux of sorafenib away from sensitized and responsive HCC cells: (1) ABC (ATP-Binding Box) efflux pumps and (2) Exosome-mediated mechanisms. Several tyrosine-kinase inhibitors (TKIs) including sorafenib are shown to interact with ABC-pumps which might have several mechanistic and clinical relevance in tackling resistant HCC [89, 90]. Surprisingly, this facet remains unclear and demands more work to understand the role of such transporters and their interaction with TKIs in HCC.

Tumor secretomes constitute a wide range of cellular secretions which include growth factors, immunomodulant substances, microRNAs (miRNAs), long noncoding RNAs (lncRNAs), and other cargos derived from tumoral cells, or surrounding cells such as the stromal cells that are in continuous circulation both at intra-tumoral as well as inter-tumoral levels. The limited research available in this regard has shown that such extra vesicular (EV) cargo involving cargo such as miRNAs through exosomes can modulate sorafenib resistance in HCC [91, 92] through different processes like EMT [93].

3.2.4. *Alterations in cellular homeostasis mechanisms*

3.2.4.1. Autophagy

In terms of sorafenib resistance, autophagy is considered to be a key upregulated process, and the inhibition of autophagy is considered a promising way to address sorafenib resistance. As discussed previously in section 2.3, several factors like ER stress can induce UPR, promoting autophagic response as an alternative to cell death. Sorafenib is shown to induce IRE-1, an ER-associated autophagy sensor, and it is shown that inhibitors of auto-phagolysosome formation like chloroquine (CLQ) can enhance sorafenib action in HCC pre-clinical models [29]. It is further correlated that higher expression of ATG7 and an active state of autophagy correlates with poor prognosis post-sorafenib treatment [94]. Additionally, Lin et al. identified methyltransferase-like 3 (METTL3), a key enzyme for RNA modification of target mRNAs like FOXO3 through N6-methyladenosine (m6 A) modification. METTL3 was observed to be downregulated in HCC patients affecting the stability of FOXO3 transcripts in sorafenib-resistant HCC by activating autophagy-promoting proteins [95]. Also, METTL3 knockdown enhanced sorafenib resistance through FOXO3 depletion in sorafenib-resistant HCC. A study involving patient-derived HCC xenografts (PDXs) showed that annexin A3 (ANXA3) upregulation to be associated with sorafenib resistance which was reported to be modulated by inhibiting the protein kinase C (PKCδ)/p38-mediated apoptotic pathway and that a combination of anti-ANXA3 with sorafenib/regorafenib improved the survival [96].

3.2.4.2. Ferroptosis

Ferroptosis refers to a regulated cell death process in which iron complexes and iron ions mediate abnormal metabolism of lipid oxides [97]. Mechanistically, metallothionein-1G (MT-1G) was found to be induced by sorafenib which subsequently evaded ferroptosis and enhanced the resistance in HCC [98]. A recent study reported that the chelator-mediated depletion of intracellular iron through the iron chelator deferoxamine (DFX), protected cancer cells from the cytotoxic effects of sorafenib, demonstrating that the depletion of intracellular iron stores prevented sorafenib from inducing oxidative stress in HCC cells [99]. These studies further point toward the possible induction of ferroptosis in addressing sorafenib resistance in HCC.

3.2.5. *Metabolome-mediated sorafenib resistance mechanisms*

Metabolic switching and reprogramming of its associated genes are a common mechanism encountered in tumor metabolome through which the energy-craving tumor cells meet their energy demands fueling their progression and spread. Glucose uptake and lactose export are reported to be enhanced in response to sorafenib treatment in HCC patients [100]. Key glycolytic enzymes such as PFKFB3, HK2, and PKM2 are reported as upregulated in sorafenib-resistant HCC cell lines [101]. CSCs are known to have a pronounced glucose metabolism mediated by low AMPK levels favoring oxidative phosphorylation. This metabolic switch in glucose metabolism in sorafenib-resistant stem-like HCC cells is shown to promote the expression of stemness-related genes through HIF-1α regulation.

A metabolic symbiosis between lactate and glucose metabolism is an increasingly studied facet of tumor metabolomics. It is now appreciated that the CAFs in the TME secrete various growth factors in response to the lactose efflux from the tumor cells as a metabolite through a lactate shuttle system [102]. Although, there is no such evidence of the existence of such a shuttle between CAFs and sorafenib-resistant HCC cells, existence of such export system cannot be completely ruled out.

Readers should note that when sorafenib sensitivity concerning oxidative stress response is being addressed, ROS is induced by sorafenib through ETC targeting [103]. ROS control is mediated by several antioxidant enzymes including glutathione (GSH). B-catenin and c-Myc are proven to be the major mediators in the maintenance of GSH-dependent stemness and sorafenib resistance of cancer cells [104]. Supplementing to this it was further observed that glutamine synthetase (GS) mediated glutaminolysis enhanced sorafenib sensitivity in HCC [105]. It was further noticed that the activation of the p62/Keap1/NRF2 pathway protected against sorafenib-induced ferroptosis in HCC [106]. As a master regulator gene of redox balance and homeostasis, NRF2 induction is known to activate several of the antioxidant genes including TXNRD1, MTIG MTHFD1L, and NADPH, all of which are known to improve the survival in sorafenib-induced oxidative stress [98, 107–109]. In short, sorafenib induces ROS-induced apoptosis, and a counterbalance system mediated by ROS-antioxidant machinery can inhibit sorafenib-mediated cell death in cancer cells. Figure 7 details the various metabolomic and cellular homeostatic pathways involved in sorafenib-induced resistance in HCC.

3.2.6. *Epigenetic mechanisms and sorafenib resistance*

Epigenetic processes constituting DNA methylation, histone modifications, and regulation by noncoding RNAs like miRNAs are known

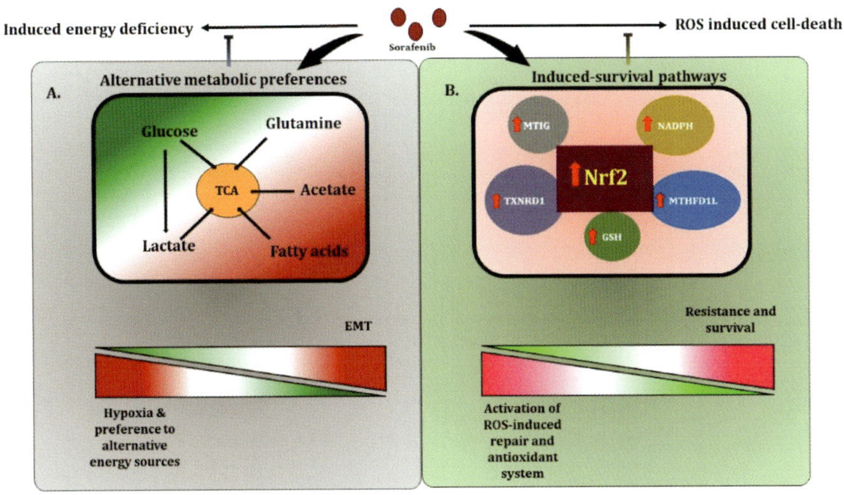

Figure 7: Metabolomic and cellular homeostatic (autophagy) pathways involved in sorafenib-induced resistance in HCC

to orchestrate the balance between HCC sensitivity and resistance toward sorafenib administration. While the role of these mechanisms is yet to be potentiated to its full extent, a few studies have linked their functions to HCC development and acquired sorafenib resistance. A study that links histone methyltransferases (HMTs) to sorafenib resistance demonstrated that HMTs like EZH2 played an important role in silencing specific genes and promoted cell survival, growth, and resistance toward sorafenib [110]. Further, it was also shown that EZH2 knockdown/inhibition promoted sorafenib-induced apoptosis. DNA methylation refers to the catalytic transfer of methyl groups from methyl-group donors such as S-adenosyl methionine (SAM) to specific cytosine groups on the double-stranded DNA. Wang et al. reported that MORC2 forms complex with with DNA methyl transferase, DNMT3A and causes hypermethylation of NF2 and KIBRA promoter, mitigating resistance and cancer stemness in HCC through repression of Hippo signaling [111].

The role of miRNAs in imparting resistance toward sorafenib treatment in HCC is an indispensable facet of epigenetic regulation in drug resistance in HCC. Several studies (Table 4) have elaboratively

Table 4: List of miRNAs up/downregulated and their downstream targets/pathways in sorafenib-resistant HCC

miRNA	Expression in HCC	Effects	Molecular Pathway/Process	Reference
miR-27a	Upregulated	Sorafenib efficacy is improved upon inhibition of miR-27a through FOXO1 and PPARγ expression	—	[112]
miR-19a-3p	Upregulated	Promotes chemoresistance and metastasis through PTEN/AKT activation	PTEN/AKT	[113]
miR-199a-3p	Upregulated	Repression of FOXO1 by upregulating mTOR/p21-activated kinase 4	mTOR/PAK4	[114]
miR-494	Upregulated	miRNA overexpression promotes sorafenib resistance through mTOR signaling	mTOR	[115]
miR-221	Upregulated	Sorafenib resistance mediation through caspase-3-mediated apoptosis	—	[116]
miR-125a-5p	Upregulated	Inhibition of miR-125a reduces sorafenib efficacy by interfering with the expressions of matrix metalloproteinase 11, Zbtb7a proto-oncogene, and c-Raf in HCC	—	[117]
miR-181a	Upregulated	Induces sorafenib resistance through RASSF1 expression	MAPK	[118]
miR-423-5p	Upregulated	Patients treated with sorafenib exhibited higher expression in serum and the miRNA was shown to enhance autophagy	—	[119]
miR-21	Upregulated	Inhibition of miR-21 expression improvised sorafenib efficacy in sorafenib-resistant HCC	AKT/PTEN	[120]
miR-137	Downregulated	miRNA upregulation reverts resistance, rescues cellular transformation through ANT-2 mediated cancer-initiating phenotype	—	[121]

miR-367-3p	Downregulated	Improves sorafenib efficacy via androgen receptor-mediated signal modulation	AKT/ERK	[122]
miR-591	Downregulated	Sorafenib resistance is dampened through overexpression of miR-591 and FBP2 expression and subsequent blockade of PI3/AKT signaling	PI3/AKT	[123]
miR-622	Downregulated	This miRNA targets KRAS signaling, and its inhibition resensitized sorafenib-resistant cells through suppression of RAF/ERK and PI3/AKT pathways	RAF/ERK and PI3/AKT	[124]
miR-7	Downregulated	Downregulation resulted in TYRO3 under-expression and evasion of growth arrest checkpoints promoting migration and invasion	PI3/AKT	[125]
miR-374b	Downregulated	Overexpression improved resensitization through antagonization of PKM2-mediated glycolytic pathway	Glycolysis	[126]
miR-375	Downregulated	Upregulates MDR-related genes like MRP-1 and p-glycoprotein, and AEG-1 upregulation	Angiogenesis	[127]
miR-122	Downregulated	Upregulates IGF-1R expression, promoting sorafenib resistance. Forced expression of miR-122 resensitized resistant cells	EMT	[92]
miR-30a-5p	Downregulated	Downregulation results in direct overexpression of corticotrophin-like cytokine factor 1 (CLCF1) that promotes glycolysis through the PI3/AKT pathway, promoting a survival edge in resistant cells	CLCF1/PI3K/AKT cascade Glycolysis PI3/AKT	[128]

worked on the mediation and functional regulation of sorafenib resistance through these short noncoding RNAs.

4. Phytochemicals to Tackle Sorafenib Resistance

Several phytochemical components from several sources are shown to improve sorafenib resistance in HCC. Now that we have understood the different mechanisms underlying sorafenib resistance in HCC, we as authors hope that our readers can appreciate the biology and various mechanisms the cancer cells adapt to when exposed to treatments like chemotherapy, and we hope to convince our readers further on the alternatives such as combinatorial therapy or as individual therapeutic regimens mediated through phytoconstituents and phytochemicals might help clinicians address the sorafenib resistance in HCC.

Anti-VEGF-A therapeutic strategy through phytochemicals forms a promising approach in combating HCC as well as overcoming sorafenib resistance. Several classes of phytochemicals, including flavonoids, terpenoids, alkaloids, coumarins, phenols, and glycosides in anti-VEGF-A therapy in HCC, and the subsequent hurdles faced in the clinical transformation of these phytochemicals in immunotherapy have been discussed in detail previously by Ayana et al. [129]. Quercetin, a naturally occurring flavonoid, was shown to overcome acquired sorafenib resistance through EGF inactivation in resistant HCC cells [130]. Further, Abdu et al. reported that quercetin alone or in combination with sorafenib downregulated key genes involved in proliferation, inflammation, and angiogenesis, such as TNF-α, VEGF-A, P53, and NF-κB [131].

Likewise, pterostilbene, a naturally occurring dimethyl derivative of resveratrol abundantly found in blueberries and grapes, was shown to interfere with the DNA synthesis machinery through ribonucleotide reductase (RR) [132]. Specifically, the phyto-component was shown to interact with RR small subunit M2 (RRM2), significantly affecting the HCC proliferation and HBV replication. However, further studies are required for the validation of pterostilbene against viral-reactivation-mediated sorafenib resistance in HCC. Further, a study by Tang et al. demonstrated that conditionally reprogrammed patient-derived-primary hepatocellular carcinoma cells (CRHCs) derived from patients treated with sorafenib and pristimerin [133] showed that pristimerin works synergistically on CRHCs alongside sorafenib, improved sorafenib sensitization, and had an anti-cancer effect which was mediated through ROS-induced apoptosis and subsequent inhibition of phosphorylation of AKT and upregulation of FOXO1 and $p27^{kip}$.

Giacomo et al. reported that two naturally occurring sesquiterpenes, namely, β-caryophyllene (CRY) and β-caryophyllene oxide (CRYO), could chemosensitize resistant HCC cells by inhibiting sorafenib efflux through ABC-pumps both in *in-vivo* and *in-vitro* conditions [134]. Wu et al. reported that a combination of carnosic acid, a polyphenol, and a Vit-D2 analog reduced autophagy markers such as Beclin1, Atg3, and LC3 in sorafenib-resistant HCO2 cells by promoting sorafenib-induced apoptosis and inhibition of autophagolysosome formation [135].

Withaferin-A (Wit-A) is a well-known steroidal lactone derived from *Withania somnifera*. Wit-A has been previously shown to inhibit NF-αB activated downstream target genes through the activation of liver X receptor (LXR) [136]. Akol et al. demonstrated that Wit-A reduced the expression of vimentin, a major mesenchymal marker which in turn downregulated the expression of ABCG2 transporter expression in sorafenib-resistant HepG2 cells [137].

Wang Y et al. demonstrated that polyphyllin D accelerates lysosomal damage by promoting sphingomyelinase-1 (SMPD-1), resulting in irreversible damage mediated through autophagy blockade and release of lytic contents and entrapped within the hypertrophic lysosomes in sorafenib-resistant HCC cells [138]. Another study by Yao et al. reported that a novel natural CCR2 antagonist named compound-747 potentiated the antitumor ability of sorafenib at lower dosages by relieving the immune suppression mediated by TAMs and increasing $CD8^+$ T-cell-mediated cytotoxicity of the tumor cells under *in-vitro* conditions [139]. Several other phytoactive compounds have already been demonstrated to act synergistically with sorafenib treatment in HCC. For example, compounds such as berberine [140], ocoxin [141], and lectin [142] are shown to promote antitumor effect in various HCC models through sorafenib-sensitization-in

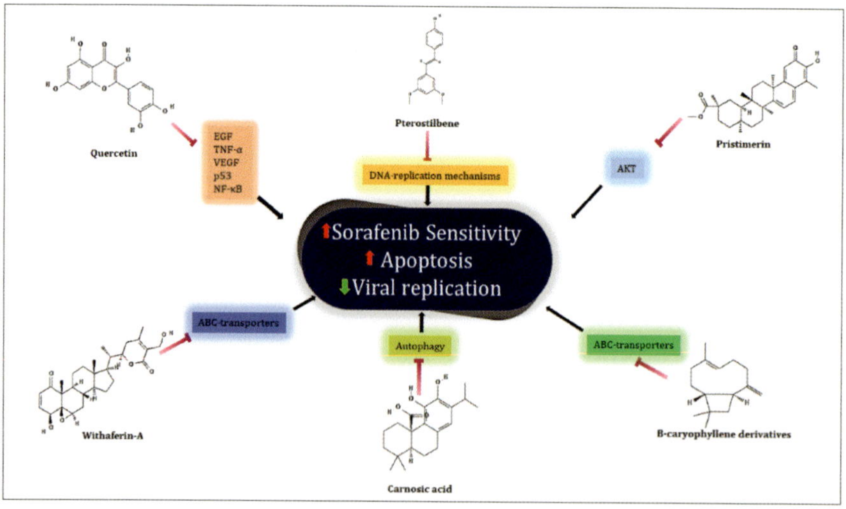

Figure 8: Sorafenib-sensitivity-related mechanisms mediated through various phytochemical active constituents

sorafenib-sensitive HCC cells. However, the ability of these plant-derived compounds to sensitize and act on sorafenib-resistant HCC cells remains open for further examination. Figure 8 depicts the possible mechanisms involved in improving sorafenib sensitivity through various phytochemical active constituents.

5. Summary

HCC is a rapidly evolving disease of concern the world over. While the molecular mechanisms underlying the causation, progression, and spread of this aggressive cancer remain elusive, the emergence of resistance for the only FDA-approved drug is alarming and requires rigorous monitoring and understanding of its possible mechanisms will help combat the emergence of sorafenib resistance in HCC. In the limelight of the same, we have tried to compile the existing knowledge on sorafenib resistance in HCC. As the basic understanding goes, to better understand the mechanisms of sorafenib resistance, we have tried catering to the possible mechanisms of action of the chemotherapeutic agent in leading cellular processes such as apoptosis, immunomodulation, and autophagy.

Sorafenib resistance which can be of primary or acquired resistance can be caused by a wide range of factors and mechanisms at different cellular and molecular levels spanning across different cellular and extracellular niches. These include the changes in the TMEs, reactivation of oncogenic virus, hypoxic stress, stromal cells and their secretions, epigenetic cues, abnormalities in drug transport, and homeostasis mechanisms.

The need of the hour is to find suitable alternatives for sorafenib for the clinical management of HCC. In this direction, phytochemicals and phytoconstituents play an indispensable role. Such bioactive molecules help either sensitizing HCC cells that are resistant to sorafenib and improve the drug-mediated antitumor effect or in general known to act synergistically along with sorafenib in non-resistant HCC. This opens a wide range of opportunities for researchers to evaluate the effectiveness of various phyto-constituents and phytochemicals in addressing sorafenib-resistant HCC.

Acknowledgment

The authors thank DBT-Ramalingaswami Re-Entry Fellowship granted to Prasanna Kumar Santhekadur, UGC-SJSGC Fellowship for Varsha Dilip Shiragannavar, ICMR-SRF Fellowship to Nirmala Gollarahalli Sannappa Gowda, and Lady-Tata Memorial Trust Junior Research Scholarship for Shreyas Hulusemane Karunakara.

Conflict of Interest

All the authors have thoroughly proofread the manuscript and have no conflicts of interest to declare.

References

1. Hsieh, JJ., et al., Renal cell carcinoma. *Nat Rev Dis Primers*, 2017. **3**(1): p. 1–19.

2. Brose, MS., et al., Sorafenib in radioactive iodine-refractory, locally advanced or metastatic differentiated thyroid cancer: a randomised, double-blind, phase 3 trial. *Lancet*, 2014. **384**(9940): p. 319–328.
3. Bruix, J., et al., Adjuvant sorafenib for hepatocellular carcinoma after resection or ablation (STORM): a phase 3, randomised, double-blind, placebo-controlled trial. *Lancet Oncol*, 2015. **16**(13): p. 1344–1354.
4. Wilhelm, SM., et al., BAY 43-9006 Exhibits broad spectrum oral anti-tumor activity and targets the RAF/MEK/ERK pathway and receptor tyrosine kinases involved in tumor progression and angiogenesis. *Cancer Res*, 2004. **64**(19): p. 7099–7109.
5. Liu, L., et al., Sorafenib blocks the RAF/MEK/ERK pathway, inhibits tumor angiogenesis, and induces tumor cell apoptosis in hepatocellular carcinoma model PLC/PRF/5. *Cancer Res*, 2006. **66**(24): p. 11851–11858.
6. Cervello, M., et al., Molecular mechanisms of sorafenib action in liver cancer cells. *Cell Cycle*, 2012. **11**(15): p. 2843–2855.
7. Abeni, E., Salvi, A., Marchina, E., Traversa, M., Arici, B., De Petro, G. Sorafenib induces variations of the DNA methylome in HA22T/VGH human hepatocellular carcinoma-derived cells. *Int J Oncol*, 2017. **51**(1): p. 128–144.
8. Li, Q., et al., HIF-1α-induced expression of m6A reader YTHDF1 drives hypoxia-induced autophagy and malignancy of hepatocellular carcinoma by promoting ATG2A and ATG14 translation. *Signal Transduct Target Ther*, 2021. **6**(1): p. 76.
9. Bao, MHR. and Wong, CCL. Hypoxia, metabolic reprogramming, and drug resistance in liver cancer. *Cells*, 2021. **10**(7): p. 1715.
10. Suthen, S., et al., Hypoxia-driven immunosuppression by Treg and type-2 conventional dendritic cells in HCC. *Hepatology*, 2022. **76**(5): p. 1329–1344.
11. Xu, M., et al., Sorafenib blocks the HIF-1α/VEGFA pathway, inhibits tumor invasion, and induces apoptosis in hepatoma cells. *DNA Cell Biol*, 2014. **33**(5): p. 275–281.
12. Wang, GL., et al., Hypoxia-inducible factor 1 is a basic-helix-loop-helix-PAS heterodimer regulated by cellular O_2 tension. *Proc Natl Acad Sci USA*, 1995. **92**(12): p. 5510–5514.

13. Wang, GL. and Semenza, GL. Purification and characterization of hypoxia-inducible Factor 1. *J Biol Chem*, 1995. **270**(3): p. 1230–1237.
14. Liu L-p., et al., Sorafenib inhibits hypoxia-inducible factor-1α synthesis: implications for antiangiogenic activity in hepatocellular carcinoma. *Clin Cancer Res*, 2012. **18**(20): p. 5662–5671.
15. Horwitz, E., et al., Human and mouse VEGFA-amplified hepatocellular carcinomas are highly sensitive to sorafenib treatment. *Cancer Discov*, 2014. **4**(6): p. 730–743.
16. Hage, C., et al., Sorafenib induces pyroptosis in macrophages and triggers natural killer cell–mediated cytotoxicity against hepatocellular carcinoma. *Hepatology*, 2019. **70**(4): p. 1280–1297.
17. Ahmadzadeh, M., et al., Tumor antigen-specific CD8 T cells infiltrating the tumor express high levels of PD-1 and are functionally impaired. *Blood*, 2009. **114**(8): p. 1537–1544.
18. Mumprecht, S., et al., Programmed death 1 signaling on chronic myeloid leukemia-specific T cells results in T-cell exhaustion and disease progression. *Blood*, 2009. **114**(8): p. 1528–1536.
19. Zhang, L., Gajewski, TF. and Kline, J. PD-1/PD-L1 interactions inhibit antitumor immune responses in a murine acute myeloid leukemia model. *Blood*, 2009. **114**(8): p. 1545–1552.
20. Sakaguchi, S. Naturally arising CD4$^+$ regulatory T cells for immunologic self-tolerance and negative control of immune responses. *Ann Rev Immunol*, 2004. **22**(1): p. 531–562.
21. Chen, ML., et al., Sorafenib relieves cell-intrinsic and cell-extrinsic inhibitions of effector T cells in tumor microenvironment to augment antitumor immunity: sorafenib treatment enhances antitumor immunity in tumor milieu. *Int J Cancer*, 2014. **134**(2): p. 319–331.
22. Tanida, I. Autophagy basics. *Microbiol Immunol*, 2011. **55**(1): p. 1–11.
23. Dikic, I. and Elazar, Z. Mechanism and medical implications of mammalian autophagy. *Nat Rev Mol Cell Biol*, 2018. **19**(6): p. 349–364.
24. Mizushima, N. The role of the Atg1/ULK1 complex in autophagy regulation. *Curr Opin Cell Biol*, 2010. **22**(2): p. 132–139.
25. Yuan, HX., Russell, RC. and Guan, KL. Regulation of PIK3C3/VPS34 complexes by MTOR in nutrient stress-induced autophagy. *Autophagy*, 2013. **9**(12): p. 1983–1995.

26. van der Veen, AG. and Ploegh, HL. Ubiquitin-like proteins. *Ann Rev Biochem*, 2012. **81**(1): p. 323–357.
27. Sou, Y., et al., The Atg8 conjugation system is indispensable for proper development of autophagic isolation membranes in mice. *MBoC*, 2008. **19**(11): p. 4762–4775.
28. Shimizu, S., et al., Inhibition of autophagy potentiates the antitumor effect of the multikinase inhibitor sorafenib in hepatocellular carcinoma. *Int J Cancer*, 2012. **131**(3): p. 548–557.
29. Shi, YH., et al., Targeting autophagy enhances sorafenib lethality for hepatocellular carcinoma via ER stress-related apoptosis. *Autophagy*. 2011. 7(10): p. 1159–1172.
30. Prieto-Domínguez, N., et al., Modulation of autophagy by sorafenib: effects on treatment response. *Front Pharmacol*, 2016. 7: p. 151.
31. Neufeld, TP. TOR-dependent control of autophagy: biting the hand that feeds. *Curr Opin Cell Biol*, 2010. **22**(2): p. 157–168.
32. Sarkar, S. Regulation of autophagy by mTOR-dependent and mTOR-independent pathways: autophagy dysfunction in neurodegenerative diseases and therapeutic application of autophagy enhancers. *Biochem Soc Trans*, 2013. **41**(5): p. 1103–1130.
33. Yang, Z. and Ming, XF. mTOR signalling: the molecular interface connecting metabolic stress, aging and cardiovascular diseases. *Obes Rev*, 2012. **13**(2): p. 58–68.
34. Zhang, C., et al., Sorafenib inhibits liver cancer growth by decreasing mTOR, AKT, and PI3K expression. *J BUON*, 2015. **20**(1): p. 218–222.
35. Zhai, B., et al., Inhibition of Akt reverses the acquired resistance to sorafenib by switching protective autophagy to autophagic cell death in hepatocellular carcinoma. *Mol Cancer Ther*, 2014. **13**(6): p. 1589–1598.
36. Jheng, JR., Ho, JY. and Horng, JT. ER stress, autophagy, and RNA viruses. *Front Microbiol*, 2014. **5**: p. 388.
37. Crespo, I., et al., Glutamine treatment attenuates endoplasmic reticulum stress and apoptosis in TNBS-induced colitis. *PLoS One*, 2012. 7(11): p. e50407.
38. Yi, P., et al., Sorafenib-mediated targeting of the AAA$^+$ ATPase p97/VCP leads to disruption of the secretory pathway, endoplasmic

reticulum stress, and hepatocellular cancer cell death. *Mol Cancer Ther*, 2012. **11**(12): p. 2610–2620.

39. Rahmani, M., et al., The kinase inhibitor sorafenib induces cell death through a process involving induction of endoplasmic reticulum stress. *Mol Cell Biol*, 2007. **27**(15): p. 5499–5513.
40. Kania, E., et al., Calcium homeostasis and ER stress in control of autophagy in cancer cells. *Biomed Res Int*, 2015. 2015:352794.
41. Ajoolabady, A., et al., Endoplasmic reticulum stress in liver diseases. *Hepatology*, 2023. 77(2): p. 619–639.
42. Llovet, JM., et al., Sorafenib in advanced hepatocellular carcinoma. *N Engl J Med*, 2008. **359**(4): p. 378–390.
43. O'Connor, R., et al., Drug resistance in cancer-searching for mechanisms, markers and therapeutic agents. *Expert Opin Drug Metab Toxicol*, 2007. **3**(6): p. 805–817.
44. Xia, S., et al., The microenvironmental and metabolic aspects of sorafenib resistance in hepatocellular carcinoma. *EBioMedicine*, 2020. **51**: p. 102610.
45. Ito, Y., et al., Expression and clinical significance of erb-B receptor family in hepatocellular carcinoma. *Br J Cancer*, 2001. **84**(10): p. 1377–1383.
46. Zhang, Z., et al., Phosphorylated ERK is a potential predictor of sensitivity to sorafenib when treating hepatocellular carcinoma: evidence from an in vitro study. *BMC Med*, 2009. 7: p. 41.
47. D'souza, S., et al., Molecular mechanisms of viral hepatitis induced hepatocellular carcinoma. *World J Gastroenterol*, 2020. **26**(38): p. 5759–5783.
48. D'Angelo, S., et al., Sorafenib and entecavir: the dioscuri of treatment for advanced hepatocellular carcinoma? *World J Gastroenterol*, 2013. **19**(14): p. 2141–2143.
49. Pattullo, V. Hepatitis B reactivation in the setting of chemotherapy and immunosuppression-prevention is better than cure. *World J Hepatol*. 2015. 7(7): p. 954–967.
50. Descamps, V., et al., The kinase-inhibitor sorafenib inhibits multiple steps of the hepatitis C virus infectious cycle in vitro. *Antiviral Res*. 2015. **118**: p. 93–102.

51. Cabrera, R., et al., The antiviral effect of sorafenib in hepatitis C-related hepatocellular carcinoma. *Aliment Pharmacol Ther*, 2013. **37**(1): p. 91–97.
52. Himmelsbach, K. and Hildt, E. The kinase inhibitor sorafenib impairs the antiviral effect of interferon α on hepatitis C virus replication. *Eur J Cell Biol*, 2013. **92**(1): p. 12–20.
53. Zhang, QB., et al., Suppression of natural killer cells by sorafenib contributes to prometastatic effects in hepatocellular carcinoma. *PLoS One*. 2013. **8**(2): p. e55945.
54. Witt-Kehati, D., et al., Inhibition of pMAPK14 overcomes resistance to sorafenib in hepatoma cells with hepatitis b virus. *Transl Oncol*, 2018. **11**(2): p. 511–517.
55. Binnewies, M., et al., Understanding the tumor immune microenvironment (TIME) for effective therapy. *Nat Med*, 2018. **24**(5): p. 541–50.
56. Zhang, T., et al., Targeting the tumor biophysical microenvironment to reduce resistance to immunotherapy. *Adv Drug Deliv Rev*, 2022. **186**: p. 114319.
57. Mao, X., et al., Crosstalk between cancer-associated fibroblasts and immune cells in the tumor microenvironment: new findings and future perspectives. *Mol Cancer*, 2021. **20**(1): p. 131.
58. Richards, KE., et al., Cancer-associated fibroblast exosomes regulate survival and proliferation of pancreatic cancer cells. *Oncogene*, 2017. **36**(13): p. 1770–1778.
59. Cooke, VG., et al., Pericyte depletion results in hypoxia-associated epithelial-to-mesenchymal transition and metastasis mediated by met signaling pathway. *Cancer Cell*, 2012. **21**(1): p. 66–81.
60. Liang, Y., et al., Hypoxia-mediated sorafenib resistance can be overcome by EF24 through Von Hippel-Lindau tumor suppressor-dependent HIF-1α inhibition in hepatocellular carcinoma. *Hepatology*, 2013. **57**(5): p. 1847–1857.
61. Méndez-Blanco, C., et al., Sorafenib resistance in hepatocarcinoma: role of hypoxia-inducible factors. *Exp Mol Med*, 2018. **50**(10): p. 1–9.
62. Dong, XF., et al., COX-2/PGE2 axis regulates HIF2α activity to promote hepatocellular carcinoma hypoxic response and reduce the

sensitivity of sorafenib treatment. *Clin Cancer Res*, 2018. **24**(13): p. 3204–3216.
63. Song, Z., et al., HIF-1α-induced RIT1 promotes liver cancer growth and metastasis and its deficiency increases sensitivity to sorafenib. *Cancer Lett*, 2019. **460**: p. 96–107.
64. Ma, L., et al., 2-Methoxyestradiol synergizes with sorafenib to suppress hepatocellular carcinoma by simultaneously dysregulating hypoxia-inducible factor-1 and -2. *Cancer Lett*, 2014. **355**(1): p. 96–105.
65. Liu, F., et al., Targeting hypoxia-inducible factor-2α enhances sorafenib antitumor activity via β-catenin/C-Myc-dependent pathways in hepatocellular carcinoma. *Oncol Lett*, 2015. **10**(2): p. 778–784.
66. Zhu, Z., et al., Yin-yang effect of tumour cells in breast cancer: from mechanism of crosstalk between tumour-associated macrophages and cancer-associated adipocytes. *Am J Cancer Res*, 2020. **10**(2): p. 383–392.
67. Wei, X., et al., Tumor-associated macrophages promote the proliferation and migration as well as invasion of sorafenib-resistant hepatocellular carcinoma cells. *Xi Bao Yu Fen Zi Mian Yi Xue Za Zhi*, 2017. **33**(5): p. 617–622.
68. Wu, FQ., et al., ADRB2 signaling promotes HCC progression and sorafenib resistance by inhibiting autophagic degradation of HIF1α. *J Hepatol*, 2016. **65**(2): p. 314–324.
69. Fan, QM., et al., Tumor-associated macrophages promote cancer stem cell-like properties via transforming growth factor-beta1-induced epithelial-mesenchymal transition in hepatocellular carcinoma. *Cancer Lett*, 2014. **352**(2): p. 160–168.
70. Multhaupt, HAB., et al., Extracellular matrix component signaling in cancer. *Adv Drug Deliv Rev*, 2016. **97**: p. 28–40.
71. Pein, M., et al., Metastasis-initiating cells induce and exploit a fibroblast niche to fuel malignant colonization of the lungs. *Nat Commun*, 2020. **11**(1): p. 1494.
72. Liu, J., et al., Cancer-associated fibroblasts provide a stromal niche for liver cancer organoids that confers trophic effects and therapy resistance. *Cell Mol Gastroenterol Hepatol*, 2021.**11**(2): p. 407–431.

73. Gao, L., et al., The BAFF/NFκB axis is crucial to interactions between sorafenib-resistant HCC cells and cancer-associated fibroblasts. *Cancer Sci*, 2021. **112**(9): p. 3545–3554.
74. Peng, H., et al., Cancer-associated fibroblasts enhance the chemoresistance of CD73^{+} hepatocellular carcinoma cancer cells via HGF-Met-ERK1/2 pathway. *Ann Transl Med*, 2020. **8**(14): p. 856.
75. Strauss, L., et al., Implications of metabolism-driven myeloid dysfunctions in cancer therapy. *Cell Mol Immunol*, 2021. **18**(4): p. 829–841.
76. Bruix, J., et al., Prognostic factors and predictors of sorafenib benefit in patients with hepatocellular carcinoma: analysis of two phase III studies. *J Hepatol*, 2017. **67**(5): p. 999–1008.
77. Li, YW., et al., Intratumoral neutrophils: a poor prognostic factor for hepatocellular carcinoma following resection. *J Hepatol*, 2011. **54**(3): p. 497–505.
78. Zhou, SL., et al., Tumor-associated neutrophils recruit macrophages and T-regulatory cells to promote progression of hepatocellular carcinoma and resistance to sorafenib. *Gastroenterology*, 2016. **150**(7): p. 1646–1658.e17.
79. Deng, X., et al., Myeloid-derived suppressor cells promote tumor growth and sorafenib resistance by inducing FGF1 upregulation and fibrosis. *Neoplasia*, 2022. **28**: p. 100788.
80. Gao, Y., et al., Intratumoral stem-like CCR4^{+} regulatory T cells orchestrate the immunosuppressive microenvironment in HCC associated with hepatitis B. *J Hepatol*, 2022. **76**(1): p. 148–159.
81. Shrestha, R., et al., Combined inhibition of TGF-β1-induced EMT and PD-L1 silencing re-sensitizes hepatocellular carcinoma to sorafenib treatment. *J Clin Med*, 2021. **10**(9): p. 1889.
82. Ungerleider, N., et al., TGFβ signaling confers sorafenib resistance via induction of multiple RTKs in hepatocellular carcinoma cells. *Mol Carcinog*. 2017. **56**(4): p. 1302–1311.
83. Bhagyaraj, E., et al., TGF-β induced chemoresistance in liver cancer is modulated by xenobiotic nuclear receptor PXR. *Cell Cycle*, 2019. **18**(24): p. 3589–3602.
84. Liu, J., et al., Targeting the PD-L1/DNMT1 axis in acquired resistance to sorafenib in human hepatocellular carcinoma. *Oncol Rep*, 2017. **38**(2): p. 899–907.

85. Xu, GL., et al., Upregulation of PD-L1 expression promotes epithelial-to-mesenchymal transition in sorafenib-resistant hepatocellular carcinoma cells. *Gastroenterol Rep (Oxf)*, 2020. **8**(5): p. 390–398.
86. Xu, R., c-Met up-regulates the expression of PD-L1 through MAPK/NF-κBp65 pathway. *J Mol Med (Berl)*, 2022. **100**(4): p. 585–598.
87. Lai, SC., et al., DNMT3b/OCT4 expression confers sorafenib resistance and poor prognosis of hepatocellular carcinoma through IL-6/STAT3 regulation. *J Exp Clin Cancer Res*, 2019. **38**(1): p. 474.
88. Ren, Y., et al., CXCR3 confers sorafenib resistance of HCC cells through regulating metabolic alteration and AMPK pathway. *Am J Transl Res*, 2020. **12**(3): p. 825–836.
89. Durmus, S., et al., Apical ABC transporters and cancer chemotherapeutic drug disposition. *Adv Cancer Res*, 2015. **125**: p. 1–41.
90. Beretta, GL., et al., Overcoming ABC transporter-mediated multidrug resistance: the dual role of tyrosine kinase inhibitors as multitargeting agents. *Eur J Med Chem*, 2017. **142**: p. 271–289.
91. Tian, XP., et al., Acidic microenvironment up-regulates exosomal miR-21 and miR-10b in early-stage hepatocellular carcinoma to promote cancer cell proliferation and metastasis. *Theranostics*, 2019. **9**(7): p. 1965–1979.
92. Lou, G., et al., Exosomes derived from miR-122-modified adipose tissue-derived MSCs increase chemosensitivity of hepatocellular carcinoma. *J Hematol Oncol*, 2015. **8**: p. 122.
93. Qu, Z., et al., Exosomes derived from HCC cells induce sorafenib resistance in hepatocellular carcinoma both in vivo and in vitro. *J Exp Clin Cancer Res*, 2016. **35**(1): p. 159.
94. Luo, T., et al., PSMD10/gankyrin induces autophagy to promote tumor progression through cytoplasmic interaction with ATG7 and nuclear transactivation of ATG7 expression. *Autophagy*, 2016. **12**(8): p. 1355–1371.
95. Lin, Z., et al., RNA m6 A methylation regulates sorafenib resistance in liver cancer through FOXO3-mediated autophagy. *EMBO J*. 2020. **39**(12): p. e103181.
96. Tong, M., et al., Efficacy of annexin A3 blockade in sensitizing hepatocellular carcinoma to sorafenib and regorafenib. *J Hepatol*, 2018. **69**(4): p. 826–839.

97. Lee, JY., et al., Lipid metabolism and ferroptosis. *Biology*, 2021. **10**(3): p. 184.
98. Sun, X., et al., Metallothionein-1G facilitates sorafenib resistance through inhibition of ferroptosis. *Hepatology*, 2016. **64**(2): p. 488–500.
99. Louandre, C., et al., Iron-dependent cell death of hepatocellular carcinoma cells exposed to sorafenib. *Int J Cancer*, 2013. **133**(7): p. 1732–1742.
100. Huang, Q., et al., CD147 promotes reprogramming of glucose metabolism and cell proliferation in HCC cells by inhibiting the p53-dependent signaling pathway. *J Hepatol*, 2014. **61**(4): p. 859–866.
101. Wong, TL., et al., CRAF methylation by PRMT6 regulates aerobic glycolysis-driven hepatocarcinogenesis via ERK-dependent PKM2 nuclear relocalization and activation. *Hepatology*, 2020. **71**(4): p. 1279–1296.
102. Fiaschi, T., et al., Reciprocal metabolic reprogramming through lactate shuttle coordinately influences tumor-stroma interplay. *Cancer Res*, 2012. **72**(19): p. 5130–5140.
103. Zhang, C., et al., Sorafenib targets the mitochondrial electron transport chain complexes and ATP synthase to activate the PINK1-Parkin pathway and modulate cellular drug response. *J Biol Chem*, 2017. **292**(36): p. 15105–15120.
104. Liao, J., et al., Regulation of stem-like cancer cells by glutamine through β-catenin pathway mediated by redox signaling. *Mol Cancer*, 2017. **16**(1): p. 51.
105. Sohn, BH., et al., Glutamine synthetase mediates sorafenib sensitivity in β-catenin-active hepatocellular carcinoma cells. *Exp Mol Med*, 2018. **50**(1): p. e421.
106. Sun, X., et al., Activation of the p62-Keap1-NRF2 pathway protects against ferroptosis in hepatocellular carcinoma cells. *Hepatology*, 2016. **63**(1): p. 173–184.
107. Lee, D., et al., Induction of oxidative stress through inhibition of thioredoxin reductase 1 is an effective therapeutic approach for hepatocellular carcinoma. *Hepatology*, 2019. **69**(4): p. 1768–1786.
108. Lee, D., et al., Folate cycle enzyme MTHFD1L confers metabolic advantages in hepatocellular carcinoma. *J Clin Invest*, 2017. **127**(5): p. 1856–1872.

109. Xu, IMJ., et al., Transketolase counteracts oxidative stress to drive cancer development. *Proc Natl Acad Sci USA*, 2016. **113**(6): p. 725–734.
110. Wang, S., et al., Sorafenib suppresses growth and survival of hepatoma cells by accelerating degradation of enhancer of zeste homolog 2. *Cancer Sci*, 2013. **104**(6): p. 750–759.
111. Wang, T., et al., Epigenetic restriction of Hippo signaling by MORC2 underlies stemness of hepatocellular carcinoma cells. *Cell Death Differ*, 2018. **25**(12): p. 2086–2100.
112. Wang, Z., et al., Anti-GPC3 antibody tagged cationic switchable lipid-based nanoparticles for the co-delivery of anti-miRNA27a and sorafenib in liver cancers. *Pharm Res*, 2019. **36**(10): p. 145.
113. Jiang, XM., et al., microRNA-19a-3p promotes tumor metastasis and chemoresistance through the PTEN/Akt pathway in hepatocellular carcinoma. *Biomed Pharmacother*, 2018. **105**: p. 1147–1154.
114. Callegari, E., et al., miR-199a-3p modulates MTOR and PAK4 pathways and inhibits tumor growth in a hepatocellular carcinoma transgenic mouse model. *Mol Ther Nucleic Acids*, 2018. **11**: p. 485–493.
115. Pollutri, D., et al., The epigenetically regulated miR-494 associates with stem-cell phenotype and induces sorafenib resistance in hepatocellular carcinoma. *Cell Death Dis*, 2018. **9**(1): p. 4.
116. Pollutri, D., et al., In hepatocellular carcinoma miR-221 modulates sorafenib resistance through inhibition of caspase-3-mediated apoptosis. *Clin Cancer Res*, 2017. **23**(14): p. 3953–3965.
117. Potenza, N., et al., MicroRNA-125a-5p is a downstream effector of sorafenib in its antiproliferative activity toward human hepatocellular carcinoma cells. *J Cell Physiol*, 2017. **232**(7): p. 1907–1913.
118. Azumi, J., et al., miR-181a induces sorafenib resistance of hepatocellular carcinoma cells through downregulation of RASSF1 expression. *Cancer Sci*, 2016. **107**(9): p. 1256–1262.
119. Stiuso, P., et al., MicroRNA-423-5p promotes autophagy in cancer cells and is increased in serum from hepatocarcinoma patients treated with sorafenib. *Mol Ther Nucleic Acids*, 2015. **4**: p. e233.
120. He, C., et al., MiR-21 mediates sorafenib resistance of hepatocellular carcinoma cells by inhibiting autophagy via the PTEN/Akt pathway. *Oncotarget*, 2015. **6**(30): p. 28867–28881.

121. Lu, AQ., et al., Upregulation of miR-137 reverses sorafenib resistance and cancer-initiating cell phenotypes by degrading ANT2 in hepatocellular carcinoma. *Oncol Rep*, 2017. **37**(4): p. 2071–2078.
122. Xu, J., et al., The miR-367-3p increases sorafenib chemotherapy efficacy to suppress hepatocellular carcinoma metastasis through altering the androgen receptor signals. *EBioMedicine*, 2016. **12**: p. 55–67.
123. Wang, H., et al., MicroRNA-591 functions as a tumor suppressor in hepatocellular carcinoma by lowering drug resistance through inhibition of far-upstream element-binding protein 2-mediated phosphoinositide 3-kinase/Akt/Mammalian target of rapamycin axis. *Pharmacol*, 2019. **104**(3–4): p. 173–186.
124. Dietrich, P., et al., Wild type Kirsten rat sarcoma is a novel microRNA-622-regulated therapeutic target for hepatocellular carcinoma and contributes to sorafenib resistance. *Gut*, 2018. **67**(7): p. 1328–1341.
125. Kabir, TD., et al., A microRNA-7/growth arrest specific 6/TYRO3 axis regulates the growth and invasiveness of sorafenib-resistant cells in human hepatocellular carcinoma. *Hepatology*, 2018. **67**(1): p. 216–231.
126. Zhang, M., et al., MiR-374b re-sensitizes hepatocellular carcinoma cells to sorafenib therapy by antagonizing PKM2-mediated glycolysis pathway. *Am J Cancer Res*, 2019. **9**(4): p. 765–778.
127. Li, D., et al., MicroRNA-375 represses tumor angiogenesis and reverses resistance to sorafenib in hepatocarcinoma. *Cancer Gene Ther*, 2021. **28**(1–2): p. 126–140.
128. Zhang, Z., et al., The miR-30a-5p/CLCF1 axis regulates sorafenib resistance and aerobic glycolysis in hepatocellular carcinoma. *Cell Death Dis*, 2020. **11**(10): p. 902.
129. Kumar, AR., et al., Anti-VEGF mediated immunomodulatory role of phytochemicals: scientific exposition for plausible HCC treatment. *CDT*, 2021. **22**(11): p. 1288–1316.
130. Zhang, Z., et al., Dietary antioxidant quercetin overcomes the acquired resistance of Sorafenib in Sorafenib-resistant hepatocellular carcinoma cells through epidermal growth factor receptor signaling inactivation. *Naunyn Schmiedebergs Arch Pharmacol*, 2023. **397**: p. 559–574.

131. Abdu, S., et al., Effects of sorafenib and quercetin alone or in combination in treating hepatocellular carcinoma: in vitro and in vivo approaches. *Molecules*, 2022. **27**(22): p. 8082.
132. Wang, R., et al., Pterostilbene inhibits hepatocellular carcinoma proliferation and HBV replication by targeting ribonucleotide reductase M2 protein. *Am J Cancer Res*, 2021. **11**(6): p. 2975–2989.
133. Tang, Y., et al., Pristimerin synergistically sensitizes conditionally reprogrammed patient derived-primary hepatocellular carcinoma cells to sorafenib through endoplasmic reticulum stress and ROS generation by modulating Akt/FoxO1/p27kip1 signaling pathway. *Phytomedicine*, 2021. **86**: p. 153563.
134. Di Giacomo, S., et al., Chemosensitization of hepatocellular carcinoma cells to sorafenib by β-caryophyllene oxide-induced inhibition of ABC export pumps. *Arch Toxicol*, 2019. **93**(3): p. 623–634.
135. Wu, Q., et al., Enhancement of sorafenib-mediated death of Hepatocellular carcinoma cells by carnosic acid and vitamin D2 analog combination. *J Steroid Biochem Mol Biol*, 2020. **197**: p. 105524.
136. Shiragannavar, VD., et al., Withaferin A acts as a novel regulator of liver X receptor-α in HCC. *Front Oncol*, 2020. **10**: p. 628506.
137. Makol, A., Vimentin as a potential therapeutic target in sorafenib resistant HepG2, a HCC model cell line. *Clin Mol Hepatol*, 2020. **26**(1): p. 45–53.
138. Wang, Y., et al., Polyphyllin D punctures hypertrophic lysosomes to reverse drug resistance of hepatocellular carcinoma by targeting acid sphingomyelinase. *Mol Ther*, 2023. **31**(7): p. 2169–2187.
139. Yao, W, et al., A natural CCR2 antagonist relieves tumor-associated macrophage-mediated immunosuppression to produce a therapeutic effect for liver cancer. *EBioMedicine*, 2017. **22**: p. 58–67.
140. Huang, Y., et al., Berberine, a natural plant alkaloid, synergistically sensitizes human liver cancer cells to sorafenib. *Oncol Rep*, 2018. **40**(3): p. 1525–1532.
141. Benedicto, A., et al., Ocoxin as a complement to first line treatments in cancer. *Int J Med Sci*, 2021. **18**(3): p. 835–845.
142. Zhang, CZ., et al., *Momordica charantia* lectin exhibits antitumor activity towards hepatocellular carcinoma. *Invest New Drugs*, 2015. **33**(1): p. 1–11.

https://doi.org/10.1142/9789811293320_0006

Chapter 6

Phytochemicals as Chemosensitizers in the Management of Hepatocellular Carcinoma

Silpa Prabha[1], Anju Jose[1], Aleena Mariya Davis[1] and Kanjoormana Aryan Manu[1,*]

[1]*Deptartment of Immunology, Amala Cancer Research Centre, Amala Nagar, Thrissur, Kerala 680555, India*

Table of Contents:

*Corresponding author: E-mail address: manu.aryan@amalaims.org or manukanjoor @gmail.com

Abbreviations:

5-FU — 5-fluorouracil
ABCB1 — ATP-binding cassette subfamily B member 1
ABCC1 — ATP-binding cassette subfamily C member 1
ABCG2 — ATP-binding cassette subfamily G member 2
Akt — Ak strain transforming 1
AMPK — AMP-activated protein kinase
APC — antigen-presenting cell
APG — Apigenin
ARID — AT-rich interactive domain-containing protein
ASCT2 — Alanine, serine, cysteine transporter 2
ATG7 — Autophagy-related gene 7
ATM — Ataxia telangiectasia mutated
ATP — Adenosine Triphosphate
AXIN1/2 — Axis inhibition protein 1/2
Bax — Bcl-2-associated X protein
Bcl-2 — B-cell lymphoma 2
Bcl-xl — B-cell lymphoma-extra large
BMPs — Bone morphogenic proteins
CCL2-MCP-1/chemokine (c-c motif)ligand 2
CD133 — Cluster of differentiation 133
CD13 — Cluster of differentiation 13
CD24 — Cluster of differentiation 24
CD44 — Cluster of differentiation 44
CD47 — Cluster of differentiation 47
CD90 — Cluster of differentiation 24
CDC25A — Cell division cycle 25 homolog A
CDK2 — Cyclin-dependent kinase 2

CDK4/6 — Cyclin-dependent kinase 4 and 6
CDK — Cyclin-dependent kinases
CDKN2B (p15INK4b) — Cyclin-dependent kinase 4 inhibitor B
CGA — Chlorogenic acid
CIN — Chromosomal instability
CIN — mitotic error-mediated chromosomal instability
Cisplatin (cis-diamminedichloroplatinum (II) or cisplatin), or CDDP
c-KIT-Receptor tyrosine kinase inhibitors
CKLF1 — chemokine-like-factor 1
c-Met — mesenchymal-epithelial transition factor
c-Myc — Cellular Myc
COX-2 — Cyclooxygenase 2
CSCs — Cancer stem cells
c-Src — Cellular Src
CTD — Cantharidin
CTLA4 — Cytotoxic T-lymphocyte associated protein 4
CTNNB1 — Catenin beta 1
CYP3A4 — Cytochrome P450 3A4
DEN — Diethylnitrosamine
Dios-DOX-LP — Diosgenin-based liposome loaded with DOX
DLK1 — Protein delta homolog 1
DPD — Dihydropyrimidine dehydrogenase
DPYS — Dihydropyrimidinase
eEF2K — Eukaryotic elongation factor 2 kinase
EGCG — Epigallocatechin-3-O-gallate
EGF — Epidermal growth factor
EGFR — Epidermal growth factor receptor
EMT — Epithelial-mesenchymal transition
EpCAM — Epithelial cell adhesion molecule
ErbB/HER — Epidermal growth factor receptor family/human epidermal growth factor receptor
ERK — Extracellular signal-regulated kinases
FBAL α — Fluoro-alanine
FdUMP — Fluorodeoxyuridine monophosphate
FdUTP — Fluorodeoxyuridine triphosphate

FGF19 — Fibroblast growth factor 19
FGF1 — Fibroblast growth factor 1
FGF — Fibroblast growth factor
FGFR1–4 — Fibroblast growth factor receptor 1–4
FLT-3 — FMS-like tyrosine kinase 3
FOXO1 — Forkhead box protein O1
FUPA-α-fluoro-β-ureidopropionic acid
FUTP — fluorouridine triphosphate
FZD — Frizzled receptor
FZD7 — frizzled class receptor 7
GNT — Genistein
GSK-3β — Glycogen synthase kinase-3 beta
H3K36me3 — Histone H3 trimethylation at lysine 36
HBV — Hepatitis B virus
HCC — Hepatocellular carcinoma
HCV — Hepatitis C virus
HGF — Hepatocyte growth factor
HIF-1α — Hypoxia-inducible factor-1alpha
YAP — Hippo/yes associated protein
ICAM 1 — Intercellular adhesion molecule 1
ICI — Immune checkpoint inhibitors
IGF-1R-Type 1 insulin-like growth factor receptor
IL-33 — Interleukin 33
IL-6 — Interleukin 6
JAK 1 — Janus kinase 1
JAK 2 — Janus kinase 2
JNK — Jun N-terminal kinase
KDM4A — Lysine-specific demethylase 4A
KIT-Receptor tyrosine kinase type III
LC3-II-LC3-phosphatidylethanolamine conjugate (LC3-II)
LDL — low-density lipoprotein cholesterol
LVN — Lenvatinib
Lgr5 — Leucine-rich repeat containing G protein-coupled receptor
Lin28B — Lin-28 homolog B
LT — Liver transplantation

MAPK — Mitogen-activated protein kinase
Mcl-1 — Myeloid cell leukemia-1
MDR1 — Multidrug resistance protein 1
MEK — MAP kinase
MMP-9 — Matrix metalloproteinase-9
MRP1-4 — Multidrug resistance proteins 1-4
mTOR — Mammalian target of rapamycin
MDR — Multidrug resistance
N-cadherin — Neural cadherin
NF-κB — Nuclear factor kappa B
Nrf2 — nuclear factor erythroid 2–related factor 2
NRP2 — Neuropilin 2
NSCLC — Non-small-cell lung cancer
OV6 — Oval cell marker
PARP — Poly (ADP-ribose) polymerases
PCNA — Proliferating cell nuclear antigen
PD1 — programmed death-ligand 1
PDGFR — platelet-derived growth factor receptors
PDGFR α — Platelet-derived growth factor receptor alpha
PDGFR β — Platelet-derived growth factor receptor beta
PDGFβ — Platelet-derived growth factor beta
PDL1 — programmed cell death protein 1
PGE2 — Prostaglandin E2
P-gp — permeability glycoprotein 1
PI3K — phosphoinositide 3-kinase
PKA — Protein kinase A
PPD-20(S)-protopanaxadiol
PPT-20(S)-protopanaxatriol
PTEN — Phosphatase and tensin homolog
QE — Quercetin
RAF-1-Apurinic/apyrimidinic endonuclease/redox factor-1
RAF — rapidly accelerated fibrosarcoma
Ras — Rat sarcoma virus
REF — Restriction endonuclease fingerprinting
RET — Rearranged during transfection
ROS — Reactive oxygen species

SGLT2 — Sodium-glucose cotransporter-2
SHP-1 — Src homology region 2 domain-containing phosphatase-1
SOR — Sorafenib
STAT3 — Signal transducer and activator of transcription 3
TACE — Transarterial chemoembolization
TCF/LEF — T cell factor/lymphoid enhancer factor family
TERT — Telomerase reverse transcriptase
TGFBR2 — Transforming growth factor beta receptor type 2
TGF-β — Transforming growth factor beta
THOC1 — THO complex subunit 1
TKI — Tyrosine kinase inhibitors
TKs — Tyrosine kinase substrate
TNF — Tumor necrosis factor
TNF-α — Tumor necrosis factor-alpha
TOP2A-DNA topoisomerase IIα
TRAIL — TNF-related apoptosis inducing ligand
TEAD — Transcriptional coactivator transcription enhanced associate domain
TS — Thymidine synthetase
UGT1A9 — UDP glucuronosyltransferase family 1 member A9
UPB1-β-ureidopropionase
VEGF — Vascular endothelial growth factor
VEGFR2 — Vascular endothelial growth factor 2
VEGFR — Vascular endothelial growth factor
VEGFR3 — vascular endothelial growth factor 3

Abstract

Hepatocellular carcinoma is the most common type of liver cancers with a highest incidence rate in Asia and Africa. Even though surgical resection or hepatectomy and liver transplantation are major treatment strategies, chemotherapy is inevitable for the patients either with possible metastasis or not eligible for surgery. Resistance to the chemotherapy is a major concern for cancer patients, and use of drugs in combination is a common possible strategy to tackle the resistance. It has been reported that various signal transduction pathways are involved in developing chemotherapy resistance.

Targeting these pathways is a useful strategy to overcome the resistance. Plant-derived compounds and plant extracts are known to be highly dependable as a source for anticancer drugs. Today it is estimated that 25%–28% of all modern medicines are directly or indirectly derived from plant sources. They are also known to target many molecular signaling that contribute to chemotherapy resistance. This review consolidates various findings that underline the possible use of plant-derived substances as chemosensitizers with its molecular mechanisms. The review also demands a focused approach to bring plant-derived drugs to clinics for making a cheaper and effective strategy to overcome the therapy resistance against HCC.

1. Introduction

Hepatocellular carcinoma (HCC) is a prominent liver malignancy worldwide. Aflatoxin ingestion, HBV and HCV infections, and alcoholic and non-alcoholic fatty liver disease are the main risk factors associated with the development of HCC [1, 2]. Depending on the stage of HCC, curative and palliative treatment methods were chosen. Liver transplantation (LT), local ablation, and hepatic resection are beneficial for treating early-stage HCC while transarterial chemoembolization (TACE) and systemic therapy (chemotherapy, targeted therapy, and immunotherapy) are for intermediate and advanced stages [3–5].

LT is a good therapeutic option for early-stage HCC since it replaces a damaged liver that might in the future become the source of HCC in addition to removing the tumor lesions [6]. As LT corrects the underlying hepatic insufficiency, it is thought to be the best treatment option for cirrhotic patients who have early-stage HCC. Milan criteria is used as the reference criteria for selecting LT patients, and with this criterion, there is a 75% of 5-year overall survival rate and a less than 15% of tumor recurrence rate [4, 5]. Hepatic resection can be done for treating early-stage HCC. A small percentage of individuals with single nodules, normal liver function, and no underlying cirrhosis can be treated with surgical resection [2]. Benefits of LT clearly outweigh those of liver resection because the danger of developing new HCC remains with the residual liver tissue. Although surgical resection patients have a 5-year survival rate of approximately 70%, they are at a high risk of HCC recurrence [4].

For treating early-stage HCC, image-guided percutaneous ablation is used as the most effective method. It is advantageous that percutaneous ablation is curative, barely invasive, and repeatable during cancer recurrences [7]. Patients who cannot have LT or surgical resection benefit most from ablative treatments. Earlier ethanol injection, the inexpensive and easy method of ablation, was mostly used for small HCC treatment [7, 8]. Other methods are microwave ablation, radiofrequency ablation (commonly used), irreversible electroporation, and cryoablation [9–12].

For intermediate-stage HCC patients, TACE is used as first-line treatment. It involves catheterization for delivering a very high dosage of chemotherapy along with an embolizing agent to the hepatic portal vein that supplies blood to the tumor. Embolization of the tumor microcirculation causes prolonged cytotoxic effects and reduced systemic toxicity compared to chemotherapy [13]. A combination of TACE and ICI can be employed for treating even advanced stages of HCC. TACE treatment with immune checkpoint inhibitor Camrelizumab showed a favorable safety profile and promising efficacy against unresectable HCC [14]. TACE combined with sorafenib plus immune checkpoint inhibitors was highly efficient and safe for treating intermediate and advanced stages of HCC [15]. Advanced HCC can be treated effectively with checkpoint inhibitors that target PD1, PDL1, and CTLA4. First-line treatment using a combination of PDL1 blockade with atezolizumab and VEGF blockade with bevacizumab is found to be highly effective for advanced HCC [16].

Chemotherapy is the most widely used treatment modality for treating advanced HCC [17]. Sorafenib has been the gold standard first-line systemic chemotherapeutic for advanced HCC since 2007. Other nonspecific cytotoxic drugs such as 5-fluorouracil (5-FU), doxorubicin (DOX), cisplatin, and so on are also used against HCC. Chemotherapeutics mainly targets rapidly dividing cancer cells.

The prolonged use of these cytotoxic drugs eventually develops chemoresistance which makes chemotherapy less efficient with a higher chance of tumor recurrence [18].

2. Common Chemotherapeutics Against HCC

2.1. *Sorafenib*

This multi-target tyrosine kinase inhibitor suppresses the activity of several kinases including EGFR, VEGFR, PDGFR, RAF kinases, and so on which is extended the total median survival in advanced HCC patients through its antiproliferation and antiangiogenesis properties [19, 20]. Usually, sorafenib is administered twice daily at a dosage of 400 mg with 25–48 hours of average half-life and 38%–49% of mean bioavailability. This anticancer agent is metabolized in liver by CYP3A4 and UGT1A9 in the liver [21].

Sorafenib inhibits the proliferation of cancer cells via Ras/Raf/MEKERK signaling pathways by suppressing the activity of Raf serine/threonine kinase isoforms. This anticancer agent inhibits tumor angiogenesis by targeting various receptors including c-KIT, VEGFR2, VEGFR3, RET, PDGFR β, and FLT-3 [20, 22]. Several adverse effects, including physical, gastrointestinal, and skin problems (hand and foot skin responses, weight loss, and diarrhea), are seen in sorafenib-treated patients, which leads to discontinuation of treatment [23, 24]. Sorafenib is effective in about 30% of HCC patients; unfortunately, this group develops therapy resistance within 6 months of treatment. Recent studies suggest that epigenetics, controlled cell death, the tumor microenvironment, and transport pathways are involved in sorafenib resistance in HCC [20].

2.2. *5-fluorouracil*

5-fluorouracil or 5-FU, a first-line cytotoxic anticancer drug, is predominantly used in the treatment of rectal, colon, gastric, breast, pancreatic, bladder, ovarian, and liver cancers. The FDA approved this heterocyclic organic aromatic medication as an antineoplastic agent, after Heidelberger introduced it in the 1950s. 5-FU is a uracil analog where the hydrogen at C5 position is replaced with fluorine atom. This structure causes 5-FU to block cell division and interfere with nucleotide synthesis [25].

In cancer cells, only 1%–3% of initial dosage of 5-FU mediates its cytotoxic effects through anabolic activities. In the liver, dihydropyrimidine dehydrogenase (DPD) catabolizes the remaining 80%–85% of 5-FU into inactive 5,6-dihydro-5-fluorouracil (DHFU) [26]. Further, DHFU is converted into α-fluoro-β-ureidopropionic acid (FUPA) and finally to α-fluoro-alanine (FBAL) by dihydropyrimidinase (DPYS) and β-ureidopropionase (UPB1), respectively through decarboxylation, and deamination reactions [27]. The active final metabolites of 5-FU are fluorouridine triphosphate (FUTP), fluorodeoxyuridine monophosphate (FdUMP), and fluorodeoxyuridine triphosphate (FdUTP), these metabolites inhibit proliferation of cancer cells in a unique way [28]. Among these, FdUMP induces indirect DNA damage by inhibiting thymidine synthetase (TS), which creates deoxynucleotide imbalances. On the other hand, FdUT causes direct damage to DNA by misincorporation, and FUTP causes significant damage to RNA by integrating into this molecule. Among these, the misincorporation of FdUMP into DNA or RNA has been proposed as the chief mechanism of 5-FU's cytotoxicity, which inhibits the activity of TS and eventually leads to apoptosis [29, 30].

5-FU is an optimal drug for HCC treatment. In advanced-stage HCC patients, 5-FU monotherapy is not very effective. In the present time, the therapeutic usage of 5-FU has been restricted due to acquired resistance, inherent cytotoxicity to normal cells, minimal bioavailability, and short half-life [31]. Several mechanisms are reported to be associated with 5-FU resistance in HCC. In them, existence of cancer stem cells (CSCs) and high expression of ABC transporters are the key factors contributing to 5-FU resistance [32].

2.3. *Doxorubicin*

Doxorubicin (DOX, also known as adriamycin) has been employed as a first-line chemotherapy agent in the management of a number of cancers, including HCC, since 1974 [33]. This anthracycline derivative was isolated from the actinobacteria *Streptomyces peucetius* in the late 1960s. The structure of DOX is composed of 14-hydroxydaunomycinone (tetracyclic quinoid aglycone adriamycinone) that is connected to daunosamine, an amino-sugar. In the native form, about 50% of administrated DOX is removed from the body. The hepatic enzymes including the aldo/keto reductase superfamily, carbonyl reductase, and CYP450 metabolize DOX into DOXol, DOX hydroxyaglycone, DOX deoxyaglycone, and DOX-semiquinone. In them, 7-deoxydoxorubicinone and DOXol have been reported to be associated with the cardiotoxicity of DOX [34].

Multiple strategies are used by DOX to kill cancer cells by causing DNA damage, including DOX intercalating into DNA and thus disrupting topoisomerase II. This anticancer drug inhibits topoisomerase II, which overwinds DNA during transcription, thereby preventing the double strand of DNA from being recombined and halting DNA replication [35, 36]. As with other anticancer drugs, DOX promotes apoptosis of cancer cells [34]. In addition, DOX generates a significant amount of free radicals which induces cell death by activating ataxia telangiectasia mediated (ATM) autophosphorylation as well as ATM-dependent phosphorylation of Chk1, SMC1, Nbs1, and Chk2 [37–39].

The clinical utility of this anthracycline drug is limited in the present day due to its low response rate (15% in advanced HCC), therapy resistance, and multiple adverse effects, including immunosuppression, myelosuppression, as well as irreversible cardiotoxicity [40]. Resistance to DOX has emerged as a central problem that limits its therapeutic utility in HCC patients. Decreased expression of TOP2A and an increase in the dependency on topoisomerase II beta isoform, overexpression of ABC transporters and presence of stem cells are suggested as potential mechanisms of DOX resistance [41, 42].

2.4. *Cisplatin*

Cisplatin (cis-diamminedichloroplatinum (II) or cisplatin, or CDDP) is another well-known antineoplastic drug predominantly used in the treatment of malignancies of head, neck, ovary, cervix, testicles, lung, and bladder. In the 1970s, the FDA approved this platinum substance as an anticancer medication. The primary target of cisplatin is genomic DNA. This platinum anticancer drug binds to DNA, inducing reversible adenine and guanine alkylation that results in DNA lesions and ultimately prevents transcription and replication. If these cisplatin-induced DNA damages are not effectively repaired, cancer cells undergo apoptosis [43, 44].

The therapeutic value of cisplatin is currently inadequate due to two inherent challenges such as side effects and therapy resistance. Although cisplatin is a potent anticancer drug, it also has adverse effects on varieties of organs including ototoxicity (75%–100%), nephrotoxicity (72%), hepatotoxicity (36%), and cardiotoxicity (6%). The other cisplatin adverse effects include myelosuppression, immunosuppression, peripheral neuropathy, nausea, and vomiting. The toxicity of cisplatin is time and dose dependent, which is connected with excessive ROS production and concurrent decrease of the antioxidant defense system [45].

Resistance to cisplatin is mediated by a number of mechanisms, including decreased accumulation of cisplatin by increased efflux by ABC transporters, enhanced DNA damage repair, activation or inactivation of EMT, presence of CSCs changes in DNA methylation levels, altering membrane protein transport, and expression of stress-response chaperones [46–49].

2.5. *Lenvatinib*

Lenvatinib (LVN), a multikinase inhibitor, was approved in 2018 as a first-line treatment for unresectable HCC according to the outcomes of phase III clinical trial [50]. Previously, LVN was mainly used in the treatment of advanced endometrial cancer and papillary differentiated thyroid carcinoma. This multikinase inhibitor acts as the inhibitor of KIT, RET, mutated oncogenes, PDGFRα, VEGFR1–3, and FGFR1–4 [51]. In unresectable HCC patients, LVN provides better survival and tumor responses than sorafenib, with a comparable incidence of side effects [52]. The extensive use of LVN is sufficient to illustrate its key therapeutic role, but drug resistance has not much been reported clinically [53]. Despite this, enhanced activation of EGFR induces LVN resistance possibly through accumulation of ROS [54].

2.6. *Sunitinib*

Sunitinib is an orally administered tyrosine kinase inhibitor that targets PDGFR-α, PDGFR-β, VEGFR1–3, and other related TKs. Sunitinib inhibits angiogenesis by inhibiting the tyrosine kinase activation. Only one phase III trial of sunitinib is carried out to evaluate the effectiveness of sunitinib as a first-line medication for HCC [55]. Compared to sorafenib, sunitinib was less effective in terms of overall survival. Constitutive activation of IGF signaling pathways is one of the key contributors of sunitinib resistance in HCC [56].

2.7. *Regorafenib*

Regorafenib, an oral multikinase inhibitor, suppresses the activation of numerous kinases including VEGFR1–3, PDGFβ, FGF1, REF, RAS, MAPK, RAF-1, and KIT that are involved in angiogenesis, proliferation, tumor microenvironment, and metastasis. This multikinase was approved as a systemic therapy for the treatment of metastatic/advanced HCC by USFDA in April 2017. Regorafenib has a higher pharmacological impact than sorafenib that targets a wide range of kinases associated with tumor growth, and angiogenesis [56]. In unresectable HCC patients, regorafenib was the first medication that showed a positive survival advantage as a second-line therapy, who had failed to sorafenib treatment previously. Treatment with regorafenib has prolonged the overall survival of HCC patients to almost 3 months [57]. Currently, the efficacy of regorafenib was reduced markedly due to acquired resistance [58].

2.8. *Erlotinib*

Erlotinib is another effective drug in the treatment of advanced HCC. This anticancer agent inhibits EGFR tyrosine kinase by binding with

ATP site in the TK domain of EGFR. This binding prevents the trans-autophosphorylation of EGFR and restrict the activation of the downstream signaling pathways associated with cell proliferation, cell cycle progression, and angiogenesis [59]. FDA approved erlotinib for the treatment of metastatic pancreatic cancer, and NSCLC in 2004. In HCC cells, erlotinib induces apoptosis and cell cycle arrest at G1/S transition by suppressing EGFR-TK [60].

2.9. *Cabozantinib*

Cabozantinib, a small molecule ATP-competitive inhibitor of c-Met, and VEGFR2. This drug was reported to be effective against HCC, and medullary thyroid cancer. Cabozantinib has been shown to suppress the phosphorylation and activation of c-Met and downstream signaling pathways in preclinical studies, resulting in the reduction of cell proliferation and tumor formation [61]. In 2019, FDA approved this ATP-competitive inhibitor as a second-line treatment option for HCC. Hypertension, diarrhea, hand-foot syndrome, fatigue, and palmar-plantar erythrodysesthesia are the common side effects of cabozantinib. Besides, this drug has many advantages over other antineoplastic agents used in HCC treatment including tolerance of adverse effects, ability to overcome P-gp overexpression, and high bioavailability. But the efficacy of this ATP inhibitor is often compromised by drug resistance [62].

3. Genes and Pathways Involved in HCC Chemoresistance

Chemoresistance remains a serious limitation in chemotherapy-based cancer treatment against HCC. Major signaling pathways responsible for the chemoresistance are as follows:

3.1. *PI3K/AKT/mTOR pathway*

mTOR is a serine/threonine protein kinase included in PI3K-associated kinase protein family [63]. Its function is to regulate cell growth and proliferation via dietary signals. Akt activation enhances tumor cell proliferation, and resistance to apoptosis, thus inhibiting Akt activity in HCC overcomes acquired resistance to sorafenib [64]. PI3K/AKT/mTOR pathway is abnormally active in nearly 50% of HCC patients [65]. Enhanced mTOR expression is seen in advanced stages of HCC [66]. The abnormal activation of PI3K/AKT/mTOR pathway stops cancer cells from undergoing apoptosis induced by sorafenib, leading to drug resistance [67].

3.2. *The Hippo/yes associated protein (YAP) pathway*

YAP is another crucial signaling pathway for organogenesis and organ size development, controlling cell proliferation and differentiation [68, 69]. In HCC tumors, YAP is involved in a number of chemoresistance problems. Increased YAP expression was noted in numerous HCC patients. Non-phosphorylated YAP moves into the nucleus where it interacts with a transcriptional coactivator transcription enhanced associate domain (TEAD) to encourage metastasis, cell growth, prevention of autophagy, and apoptosis [70]. In adriamycin-resistant HCC cells, YAP1 promoted the expression of ABC transporters, and various stem cell markers. After TACE therapy, YAP1 is markedly increased in the recurrent HCC [71]. It negatively affects survival of patients by inducing tumor cell immune escape, and enriching regulatory T cells in HCC tissue [72]. It promotes TGFBR2 transcription, recruits M2 macrophages, and upregulates CCL2 expression in hepatocytes, promoting HCC development [73]. YAP1 is overexpressed in hepatoblastoma and cholangiocarcinoma, interacting with β-catenin, and promoting rapid tumor development [74].

3.3. *Janus kinases (JAK)/STAT3 signaling*

STAT3 signaling plays a critical role in various physiological activities, including cell division, growth, and immunological control [75]. Inflammatory cytokines, interleukins, HGF, TNF, EGF, and TGF-β activate the JAK/STAT3 pathway [76, 77]. These extracellular ligands bind to the common receptor gp130 (Gp130 is the common β-receptor for all cytokines of the IL-6 family) and a ligand-specific receptor and activate Janus kinases leading to phosphorylation, dimerization and nuclear translocation of STAT3 [78].

Due to its interactions with numerous networks and molecular signaling pathways, STAT3 has a broad range of functions in HCC. These effects are caused by the elevated expression of various target genes, including cyclin D, c-Myc, Bcl-xL, Bcl-2, and Mcl1. HCC may acquire radio and chemoresistance as a result of elevated STAT3 levels. Therapeutic STAT3 signaling inhibition may reduce the growth and make tumor cells more susceptible to treatment. In HCC cells, STAT3 and ABCB1 have some interactions. The development of drug resistance may result from the exocytosis of envatinib from HCC cells caused by high expression of ABCB1, leading to the development of chemoresistance [79]. DOX is used to treat HCC with the intention of inducing tumor cell death. Due to the activation of the IL-6/STAT3 axis, the high expression level of CKLF1 can inhibit apoptosis in HCC cells exposed to DOX [80].

3.4. *Wnt pathway*

The Wnt signaling system plays a pivotal role in cell proliferation, angiogenesis, embryonic patterning, and differentiation [81, 82]. In the canonical pathway, proteasome complex (consisting of APC protein, axin, and GSK-3) dissolves when Wnt ligands bind to its transmembrane receptor — Wnt/FZD-related protein and LDL receptor. Typically, this APC complex mediates the destruction of β-catenin. β-catenin accumulates in the cytoplasm once this complex is broken down, and it then moves to the nucleus, where it interacts to the transcription factor, the LEF/TCF proteins. This complex controls the transcription of target genes associated with cell proliferation, cancer stemness, metastasis, and therapy resistance [83, 84]. β-catenin signaling can act as upstream mediator of ABC transporters; hence the suppression of this pathway downregulates ABC transporters, thereby improving drug sensitivity [85]. In HCC cells, FZD7 stimulates Wnt/-catenin signaling to elevate the levels of various ABC transporters, including ABCB1, ABCC1, as well as ABCC2 that induce DOX and rhodamine resistance. β-catenin and AXIN1/2 mutations induce the aberrant activation of the Wnt/β-catenin pathway [81]. Approximately 11%–41% of liver malignancies have CTNNB1 activating mutations [86, 87]. The destruction complex's APC and Axin have loss-of-function mutations that increase β-catenin and allow oncogenic transcription [87, 88]. Around 5%–19% of liver cancer cases have AXIN1 mutations which regulate Wnt/β-catenin signaling [86, 89, 90].

3.5. *P53 — Tumor suppressor pathway*

The TP53 gene on human chromosome 17 encodes the protein p53 [91]. The p53 function as a tumor suppressor gene (guardian of the genome) is crucial in the development of HCC, regulating cell division and preventing cancer formation [92]. In HCC, aflatoxin B1, a mycotoxin, induces mutations in p53 by causing G:C to T:A transversions at the third base in codon [93]. While oxyradical illnesses, chronic HCV, and HBV infections also alter TP53 [94]. The viral protein, HBx, can inhibit p53's DNA binding activity, leading to hepatocellular carcinogenesis [94, 95]. Other genetic changes, epigenetic silencing, and viral infections can also target the p53 pathway [96]. Dysregulation of p53 function can allow aneuploid cell survival or propagation and produce centrosome amplification and CIN (mitotic error-mediated chromosomal instability) [97–99]. CAN-03-3908, with high CIN in HCC associated with p53 mutation and hepatitis virus infection, while low CIN is associated with β-catenin mutation [100]. Mutant p53 increases DOX resistance, and inhibition of p53 activation can reduce sensitivity [101, 102]. In addition to DOX resistance, p53 inactivation and mutation are associated with 5-FU and vincristine resistance in HCC cells [103].

3.6. *Autophagy pathways*

Autophagy is a lysosome-dependent type II cell death initiated by self-degradation of cells, and autophagosome [104]. It is essential in the process of removing harmful proteins and defective organelles during the aging process [105]. In late stages of HCC, autophagy promotes metastasis, EMT, and survival of cells through activation of TGF-β pathway, degradation of P53, as well as resistance to chemotherapy, while inhibitors of MAPK/ERK, PI3K/Akt and JAK/STAT3 signaling pathways can cause cell death, and autophagy [106, 107]. Autophagy regulates stem cell development in HCC and makes cancer cells resistant to chemotherapy and radiotherapy [108].

3.7. *Ras*

Ras (rat sarcoma virus protein) is an oncogene that undergoes a variety of mutations during hepatocarcinogenesis. Among the various signaling pathways, the Ras pathway is pivotal signaling network that promotes cell proliferation. Growth factors such as EGF and IGF-1 when bound to their respective receptors (e.g., EGFR, IGF-1R) activate Ras, which in turn stimulates c-raf, MEK, and ERK [109]. Overactive MAPK signaling is linked to HCC development by inducing cellular proliferation while suppressing apoptosis [110]. In HCC, levels of MAPK and Ras/Raf/MEK/ERK pathway influence sorafenib sensitivity [111].

3.8. *AT-rich interactive domain-containing protein (ARID)*

ARID1A (BAF250a) and ARID2/ARID1B (BAF200) belong to SWI/SNF family which controls the transcription of specific genes by altering the surrounding gene's chromatin structure [112]. They can induce apoptosis by regulating the target genes — Bcl-2 and cyclin D1 [113]. ARID1A mutation was detected in 9.35% (33/353) of HCC cases that were sequenced [114]. It is considered to be a tumor suppressor, responds to DNA damage, regulates gene transcription, and influences the tumor immune microenvironment as well as signaling pathways [115, 116]. Existence of driver mutations in ARID1A is one major obstacle to TKI-based therapy [117]. Advanced HCC patients lacking ARID1A had increased sorafenib sensitivity while stimulating angiopoietin-2-dependent angiogenesis and tumor growth [118]. In addition to this, ARID2/ARID1B mutations are common in HCV-related HCC, while HCC caused by alcohol consumption is likely to have ARID1A alterations [119]. ARID1B, a homolog of ARID1A, shares high sequence similarity but has a lower mutation rate than ARID1A [120].

3.9. *Ataxia telangiectasia mutated (ATM)*

The ATM protein is a member of the PI3K family, with a conserved COOH-terminal phosphatidylinositol 3-kinase domain [121, 122]. It involves in repair, and DNA damage checkpoint [123]. Damages in DNA trigger the activation of ATM, which phosphorylates p53 and other downstream target proteins that regulate cell cycle checkpoints. HCC alters the expression of the ATM protein kinase. Blocking of ATM activity improves sorafenib's anticancer impact via inhibiting the Akt pathway (MOC-5) in HCC cells [124].

3.10. *CDKN2B*

p15INK4b is a CDK inhibitor encoded by CDKN2B gene. This CDK inhibitor controls the proliferation of cells via inhibiting CDK4/6 kinase activation. This gene is therapeutically significant since the lower CDKN2B expression is linked to the worse treatment outcome in HCC patients treated with sorafenib [125].

3.11. *Transporter pump*

In cancer chemotherapy, multidrug resistance (MDR) is a prevalent issue. Overexpression of the MDR1 gene is linked with HCCs' chemoresistance. ABC transporters are transmembrane proteins that transport substances like lipids, metabolic products, sterols, and drugs via membranes of cells [126]. In tumor cells, the P-glycoprotein or P-gp or ABCB1 is an ATP-binding cassette transporter that expels chemotherapeutic drugs from cells, reducing drug efficacy.

This transporter proteins affects caspase-3 activity, decreasing cellular apoptosis, and reversing sorafenib resistance in liver cancer cells [127, 128]. ABCG2 expression is high in HCC, and increases following chemotherapy in hepatoblastoma patients [129, 130]. In Sorafenib-resistant HCC cells HepG2, and Huh7 overexpress P-gp, to some extent, it is influenced by EMT and Akt activation.

3.12. *TERT*

TERT or the telomerase reverse transcriptase encodes the catalytic subunit of telomerase that preserves the integrity of chromosome length and telomeric DNA length [131]. TERT is activated by mutations in TERT promoter which functions as a gatekeeper during the malignant transition [132]. Activated TERT was reported to induce Cisplatin resistance. Mitochondrial translocation of hTERT has a role in resistance to drugs of human HCC cells [133]. The mutation rate for hTERT (including the promoter region) in HCC is 60%, and playing a crucial role in early carcinogenesis [133, 134].

3.13. *TGF-β*

TGF-β is a cytokine and growth factor family encoded by 32 genes that can be classified into two groups: TGF-βs and bone morphogenic proteins (BMPs) [135]. TGF-β1, β2, and β3 are the three isoforms of TGF-β in mammals [136]. It is a key regulator of liver fibrosis and EMT in various cancers and acts as tumor suppressor or promoter [137, 138]. In a number of cancers, including HCC, TGF-β signaling activity has been associated with drug resistance [139].

3.14. *Epidermal growth factor (EGF)*

EGFR belongs to the ErbB/HER family of transmembrane RTKs. In HCC, EGF pathway is activated abnormally through autocrine or paracrine secretion that promotes cancer cell proliferation and migration [140]. Proteins including NF-kB, MAPK/ERK, PI3K/Akt, and

P38/MAPK are activated when it attaches to EGF receptors [141, 142]. HER-3 or ErbB-3 is the major dimerization partner of EGFR, and both its expression and activity are usually dysregulated in HCC [143]. Dysregulation of the EGFR/HER-3 signaling pathway limits the efficacy of sorafenib in resistant HCC cells due to. Through the reduction of initial resistance, anti-EGFR treatment may increase the therapeutic efficacy of sorafenib [144].

3.15. *VEGF*

VEGF, or vascular endothelial growth factor, is essential for tumor angiogenesis [145]. VEGF also appears to play a function in chemoresistance through modulating autophagy via NRP2 and mTOR [146]. Resistance to the VEGFR inhibitor sorafenib in advanced HCC may be explained in part by the synergy between the FGF and VEGF pathways [147, 148].

3.16. *FGF*

The fibroblast growth factor (FGF) family is a group made up of 18 ligands and four homologous factors. Four to six percent of individuals with HCC had a mutation in FGF19, which impacts the PI3K-Akt-mTOR pathway [149, 150]. Resistance to sorafenib-induced apoptosis in HCC has been connected to aberrant FGF19 signaling through its receptor FGFR4. It is caused by blocking the drug-induced production of ROS and promoting epithelial-mesenchymal transition via E-cadherin downregulation [148].

3.17. *c-Myc*

c-Myc, an oncogene, is a member of the Myc family. This transcription factor binds to CACGTG, the enhancer box sequence and regulates the expression of more than 15% of human genes related to metabolism, differentiation, cell proliferation, apoptosis, and tumorigenesis. c-Myc signaling has a vital role in drug resistance [151, 152].

Furthermore, c-Myc inhibition increases the sensitivity of chemotherapeutic drugs to HCC [153].

3.18. *Cancer stem cell markers*

A distinct population of cancer cells known as cancer stem cells (CSCs) that continuously renew and differentiate themselves [154]. Drug resistance is one of the hallmarks of CSCs. CSCs are also important in the maintenance and promotion of HCC's malignant features, such as plasticity, heterogeneity, EMT, angiogenesis, and vascular mimicry. In liver cancer, various CSC markers, including CD90, CD133, oval cell marker OV6, CD13, CD44, CD47, DLK1, Lgr5, EpCAMCD24, ICAM-1, and keratin19 have been identified [155, 156]. It can control the expression of DNA repair genes, resulting in radioresistance [157]. MEK, JNK, Hedgehog, NF-κB/snail, IL-33/p38, and ERK1/2 are reported to regulate CSC features [158–163].

4. Phytochemicals as Chemosensitizers in the Management of HCC

There are still certain issues that need to be tackled even if traditional therapeutic strategies and diagnostic equipment are getting more effective every day. High cost of treatments and tumor relapse are the chief reasons for treatment failure and tumor relapses, particularly in the case of MDR, which results in a worse prognosis. Chemotherapy is one of the golden standards of cancer treatment; hence overcoming chemoresistance has the greatest importance in cancer research. Many compounds from nature show promising anticancer activities. When combined with conventional chemotherapeutics, these compounds help to overcome the chemoresistance and avoid its side effects due to selectivity, cyto-friendly nature and multiple specificity. Numerous studies have demonstrated the safety, effectiveness, and mode of action of phytochemicals, justifying their inclusion in the current chemotherapies (Table 1). The combination of phytochemicals in cancer

Table 1: List of phytochemicals with Chemosensitisation property in HCC

No.	Phytochemical Compound	Class	Structure	Molecular Targets	References
1	Curcumin	Polyphenol	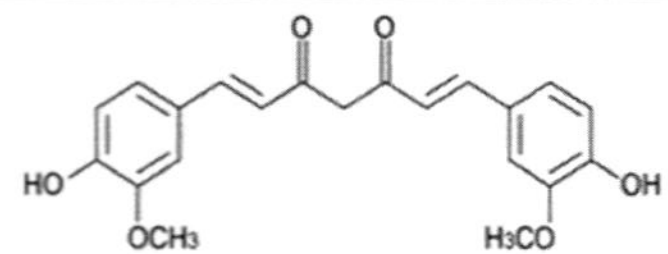	Caspase-3, Bcl-2, c-Myc, PCNA, VEGF, MDR1, HIF-1α, COX-2, NF-κB, GLUT-1, MCT-1, MCT-4, HCAR-1, p53, SDH, IDH3a, GAPDH, FASN, PKM2, LDH-A, Lin28B	[168–170, 172, 173]
2	Apigenin	Flavonoid	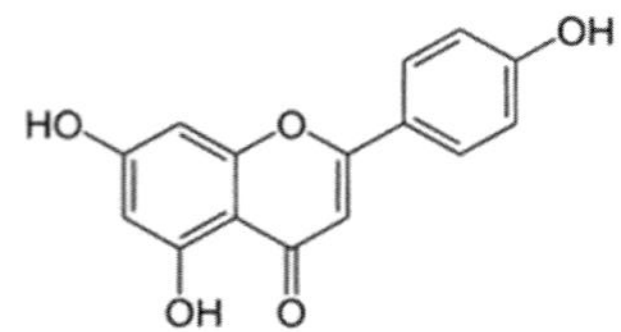	miR-520b, ATG7, PARP, Bcl-2	[178, 179]
3	Epigallocatechin-3-O-gallate	Polyphenol	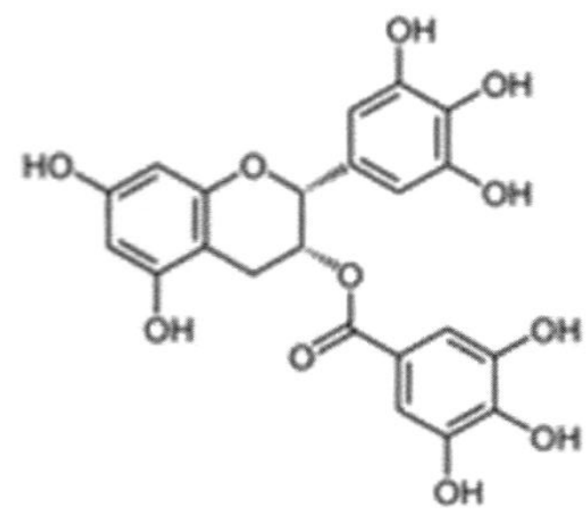	PI3K/Akt, MEK/ERK, ABCB1, LC3, COX-2, PGE2	[184–186]

4	Allicin	Organosulphur compound	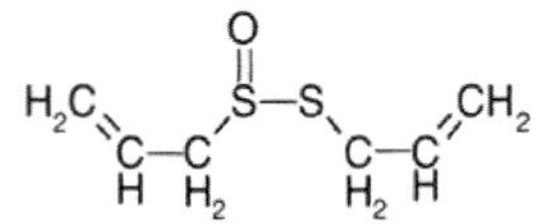	Caspase-3, PARP, Bcl-2	[189]
5	Resveratrol	Stillbenoid	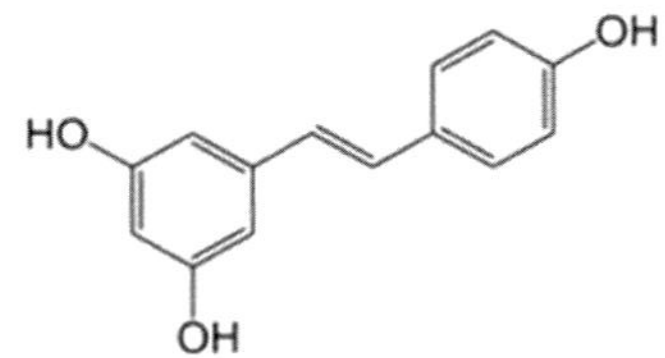	CDC25A, CDK2, eEF2K, p-AMPK, Caspase-3, Caspase-8, Caspase-9, Cyclin A, ASCT2	[191–193]
6	Chlorogenic acid	Polyphenol	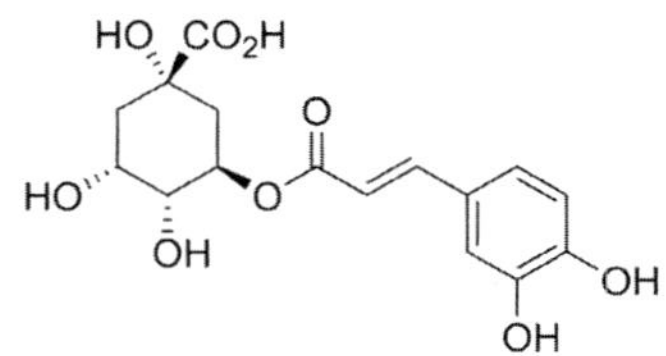	Bax, Caspase-3, Caspase-7, MAPK, PI3K/Akt/mTORC, ERK1/2	[194, 195]
7	Capsaicin	Vanilloid	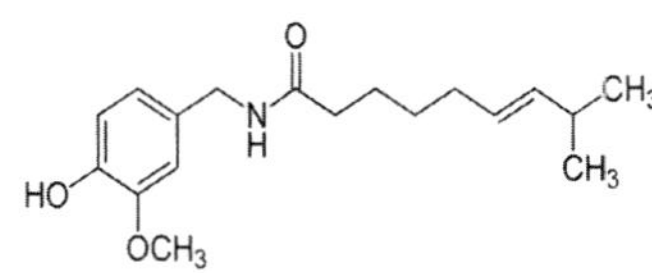	Bax, Caspase-3, PARP, Bcl-2, LC3AB II, Beclin-1, E-cadherin, vimentin, N-cadherin, MMP2, MMP9	[199]

(*Continued*)

Table 1: (*Continued*)

No.	Phytochemical Compound	Class	Structure	Molecular Targets	References
8	Quercetin	Flavonoid	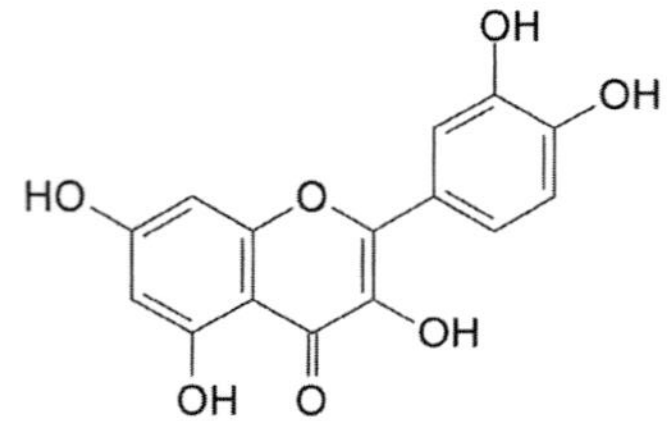	TNF-α, VEGF, p53, NF-κB, p16, MDR1, HIF-1α, ABCB1, ABCC2, ABCC1, FZD7/β-catenin	[201–204]
9	Baicalein	flavonoid	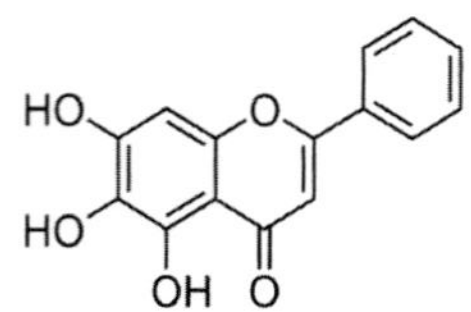	P-gp, Bcl-xl	[211]
10	Wogonin	flavonoid	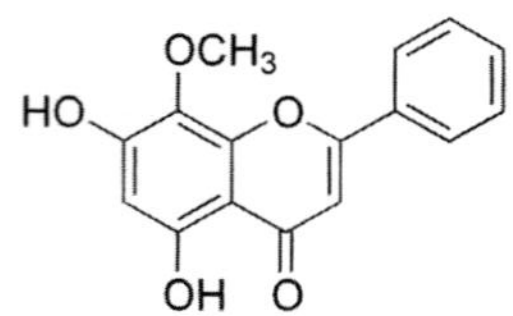	Nrf2, LC3-II, PARP, MRP1-4, ABCG2	[216–218]

11	Caffeine	methylxanthine	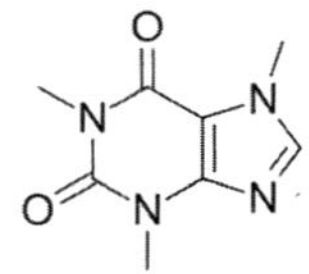	PARP, BCl-2, Bcl-xL	[222]
12	Beta-escin	Triterpenoid	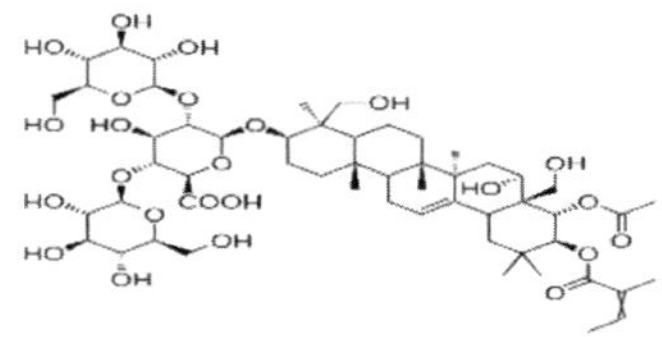	STAT3, Cyclin D1, Bcl-2, Bcl-xL, Survivin, Mcl-1, VEGF, Caspase-3, Caspase-8, Caspase-9	[225, 226]
13	Phloretin	Dihydrochalcone flavonoid	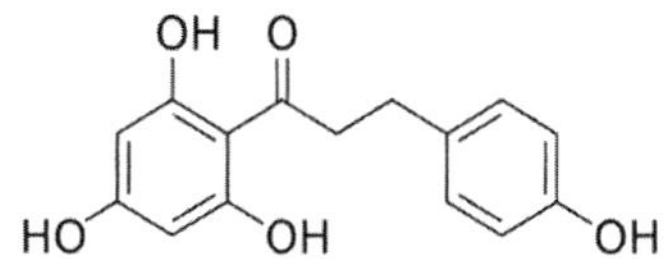	SHP-1, STAT3, AKt/VEGFR	[227]
14	Ginsenoside PPD	Triterpene saponins	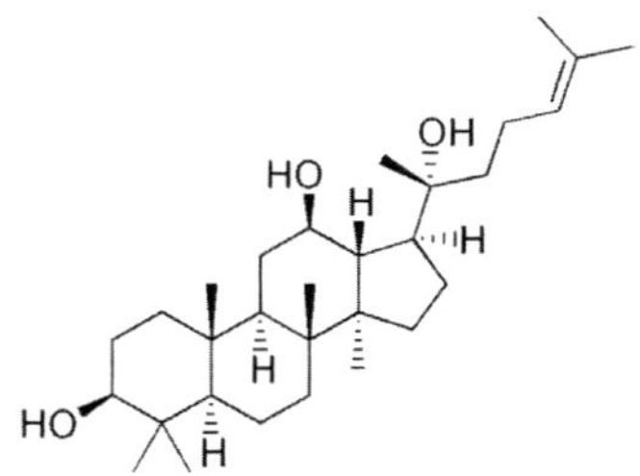	STAT3-Twist signaling pathway	[229]

(*Continued*)

Table 1: (*Continued*)

No.	Phytochemical Compound	Class	Structure	Molecular Targets	References
15	Ginsenoside Rg3	Triterpene saponins	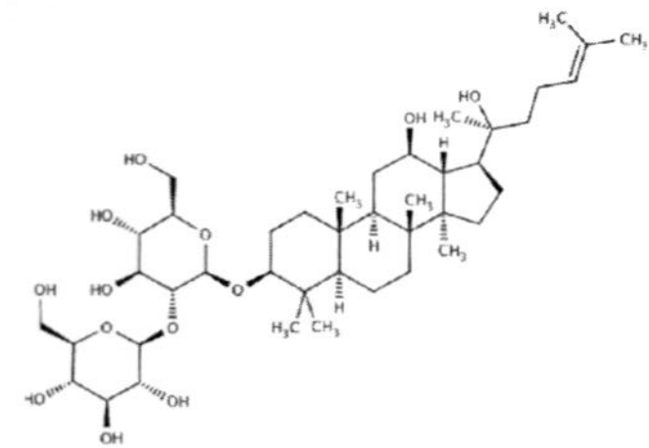	PTEN/Akt signaling pathway, PCNA, Cyclin D1, mTORC1	[231, 233]
16	Genistein	Isoflavone	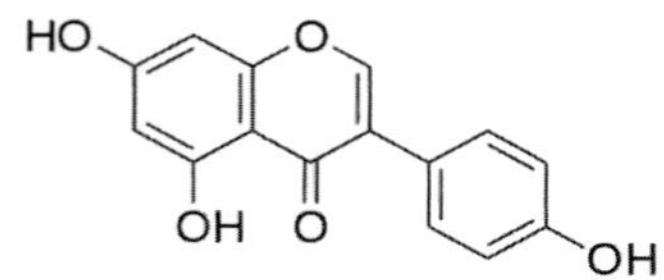	EGFR, Akt/Erk/mTOR	[242]
17	Luteolin	Flavonoid	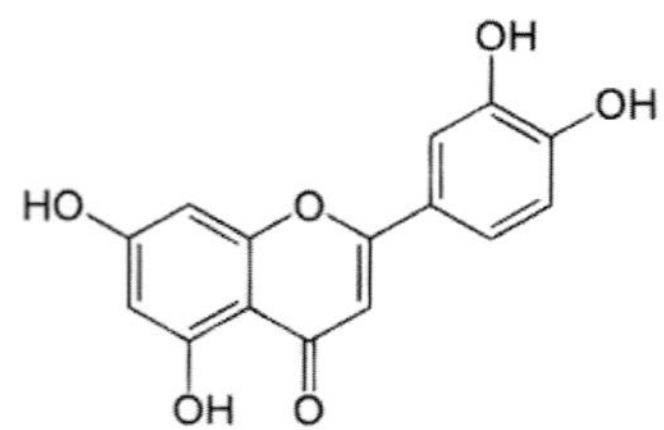	THOC1, JNK, Caspase-3, Bcl-2, p53	[245–247]

18	Cantharidin	Mono-terpenoid	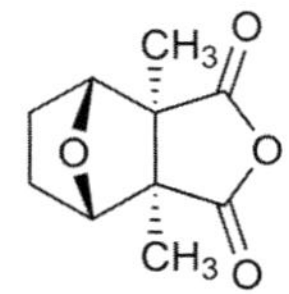	KDM4A, H3K36me3	[251]
19	Dioscin	Steroidal saponin	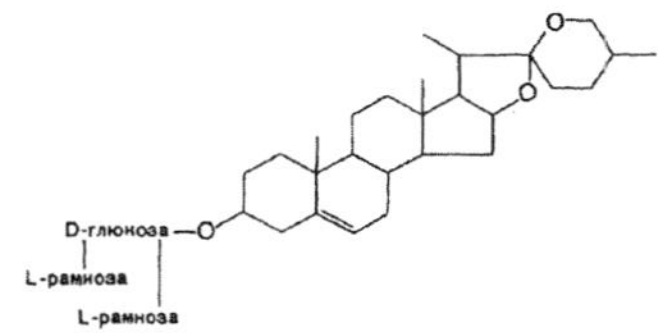	P-gp	[262]
20	Diosgenin	Steroid sapogenin	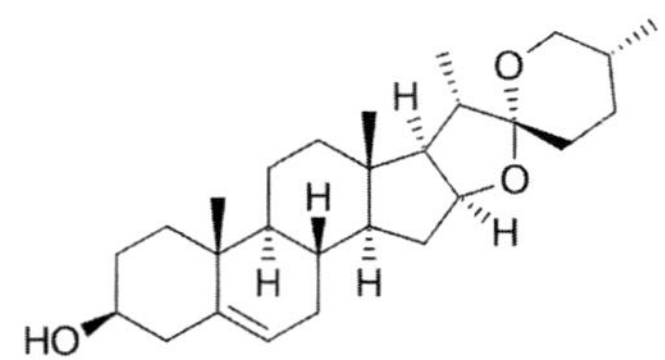	STAT3, c-Src, JAK 1, JAK 2	[264]

therapy needs further validations to ensure its effectiveness in cancer treatment strategy.

4.1. *Curcumin*

Curcumin is a polyphenol extracted from *Curcuma longa*. Curcumin shows anti-angiogenic, antioxidant, and anticancer properties in HCC with low cytotoxicity [164–166]. In combination therapies, curcumin can enhance the efficacy of chemotherapeutic drugs. Nanocarriers are used for delivering chemotherapeutics along with chemosensitizers like curcumin for HCC treatment. Cisplatin co-loaded with curcumin in nanoliposomes enhanced HCC sensitivity to cisplatin. These curcumin nanoliposomes improved anticancer properties of cisplatin in mouse hepatoma H22, human HCC HepG2 xenograft models and *in vitro* studies [167]. Lipid nanoparticles co-loaded with DOX and curcumin used for HCC treatment have shown a synergistic effect on inhibiting proliferation (decreased c-Myc, PCNA expressions), angiogenesis (decreased VEGF expression), reversing multidrug resistance (decreased MDR1, Bcl-2 and HIF-1α expressions), and inducing apoptosis (enhanced Bax/Bcl-2 ratio, and caspase-3) in diethylnitrosamine-induced HCC in mice [168]. Similarly, treatment with curcumin and sorafenib co-loaded lactosylated pH-responsive nanoparticles has shown high degree of tumor inhibition with low systemic toxicity in HepG2 cells and HCC tumor xenograft models [169]. 5-FU in combination with curcumin shows enhanced antitumor effects via regulating NF-κB, and COX-2 expression in SMMC-7721 cells and in mice bearing tumor xenograft [170]. In addition to this, curcumin also inhibits chemoresistance in HepG2 cells induced by high glucose by inhibiting the expression of certain enzymes, receptors and transporters which were elevated in high glucose conditions [171]. Curcumin reversing paclitaxel-induced chemoresistance in Hep3B and HepG2 cells by suppressing Lin28B and its upstream protein NF-κB [172]. By suppressing radiation-induced NF-κB activity, curcumin sensitizes HCC to radiation as well in HepG2 cells [173].

4.2. *Apigenin*

Apigenin (APG or 4′,5,7-trihydroxyflavone) is a naturally occurring flavonoid present in a variety of herbs, fruits, vegetables, nuts, and tea. It has various health benefits, including antioxidant, anti-telomerase, antidepressant, anti-inflammatory, antiviral, antibacterial, and chemopreventive actions [174]. Besides these, APG induces cell cycle arrest, apoptosis, and autophagy, inhibiting migration, invasion, cell proliferation, and angiogenesis in different cancer cells [175, 176]. Numerous studies have shown that apigenin combination treatment improves the effectiveness of chemotherapy in various cancers. Apigenin enhances the cytotoxicity of 5-FU in BEL-7402 and SK-Hep-1 cells. In this study, APG suppresses drug resistance mediated by ROS in HCC cells with subsequent activation of the mitochondrial apoptotic pathways. The combined treatment of 5-FU and APG decreases the growth of HCC xenograft [177]. In another study, APG increased the expression of miR-520b and suppressed ATG7-dependent autophagy to render BEL-7402/ADM cells (DOX-resistant HCC cell line) more susceptible to DOX. It also reduced the xenograft growth in nude mice through inhibition of ATG7 as well as upregulation of miR-520b [178]. Furthermore, combined treatment of apigenin and sorafenib has been shown to arrest cell cycle, reduce cell viability, migration and invasion, as well as induce apoptotic gene expression in HepG2 cells [179].

4.3. *Epigallocatechin-3-O-gallate*

(-)-Epigallocatechin-3-O-gallate or EGCG is the abundant polyphenol in the dried fresh leaves of *Camellia sinensis* L.Ktze.) (Green tea) that contributes various beneficial health effects. Several studies have reported that EGCG exhibits antioxidant, anti-inflammatory, antiaging, neuroprotective, antifibrotic, and cardioprotective activities [180]. Succeeding evidence suggests that EGCG acts as a potent anticancer agent that inhibits the proliferation of cancers of the esophagus, liver, stomach, colon, prostate, bladder, skin, lung, pancreas, and breast. In addition to this, combination of EGCG synergistically enhances the anticancer potential of conventional chemotherapeutics in various cancers including HCC [181]. EGCG downregulates the expression of ABC transporters that contribute to MDR by expelling chemotherapeutics from cancer cells [182]. EGCG reduces DOX-induced P-gp overexpression via coordinately suppressing PI3K/Akt and MEK/ERK signaling pathways [183]. EGCG acts as chemotherapeutic augmenter that synergistically enhances anticancer effects of DOX in Hep3B cells through inhibition of autophagy [184]. According to Yang et al. (2012), EGCG sensitizes HCC cells to 5-FU by eliminating 5-FU-induced overexpression of COX-2, and secretion of PGE2 [185]. Additionally, EGCG enhances the anticancer effect of DOX through reversing the MDR mechanisms such as the downregulation of MDR-1, decreasing the activity of P-gp efflux pump, and enhancing DOX accumulating within HCC cells [186].

4.4. *Allicin*

Allicin is a volatile compound that is widely found in cruciferous vegetables, asparagus, onion, and Allium family of plants which includes alpine leek (*Allium victorialis* L), wild garlic (*Allium ursinum* L), white garlic (*Allium sativum* L), elephant garlic (*Allium ampeloprasum* L), and field garlic (*Allium vineale* L) and [187]. It is one of the main bioactive sulfur-containing compounds that gives Allium species their very strong taste and odor. Numerous biological benefits of allicin are demonstrated, such as antibacterial, anti-inflammatory, cardiovascular protective, and immunomodulatory actions [188]. In addition to this, allicin prevents the proliferation of some cancer cells, including glioblastoma, gastric, breast, liver, lung, prostate, renal, cervical, and colon cancer. The combination of allicin and 5-FU is thought to be a novel therapy strategy for HCC as allicin sensitizes HCC cells to 5-FU-mediated apoptosis via ROS-mediated mitochondrial pathway. When allicin and 5-FU are combined, the intracellular amount of ROS is increased, mitochondrial membrane potential is decreased, the genes for caspase-3 and PARP are induced to express, and Bcl-2 is downregulated [189].

4.5. *Resveratrol*

Resveratrol or trans 3′,4′,5′-trihydroxystilbene is a naturally occurring stilbenoid polyphenol that has antioxidant, anti-inflammatory, immunomodulatory, hepatoprotective, cardioprotective, antidiabetic, and anti-tumorigenic characteristics that can be used in the treatment of various chronic disorders. Red wine, berries, peanuts, grapes, and medicinal plants like Japanese knotweed are the main sources of resveratrol [190]. *In vitro* studies have shown that resveratrol sensitized HepG2 and Huh7 cells to sorafenib through PKA/AMPK/eEF2K pathway. This combination treatment leads to the decreased protein levels of CDC25A, CDK2, eEF2K, and p-AMPK with concomitant enhancement in caspase-3, caspase-8, caspase-9, and cyclin A. Furthermore, sorafenib and resveratrol combination treatment also reduces the growth of HepG2 xenograft tumor in mice, suggesting a promising therapeutic approach to enhance the anticancer response of sorafenib in the future [191]. In another *in vitro* study, resveratrol sensitizes human hepatoma cells — C3A and SMCC7721 to cisplatin through ROS generation and apoptosis-dependent mechanisms. In addition to this, resveratrol reduces glutathione and glutamine content by decreasing the ASCT2, glucose transporter expression [192]. Resveratrol causes S-phase arrest in H22 murine hepatoma cells. Furthermore, resveratrol elevates the antitumor effect of 5-FU in mice bearing hepatoma induced by H22 cells [193].

4.6. *Chlorogenic acid*

Chlorogenic acid (CGA) is a prevalent polyphenol found in coffee beans, potatoes, eggplants, plums, and apples. It is a quinic acid and caffeic acid ester formed when acid part of caffeic acid is attached to the hydroxyl group of quinic acid at the fifth position. Coffee is a prevalent dietary source of CGA; it possesses various biological effects such as anti-inflammatory, antioxidant, anticancer, and antiviral activity. CGA synergistically enhances the anticancer effect of regorafenib in HepG2 cells by potentiating apoptosis. Chlorogenic acid modulates the apoptotic action of regorafenib in HCC cells via activating proapoptotic proteins (Bax, caspase-7, and caspase-3) with concomitant inhibition of anti-apoptotic (Bcl-xL and Bcl2) proteins. Regorafenib and CGA combination can potentiate enhanced inhibition of MAPK, and PI3K/Akt/mTORC signaling [194]. In another *in vitro* study, chlorogenic acid works as a powerful chemosensitizer in HCC, where it makes human HCC cells (HepG2 and Hep3B cells) more sensitive to 5-FU by suppressing the activation of ERK1/2 and excessive production of ROS [195].

4.7. *Capsaicin*

Capsaicin or N-vanillyl-8-methyl-1-nonenamide is an odorous ingredient of hot peppers that exhibits antiproliferative activity in many cancers. In HCC cells, capsaicin-induced apoptosis by inhibiting ROS-STAT3-dependent autophagy, levels of intracellular calcium, heme oxygenase-1 expression, ROS production, and caspase-3 activation [196–198]. Capsaicin could be used as a potential therapeutic target in combination therapy for the HCC treatment. It synergistically improves the sorafenib's anticancer properties in human HCC cells (LM3, Hep3B, and HuH7). This study shows the combined treatment of capsaicin, and sorafenib induces apoptosis by enhancing proapoptotic proteins (PARP, caspase-3, and Bax) with blocking Bcl-2, an antiapoptotic protein. This combination treatment induces autophagy in HCC cells by upregulating LC3AB II and beclin-1 levels, suppresses cell invasion as well as metastasis through E-cadherin upregulation as well as MMP2/9, vimentin, and N-cadherin downregulation. In addition to this, capsaicin's synergistic anticancer effect can possibly be inhibited by EGFR and PI3K/Akt/mTOR signaling pathways [199].

4.8. *Quercetin*

Quercetin (QE) or 3,3′,4′,5,7-pentahydroflavone is a polyphenolic flavonoid. It is widely distributed in many plants, vegetables, and fruits. It has various biological effects, such as antioxidant, anti-inflammatory, immunomodulatory, anticancer, antiviral, and vasodilating properties [200]. According to various *in vitro* studies, quercetin synergistically enhances the anticancer properties of conventional chemotherapeutics in several cancers including HCC. Quercetin functions as a natural sensitizer that reduces chemoresistance and reverses multidrug resistance in HCC cells. According to Abdu et al. (2022), QE, and sorafenib combination is a promising treatment strategy to improve treatment outcome of HCC. In this study, quercetin enhances the anticancer effect of sorafenib as evidenced from reduced the proliferation of HepG2, induced cell cycle arrest, and apoptosis as well as downregulated the expression of proliferation, inflammation, and angiogenesis (TNF-α, NF-κB, VEGF, and p53) associated genes. The combination treatment was more effective in restoring liver enzymes, lipid profile, and inflammation than QE or sorafenib alone in Wistar rats bearing HCC induced by diethylnitrosamine (DEN) [201]. In another *in vitro* study, QE potentiates the cytotoxicity of DOX by downregulating the MDR1, and HIF-1α gene expressions in HepG2 cells [202]. QE decreased the ABCB1, ABCC2, and ABCC1 expressions as well as increased the sensitivity of BEL/5-FU to 5-FU by 1.63–3.41 times through the FZD7/β-catenin pathway [203]. Furthermore, QE synergistically enhances the anticancer effects of cisplatin in HepG2 cells. In this study, QE suppresses the HepG2 cell proliferation through p16-mediated cell cycle arrest as well as apoptosis [204].

4.9. *Baicalein*

Plant-derived flavonoid baicalein or 5,6,7-trihydroxy-2-phenyl-4H-1-benzopyran-4-one is extracted from the roots of *Scutallaria radix.* Baicalein known to have antioxidant, anti-inflammatory, and antiviral properties [205]. Succeeding evidences has shown that baicalein can be used as a potential candidate for HCC treatment. Through the mitochondrial-dependent caspase activation pathway it induces apoptosis in HCC cells. Baicalein downregulates CD24 thereby suppresses the growth and survival of HCC cells, induces cell cycle arrest at the G0/G1 phase through regulating cyclin D1 transcription, triggers autophagy via ER stress as well as inhibits Akt/mTOR pathway

[206–210]. In an *in vitro* study, baicalein sensitizes Bel7402/5-FU cells (multidrug-resistant HCC cell) to epirubicin and 5-FU by reversing drug efflux mediated by P-gp protein and inducing apoptosis by enhancing Bcl-xl level. Baicalein might be effective for the treatment of drug-resistant HCC [211].

4.10. *Wogonin*

Wogonin or 5,7-dihydroxy-8-methoxyflavone is a natural flavonoid derived from a Chinese herb, *Scutellaria baicalensis.* Several studies revealed the remarkable anti-inflammatory, antimicrobial, chemopreventive, and anticarcinogenic effects of this compound [212, 213]. Wogonin has been reported to exert a significant anticancer effect in HCC that diminishes the metastatic ability of HCC by suppressing the activity of MMP-9 [214]. It induces the cell cycle by activating GSK-3β and activates the unfolded protein response as well as the inactivation of Akt [213, 215]. Numerous studies have reported the sensitization effect of wogonin in combination with conventional chemotherapeutics. Wogonin enhanced the therapeutic potential of sorafenib by inhibiting sorafenib-induced autophagy and apoptosis in human HCC cells (Hep3B and Bel-7402). In this study, wogonin markedly inhibited sorafenib-induced autophagy by suppressing LC3-II expression. Increased level of PARP protein, caspase-3 substrate was found to be elevated in HCC cells co-treated with sorafenib, and wogonin [216]. Additionally, wogonin acts as a cisplatin sensitizer for cancer therapy, which causes cisplatin-induced apoptosis through the accumulation of intracellular ROS [217]. In this study, wogonin enhances the cytotoxic potential of chemotherapeutic drugs in HepG2 cells by suppressing Nrf2 level via regulating c-Myc and p53 expression. In addition to this, wogonin also enhances drug level in cancer cells by inhibiting MRP1-4 and ABCG2 [218].

4.11. *Caffeine*

Caffeine or 1,3,7-trimethylxanthine is found abundantly in cocoa, coffee beans, and certain types of tea. It is a naturally occurring methylxanthine derivative used as an additive in energy and soft drinks. Caffeine is mostly consumed to fight fatigue and sleepiness; hence, it is the widely consumed psychoactive chemical in the world. Intake of caffeine causes a number of physiological effects, such as stimulation of the neurological and musculoskeletal systems, relaxation of smooth muscles in the bronchi and arteries, stimulation of intestinal motility, and diuresis [219]. In addition to this, caffeine has been reported to have anti-inflammatory, antidiabetic, antioxidant, and neuroprotective activities, as well as plays a crucial role in the regulation of lipid metabolism [220, 221]. Several epidemiological and experimental studies have suggested that caffeine may have potential as an anticancer agent that inhibits cell growth and triggers apoptosis in cancers of the esophagus, breast, liver, and brain through various oncogenic pathways, such as PTEN, PI3K/Akt, p53, and mTOR pathways [219]. Additionally, it has recently been established that combining several anticancer medications with caffeine might boost their effectiveness. The *in vitro* study conducted by Wang et al. (2019) reported that caffeine sensitizes human HCC cells (Hep3B and SMMC-7721) to 5-FU. In this study, the combination treatment of caffeine and 5-FU suppressed the HCC cell proliferation and induced apoptosis by regulating intracellular ROS production. Bcl-xL and Bcl-2 protein levels are found to be downregulated, while upregulated cleaved PARP level was observed after the combination treatment in comparison with caffeine or 5-FU monotherapy [222].

4.12. *Beta-escin*

The primary active ingredient of horse chestnut (*Aesculus hippocastanum*) seed extracts is beta-escin, a pentacyclic triterpenoid. Over 30 escin isomers have been identified and analyzed [223]. It has shown anti-inflammatory as well as antitumor activities in various cancers such as lung cancer, colon cancer, cholangiocarcinoma, leukemia, liver cancer, and so on. Beta-escin inhibits tumor development and metastasis in various *in vivo* models. Escin promotes induction of apoptosis and inhibition of cell proliferation [224]. In a dose-and time-dependent manner, escin can inhibit STAT3 activation in HCC cells, thereby downregulating the expression of STAT3-controlled genes such as Bcl-2, Bcl-xL, cyclin D1, Mcl-1, VEGF and survivin, resulting in HCC chemosensitization to paclitaxel and DOX. In HCC cells, escin enhances the apoptotic effects of paclitaxel and DOX [225]. Combination of beta-escin and 5-FU has shown a synergistic effect in the inhibition of SMMC-7721 cell proliferation through inducing cell cycle arrest, apoptosis, activation of expression of caspases-3, 8 and 9, and downregulation of Bcl-2 expression [226]. Escin also enhances the effects of currently available chemotherapeutic drugs, suggesting the use of escin as an adjunct or alternative anticancer therapy.

4.13. *Phloretin*

Phloretin (2′,4,4′,6′-tetrahydroxy-dihydroxychalcone) is a dihydrochalcone flavonoid mainly present in Manchurian apricots and leaves, fruit, and roots of apple trees. Phloretin displays several physiological effects, including antiosteoclastogenic, antiviral, anti-inflammatory, antidiabetic, antibacterial, antifungal, and estrogenic properties. It is a potent inhibitor of sodium-glucose cotransporter-2 (SGLT2). This natural polyphenolic compound is capable of inhibiting the progression of liver, colon, gastric, esophageal, oral, breast, cervical, and lung cancers in various preclinical studies. Phloretin is reported to act as proapoptotic, antiangiogenesis, antimetastatic, and antiproliferative as well as modulating various intracellular signal pathways that make it a promising anticancer agent [226]. The co-treatment with phloretin sensitizes various cancer cells to conventional chemotherapeutics. Saraswati et al. (2019) conducted an *in vitro* and *in vivo* study that revealed the targeting of SHP-1 by phloretin may help to overcome sorafenib resistance in HCC. The combination of sorafenib and phloretin inhibits the proliferation and induces apoptosis in both SOR-resistant (HepG2R and Huh7SR) and SOR-sensitive (HepG2, Hep3B21-7, PLC-5, SK-Hep1, and Huh-7) HCC cells than SOR or phloretin alone indicating its synergistic effect on anticancer activity of sorafenib. Phloretin upregulates the expression of SHP-1, downregulates STAT3 expression, and eventually blocks pAKT/pERK signaling. In addition to this, phloretin markedly suppresses the tumor growth in both SOR-resistant and SOR-sensitive *in vivo* xenograft by inducing apoptosis, inhibiting cell proliferation, impairing angiogenesis via targeting SHP-1/STAT3 signaling pathway [227].

4.14. *Ginsenosides*

Ginsenosides belong to the class of triterpene saponins extracted from *Panax ginseng*, an important herb of Chinese medicine. More than 30 reported ginsenosides have been divided into two groups: the 20(S)-protopanaxadiol (PPD) (Rb1, Rb2, Rb3, Rc, Rd, Rg3, Rh2, Rs1) and the 20(S)-protopanaxatriol (PPT) (Re, Rf, Rg1, Rg2, Rh1). Carboxyl group attached to the C-6 position of PPDs forms PPT [228]. Protopanaxadiol (PPD), a diol-type ginsenoside, was reported to have excellent antitumor activity by inhibiting HCC proliferation. Through the STAT3-Twist signaling pathway, it also inhibits the HCC cell migration, invasion, and EMT. PPD enhances sensitivity of HCC to oxaliplatin and causes the prevention of the lung metastasis of tumors in the mouse xenograft model [229]. Rg3 acts as an inhibitor of cell growth and inducer of apoptosis [230]. It has shown antitumor activities in HCC. It also enhances the efficacy of chemotherapeutics used for HCC treatment. 20(S)-Ginsenoside Rg3 and Sorafenib have shown synergistic anticancer activity in HCC by regulating PTEN/Akt signaling pathway [231]. In HCC cells, Rg3's suppression of autophagy substantially boosts the cell death caused by DOX both *in vitro* and *in vivo* [232]. By suppressing PCNA and Cyclin D1 expressions, oxaliplatin combined with Rg3 inhibits the proliferation and promotes apoptosis of HCC cells [233]. In several HCC cell lines, Rg3 can promote TRAIL-induced apoptosis. It also increases the therapeutic efficacy of TRAIL in mouse xenograft models and acts as a chemosensitizer *in vivo* [234]. However, the pro-apoptotic and anti-proliferative effects require high concentrations of Rg3. At low concentrations, Rg3 enhances cell proliferation by activating mTORC1 [235].

4.15. *Genistein*

Genistein (GNT), also known as 5,7,4′-trihydroxyisoflavone, is an isoflavone found in Glycine max that has been shown to lower the chance of developing liver, lung, and breast cancer [236, 237]. It is consumed as a dietary supplement or as a vegetable (e.g., lupins, soy beans, fava beans) [128]. Genistein is reported to have anticarcinogenic and antioxidant properties [238, 239]. Genistein therapy decreased proliferation while inducing death in hepatoma cells and inhibited EGFR activation [240, 241]. When combined with gefitinib, genistein could decrease Hep3B cell proliferation and promote apoptosis more effectively than either agent alone. This effect could be due to the suppression of the Akt/Erk/mTOR pathway [242].

4.16. *Luteolin*

Luteolin or 3,4,5,7-tetrahydroxy flavone is a flavonoid compound that is widely distributed in celery, onion leaves, broccoli, chrysanthemum flowers, carrots, sweet bell peppers, and parsley. In Chinese medicine, luteolin-rich plants have been widely used to treat various pathological conditions such as inflammatory disorders and hypertension. Additionally, luteolin exerts several health-beneficial effects, including anti-allergy, anti-inflammatory, and anticancer properties. This flavonoid exerts strong anticancer properties both *in vitro* and *in vivo* [243]. In SMMC-7721 cells (human liver cancer cells), luteolin promoted apoptosis partially by autophagy, and it can be employed as an autophagy regulator in the therapy of HCC [244]. Treatment of luteolin has been proven to be effective against diverse cancer cells. Furthermore, numerous studies highlight the synergistic effect of this flavonoid with conventional anticancer medications, opening up new therapeutic possibilities. Luteolin in combination with cisplatin effectively suppresses the growth of HCC cells. In this study, suppression of THOC1 (THO complex 1) by luteolin potentiates the anticancer effect of cisplatin in SK-Hep1, PLC/PRF/5, HepG2, and Hep3B. Additionally, the combined treatment of cisplatin and luteolin enhances the antineoplastic effect of cisplatin in BALB/c nu/nu mice injected with PLC/PRF/5 cells by targeting THOC1 [245]. Besides this, the combination of luteolin and sorafenib acts synergistically in human HCC (SMMC-7721 and Hep3B) cells. In this study, luteolin potentiates HCC cells toward sorafenib by enhancing apoptosis and activating JNK, suggesting that luteolin may be an ideal candidate for enhancing the anticancer activity of sorafenib in liver cancer treatment [246]. In another study, luteolin increases the antineoplastic effect of 5-FU in Bel7402, and HepG2 cells via inducing apoptosis. The synergistic potential of this combined treatment was evident from induced PARP cleavage, enhanced expression of p53, and Bax/Bcl-2 ratio [247]. Hence, combining this natural flavonoid with conventional chemotherapeutics may be developed to reduce the effective doses of antineoplastic agents, as well as to alleviate the associated adverse side effects.

4.17. *Cantharidin*

Cantharidin (CTD) is a mono-terpene derived from Mylabris (*Mylabris phalerata Pallas* or *Mylabris sichorii Linnaeus*). It has been proven to have anticancer action in diverse cancers, particularly HCC. CTD is in use as cancer medicine for its antitumor properties preventing tumor cell proliferation, suppression of cell cycle, apoptosis induction, and altering multidrug resistance in China [248–250]. CTD induces DNA by upregulating KDM4A and downregulating H3K36me3 expression. It sensitizes HCC to sorafenib in HepG2 and SMMC-7721 cells through the induction of DNA damage [251]. Recently, CTD derivative-related medicines, such as magnesium demethylcantharidate, norcantharidin, and methyl-cantharidimide with lower toxicity and anticancer activity, have recently been discovered [252–254]. Norcantharidin induces cell death in HCC via inhibition of c-Met-mTOR signaling [255]. When magnesium demethylcantharidate and sorafenib are combined, FOXO1 is activated that subsequently inhibited metastasis and invasion in cancer cells [252]. Methyl-cantharidimide is essential for lowering cisplatin resistance in cancer cells overexpressing ABCB1 and ABCG2 [256].

4.18. *Dioscin*

Dioscin or diosgenyl 2,4-di-O-L-rhamnopyranosyl-β-D-glucopyranoside is a steroidal saponin with a steroid aglycone moiety that is found in a wide range of vegetables and herbs belonging to the Dioscoreaceae, Liliaceae and Solanaceae family. It is a derivative of diosgenin, whose position 3 was attached by a spirostanyl glycoside [257]. Dioscin is one of the prevalent steroidal saponins in plants with immunostimulatory, antiviral, antifungal, hepatoprotective, lipid-lowering, antitumor and anti-inflammatory activities [258]. Dioscin has anticancer properties in a variety of cancer cells, including human leukemia K562, human lung cancer A549 and HCC [259]. This steroidal saponin induces apoptosis and inhibits division, invasion, and migration of liver cancer cells [260, 261]. Additionally, dioscin reverses multidrug resistance in resistant HepG2 cells (HepG2/adiamycin) *in vitro.* This steroidal saponin elevates the accumulation of adriamycin or DOX by inhibiting P-gp expression [262].

4.19. *Diosgenin*

Diosgenin (3β-hydroxy-5-spirostene) is a steroid sapogenin and acts as precursor in steroid hormone synthesis. Diosgenin is found abundantly in fenugreek seeds and roots of yam. Several studies have documented the beneficial effects of diosgenin in the management of diverse human malignancies, such as leukemia, colon cancer, liver cancer, glioma, prostate cancer, cervical cancer, lung cancer, breast cancer, and pancreatic cancer. It inhibits proliferation of cancer cells, invasion and metastasis. In addition to that, diosgenin induces cell cycle arrest, autophagy, and apoptosis [263]. Furthermore, diosgenin sensitizes HCC cells to DOX and paclitaxel by downregulating the expression of STAT3 and STAT3 regulated downstream targets including c-Src, JAK 1, and JAK 2 [264]. DOX Dios-DOX-LP (diosgenin-based liposome loaded with DOX) can be used as an adjuvant of DOX for the combination treatment of HCC. This complex is a targeted delivery system in which chemotherapeutics combined with natural products help to fight against cancers with fewer toxicity and better efficiency. Studies have shown that Dios-DOX-LP complex enhances the antineoplastic effect of DOX *in vivo* systems [265].

5. Conclusion

Chemoresistance is the major problem for management of HCC. Development of resistance against the chemotherapeutics limits the success of treatment and life expectancy of the patient. Even though many targeted therapies shows survival benefits in some HCC patients either treated alone or in combination, many of such medicines may not be available for a large population due to higher cost. Almost 40% of all drugs in market are from plant source. This chapter discusses the possible use of the some of the naturally occurring compounds which shown chemo sensitization effect in HCC. These compounds are mostly isolated from various plant sources which can be isolated at a lesser cost. Due to various reasons, most of these compounds are still not reached to the clinical trials. More effort should be required in order to validate the clinical usage of these compounds which may benefit a large number of patients as a better affordable therapy.

References

1. Tunissiolli, N.M., et al. Hepatocellular carcinoma: a comprehensive review of biomarkers, clinical aspects, and therapy. *Asian Pac J Cancer Prev*, 2017. **18**(4): p. 863–872.
2. Shannon, A.H., S.M. Ruff, and T.M. Pawlik. Expert insights on current treatments for hepatocellular carcinoma: clinical and molecular approaches and bottlenecks to progress. *J Hepatocell Carcinoma*, 2022. **9**: p. 1247–1261.
3. Sidali, S., et al. New concepts in the treatment of hepatocellular carcinoma. *United Eur Gastroenterol J*, 2022. **10**(7): p. 765–774.
4. Raza, A., and G.K. Sood. Hepatocellular carcinoma review: current treatment, and evidence-based medicine. *World J Gastroenterol*, 2014. **20**(15): p. 4115–4127.
5. Kumari, R., et al. Hepatocellular carcinoma treatment: hurdles, advances and prospects. *Hepat Oncol*, 2018. **5**(2): p. 2018–0002.

6. Shimamura, T., et al. Liver transplantation for hepatocellular carcinoma: how should we improve the thresholds? *Cancers*, 2022. **14**(2).
7. Akkız, H. Hepatocellular carcinoma: from molecular basis to novel treatment approaches. *Can J Gastroenterol Hepatol*, 2019 Mar 3. **2019**: p. 4970731. doi: 10.1155/2019/4970731. eCollection 2019.
8. Livraghi, T., et al. Small hepatocellular carcinoma: percutaneous alcohol injection--results in 23 patients. *Radiology*, 1988. **168**(2): p. 313–317.
9. Seki, T., et al. Ultrasonically guided percutaneous microwave coagulation therapy for small hepatocellular carcinoma. *Cancer*, 1994. **74**(3): p. 817–825.
10. Rossi, S., et al. Percutaneous radiofrequency interstitial thermal ablation in the treatment of small hepatocellular carcinoma. *Cancer J Sci Am*, 1995. **1**(1): p. 73–81.
11. Zimmerman, A., D. Grand, and K.P. Charpentier. Irreversible electroporation of hepatocellular carcinoma: patient selection and perspectives. *J Hepatocell Carcinoma*, 2017. **4**: p. 49–58.
12. Kim, D.K., et al. Percutaneous cryoablation in early stage hepatocellular carcinoma: analysis of local tumor progression factors. *Diagn Interv Radiol*, 2020. **26**(2): p. 111–117.
13. Kotsifa, E., et al. Transarterial chemoembolization for hepatocellular carcinoma: why, when, how? *J Pers Med*, 2022. **12**(3).
14. Zhang, J.X., et al. Safety and efficacy of transarterial chemoembolization and immune checkpoint inhibition with camrelizumab for treatment of unresectable hepatocellular carcinoma. *J Hepatocell Carcinoma*, 2022. **9**: p. 265–272.
15. Zheng, L., et al. Efficacy and safety of TACE combined with sorafenib plus immune checkpoint inhibitors for the treatment of intermediate and advanced TACE-refractory hepatocellular carcinoma: a retrospective study. *Front Mol Biosci*, 2021. **7**: p. 609322.
16. Sangro, B., et al. Advances in immunotherapy for hepatocellular carcinoma. *Nat Rev Gastroenterol Hepatol*, 2021. **18**(8): p. 525–543.
17. Ikeda, M., et al. Chemotherapy for hepatocellular carcinoma: current status and future perspectives. *Jpn J Clin Oncol*, 2018. **48**(2): p. 103–114.

18. Lohitesh, K., R. Chowdhury, and S. Mukherjee. Resistance a major hindrance to chemotherapy in hepatocellular carcinoma: an insight. *Cancer Cell Int*, 2018. **18**: p. 44.
19. Tian, X., et al. Link of sorafenib resistance with the tumor microenvironment in hepatocellular carcinoma: mechanistic insights. *Front Pharmacol*, 2022. **13**: p. 991052.
20. Tang, W., et al. The mechanisms of sorafenib resistance in hepatocellular carcinoma: theoretical basis and therapeutic aspects. *Signal Transduct Target Ther*, 2020. **5**(1): p. 87.
21. Ben Mousa, A. Sorafenib in the treatment of advanced hepatocellular carcinoma. *Saudi J Gastroenterol*, 2008. **14**(1): p. 40–42.
22. Bruix, J., et al. Efficacy and safety of sorafenib in patients with advanced hepatocellular carcinoma: subanalyses of a phase III trial. *J Hepatol*, 2012. **57**(4): p. 821–829.
23. Zeng, Z., et al. Effect of the hypoxia inducible factor on sorafenib resistance of hepatocellular carcinoma. *Front Oncol*, 2021. **11**: p. 641522.
24. Zhu, Y.-J., et al. New knowledge of the mechanisms of sorafenib resistance in liver cancer. *Acta Pharmacologica Sinica*, 2017. **38**(5): p. 614–622.
25. Hu, Z., et al. Enhancement of anti-tumor effects of 5-fluorouracil on hepatocellular carcinoma by low-intensity ultrasound. *J Exp Clin Cancer Res*, 2016. **35**(1): p. 71.
26. Miura, K., et al. 5-FU metabolism in cancer and orally-administrable 5-FU drugs. *Cancers*, 2010. **2**(3): p. 1717–1730.
27. Azwar, S., et al. Recent updates on mechanisms of resistance to 5-fluorouracil and reversal strategies in colon cancer treatment. *Biology*, 2021. **10**(9): p. 854.
28. Ghafouri-Fard, S., et al. 5-fluorouracil: a narrative review on the role of regulatory mechanisms in driving resistance to this chemotherapeutic agent. *Front Oncol*, 2021. **11**: p. 658636.
29. Yan, Y., et al. Chlorogenic acid enhances the effects of 5-fluorouracil in human hepatocellular carcinoma cells through the inhibition of extracellular signal-regulated kinases. *Anti-Cancer Drugs*, 2015. **26**(5): p. 540–546.

30. Longley, D.B., D.P. Harkin, and P.G. Johnston. 5-fluorouracil: mechanisms of action and clinical strategies. *Nat Rev Cancer*, 2003. **3**(5): p. 330–338.
31. Jubeen, F., et al. Anticancer potential of novel 5-fluorouracil co-crystals against MCF7 breast and SW480 colon cancer cell lines along with docking studies. *Arab J Chem*, 2022. **15**(12): p. 104299.
32. Wei, D.-D., J.-S. Wang, and L.-Y. Kong. Reversal effects of components from the fruits of Illicium simonsii on human adriamycin-resistant MCF-7 and 5-fluorouracil-resistant Bel7402 cells. *Phytother Res*, 2012. **26**(4): p. 562–567.
33. Shao, M., et al. Crizotinib and doxorubicin cooperatively reduces drug resistance by mitigating MDR1 to increase hepatocellular carcinoma cells death. *Front Oncol*, 2021. **11**: p. 650052.
34. Wang, S., et al. Doxorubicin induces apoptosis in normal and tumor cells via distinctly different mechanisms: intermediacy OF H2O2- and p53-dependent pathways*. *J Biol Chem*, 2004. **279**(24): p. 25535–25543.
35. Kciuk, M., et al. Doxorubicin — an agent with multiple mechanisms of anticancer activity. *Cells*, 2023. **12**(4): p. 659.
36. Taymaz-Nikerel, H., et al. Doxorubicin induces an extensive transcriptional and metabolic rewiring in yeast cells. *Sci Rep*, 2018. **8**(1): p. 13672.
37. Cox, J., and S. Weinman. Mechanisms of doxorubicin resistance in hepatocellular carcinoma. *Hepatic Oncol*, 2016. **3**(1): p. 57–59.
38. Berthiaume, J.M., and K.B. Wallace. Adriamycin-induced oxidative mitochondrial cardiotoxicity. *Cell Biol Toxicol*, 2007. **23**(1): p. 15–25.
39. Kurz, E.U., P. Douglas, and S.P. Lees-Miller. Doxorubicin activates ATM-dependent phosphorylation of multiple downstream targets in part through the generation of reactive oxygen species*. *J Biol Chem*, 2004. **279**(51): p. 53272–53281.
40. Liu, Y.-C., C.-T. Yeh, and K.-H. Lin. Cancer stem cell functions in hepatocellular carcinoma and comprehensive therapeutic strategies. *Cells*, 2020. **9**(6): p. 1331.
41. Nitiss, J.L. Targeting DNA topoisomerase II in cancer chemotherapy. *Nat Rev Cancer*, 2009. **9**(5): p. 338–350.

42. Shi, G.-M., et al. Identification of side population cells in human hepatocellular carcinoma cell lines with stepwise metastatic potentials. *J Cancer Res Clin Oncol*, 2008. **134**(11): p. 1155–1163.
43. Ghosh, S. Cisplatin: the first metal based anticancer drug. *Bioorg Chem*, 2019. **88**: p. 102925.
44. Rocha, C.R.R., et al. DNA repair pathways and cisplatin resistance: an intimate relationship. *Clinics*, 2018. **73**(suppl 1): p. e478s.
45. Abd Rashid, N., et al. The role of natural antioxidants in cisplatin-induced hepatotoxicity. *Biomed Pharmacother*, 2021. **144**: p. 112328.
46. Korita, P.V., et al. Multidrug resistance-associated protein 2 determines the efficacy of cisplatin in patients with hepatocellular carcinoma. *Oncol Rep*, 2010. **23**(4): p. 965–972.
47. Liedert, B., et al. Overexpression of cMOAT (MRP2/ABCC2) is associated with decreased formation of platinum-DNA adducts and decreased G2-Arrest in melanoma cells resistant to cisplatin. *J Invest Dermatol*, 2003. **121**(1): p. 172–176.
48. Mandic, A., et al. Cisplatin induces endoplasmic reticulum stress and nucleus-independent apoptotic signaling*. *J Biol Chem*, 2003. **278**(11): p. 9100–9106.
49. Holzer, A.K., G.H. Manorek, and S.B. Howell. Contribution of the major copper influx transporter CTR1 to the cellular accumulation of cisplatin, carboplatin, and oxaliplatin. *Mol Pharmacol*, 2006. **70**(4): p. 1390–1394.
50. Hatanaka, T., A. Naganuma, and S. Kakizaki. Lenvatinib for hepatocellular carcinoma: a literature review. *Pharmaceuticals*, 2021. **14**(1): p. 36.
51. Wang, S., et al. Lenvatinib as first-line treatment for unresectable hepatocellular carcinoma: a systematic review and meta-analysis. *Cancers*, 2022. **14**(22): p. 5525.
52. Wang, C.-C., et al. A bibliometric study on the utilization of lenvatinib in hepatocellular carcinoma (2014–2022). *Front Pharmacol*, 2023. **14**.
53. Bo, W., and Y. Chen. Lenvatinib resistance mechanism and potential ways to conquer. *Front Pharmacol*, 2023. **14**.
54. He, X., et al. EGFR inhibition reverses resistance to lenvatinib in hepatocellular carcinoma cells. *Sci Rep*, 2022. **12**(1): p. 8007.

55. Farasati Far, B., et al. Unresectable hepatocellular carcinoma: a review of new advances with focus on targeted therapy and immunotherapy. *Livers*, 2023. **3**(1): p. 121–160.
56. Lohitesh, K., R. Chowdhury, and S. Mukherjee. Resistance a major hindrance to chemotherapy in hepatocellular carcinoma: an insight. *Cancer Cell Int*, 2018. **18**(1): p. 44.
57. Bruix, J., et al. Regorafenib for patients with hepatocellular carcinoma who progressed on sorafenib treatment (RESORCE): a randomised, double-blind, placebo-controlled, phase 3 trial. *The Lancet*, 2017. **389**(10064): p. 56–66.
58. Grothey, A., et al. Evolving role of regorafenib for the treatment of advanced cancers. *Cancer Treat Rev*, 2020. **86**: p. 101993.
59. Tang, J., et al. Erlotinib resistance in lung cancer: current progress and future perspectives. *Front Pharmacol*, 2013. **4**.
60. Huether, A., et al. Erlotinib induces cell cycle arrest and apoptosis in hepatocellular cancer cells and enhances chemosensitivity towards cytostatics. *J Hepatology*, 2005. **43**(4): p. 661–669.
61. Lefebvre, C., et al. Involvement of the AKT pathway in resistance to erlotinib and cabozantinib in triple-negative breast cancer cell lines. *Biomedicines*, 2023. **11**(9): p. 2406.
62. Deng, S., A. Solinas, and D.F. Calvisi. Cabozantinib for HCC treatment, from clinical Back to experimental models. *Front Oncol*, 2021. **11**.
63. Pópulo, H., J.M. Lopes, and P. Soares. The mTOR signalling pathway in human cancer. *Int J Mol Sci*, 2012. **13**(2): p. 1886–1918.
64. Chen, K.F., et al. Activation of phosphatidylinositol 3-kinase/Akt signaling pathway mediates acquired resistance to sorafenib in hepatocellular carcinoma cells. *J Pharmacol Exp Ther*, 2011. **337**(1): p. 155–161.
65. Llovet, J.M., et al. Sorafenib in advanced hepatocellular carcinoma. *N Engl J Med*, 2008. **359**(4): p. 378–390.
66. Zhou, L., et al. The mTOR pathway is associated with the poor prognosis of human hepatocellular carcinoma. *Med Oncol*, 2010. **27**(2): p. 255–261.
67. Ding, X., et al. Genomic and epigenomic features of primary and recurrent hepatocellular carcinomas. *Gastroenterology*, 2019. **157**(6): p. 1630–1645.

68. Zhao, B., et al. Inactivation of YAP oncoprotein by the Hippo pathway is involved in cell contact inhibition and tissue growth control. *Genes Dev*, 2007. **21**(21): p. 2747–2761.
69. Boopathy, G.T.K., and W. Hong. Role of hippo pathway-YAP/TAZ signaling in angiogenesis. *Front Cell Dev Biol*, 2019. 7(49).
70. Valero, V., 3rd, T.M. Pawlik, and R.A. Anders. Emerging role of Hpo signaling and YAP in hepatocellular carcinoma. *J Hepatocell Carcinoma*, 2015. **2**: p. 69–78.
71. Zhu, P., et al. LncBRM initiates YAP1 signalling activation to drive self-renewal of liver cancer stem cells. *Nat Commun*, 2016. **7**: p. 13608.
72. Fan, Y., et al. YAP-1 promotes tregs differentiation in hepatocellular carcinoma by enhancing TGFBR2 transcription. *Cell Physiol Biochem*, 2017. **41**(3): p. 1189–1198.
73. Guo, X., et al. Single tumor-initiating cells evade immune clearance by recruiting type II macrophages. *Genes Dev*, 2017. **31**(3): p. 247–259.
74. Li, H., et al. Deregulation of Hippo kinase signalling in human hepatic malignancies. *Liver Int*, 2012. **32**(1): p. 38–47.
75. Zhong, Z., Z. Wen, and J.E. Darnell, Jr. Stat3: a STAT family member activated by tyrosine phosphorylation in response to epidermal growth factor and interleukin-6. *Science*, 1994. **264**(5155): p. 95–98.
76. Seif, F., et al. The role of JAK-STAT signaling pathway and its regulators in the fate of T helper cells. *Cell Commun and Signal*, 2017. **15**(1): p. 23.
77. Banerjee, S., et al. JAK–STAT signaling as a target for inflammatory and autoimmune diseases: current and future prospects. *Drugs*, 2017. 77(5): p. 521–546.
78. Huynh, J., et al. Therapeutically exploiting STAT3 activity in cancer — using tissue repair as a road map. *Nat Rev Cancer*, 2019. **19**(2): p. 82–96.
79. Hu, B., et al. Inhibition of EGFR overcomes acquired lenvatinib resistance driven by STAT3–ABCB1 signaling in hepatocellular carcinoma. *Cancer Res*, 2022. **82**(20): p. 3845–3857.
80. Crosby, E.J., et al. Stimulation of oncogene-specific tumor-infiltrating T cells through combined vaccine and αPD-1 enable sustained

antitumor responses against established HER2 breast cancer. *Clin Cancer Res*, 2020. **26**(17): p. 4670–4681.

81. Li, P., et al. Expression of Wnt-5a and β-catenin in primary hepatocellular carcinoma. *Int J Clin Exp Pathol*, 2014. 7(6): p. 3190–3195.
82. Vilchez, V., et al. Targeting Wnt/β-catenin pathway in hepatocellular carcinoma treatment. *World J Gastroenterol*, 2016. **22**(2): p. 823–832.
83. Xu, W., et al. Hypoxia activates Wnt/β-catenin signaling by regulating the expression of BCL9 in human hepatocellular carcinoma. *Sci Rep*, 2017. 7: p. 40446.
84. Wang, W., et al. Action and function of Wnt/β-catenin signaling in the progression from chronic hepatitis C to hepatocellular carcinoma. *J Gastroenterol*, 2017. **52**(4): p. 419–431.
85. Chen, Z., et al. The lncRNA-GAS5/miR-221-3p/DKK2 axis modulates ABCB1-mediated adriamycin resistance of breast cancer via the Wnt/β-Catenin signaling pathway. *Mol Ther Nucleic Acids*, 2020. **19**: p. 1434–1448.
86. Guichard, C., et al. Integrated analysis of somatic mutations and focal copy-number changes identifies key genes and pathways in hepatocellular carcinoma. *Nat Gene*, 2012. **44**(6): p. 694–698.
87. Wang, W., et al. Action and function of Wnt/β-catenin signaling in the progression from chronic hepatitis C to hepatocellular carcinoma. *J Gastroenterol*, 2017. **52**(4): p. 419–431.
88. Xu, W., et al. Hypoxia activates Wnt/β-catenin signaling by regulating the expression of BCL9 in human hepatocellular carcinoma. *Sci Rep*, 2017. 7(1): p. 40446.
89. Takai, A., H.T. Dang, and X.W. Wang. Identification of drivers from cancer genome diversity in hepatocellular carcinoma. *Int J Mol Sciences*, 2014. **15**(6): p. 11142–11160.
90. Ahn, S.-M., et al. Genomic portrait of resectable hepatocellular carcinomas: implications of RB1 and FGF19 aberrations for patient stratification. *Hepatology*, 2014. **60**(6): p. 1972–1982.
91. Marei, H.E., et al. p53 signaling in cancer progression and therapy. *Cancer Cell Int*, 2021. **21**(1): p. 703.
92. Rivlin, N., et al. Mutations in the p53 tumor suppressor gene: important milestones at the various steps of tumorigenesis. *Gene Cancer*, 2011. **2**(4): p. 466–474.

93. Aguilar, F., S.P. Hussain, and P. Cerutti. Aflatoxin B1 induces the transversion of G→T in codon 249 of the p53 tumor suppressor gene in human hepatocytes. *Proc Natl Acad Sci USA*, 1993. **90**(18): p. 8586–8590.
94. Hussain, S.P., et al. TP53 mutations and hepatocellular carcinoma: insights into the etiology and pathogenesis of liver cancer. *Oncogene*, 2007. **26**(15): p. 2166–2176.
95. Tang, H., et al. Molecular functions and biological roles of hepatitis B virus x protein. *Cancer Sci*, 2006. **97**(10): p. 977–983.
96. Nag, S., et al. The MDM2-p53 pathway revisited. *J Biomed Res*, 2013. **27**(4): p. 254–271.
97. Manning, A.L., C. Benes, and N.J. Dyson. Whole chromosome instability resulting from the synergistic effects of pRB and p53 inactivation. *Oncogene*, 2014. **33**(19): p. 2487–2494.
98. Schvartzman, J.M., et al. Mad2 is a critical mediator of the chromosome instability observed upon Rb and p53 pathway inhibition. *Cancer Cell*, 2011. **19**(6): p. 701–714.
99. Kawamura, K., et al. Induction of centrosome amplification and chromosome instability in human bladder cancer cells by p53 mutation and cyclin E overexpression. *Cancer Res*, 2004. **64**(14): p. 4800–4809.
100. Laurent-Puig, P., et al. Genetic alterations associated with hepatocellular carcinomas define distinct pathways of hepatocarcinogenesis. *Gastroenterology*, 2001. **120**(7): p. 1763–1773.
101. Chan, K.-T., and M.L. Lung. Mutant p53 expression enhances drug resistance in a hepatocellular carcinoma cell line. *Cancer Chemother Pharmacol*, 2004. **53**(6): p. 519–526.
102. Fang, F., et al. FBI-1 promotes cell proliferation and enhances resistance to chemotherapy of hepatocellular carcinoma *in vitro* and *in vivo. Cancer*, 2012. **118**(1): p. 134–146.
103. Li, S., et al. p53 and P-glycoprotein influence chemoresistance in hepatocellular carcinoma. *Front Biosci*, 2018. **10**(3): p. 461–468.
104. Yu, L., Y. Chen, and S.A. Tooze. Autophagy pathway: cellular and molecular mechanisms. *Autophagy*, 2018. **14**(2): p. 207–215.
105. Mizushima, N. Physiological functions of autophagy. *Curr Top Microbiol Immunol*, 2009. **335**: p. 71–84.

106. Yazdani, H.O., H. Huang, and A. Tsung. Autophagy: dual response in the development of hepatocellular carcinoma. *Cells*, 2019. **8**(2): p. 91.
107. Duan, Y., et al. Fucoidan induces apoptosis and inhibits proliferation of hepatocellular carcinoma via the p38 MAPK/ERK and PI3K/Akt signal pathways. *Cancer Manag Res*, 2020. **12**: p. 1713–1723.
108. Hashemi, M., et al. Targeting and regulation of autophagy in hepatocellular carcinoma: revisiting the molecular interactions and mechanisms for new therapy approaches. *Cell Commun Signal*, 2023. **21**(1): p. 32.
109. Newell, P., et al. Ras pathway activation in hepatocellular carcinoma and anti-tumoral effect of combined sorafenib and rapamycin *in vivo*. *J Hepatol*, 2009. **51**(4): p. 725–733.
110. Fernández-Medarde, A., and E. Santos. Ras in cancer and developmental diseases. *Gene Cancer*, 2011. **2**(3): p. 344–358.
111. Aksamitiene, E., A. Kiyatkin, and B.N. Kholodenko. Cross-talk between mitogenic Ras/MAPK and survival PI3K/Akt pathways: a fine balance. *Biochem Soc Trans*, 2012. **40**(1): p. 139–146.
112. Cajuso, T., et al. Exome sequencing reveals frequent inactivating mutations in ARID1A, ARID1B, ARID2 and ARID4A in microsatellite unstable colorectal cancer. *Int J Cancer*, 2014. **135**(3): p. 611–623.
113. Luo, B., et al. Highly parallel identification of essential genes in cancer cells. *Proc Natl Acad Sci U S A*, 2008. **105**(51): p. 20380–20385.
114. Meng, G.X., et al. The somatic mutational landscape and role of the ARID1A gene in hepatocellular carcinoma. *Heliyon*, 2023. **9**(3): p. e14307.
115. Hanahan, D. Hallmarks of cancer: new dimensions. *Cancer Discov*, 2022. **12**(1): p. 31–46.
116. Zhang, X., et al. ARID1A mutations in cancer development: mechanism and therapy. *Carcinogenesis*, 2023. **44**(3): p. 197–208.
117. Bouattour, M., et al. Systemic treatment for advanced hepatocellular carcinoma. *Liver Cancer*, 2019. **8**(5): p. 341–358.
118. Hu, C., et al. Arid1a regulates response to anti-angiogenic therapy in advanced hepatocellular carcinoma. *J Hepatol*, 2018. **68**(3): p. 465–475.

119. Ding, X.-X., et al. Precision medicine for hepatocellular carcinoma: driver mutations and targeted therapy. *Oncotarget*, 2017. **8**(33): p. 55715–55730.
120. Helming, K.C., et al. ARID1B is a specific vulnerability in ARID1A-mutant cancers. *Nat Med*, 2014. **20**(3): p. 251–254.
121. Shiloh, Y. ATM and related protein kinases: safeguarding genome integrity. *Nat Rev Cancer*, 2003. **3**(3): p. 155–168.
122. Abraham, R.T. Cell cycle checkpoint signaling through the ATM and ATR kinases. *Gene Dev*, 2001. **15**(17): p. 2177–2196.
123. Daugherity, E.K., et al. The DNA damage checkpoint protein ATM promotes hepatocellular apoptosis and fibrosis in a mouse model of non-alcoholic fatty liver disease. *Cell Cycle*, 2012. **11**(10): p. 1918–1928.
124. Fujimaki, S., et al. Blockade of ataxia telangiectasia mutated sensitizes hepatoma cell lines to sorafenib by interfering with Akt signaling. *Cancer Lett*, 2012. **319**(1): p. 98–108.
125. Weng, X., et al. Cyclin-dependent kinase inhibitor 2B gene is associated with the sensitivity of hepatoma cells to Sorafenib. *Onco Targets Ther*, 2019. **12**: p. 5025–5036.
126. Velamakanni, S., et al. ABCG transporters: structure, substrate specificities and physiological roles. *J Bioenerg Biomembr*, 2007. **39**(5): p. 465–471.
127. Sen, Q., W. Hai, and C. Xiaoping. Reversal of HCC drug resistance by using hammerhead ribozymes against multidrug resistance 1 gene. *J Huazhong U Sci Technol [Med Sci]*, 2005. **25**(6): p. 662–664.
128. Rigalli, J.P., et al. Regulation of multidrug resistance proteins by genistein in a hepatocarcinoma cell line: impact on sorafenib cytotoxicity. *PLoS One*, 2015. **10**(3): p. e0119502.
129. Sun, Z., et al. Relevance of two genes in the multidrug resistance of hepatocellular carcinoma: *in vivo* and clinical studies. *Tumori*, 2010. **96**(1): p. 90–96.
130. Vander Borght, S., et al. Up-regulation of breast cancer resistance protein expression in hepatoblastoma following chemotherapy: a study in patients and *in vitro*. *Hepatol Res*, 2008. **38**(11): p. 1112–1121.
131. Sarek, G., et al. Molecular basis of telomere dysfunction in human genetic diseases. Nat *Struct Mol Biol*, 2015. **22**(11): p. 867–874.

132. Nault, J.C., and J. Zucman-Rossi. TERT promoter mutations in primary liver tumors. *Clin Res Hepatol Gastroenterol*, 2016. **40**(1): p. 9–14.
133. Zucman-Rossi, J., et al. Genetic landscape and biomarkers of hepatocellular carcinoma. *Gastroenterology*, 2015. **149**(5): p. 1226–1239.
134. Torrecilla, S., et al. Trunk mutational events present minimal intra- and inter-tumoral heterogeneity in hepatocellular carcinoma. *J Hepatol*, 2017. **67**(6): p. 1222–1231.
135. Batlle, E., and J. Massagué. Transforming growth factor-β signaling in immunity and cancer. *Immunity*, 2019. **50**(4): p. 924–940.
136. Hinck, A.P., T.D. Mueller, and T.A. Springer. Structural biology and evolution of the TGF-β family. *Cold Spring Harb Perspect Biol*, 2016. **8**: p. a022103. Doi: 10.1101/cshperspect.a022103.
137. Tian, Y., et al. Epigenetic activation of Wnt/β-catenin signaling in NAFLD-associated hepatocarcinogenesis. *Cancers*, 2016. **8**(8): p. 76.
138. Rao, S., and L. Mishra. Targeting transforming growth factor beta signaling in liver cancer. *Hepatology*, 2019 Apr. **69**(4): p. 1375–1378. doi: 10.1002/hep.30426. Epub 2019 Mar 5.
139. Bhagyaraj, E., et al. TGF-β induced chemoresistance in liver cancer is modulated by xenobiotic nuclear receptor PXR. *Cell Cycle*, 2019. **18**(24): p. 3589–3602.
140. Liu, Z., et al. EGF is highly expressed in hepatocellular carcinoma (HCC) and promotes motility of HCC cells via fibronectin. *J Cell Biochem*, 2018. **119**(5): p. 4170–4183.
141. Peng, Q., et al. Mitogen-activated protein kinase signaling pathway in oral cancer. *Oncol Lett*, 2018. **15**(2): p. 1379–1388.
142. Cargnello, M., and P.P. Roux. Activation and function of the MAPKs and their substrates, the MAPK-activated protein kinases. *Microbiol Mol Biol Rev*, 2011. **75**(1): p. 50–83.
143. Negrini, S., V.G. Gorgoulis, and T.D. Halazonetis. Genomic instability--an evolving hallmark of cancer. *Nat Rev Mol Cell Biol*, 2010. **11**(3): p. 220–228.
144. Ippolito, M.R., et al. Gene copy-number changes and chromosomal instability induced by aneuploidy confer resistance to chemotherapy. *Dev Cell*, 2021. **56**(17): p. 2440–2454.

145. Zhang, L., et al. VEGF is essential for the growth and migration of human hepatocellular carcinoma cells. *Mol Biol Rep*, 2012. **39**(5): p. 5085–5093.
146. Amini, A., et al. The critical role of vascular endothelial growth factor in tumor angiogenesis. *Curr Cancer Drug Targets*, 2012. **12**(1): p. 23–43.
147. Lieu, C., et al. Beyond VEGF: inhibition of the fibroblast growth factor pathway and antiangiogenesis. *Clin Cancer Res*, 2011. **17**(19): p. 6130–6139.
148. Gao, L., et al. FGF19/FGFR4 signaling contributes to the resistance of hepatocellular carcinoma to sorafenib. *J Exp Clin Cancer Res*, 2017. **36**(1): p. 8.
149. Sawey, E.T., et al. Identification of a therapeutic strategy targeting amplified FGF19 in liver cancer by oncogenomic screening. *Cancer Cell*, 2011. **19**(3): p. 347–358.
150. Guichard, C., et al. Integrated analysis of somatic mutations and focal copy-number changes identifies key genes and pathways in hepatocellular carcinoma. *Nat Genet*, 2012. **44**(6): p. 694–698.
151. Liu, R., et al. Gankyrin drives metabolic reprogramming to promote tumorigenesis, metastasis and drug resistance through activating β-catenin/c-Myc signaling in human hepatocellular carcinoma. *Cancer Lett*, 2019. **443**: p. 34–46.
152. Wang, J.W., et al. RCN1 induces sorafenib resistance and malignancy in hepatocellular carcinoma by activating c-MYC signaling via the IRE1α-XBP1s pathway. *Cell Death Discov*, 2021. **7**(1): p. 298.
153. Lin, C.P., et al. Small-molecule c-Myc inhibitor, 10058-F4, inhibits proliferation, downregulates human telomerase reverse transcriptase and enhances chemosensitivity in human hepatocellular carcinoma cells. *Anticancer Drug*, 2007. **18**(2): p. 161–170.
154. Shukla, G., et al. Therapeutic potential, challenges and future perspective of cancer stem cells in translational oncology: a critical review. *Curr Stem Cell Res Ther*, 2017. **12**(3): p. 207–224.
155. Ma, S., et al. Identification and characterization of tumorigenic liver cancer stem/progenitor cells. *Gastroenterology*, 2007. **132**(7): p. 2542–2556.

156. Kawai, T., et al. Keratin 19, a cancer stem cell marker in human hepatocellular carcinoma. *Clin Cancer Res*, 2015. **21**(13): p. 3081–3091.
157. Desai, A., B. Webb, and S.L. Gerson. CD133+ cells contribute to radioresistance via altered regulation of DNA repair genes in human lung cancer cells. *Radiother Oncol*, 2014. **110**(3): p. 538–545.
158. Cheng, J., et al. MEK1 signaling promotes self-renewal and tumorigenicity of liver cancer stem cells via maintaining SIRT1 protein stabilization. *Oncotarget*, 2016. **7**(15): p. 20597–20611.
159. Tong, M., et al. ANXA3/JNK signaling promotes self-renewal and tumor growth, and its blockade provides a therapeutic target for hepatocellular carcinoma. *Stem Cell Rep*, 2015. **5**(1): p. 45–59.
160. Jeng, K.S., et al. Activation of the sonic hedgehog signaling pathway occurs in the CD133 positive cells of mouse liver cancer Hepa 1–6 cells. *Onco Targets Ther*, 2013. **6**: p. 1047–1055.
161. Nikolaou, K.C., et al. Spontaneous development of hepatocellular carcinoma with cancer stem cell properties in PR-SET7-deficient livers. *Embo J*, 2015. **34**(4): p. 430–447.
162. Xie, C., et al. Tobacco smoke induced hepatic cancer stem cell-like properties through IL-33/p38 pathway. *J Exp Clin Cancer Res*, 2019. **38**(1): p. 39.
163. Mahati, S., et al. TMPRSS4 promotes cancer stem cell traits by regulating CLDN1 in hepatocellular carcinoma. *Biochem Biophys Res Commun*, 2017. **490**(3): p. 906–912.
164. Pan, Z., et al. Curcumin inhibits hepatocellular carcinoma growth by targeting VEGF expression. *Oncol Lett*, 2018. **15**(4): p. 4821–4826.
165. Elkhamesy, A., et al. Diminished CCl(4)-induced hepatocellular carcinoma, oxidative stress, and apoptosis by co-administration of curcumin or selenium in mice. *J Food Biochem*, 2022. **46**(4): p. 6.
166. Hu, P., et al. Both glypican-3/Wnt/β-catenin signaling pathway and autophagy contributed to the inhibitory effect of curcumin on hepatocellular carcinoma. *Dig Liver Dis*, 2019. **51**(1): p. 120–126.
167. Cheng, Y., et al. Cisplatin and curcumin co-loaded nano-liposomes for the treatment of hepatocellular carcinoma. *Int J Pharm*, 2018. **545**(1–2): p. 261–273.
168. Zhao, X., et al. Doxorubicin and curcumin co-delivery by lipid nanoparticles for enhanced treatment of diethylnitrosamine-induced

hepatocellular carcinoma in mice. *Eur J Pharm Biopharm*, 2015. **93**: p. 27–36.

169. Bian, Y., and D. Guo. Targeted therapy for hepatocellular carcinoma: co-delivery of sorafenib and curcumin using lactosylated pH-Responsive nanoparticles. *Drug Des Devel Ther*, 2020. **14**: p. 647–659.
170. Xu, T., et al. Synergistic effects of curcumin and 5-fluorouracil on the hepatocellular carcinoma *in vivo* and *vitro* through regulating the expression of COX-2 and NF-κB. *J Cancer*, 2020. **11**(13): p. 3955–3964.
171. Soni, V.K., et al. Counteracting action of curcumin on high glucose-induced chemoresistance in hepatic carcinoma cells. *Front Oncol*, 2021. **11**: p. 738961.
172. Tian, N., et al. Lin28b is involved in curcumin-reversed paclitaxel chemoresistance and associated with poor prognosis in hepatocellular carcinoma. *J Cancer*, 2019. **10**(24): p. 6074–6087.
173. Hsu, F.T., et al. Curcumin sensitizes hepatocellular carcinoma cells to radiation via suppression of radiation-induced NF-κB activity. *Biomed Res Int*, 2015. **363671**(10): p. 11.
174. Abid, R., et al. Pharmacological properties of 4', 5, 7-trihydroxyflavone (Apigenin) and its impact on cell signaling pathways. *Molecules*, 2022. **27**(13): p. 4304.
175. Ganai, S.A. Plant-derived flavone apigenin: the small-molecule with promising activity against therapeutically resistant prostate cancer. *Biomed Pharmacother*, 2017. **85**: p. 47–56.
176. Ashrafizadeh, M., et al. Apigenin as tumor suppressor in cancers: biotherapeutic activity, nanodelivery, and mechanisms with emphasis on pancreatic cancer. *Front Chem*, 2020. **8**: p. 829.
177. Hu, X.Y., et al. 5-fluorouracil combined with apigenin enhances anticancer activity through mitochondrial membrane potential ($\Delta\Psi$m)-mediated apoptosis in hepatocellular carcinoma. *Clin Exp Pharmacol Physiol*, 2015. **42**(2): p. 146–153.
178. Gao, A.M., et al. Apigenin sensitizes hepatocellular carcinoma cells to doxorubic through regulating miR-520b/ATG7 axis. *Chem Biol Interact*, 2018. **280**: p. 45–50.
179. Şirin, N., et al. Investigation of possible effects of apigenin, sorafenib and combined applications on apoptosis and cell cycle in hepatocellular cancer cells. *Gene*, 2020. **737**(144428): p. 8.

180. Mokra, D., M. Joskova, and J. Mokry. Therapeutic effects of green tea polyphenol (−)-epigallocatechin-3-Gallate (EGCG) in relation to molecular pathways controlling inflammation, oxidative stress, and apoptosis. *Int J Mol Sci*, 2022. **24**(1): p. 340.
181. Kojima-Yuasa, A., X. Huang, and I. Matsui-Yuasa. Synergistic anticancer activities of natural substances in human hepatocellular carcinoma. *Diseases*, 2015. **3**(4): p. 260–281.
182. Li, D., et al. The potential of epigallocatechin gallate in the chemoprevention and therapy of hepatocellular carcinoma. *Front Pharmacol*, 2023. **14**: p. 1201085.
183. Satonaka, H., et al. *(-)-Epigallocatechin-3-gallate down-regulates doxorubicin-induced overexpression of p-glycoprotein through the coordinate inhibition of PI3K/Akt and MEK/ERK signaling pathways. Anticancer Res*, 2017. **37**(11): p. 6071–6077.
184. Chen, L., et al. Autophagy inhibition contributes to the synergistic interaction between EGCG and doxorubicin to kill the hepatoma Hep3B cells. *PLoS One*, 2014. **9**(1): p. e85771.
185. Yang, X.W., et al. Green tea polyphenol epigallocatechin-3-gallate enhances 5-fluorouracil-induced cell growth inhibition of hepatocellular carcinoma cells. *Hepatol Res*, 2012. **42**(5): p. 494–501.
186. Liang, G., et al. Green tea catechins augment the antitumor activity of doxorubicin in an *in vivo* mouse model for chemoresistant liver cancer. *Int J Oncol*, 2010. **37**(1): p. 111–123.
187. Sarvizadeh, M., et al. Allicin and digestive system cancers: from chemical structure to its therapeutic opportunities. *Front Oncol*, 2021. **11**: p. 650256.
188. Ţigu, A.B., et al. The synergistic antitumor effect of 5-fluorouracil combined with allicin against lung and colorectal carcinoma cells. *Molecules*, 2020. **25**(8): p. 1947.
189. Zou, X., et al. Allicin sensitizes hepatocellular cancer cells to antitumor activity of 5-fluorouracil through ROS-mediated mitochondrial pathway. *J Pharmacol Sci*, 2016. **131**(4): p. 233–240.
190. Meng, X., et al. Health benefits and molecular mechanisms of resveratrol: a narrative review. *Foods*, 2020. **9**(3): p. 340.
191. Gao, M., C. Deng, and F. Dang. Synergistic antitumor effect of resveratrol and sorafenib on hepatocellular carcinoma through PKA/AMPK/eEF2K pathway. *Food Nutr Res*, 2021. **13**: p. 65.

192. Liu, Z., et al. Resveratrol enhances cisplatin-induced apoptosis in human hepatoma cells via glutamine metabolism inhibition. *BMB Rep*, 2018 Sep. **51**(9): p. 474–479. doi: 10.5483/BMBRep.2018.51.9.114.
193. Wu, S.L., et al. Effect of resveratrol and in combination with 5-FU on murine liver cancer. *World J Gastroenterol*, 2004. **10**(20): p. 3048–3052.
194. Refolo, M.G., et al. Chlorogenic acid improves the regorafenib effects in human hepatocellular carcinoma cells. *Int J Mol Sci*, 2018. **19**(5): p. 1518.
195. Yan, Y., et al. Chlorogenic acid enhances the effects of 5-fluorouracil in human hepatocellular carcinoma cells through the inhibition of extracellular signal-regulated kinases. *Anticancer Drug*, 2015. **26**(5): p. 540–546.
196. Chen, X., et al. Inhibiting ROS-STAT3-dependent autophagy enhanced capsaicin-induced apoptosis in human hepatocellular carcinoma cells. *Free Radic Res*, 2016. **50**(7): p. 744–755.
197. Joung, E.J., et al. Capsaicin induces heme oxygenase-1 expression in HepG2 cells via activation of PI3K-Nrf2 signaling: NAD(P)H:quinone oxidoreductase as a potential target. *Antioxid Redox Signal*, 2007. **9**(12): p. 2087–2098.
198. Bort, A., et al. Capsaicin exerts synergistic antitumor effect with sorafenib in hepatocellular carcinoma cells through AMPK activation. *Oncotarget*, 2017. **8**(50): p. 87684–87698.
199. Dai, N., et al. Capsaicin and sorafenib combination treatment exerts synergistic anti-hepatocellular carcinoma activity by suppressing EGFR and PI3K/Akt/mTOR signaling. *Oncol Rep*, 2018. **40**(6): p. 3235–3248.
200. Mirazimi, S.M.A., et al. Application of quercetin in the treatment of gastrointestinal cancers. *Front Pharmacol*, 2022. **13**: p. 860209.
201. Abdu, S., et al. Effects of sorafenib and quercetin alone or in combination in treating hepatocellular carcinoma: *in vitro* and *in vivo* approaches. *Molecules*, 2022. **27**(22): p. 8082.
202. Hassan, S., et al. Quercetin potentializes the respective cytotoxic activity of gemcitabine or doxorubicin on 3D culture of AsPC-1 or HepG2 cells, through the inhibition of HIF-1α and MDR1. *PLoS One*, 2020. **15**(10): p. e0240676.

203. Chen, Z., et al. Reversal effect of quercetin on multidrug resistance via FZD7/β-catenin pathway in hepatocellular carcinoma cells. *Phytomedicine*, 2018. **43**: p. 37–45.
204. Zhao, J.L., J. Zhao, and H.J. Jiao. Synergistic growth-suppressive effects of quercetin and cisplatin on HepG2 human hepatocellular carcinoma cells. *Appl Biochem Biotechnol*, 2014. **172**(2): p. 784–791.
205. Liu, H., et al. The fascinating effects of baicalein on cancer: a review. *Int J Mol Sci*, 2016. **17**(10): p. 1681.
206. Kuo, H.M., et al. Mitochondrial-dependent caspase activation pathway is involved in baicalein-induced apoptosis in human hepatoma J5 cells. *Int J Oncol*, 2009. **35**(4): p. 717–724.
207. Han, Z., et al. Baicalein inhibits hepatocellular carcinoma cells through suppressing the expression of CD24. *Int Immunopharmacol*, 2015. **29**(2): p. 416–422.
208. Zheng, Y.H., et al. Anticancer effects of baicalein on hepatocellular carcinoma cells. *Phytother Res*, 2014. **28**(9): p. 1342–1348.
209. Wang, Z., et al. Baicalein induces apoptosis and autophagy via endoplasmic reticulum stress in hepatocellular carcinoma cells. *Biomed Res Int*, 2014. **732516**(10): p. 3.
210. Wang, Y.F., et al. Baicalein triggers autophagy and inhibits the protein kinase B/Mammalian target of rapamycin pathway in hepatocellular carcinoma HepG2 cells. *Phytother Res*, 2015. **29**(5): p. 674–679.
211. Li, J., et al. Baicalein sensitizes hepatocellular carcinoma cells to 5-FU and Epirubicin by activating apoptosis and ameliorating P-glycoprotein activity. *Biomed Pharmacother*, 2018. **98**: p. 806–812.
212. Chen, M., et al. Combination of wogonin and artesunate exhibits synergistic anti-hepatocellular carcinoma effect by increasing DNA-Damage-inducible alpha, tumor necrosis factor α and tumor necrosis factor receptor-associated factor 3-mediated apoptosis. *Front Pharmacol*, 2021. **12**: p. 657080.
213. Hong, M., et al. Wogonin inhibits cell cycle progression by activating the glycogen synthase kinase-3 beta in hepatocellular carcinoma. *Phytomedicine*, 2020. **68**(153174): p. 18.
214. Hong, M., et al. Wogonin suppresses the activity of matrix metalloproteinase-9 and inhibits migration and invasion in human hepatocellular carcinoma. *Molecules*, 2018. **23**(2): p. 384.

215. Xu, M., et al. Wogonin induced cytotoxicity in human hepatocellular carcinoma cells by activation of unfolded protein response and inactivation of AKT. *Hepatol Res*, 2013. **43**(8): p. 890–905.
216. Rong, L.W., et al. Combination of wogonin and sorafenib effectively kills human hepatocellular carcinoma cells through apoptosis potentiation and autophagy inhibition. *Oncol Lett*, 2017. **13**(6): p. 5028–5034.
217. He, F., et al. Wogonin potentiates cisplatin-induced cancer cell apoptosis through accumulation of intracellular reactive oxygen species. *Oncol Rep*, 2012. **28**(2): p. 601–605.
218. Qian, C., et al. Wogonin-enhanced reactive oxygen species-induced apoptosis and potentiated cytotoxic effects of chemotherapeutic agents by suppression Nrf2-mediated signaling in HepG2 cells. *Free Radic Res*, 2014. **48**(5): p. 607–621.
219. Liu, H., Y. Zhou, and L. Tang. Caffeine induces sustained apoptosis of human gastric cancer cells by activating the caspase-9/caspase-3 signalling pathway. *Mol Med Rep*, 2017. **16**(3): p. 2445–2454.
220. Ikram, M., et al. Antioxidant and neuroprotective effects of caffeine against Alzheimer's and Parkinson's disease: insight into the role of Nrf-2 and A2AR signaling. *Antioxidants*, 2020. **9**(9): p. 902.
221. Xu, H., et al. Caffeine inhibits the anticancer activity of paclitaxel via down-regulation of α-tubulin acetylation. *Biomed Pharmacother*, 2020. **129**(110441): p. 21.
222. Wang, Z., et al. Caffeine enhances the anti-tumor effect of 5-fluorouracil via increasing the production of reactive oxygen species in hepatocellular carcinoma. *Med Oncol*, 2019. **36**(12): p. 97.
223. Fazliev, S., et al. Escin's multifaceted therapeutic profile in treatment and post-treatment of various cancers: a comprehensive review. *Biomolecules*, 2023. **13**(2): p. 315.
224. Huang, G.L., et al. β-escin reverses multidrug resistance through inhibition of the GSK3β/β-catenin pathway in cholangiocarcinoma. *World J Gastroenterol*, 2015. **21**(4): p. 1148–1157.
225. Tan, S.M., et al. Identification of beta-escin as a novel inhibitor of signal transducer and activator of transcription 3/Janus-activated kinase 2 signaling pathway that suppresses proliferation and induces apoptosis in human hepatocellular carcinoma cells. *J Pharmacol Exp Ther*, 2010. **334**(1): p. 285–293.

226. Ming, Z.J., et al. Synergistic effects of beta-aescin and 5-fluorouracil in human hepatocellular carcinoma SMMC-7721 cells. *Phytomedicine*, 2010. **17**(8-9): p. 575–580.
227. Saraswati, S., et al. Phloretin attenuates STAT-3 activity and overcomes sorafenib resistance targeting SHP-1-mediated inhibition of STAT3 and Akt/VEGFR2 pathway in hepatocellular carcinoma. *Cell Commun Signal*, 2019. **17**(1): p.127.
228. Leung, K.W., and A.S. Wong. Pharmacology of ginsenosides: a literature review. *Chin Med*, 2010. **5**(20): p. 1749–8546.
229. Yang, L., et al. Protopanaxadiol inhibits epithelial-mesenchymal transition of hepatocellular carcinoma by targeting STAT3 pathway. *Cell Death Dis*, 2019. **10**(9): p. 630.
230. Kim, B.M., et al. Ginsenoside Rg3 inhibits constitutive activation of NF-κB signaling in human breast cancer (MDA-MB-231) cells: ERK and Akt as potential Upstream targets. *J Cancer Prev*, 2014. **19**(1): p. 23–30.
231. Lu, M., Z. Fei, and G. Zhang. Synergistic anticancer activity of 20(S)-Ginsenoside Rg3 and Sorafenib in hepatocellular carcinoma by modulating PTEN/Akt signaling pathway. *Biomed Pharmacother*, 2018. **97**: p. 1282–1288.
232. Kim, D.G., et al. 20(S)-Ginsenoside Rg3 is a novel inhibitor of autophagy and sensitizes hepatocellular carcinoma to doxorubicin. *Oncotarget*, 2014. **5**(12): p. 4438–4451.
233. Shan, K., et al. Ginsenoside Rg3 combined with oxaliplatin inhibits the proliferation and promotes apoptosis of hepatocellular carcinoma cells via downregulating PCNA and cyclin D1. *Biol Pharm Bull*, 2019. **42**(6): p. 900–905.
234. Lee, J.Y., et al. Sensitization of TRAIL-induced cell death by 20(S)-ginsenoside Rg3 via CHOP-mediated DR5 upregulation in human hepatocellular carcinoma cells. *Mol Cancer Ther*, 2013. **12**(3): p. 274–285.
235. Liu, W., et al. Ginsenoside Rg3 promotes cell growth through activation of mTORC1. *Front Cell Dev Biol*, 2021. **9**: 730309.
236. Akiyama, T., et al. Genistein, a specific inhibitor of tyrosine-specific protein kinases. *J Biol Chem*, 1987. **262**(12): p. 5592–5595.
237. Banerjee, S., et al. Multi-targeted therapy of cancer by genistein. *Cancer Lett*, 2008. **269**(2): p. 226–242.

238. Barone, M., et al. Dietary, endocrine, and metabolic factors in the development of colorectal cancer. *J Gastrointest Cancer*, 2012. **43**(1): p. 13–19.
239. Barnes, S. Effect of genistein on *in vitro* and *in vivo* models of cancer. *J Nutr*, 1995. **125**(3 Suppl): 777S–783S.
240. Li, S., et al. Genistein suppresses aerobic glycolysis and induces hepatocellular carcinoma cell death. *Br J Cancer*, 2017. **117**(10): p. 1518–1528.
241. Gruca, A., et al. Synthetic genistein glycosides inhibiting EGFR phosphorylation enhance the effect of radiation in HCT 116 colon cancer cells. *Molecules*, 2014. **19**(11): p. 18558–18573.
242. Tong, Y., et al. Inhibitory effects of genistein in combination with gefitinib on the hepatocellular carcinoma Hep3B cell line. *Exp Ther Med*, 2019. **18**(5): p. 3793–3800.
243. Imran, M., et al. Luteolin, a flavonoid, as an anticancer agent: a review. *Biomed Pharmacother*, 2019. **112**(108612): p. 21.
244. Cao, Z., et al. Luteolin promotes cell apoptosis by inducing autophagy in hepatocellular carcinoma. *Cell Physiol Biochem*, 2017. **43**(5): p. 1803–1812.
245. Cai, S., et al. Knockdown of THOC1 reduces the proliferation of hepatocellular carcinoma and increases the sensitivity to cisplatin. *J Exp Clin Cancer Res*, 2020. **39**(1): p. 135.
246. Feng, X.Q., et al. Luteolin and sorafenib combination kills human hepatocellular carcinoma cells through apoptosis potentiation and JNK activation. *Oncol Lett*, 2018. **16**(1): p. 648–653.
247. Klionsky, D.J., et al. Guidelines for the use and interpretation of assays for monitoring autophagy (3rd edition). *Autophagy*, 2016. **12**(1): p. 1–222.
248. Yan, J., et al. Cantharidin suppresses hepatocellular carcinoma development by regulating EZH2/H3K27me3-dependent cell cycle progression and antitumour immune response. *BMC Complement Med Ther*, 2023. **23**(1): p. 160.
249. Liu, D., and Z. Chen. The effects of cantharidin and cantharidin derivates on tumour cells. *Anticancer Agents Med Chem*, 2009. **9**(4): p. 392–396.

250. Jin, D., N.N. Huang, and J.X. Wei. Hepatotoxic mechanism of cantharidin: insights and strategies for therapeutic intervention. *Front Pharmacol*, 2023. **14**: p. 1201404.
251. Wei, C., et al. Cantharidin inhibits proliferation of liver cancer by inducing DNA damage via KDM4A-dependent histone H3K36 demethylation. *Evid Based Complement Alternat Med*, 2022. **11**: p. 2197071.
252. Liu, F., et al. Magnesium demethylcantharidate inhibits hepatocellular carcinoma cell invasion and metastasis via activation transcription factor FOXO1. *Eur J Pharmacol*, 2021. **911**(174558): p. 8.
253. Huang, X., et al. Methyl-cantharidimide inhibits growth of human hepatocellular carcinoma cells by inducing cell cycle arrest and promoting apoptosis. *Front Oncol*, 2019. **9**: p. 1234.
254. Xie, M.H., et al. A new core-shell-type nanoparticle loaded with paclitaxel/norcantharidin and modified with APRPG enhances anti-tumor effects in hepatocellular carcinoma. *Front Oncol*, 2022. **12**: p. 932156.
255. Sun, C.Y., et al. Norcantharidin alone or in combination with crizotinib induces autophagic cell death in hepatocellular carcinoma by repressing c-Met-mTOR signaling. *Oncotarget*, 2017. **8**(70): p. 114945–114955.
256. Li, Y.D., et al. Methyl-Cantharidimide (MCA) has anticancer efficacy in ABCB1- and ABCG2-Overexpressing and cisplatin resistant cancer cells. *Front Oncol*, 2020. **10**: p. 932.
257. Chen, Y., et al. Advances in the pharmacological activities and mechanisms of diosgenin. *Chin J Nat Med*, 2015. **13**(8): p. 578–587.
258. Tao, X., et al. Dioscin: a diverse acting natural compound with therapeutic potential in metabolic diseases, cancer, inflammation and infections. *Pharmacol Res*, 2018. **137**: p. 259–269.
259. Xu, X.H., et al. Saponins from Chinese medicines as anticancer agents. *Molecules*, 2016. **21**(10): p. 1326.
260. Chen, B., et al. Dioscin inhibits the invasion and migration of hepatocellular carcinoma HepG2 cells by reversing TGF-β1-Induced epithelial-mesenchymal transition. *Molecules*, 2019. **24**(12): 2222.
261. Zhang, G., et al. Dioscin suppresses hepatocellular carcinoma tumor growth by inducing apoptosis and regulation of TP53, BAX, BCL2 and cleaved CASP3. *Phytomedicine*, 2016. **23**(12): p. 1329–1336.

262. Sun, B.T., et al. Reversal effect of Dioscin on multidrug resistance in human hepatoma HepG2/adriamycin cells. *Eur J Pharmacol*, 2011. **654**(2): p. 129–134.
263. Liao, A.M., et al. Synthesis, anticancer activity and potential application of diosgenin modified cancer chemotherapeutic agent cytarabine. *Food Chem Toxicol*, 2021. **148**(111920): p. 18.
264. Li, F., et al. Diosgenin, a steroidal saponin, inhibits STAT3 signaling pathway leading to suppression of proliferation and chemosensitization of human hepatocellular carcinoma cells. *Cancer Lett*, 2010. **292**(2): p. 197–207.
265. Chen, L., et al. A novel diosgenin-based liposome delivery system combined with doxorubicin for liver cancer therapy. *Pharmaceutics*, 2022. **14**(8): 1685.

https://doi.org/10.1142/9789811293320_0007

Chapter 7

Phytomedicine in the Battle Against Liver Cancer: The Impact of Phytochemical mTOR Inhibition

Srishti Bhargav[1,#], Sumitra Patel[1,#], Shweta Shrivastava[2], Rajan Swami[3], and Manish Kumar Jeengar[1,*]

[1]*Department of Pharmacology, Amrita School of Pharmacy, Amrita Vishwa Vidyapeetham, AIMS Health Sciences Campus, Kochi, Kerala, India*

[2]*School of Pharmacy, School of Health and Allied Sciences, ARKA JAIN University, Gamharia, SeraikelaKharsawan, Jharkhand, India*

[3]*Chitkara Collage of Pharmacy, Chitkara University, Punjab, India*

[#]*Both author shares equal authorship*

Table of Contents:

---

*Corresponding author: Tel: E-mail address: manish.pharmacology@live.in, manishkumarj@pharmacy.aims.amrita.edu

Abstract

This chapter provides an in-depth analysis of the emerging role of phytomedicine in combating liver cancer, with an emphasis on phytochemical inhibitors of the mammalian target of rapamycin (mTOR) pathway. Liver cancer, a major global health concern, often presents challenges due to the limited efficacy of traditional treatments. Phytomedicine, with its basis in plant-derived compounds, presents a novel frontier for therapeutic innovation. This chapter provides an overview of the processes involved in the formation and progression of liver cancer, with a particular emphasis on the crucial role played by the mTOR signaling pathway. It delves into the capacity of phytochemicals to alter mTOR activity and its associated signaling pathways, thereby exerting anticancer effects. The therapeutic possibilities of diverse phytochemicals are examined, including their roles in apoptosis induction, angiogenesis inhibition, and metastasis suppression in liver cancer. The chapter concludes by addressing the challenges in leveraging phytochemical mTOR inhibitors in liver cancer treatment and discusses future directions, highlighting the imperative for ongoing research and clinical validation.

1. Introduction

Liver cancer stands as a formidable challenge in global health. Despite significant strides in medical research, it persists as a leading cause of oncological mortality worldwide. The disease's complexity, often marked by delayed diagnosis and constrained therapeutic options, accentuates the critical need for novel and efficacious treatment strategies. In this landscape, the field of phytomedicine — the therapeutic use of plant-derived compounds — emerges as a beacon of hope. Enriched with a longstanding history and a spectrum of pharmacological attributes, phytomedicine provides a vast reservoir of potential anticancer agents. The inherent complexity and multi-targeted actions of phytochemicals render them particularly potent in addressing the diverse challenges presented by liver cancer.

The complex association between liver cancer and the mTOR signaling pathway is explored in this chapter. This pathway is a key regulator of cell proliferation, growth, and survival. It is frequently subjected to dysregulation in several kinds of malignancies, including liver cancer, making it an important target for therapeutic intervention.

Our exploration will encompass an array of natural products that have demonstrated potential as mTOR inhibitors. We will thoroughly examine the interactions of these phytochemicals with the mTOR pathway, elucidating their mechanisms of action and evaluating the potential they harbor in enhancing existing liver cancer treatments. Furthermore, this chapter will traverse the latest advancements in this domain, encompassing clinical studies, and will engage in a discourse on the challenges and prospective avenues in the incorporation of these natural mTOR inhibitors into conventional liver cancer treatment paradigms.

2. mTOR Signaling Pathway

Mechanistic/mammalian target of rapamycin (mTOR) is a serine/threonine kinase that is an integral component of the PI3K-related protein kinase family. This kinase has a molecular weight of around

289 kDa and is also referred to as FKBP12-rapamycin associated protein (FRAP), rapamycin and FKBP12 target (RAFT1), rapamycin target (RAPT1), and sirolimus effector protein (SEP) [1, 2]. mTOR is a multi-environment integrator that is found on chromosome 1p36.2. It was first discovered in *Saccharomyces cerevisiae* as a target of the macrolide fungicide rapamycin. It integrates growth factors, hormones, nutrients, oxygen, and energy. This integration is essential for several cellular functions, such as motility, differentiation, growth, proliferation, survival, and metabolism [1, 3].

mTOR is essential for several biological processes, such as gene transcription, protein synthesis, and ribosome biogenesis. It evaluates data about nutrients and growth factors that enter the cell from the outside in order to synchronize cellular processes that control growth, multiplication, specialization, self-degradation, and cell death. The mTOR signaling system is essential for many biological processes, such as cell survival, proliferation, apoptosis, and the development of new blood vessels in tumors. The mTOR pathway has become a promising target for anticancer therapies due to its enhanced activity in a variety of human malignancies [4].

2.1. *Structure of mTOR*

One remarkable serine/threonine enzyme that is essential for controlling cellular growth and metabolism is called mTOR kinase. It plays an essential function in preventing catabolic processes like autophagy while concurrently stimulating anabolic processes including the synthesis of proteins, ribosomes, nucleotides, fatty acids, and lipids. Two distinct multi-protein complexes of mTOR are known as mTOR complex 1 (mTORC1) and mTOR complex 2 (mTORC2).

Rapamycin has a suppressive effect on the mTORC1 complex, which is made up of the mTOR enzyme, regulatory-associated protein of mTOR (RAPTOR), and mammalian lethal with sec-13 protein 8 (mLST8). However, rapamycin administered immediately has little effect on mTORC2, which is made up of mTOR, rapamycin-insensitive companion of mTOR (RICTOR), mSIN1 (also called MAPKAP1), and mLST8. The two complexes' different rapamycin sensitivity

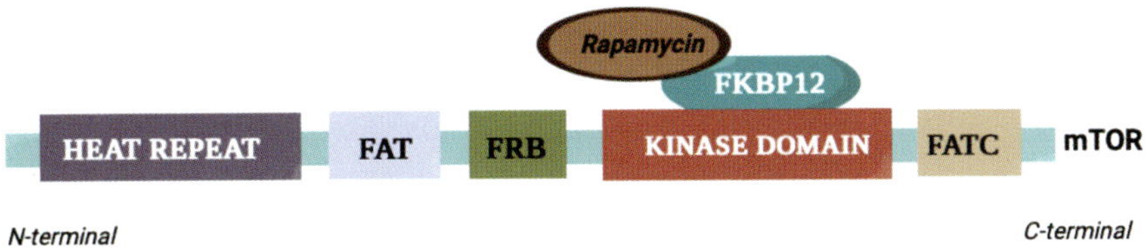

Figure 1: Displays structure of mTOR. mTOR is a protein kinase consisting of 2549 amino acids and exhibiting conserved functional domains across different species. The N-terminus is comprised of 20 consecutive HEAT repeats, which serve as domains for protein-protein interactions. The C-terminal region of mTOR consists of a kinase domain that shows sequence similarities to the catalytic domain of PI3K, a catalytic domain including a FRB domain, and a FAT domain and FATC domain. The negative regulatory domain (NRD) is situated intermediate to the catalytic and FATC domains

highlights the many regulatory roles that mTOR plays in a variety of cellular processes.

According to current knowledge, mTOR operates through two main complexes in mammalian cells: mTORC1 and mTORC2. The mTORC1 complex is composed of several components, including mTOR, mLST8 (also known as G-protein β-subunit-like protein, GβL, or mammalian lethal with sec-13 protein 8), RAPTOR, as well as two inhibitory components, PRAS40 (proline-rich Akt substrate of 40 kDa), and DEPTOR (DEP domain-containing mTOR-interacting protein). Both mTORC1 and mTORC2 are essential protein complexes that have a substantial impact on cellular regulatory systems. The mTORC2 complex is composed of mTOR, mLST8, RICTOR, mSin1 (mammalian stress-activated protein kinase-interacting protein, also known as MAPKAP1), PROTOR (protein seen with RICTOR, originally identified as PRR5, proline-rich protein 5), and DEPTOR. DEPTOR has a vital role in regulating the activity of both mTORC1 and mTORC2, acting as an inhibitor for both complexes. This highlights the crucial significance of DEPTOR in regulating the functioning of both complexes [5].

mTORC1 is crucial in regulating the phosphorylation or expression of various proteins, such as p70 S6 kinase (S6K1), eukaryotic initiation factor 4E (eIF4E) binding protein 1 (4E-BP1), lipin1, Unc-51-like autophagy activating kinase 1 (ULK1), transcription factor EB (TFEB), activating transcription factor 4 (ATF4), hypoxia-inducible factor 1 alpha (HIF1α), and others. The cell carries out several functions, including the regulation of protein synthesis/turnover, the production of lipids, and the synthesis of nucleotides. As a result, it controls cellular growth, replication, self-destruction, and metabolism [3, 6].

In contrast, mTORC2 mostly regulates the phosphorylation of essential proteins such as Akt, serum/glucocorticoid regulated kinase (SGK), and protein kinase C (PKC), hence managing their functioning. mTORC2 regulation exerts a substantial impact on cellular processes such as cell migration, death, and metabolism. These roles highlight the fundamental participation of mTOR in both normal and abnormal cellular processes. The mTOR signaling network's complexity is evident in its domain structure, consisting of six functional areas: the HEAT motifs with two tandem repeats, the focal adhesion targeting domain (FAT domain), the FKBP12 rapamycin binding

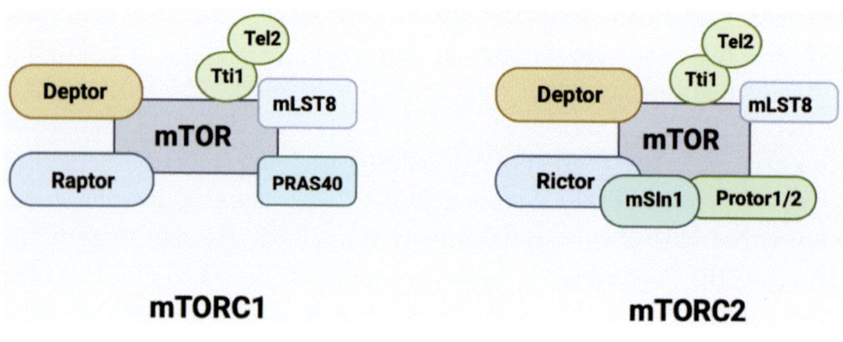

Figure 2: A schematic representation of mTORC1 and mTORC2. The mTORC1 and mTORC2 complexes share key proteins, including mTOR and mLST8, together with the Tti1/Tel2 complex and the inhibitory protein DEPTOR. The mTORC1 complex consists of two essential constituents: regulatory-associated protein of mTOR (Raptor) and the inhibitory subunit proline-rich Akt substrate of 40 kDa (PRAS40). In contrast, the mTORC2 complex consists of RICTOR, which is not affected by rapamycin, together with the regulatory proteins Protor1/2 and mSin1

domain (FRB domain), the kinase (KIN) domain, the NRD domain, and the focal adhesion targeting domain of C-terminal (FATC) domain.

The HEAT motifs within mTOR are instrumental in mediating protein-protein interactions, whereas the FRB domain functions as the binding site for the mTOR and FKBP12-rapamycin complexes. Adjacent to the FRB domain lies the KIN domain, which acts as the catalytic core of mTOR, capable of phosphorylating serine/threonine residues. Nested within the KIN domain is the NRD domain. The FAT and FATC domains, collectively forming part of the mTOR's molecular catalytic region, play a crucial role in intramolecular coordination, thereby regulating the kinase activity of mTOR. These domains collectively enable mTOR to assemble various proteins and active molecules, forming functional complexes such as mTOR-Raptor and mTOR-RICTOR, integral to a host of biological functions [7].

At the N-terminus of the mTOR protein are multiple HEAT repeats, primarily responsible for protein-protein interactions, while the C-terminus encompasses the FKBP-binding domain and a kinase domain, positioning mTOR within the phosphatidylinositol-3-kinase (PI3K) kinase family. The PI3K/Akt/mTOR signaling pathway is pivotal in controlling a variety of physiological processes, including cell cycle progression, transcription, mRNA translation, differentiation, apoptosis, autophagy, motility, and metabolism [8].

The activation of mTORC1 can precipitate several precancerous changes, such as advancement through the cell cycle, enhanced cell proliferation, and increased cell survival. Conversely, activation of mTORC2 contributes to Akt phosphorylation and modulates the functions of cytoskeletal proteins.

In the context of oncology, the Warburg effect, which promotes cancer cell growth and metastasis, is often driven by oncogenic signaling pathways like PI3K, AKT, and mTOR. The liver, being a central metabolic organ, plays a vital role in maintaining metabolic homeostasis and regulates various metabolic pathways. It has been observed that cancer cells exhibiting activated PI3K/AKT signaling tend to exhibit more aggressive behavior [9].

2.2. *Involvement of mTOR pathway in HCC*

Hepatocellular carcinoma (HCC) is the most common type of primary liver cancer. The mTOR pathway, which is important for cell growth and metabolism, plays a critical role in HCC. Upregulation of mTORC1 and mTORC2 pathways, including pRPS6, p-AKT, IGF-1R, and RICTOR, is observed in 40%–50% of HCCs. Additionally, an increase in the mTOR pathway is frequently seen in cholangiocarcinoma, which is the second most common type of primary liver cancer. Activation of the mTOR pathway in HCC is linked to less differentiated tumors, poor prognosis, and earlier recurrence, regardless of the underlying cause of liver cancer.

One study found that the most commonly mutated gene in HCC was RPS6KA3, a serine/threonine kinase that regulates PI3K/RAS signaling. This suggests that mutations in the mTOR pathway are rare in HCC and that the activation of the mTOR pathway is mainly caused by receptor activation. Previous genomic studies have identified several molecular classifications of HCC and have shown that some subgroups of patients have unique, deregulated signaling pathways. These studies have indicated that the mTOR pathway and its upstream pathways PI3K and AKT play a central role in the network of deregulated signaling pathways in HCC [10, 11].

2.3. *Activation of mTORC1*

The activation of mTORC1 is dependent on both nutrients and growth factors. mTOR is a central regulator of growth and metabolism that relies on these nutrients and growth factors. mTORC1 plays a crucial role in synthesizing proteins, lipids, glucose, and other types of biomass. Activation of mTORC1 mainly depends on the availability of nutrients such as amino acids (AAs), glucose [12], nucleotides, fatty acids, and lipids, as well as growth factors. The plasma membrane contains various AA transporters, including transporters for glutamine (SLC1A5/ASCT2) and leucine (SLC7A5/LAT1), which are associated with mTORC1 activation. These transporters are highly expressed and are undoubtedly associated with malignancies.

The most common and significant way mTORC1 is activated is through its translocation from the cytoplasm to the lysosomal surface, where it is unequivocally activated by growth factors via the PI3K-AKT signaling pathway [12].

2.4. *Nutrient-induced lysosomal translocation of mTORC1*

RHEB, a small GTPase, is a well-established regulator of mTORC1, and its activity is solely dependent on its guanine nucleotide state. Nutrients, especially AAs, play a crucial role in the lysosomal localization of mTORC1 through Ras-related GTP-binding proteins (RAGs), effectively facilitating the interaction between mTORC1 and RHEB. The available evidence strongly suggests that AAs promote the localization of mTORC1 to the lysosomal surface, and this process is mainly driven by the RAG GTPase. mTORC1activation is mediated through the engagement of small GTPases known as Ras-related GTP-binding proteins (RAGs), which form obligatory heterodimers. Mammals possess four distinct RAG protein, namely RAGA, RAGB, RAGC, and RAGD. Within mammalian cells, RAG GTPases operate as heterodimers by combining either RAGA or RAGB with RAGC or RAGD, and they play a crucial role in both the activation of mTORC1 and their own maintenance. The activation status of RAG GTPases is under the control of AA signals.

In the presence of high levels of AAs, the RAG GTPase complex becomes active. This is because RAGA or RAGB is bound to GTP, while RAGC/D is bound to GDP. Conversely, the complex is mostly inactive in the absence of high levels of AA, with RAGA or RAGB bound to GDP and RAGC/D bound to GTP. Once activated, the RAG GTPase/RAG heterodimers bind to RAPTOR and relocate mTORC1 to the lysosome's surface. This is where the active RHEB can stimulate mTORC1 kinase [13].

The current progress on the "inside-out" model asserts that the RAG GTPase is located on the lysosomal membrane and is synchronized by multiple signals to sense the AA level in the lysosomal lumen. Moreover, lysosomal AA exerts a regulatory effect on mTORC1. Studies on leucyl-tRNA synthetase (LRS) and GATOR have undeniably revealed that mTORC1 activation can respond to free AA present in the cytoplasm. GATOR is a complex that unequivocally comprises eight proteins. Its primary function is to act as a GTPase-activating protein (GAP) for RAGA/B. The complex is definitively made up of two subunits called GATOR1 and GATOR2. GATOR1 is a trimer and is composed of DEP domain-containing protein 5 (DEPDC5), Nprl2, and Nprl3. On the other hand, GATOR2 is a pentamer and decisively consists of Mios, WDR24, WDR59, Seh1L, and Sec13.

CUL3-KLHL22 is an E3 ubiquitin ligase that definitively promotes the degradation of DEPDC5, a critical component of GATOR1. GATOR1, a protein complex that is conserved across evolution, plays a crucial role in regulating mTORC1, a master regulator of cell growth and metabolism, by sensing AA levels in cells. When AA levels are low, GATOR1 unambiguously binds to RAGA/B, proteins that activate mTORC1, and acts as their GAP to definitively inhibit the localization and activation of mTORC1 in lysosomes. This is the opposite of the function of Ragulator, which definitively promotes mTORC1 localization and activation. Conversely, when AA levels are high, GATOR2 unambiguously combines with GATOR1 and definitively inhibits its GAP function, thereby positively controlling mTORC1.

The nucleotide-binding status of the RAGs is precisely regulated via specific transporters, intracellular synthesis, and protein turnover. It is an undeniable fact that leucine, arginine, and glutamine are the most powerful activators of mTORC1.

In the presence of leucine, the interaction between sestrin2 and leucine relieves the inhibition of GATOR1 by GATOR2, which subsequently activates RAGA/B and mTORC1. Leucine can also independently signal through its catabolite, acetyl-coenzyme A (acetyl-CoA), leading to the activation of mTORC1 via the acetylation of raptor at K1097, mediated by EP-300.

Currently, it seems that this method of mTORC1 activation varies depending on the cell type. Arginine, when bound to CASTOR1, also alleviates the inhibition of GATOR2 by CASTOR1, resulting in mTORC1 activation. CASTOR1 functions as an arginine sensor, whereas SLC38A9, an arginine-regulated AA transporter, serves as another sensor that modulates mTORC1 activity.

Arginine binding to SLC38A9 promotes the export of leucine. When activated by arginine, SLC38A9 alters the nucleotide state of RAGA/RAGB by facilitating the release of GDP from RAGA, providing an additional mechanism to regulate mTORC1 activation. Methionine is detected in the form of S-adenosylmethionine (SAM) by SAMTOR. Elevated SAM levels hinder the binding of SAMTOR to GATOR1, consequently boosting mTORC1 activation.

Glutamine plays a vital role in activating RAGs through the process of glutaminolysis. The conversion of glutamine to α-ketoglutarate (αKG) by glutaminase (GLS) and glutamate dehydrogenase (GDH) is a crucial step in the process. Ultimately, αKG activates mTORC1 via prolyl hydroxylases (PHDs) by promoting the GTP loading of RAGB. The regulation of glutamine uptake and efflux via SLC1A5 (ASCT2), a glutamine transporter, and the CD98 complex (SLC7A5/SLC3A2), respectively, is of utmost importance in controlling mTORC1 activity. It is worth noting that the inhibition of autophagy is linked to the process of glutaminolysis, which is also critical for RAGB GTP loading.

Leucine directly binds and activates GDH, thereby stimulating the production of αKG. Glutamine activates mTORC1 independently of RAGs through the small GTPase ADP-ribosylation factor 1 (ARF1). AAs signal through folliculin (FLCN) and its binding partners FLCN-interacting proteins 1 or 2 (FNIP1 or FNIP2), which act as GAPs for RAGC and/or RAGD. Consequently, different key AAs and their metabolites modulate mTORC1 by impacting regulatory molecules that affect mTORC1 activation and/or translocation to the lysosomes.

2.5. *Activation of mTORC1 via growth factors*

In the presence of nutrients, mTORC1 relocates from the cytoplasm to the lysosomal surface, where it is activated by growth factors via PI3K-AKT signaling. The activation process occurs when growth factors, such as insulin, phosphorylate AKT through a receptor called phosphoinositide-dependent kinase 1 (PDK1) and PI3K proteins. Two major pathways for growth signaling, phosphatidylinositol 3-kinase (PI3K)-Akt and Ras-ERK, regulate mTORC1 activity by functionally inhibiting the tumor suppressor tuberous sclerosis complex (TSC1, TSC2, and TBC1D7) through several phosphorylation events triggered by growth factor-dependent kinases [13].

Akt exerts an inhibitory effect on the TSC, which is a heterodimer complex consisting of TSC1, TSC2, and TBC1D7. This complex functions as a GAP for the RHEB GTPase, with TSC2 specifically acting as GAP to restrain RHEB GTPase activity. Consequently, when cells are exposed to growth-promoting signals, Akt hinders the association between TSC2 and TSC2 by phosphorylating the Ser939 and Thr1462 residues on TSC2. This molecular event permits the GTP-bound RHEB to directly interact with and activate mTORC1 at the lysosomal surface. As a result, cells with mutations or loss-of-function in the TSC1 or TSC2 tumor suppressor genes exhibit heightened mTORC1 activity.

mTORC2 can enhance mTORC1 signaling by phosphorylating TSC2 and other substrates involved in cell growth and metabolism, thus boosting mTOR signaling.

The Ras-ERK pathway exerts precise controls over the control of mTORC1 via inhibitory phosphorylation of TSC2 at certain locations. The interaction between growth factors, such as epidermal growth factor, and the Ras GTPases initiates a series of reactions that ultimately result in the activation of mitogen-activated protein kinases (MAPKs) like ERK. ERK1/2 phosphorylates TSC2 at Ser540 and Ser664, enabling it to assume control of the situation. In addition, ERK indirectly stimulates the activation of mTORC1 by regulating another AGC kinase called p90 ribosomal S6 kinase (RSK). RSK phosphorylates TSC2 at Ser1798, which in turn promotes mTORC1 signaling to S6K1, so establishing its control over the entire process.

Anabolic processes necessitate lipids, glucose, and nucleotides, whereas catabolic processes like autophagy are impeded by them. mTORC1 is essential for facilitating the expression of metabolic genes, including SREBP1 and SREBP2, which are key transcription factors involved in the production of fatty acids and cholesterol. Furthermore, mTORC1 enhances the production of glycolytic enzymes, such as phospho-fructo kinase (PFK), hence facilitating glucose metabolism. In addition, mTORC1 promotes the production of nucleotides, which are essential for DNA replication and the assembly of ribosomes, by upregulating the expression of methylenetetrahydrofolate dehydrogenase 2 and carbamoyl-phosphate synthetase. These two enzymes play crucial roles in the pathways responsible for synthesizing purines and pyrimidines, respectively [9, 13–15].

2.6. *Activation of mTORC2*

mTORC2 has a crucial function in regulating cell growth and viability by phosphorylating many members of the AGC protein kinase family, including AKT, PKC, and SGK kinases. The role of mTORC2 as a downstream mediator of the insulin/PI3K cascade, either directly or indirectly, has been clearly established. Upon the stimulation of mTORC2, it triggers the activation of AKT, SGK, and PKC kinases via phosphorylation. These kinases play a vital role in increasing cell survival and proliferation.

The activation of AKT by mTORC2 can subsequently activate mTORC1 by phosphorylating and inhibiting TSC1/2, resulting in a positive feedback loop between mTORC1 and mTORC2. This loop controls the regulation of cellular growth, metabolism, and survival. While the control of mTORC2 activity remains unclear, it is evident that the PI3K pathway facilitates the phosphorylation of Akt Ser473 by mTORC2 in response to growth factors. Emerging research indicates that mTORC2 can be activated by several additional cues [16, 17].

mTORC1 activation required both AAs and energy, whereas mTORC2 can be activated only through growth factor signaling, but the precise mechanism remains incompletely comprehended. Insulin and other growth factors stimulate PI3K to generate PIP3, which then interacts with mSIN1 to counteract its inhibitory impact on mTORC2. PI3K facilitates the association of mTORC2 with the ribosome, hence enhancing its activation. The activation signals of mTORC2 are less well-characterized than those of mTORC1. The influence of nutrition and growth factors on mTORC2 activation is more complex and intricate than their regulation of mTORC1.

Mammals experience an enhancement in mTORC2 activity when there is an increase in growth factor/PI3K signaling. PI3K activation generates phosphatidylinositol 3,4,5-trisphosphate (PIP3), which attaches signaling molecules to the membrane by binding to the pleckstrin homology (PH) domain in target proteins.

When PI3K signaling is activated, the Akt PH domain assists in recruiting the membrane. When PI3K is activated, mTORC2 phosphorylates Akt at Ser473 of the hydrophobic motif (HM). This phosphorylation is frequently employed as an indicator of mTORC2 activation in research investigations.PIP3 interacts with SIN1 via its PH domain, resulting in the liberation of the mTOR kinase domain from SIN1-PH suppression. This mechanism facilitates the initiation of mTORC2. Given that mTORC2 is activated by PIP3 at the membrane, it is likely that mTORC2 is regulated inside distinct membrane compartments.

Multiple investigations have unequivocally shown that the endosomal reservoirs of mTORC2 rely exclusively on PI3K signaling. Moreover, it has been demonstrated that insulin/PI3K can stimulate the activation of mTORC2 and enhance its interaction with ribosomes. It is crucial to acknowledge that the behavior of mTORC2 is greatly influenced by the intracellular nutrition or metabolite circumstances. The removal of AAs, particularly glutamine, and the deprivation of glucose in the presence of serum have been demonstrated to increase the activation of mTORC2. The activation of mTORC2 is crucial during periods of glutamine or glucose deprivation to ensure the continuous flow through the hexosamine biosynthesis pathway. This pathway is vital for biosynthesis and relies on the availability of both glucose and glutamine [17].

AMP-activated protein kinase (AMPK) directly stimulates mTORC2 activation by phosphorylating mTOR and maybe RICTOR when glucose levels are depleted. It is capable of achieving this even with little PI3K signals. The activation mechanism of mTORC2 under conditions of low glutamine levels is still not fully understood, but sestrin2 is believed to be involved in this process. Sestrin2 binding to mTORC2 results in a decrease in mTORC1 activity. These findings indicate that the activation of mTORC2 during glutamine deprivation may be linked to the suppression of mTORC1 through the utilization of sestrin2 as a means of survival. Sestrin2 enhances the catalytic activity of mTORC2, resulting in the activation of Akt Ser473. The reason for this occurrence is that sestrin2 facilitates the phosphorylation of Akt by interacting with Sestrin/GATOR2 and GATOR2/mTORC2. Thus, the activation of mTORC2 during glutamine deprivation may be associated with the suppression of mTORC1 through sestrin2. In addition, Sestrin3 interacts to RICTOR and increases mTORC2 activation when insulin and nutrients are present.

Research has demonstrated that phosphorylation of Akt Thr450 is responsive to both glucose deprivation and acute ATP depletion. This offers valuable insights into the functioning of mTORC2 under these specific circumstances. In addition, the activation of mTORC2 can occur without the involvement of PI3K through the binding of RICTOR to CD146, a cell adhesion molecule commonly referred to as melanoma cell adhesion molecule (MCAM). The interaction between RICTOR and this association shields it from being broken down by ubiquitin, therefore ensuring the continuous activation of mTORC2.

Feedback signals from mTORC1 have a significant impact on the activation of mTORC2. As the signaling of mTORC1 intensifies, it enhances the activity of S6K1, resulting in the phosphorylation of inhibitory sites on the insulin receptor substrate-1 (IRS-1). Phosphorylation of mTORC2 is inhibited by this process, leading to the suppression of subsequent signals. Nevertheless, the suppression of mTORC1 using rapamycin diminishes the activity of S6K1 toward IRS-1, thereby enhancing PI3K signaling. mTORC1 phosphorylates Grb10, leading to a detrimental effect on insulin signaling. Rapamycin, when employed as an inhibitor of mTOR, further augments the expression of growth factor receptors such as IGF1R, hence

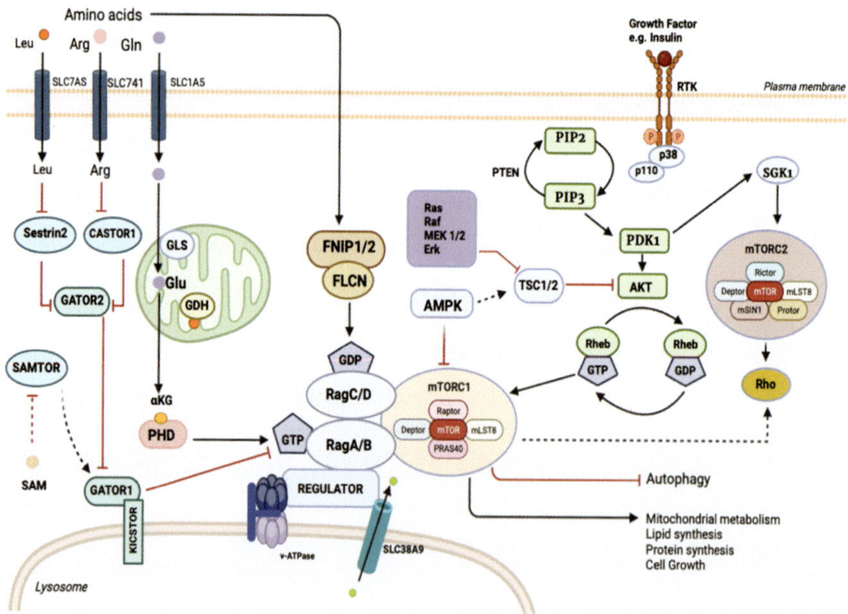

Figure 3: mTOR signaling pathway

Insulin and several growth hormones engage with receptor tyrosine kinases (RTKs), initiating a cascade of chemical reactions that eventually trigger the activation of phosphoinositide 3-kinase (PI3K). PI3K is a crucial enzyme in this pathway that catalyzes the conversion of phosphatidylinositol-4,5-bisphosphate (PIP2) into the more phosphorylated phosphatidylinositol-3,4,5-trisphosphate (PIP3). The phosphatase and tensin homolog (PTEN) exerts a pivotal role in modulating the route by dephosphorylating PIP3, hence regulating its activity. Subsequently, PIP3 serves as a site for binding, attracting, and activating phosphoinositide-dependent kinase 1 (PDK1). PDK1 is necessary for the activation of AKT, a protein kinase that selectively phosphorylates serine and threonine residues. When activated, AKT inhibits the function of the TSC, which is a GAP required for the activation of the small GTPase RHEB. RHEB, in its GTP-bound state, directly interacts with mTOR complex 1 (mTORC1), resulting in its activation.

Simultaneously, the activation of mTOR complex 2 (mTORC2) is enhanced by PIP3, which assists in the complex's interaction with mammalian stress-activated MAPK-interacting protein 1 (mSIN1). The regulation of this process is meticulously controlled by AMPK, which opposes the activity of mTORC1 by both suppressing the RAPTOR and enhancing the TSC complex. This intricate network of interactions and regulatory mechanisms underscores the complexity of cellular signaling promoting the activation of PI3K/mTORC2 signaling. Increased mTORC2 signaling also triggers a feedback process that decreases insulin signals by controlling the turnover of IRS-1, leading to the downregulation of mTORC2 [18, 19].

Figure 3: (*Continued*) pathways influenced by insulin and growth hormones, particularly in the context of mTOR pathway activation. The full activation of mTORC1 also hinges on a separate signaling pathway initiated by AAs. Specific transporters, including SLC7A1, SLC7A5, and SLC1A5, ferry AAs into the cell. These AAs then stimulate RAS-related GTP-binding proteins (RAGs), promoting the translocation of mTORC1 to the lysosome. At the lysosomal surface, ragulator, acting as a guanine nucleotide exchange factor, complexes with RAGs, facilitating their interaction with RAGA and/or RAGB. GATOR1, which normally inhibits RAGA and/or RAGB, is countered by KICSTOR, which binds to and sequesters GATOR1. Furthermore, GATOR2 plays a crucial role in mTORC1 activation, presumably by interacting with and suppressing GATOR1. The activation process of mTORC1 involves specific AA sensing mechanisms, such as leucine binding to Sestrin 2 and arginine binding to CASTOR1.

Both Sestrin 2 and CASTOR1 have the ability to alleviate the inhibition of GATOR2. Glutamine is essential for the activation of mTORC1 through two distinct mechanisms. The first mechanism involves glutaminolysis, which is dependent on the RAG protein. The second mechanism is independent of RAG and involves the small GTPase ARF1. The lysosomal transporter SLC38A9 transports vital AAs from the lysosome to the cytosol in response to arginine stimulation. AAs transmit signals via the proteins folliculin (FLCN) and FLCN-interacting protein 1 (FNIP1) or FNIP2, which function as GAPs for RAGC and/or RAGD.

S-adenosyl-methionine (SAM) has been discovered to inhibit the binding of SAMTOR to GATOR1 and KICSTOR, which act as negative regulators of mTOR signaling. The molecules that are colored red serve as negative regulators, whilst the molecules that are colored purple serve as positive regulators of mTOR signaling. The turquoise arrows symbolize the flow of metabolites, whereas the black arrows represent a sequence of signaling events. Dotted lines signify indirect activities or uncertainty regarding the need for further procedures. Furthermore, the αKG (α-ketoglutarate), GDH (glutamate dehydrogenase), GLS (glutaminase), mLST8 (mammalian lethal with sec-13 protein 8), and PHD (prolyl hydroxylase) all play a role in this process. The mTORC1 and mTORC2 complexes connect external signals and the cytoskeleton through the use of Rho GTPases.

3. PI3K/AKT/mTOR Signaling Pathway and Its Mechanism

The phosphoinositide 3-kinases (PI3Ks) represent a pivotal family of kinases that are integral in regulating cellular processes such as viability, replication, and differentiation. These kinases are categorized into four distinct classes: Class I, Class II, Class III, and Class IV. Of these, Class I PI3K is primarily implicated in oncogenesis, catalyzing the phosphorylation of phosphatidylinositol 4,5-biphosphate (PIP2) to produce phosphatidylinositol 3,4,5-triphosphate (PIP3).

Class IA PI3Ks, the most extensively studied group within the PI3K family, comprise three catalytic isoforms (p110α, p110β, and p110δ) and a regulatory subunit (p85). The p85 regulatory subunit is characterized by an inter-Src homology 2 (iSH2) domain, flanked by two Src homology (SH2) domains, which interact with the p110 catalytic subunit. In its basal state, p85 inhibits the activity of p110 through binding via the iSH2 domain. However, upon stimulation by growth factors or cytokines, which activate RTKs and G-protein-coupled receptors, PI3K is translocated to the membrane. This translocation occurs through direct or indirect interactions with activated receptors, facilitating the enzyme's access to its substrate in the lipid bilayer [20, 21].

The activation of PI3K catalyzes the formation of PIP3 from PIP2 via phosphorylation on the inositol ring in the lipid membrane. PIP3 then recruits and activates the serine-threonine kinase Akt, which is phosphorylated by phosphoinositide-dependent kinases. Once activated, Akt orchestrates a cascade of downstream signaling pathways crucial for cell survival, proliferation, cell cycle progression, migration, and angiogenesis. Additionally, Akt activation leads to the phosphorylation and subsequent activation of the mammalian target of rapamycin complex 1 (mTORC1), a serine/threonine kinase pivotal in cellular growth and metabolism regulation.

The (mTOR) protein orchestrates the phosphorylation of key downstream targets, notably the p70 S6 kinase and the eukaryotic translation initiation factor 4E-binding protein 1 (4E-BP1). These downstream effectors are crucial in modulating the translation of vital proteins that are central to cellular processes like proliferation and angiogenesis, including c-Myc, Cyclin D1, HIF-1α, and vascular endothelial growth factor (VEGF). The PI3K/Akt/mTOR signaling pathway is typically activated by various growth factors and cytokines. However, its regulation is also subject to inhibition by tumor suppressors such as PTEN (phosphatase and tensin homolog deleted on chromosome 10), which counteracts this pathway by dephosphorylating PIP3. Other negative regulators of this pathway include SH2-containing inositol phosphatase-1 (SHIP1) and PITenins (PITs).

mTOR complex 2 (mTORC2) is notably sensitive to changes in intracellular nutrients and metabolite levels. Interestingly, the activation of mTORC2 is observed to increase under conditions of AA scarcity, particularly in the absence of glutamine, and during glucose deprivation, even with serum presence. In low-glucose environments, AMPK plays a pivotal role in activating mTORC2. AMPK achieves this by phosphorylating both mTOR and potentially RICTOR, a component of the mTORC2 complex. This activation process is intriguingly independent of PI3K signaling, indicating a unique regulatory mechanism in response to cellular metabolic status [8, 12, 20, 21].

4. The Role of PI3K/AKT/mTOR Pathway in HCC

The PI3K/AKT/mTOR signaling cascade plays a crucial role in controlling essential cellular activities, such as the cell cycle, cell survival, metabolism, cell movement, and blood vessel formation, in both healthy and cancerous cells. An important characteristic of the development of tumors is the frequent disruption of the phosphatidylinositol 3-kinase (PI3K) pathway. Within the human genome, PI3K is classified into three separate classes: Class I, Class II, and Class III. Class I PI3Ks, which comprise four catalytic subunits encoded by the PIK3CA, PIK3CB, PIK3CG, and PIK3CD genes, are frequently associated with human malignancies. The p110α isoform is commonly mutated in tumors, although the p110β, p110δ, and p110γ isoforms are less frequently changed but may exhibit overexpression in malignant tissues. Elevated expression of PI3K, particularly PIK3CA, in HCC is linked to increased tumor growth and decreased cell death, which is associated with worse prognoses.

The Class II PI3Ks, which include the isoforms PI3K-C2α, PI3K-C2β, and PI3K-C2γ, have specific and separate functional functions. PI3K-C2α is involved in the processes of endocytosis, vesicular trafficking, and mitosis. On the other hand, PI3K-C2β controls cell migration and inhibits mTOR signaling. PI3K-C2γ has a role in the activation of AKT2 and the storage of glycogen. More precisely, the decrease in PI3KC2α hinders the transmission of signals and the formation of new blood vessels in HCC that are induced by VEGFA. PI3K-C2β is involved in the growth of hepatitis C virus (HCV) in liver cancer cells. PIK3C3, which is a Class III PI3K, plays a role in several cellular processes. When it is inhibited, it impacts the activation of SGK3, which promotes the growth of cancer stem cells (CSCs), as well as the activity of AMPK.

The AKT kinase family, encompassing AKT1, AKT2, and AKT3, are serine/threonine kinases implicated in a variety of diseases, most notably cancer. In hepatocytes, the expression of AKT1 and AKT2 is notable, whereas AKT3 is typically absent. A significant relationship has been established between the phosphorylation of AKT1 and the activation of the oncogene c-MYC. Notably, increased levels of AKT1 in HCC have been associated with poorer patient prognoses. While earlier studies suggest a potential role for AKT2 in influencing HCC outcomes, its primary functions include promoting cellular proliferation and invasion. The PI3K/AKT signaling pathway is frequently activated due to the loss of the tumor suppressor PTEN. The mTOR kinase, intricately involved in protein synthesis regulation, links nutrient sensing to cell proliferation and is prevalently active in cancerous conditions.

mTOR functions via two complexes: mTORC1 and mTORC2. The activation of PI3K and AKT catalyzes the activation of mTORC1, leading to the phosphorylation of ribosomal proteins S6K1 and 4E-BP1. In contrast, mTORC2, which includes the component RICTOR and is insensitive to rapamycin, phosphorylates AKT, thereby augmenting its kinase activity. A consistent feature of cancer cells is the sustained activation of the PI3K/AKT/mTOR pathway, with an observed upregulation of the mTOR pathway in approximately 50% of HCC cases, highlighting mTORC1 as a viable target for therapeutic intervention. Additionally, hepatic mTORC2 is implicated in the development of hepatosteatosis and cancer through its role in enhancing fatty acid and lipid synthesis in HCC.

The frequent aberrations in the PI3K pathway in various cancers, including HCC, arise from multiple etiological factors. These include gain-of-function mutations or amplifications in PIK3CA (p110α catalytic subunit), increased activity or expression of PIK3CB (p110β catalytic subunit), inactivation of PTEN due to gene loss, mutations, or epigenetic modifications, and alterations in the Akt isoforms, particularly Akt1 and Akt2. Additionally, the stimulation of RTK signaling pathways, such as those mediated by the EGFR family or IGF1-R, contributes to the dysregulation of the PI3K/Akt/mTOR axis.

5. Modulation of mTOR Activity by Phytochemicals

Phytochemicals, derived from a wide variety of plants, are generally categorized into different classes including flavones, diterpenes, indoles, isoflavones, polyphenols, and others. Each of these classes includes compounds with distinct capabilities in controlling the mTOR pathway, which has a crucial function in cancer biology, particularly in liver cancer. Comprehending the distinct characteristics of each category in this situation is crucial for formulating precise therapy approaches. Table 1 presents a comprehensive summary of different phytochemicals in these categories, emphasizing their distinct functions and impacts on the modulation of the mTOR pathway.

5.1. *Flavones*

5.1.1. *Apigenin*

Apigenin, a naturally occurring flavonoid, is widely distributed in a diverse array of fruits and vegetables, enhancing their nutritional value. It is found in fruits, such as grapes, oranges, cherries, and

Table 1: Phytochemicals targeting PI3K/Akt/mTOR pathway in liver cancer

Class	Phytoconstituents
Flavones	Apigenin
diterpenes	Cryptotanshinone
Indoles	3,3-diindolylmethane
Isoflavones	Genistein Deguelin
Polyphenols	Curcumin Fisetin Resveratrol Epigallocatechin (EGCG) Quercetin Gallic acid
Others	Tocotrienols Timosaponin Diosgenin

apples, and is equally abundant in vegetables including sweet green peppers, celery, onions, barley, parsley, tomatoes, and broccoli. Beyond solid foods, apigenin is also a constituent in popular beverages such as tea and wine, contributing to their health-promoting properties. This widespread presence across various dietary sources makes apigenin an integral component of a balanced diet, offering potential health benefits attributable to its flavonoid nature. This compound has attracted considerable interest due to its ability to modulate the PI3K/Akt/mTOR signaling pathway, a critical pathway in cancer biology. Research indicates that apigenin can either directly inhibit PI3K/Akt activity or indirectly stimulate the AMPK-TSC axis, thereby impacting this pathway. Apigenin is soluble in dimethylsulfoxide and to a lesser extent in acetone and alcohols. In its natural form, apigenin predominantly exists as glycoside conjugates, which undergo enzymatic breakdown into free flavonoids within the human digestive tract. Apigenin's role in inducing apoptosis and autophagy is dose-dependent. Intriguingly, inhibiting autophagy can amplify apigenin-induced cell death, suggesting that autophagy might act as a cellular defense mechanism against apigenin-induced stress. In HepG2 cells, apigenin suppresses the PI3K/Akt/mTOR signaling pathway, leading to reduced cell proliferation and the induction of apoptosis and autophagy. These effects have been validated through both *in vitro* studies and *in vivo* experiments. Moreover, apigenin has demonstrated efficacy in inhibiting tumor proliferation in a xenograft mouse model.

The function of H19 long non-coding RNA in HCC is becoming more widely understood, especially in light of its frequent overexpression in HCC and its significance in the initiation and spread of tumors. A naturally occurring flavonoid called apigenin has shown promise in blocking H19 expression and hence blocking the Wnt/β-catenin signaling pathway. The creation of innovative treatment approaches for liver cancer is particularly interested in this disruption. Apigenin has been shown to have anticancer properties beyond HCC, and its effects are being further studied in a variety of animal cancer models. These comprise head and neck squamous cell carcinoma (HNSCC), prostate, lung, pancreatic, nasopharyngeal carcinoma, and sarcoma. The consistency of these trials' findings, especially with regard to the shrinkage of tumor sizes, highlights apigenin's potential as a strong cancer treatment agent. Its adaptability is demonstrated by its broad range of action against many cancer types, which also suggests that it may play a part in future oncological therapy regimens [21–23].

5.2. *Diterpenes*

5.2.1. *Cryptotanshinone*

Cryptotanshinone, a compound found in the plant *Salvia miltiorrhiza* Bunge, exhibits potential as an anticancer substance by impeding cell growth, triggering cell demise, and obstructing the formation of blood vessels and lymphatic vessels. Nevertheless, its limited ability to be absorbed by the body has hindered its utilization in cancer treatment clinical trials. In addition, cryptotanshinone has been discovered to hinder angiogenesis and lymphangiogenesis, both of which are crucial processes in the proliferation and dissemination of malignancies. Cryptotanshinone hinders the mTORC1-induced phosphorylation of S6K1 and 4E-BP1, two proteins implicated in cellular growth and proliferation. The impact of cryptotanshinone on mTORC2-mediated Akt, a protein implicated in cell proliferation and viability, seems to differ based on the particular cell line under investigation [24].

5.2.2. *Artemisinin*

Significant anticancer effects have been shown by the ethanol extract obtained from Artemisiae Iwayomogii Herba, especially in terms of HCC cell growth and proliferation inhibition that occurs in a dose-dependent manner. A rise in the number of apoptotic cells and increased levels of cleaved caspase-3 and PARP indicate that this extract promotes apoptosis. Through the downregulation of XIAP and Mcl-1 expression, it further causes the loss of mitochondrial membrane potential. Furthermore, the extract prevents HCC cells from migrating and invading. This extract increases apoptosis and dramatically reduces tumor cell growth in an *ex vivo* mouse xenograft model. Its effectiveness is extended to HCC cell suppression of the PI3K/AKT/mTOR signaling pathway. The extract from Artemisiae Iwayomogii Herba exhibits potential as a natural therapeutic agent for the prevention and treatment of HCC due to its diverse actions, which include inducing apoptosis, inhibiting cancer cell invasion and migration, and suppressing the PI3K/AKT/mTOR pathway [25].

Parallelly, the ethanol fraction LAC117, extracted from *Artemisia capillaris*, exhibits notable anti-proliferative effects on human HCC cell lines. This suggests LAC117's potential as a viable drug candidate against HCC. The pro-apoptotic effect of LAC117 is marked by an increase in cleaved caspase-3 and PARP expression, along with a rise in TUNEL-positive cells. Because of modifications to the potential of the mitochondrial membrane, LAC117 induces apoptosis in HCC cells, which is shown by an increase in cytochrome c release and a decrease in XIAP expression. Both *in vitro* and *in vivo*, the chemical efficiently inhibits the PI3K/AKT signaling pathway in HCC. Furthermore, in both *ex vivo* and *in vivo* mice xenograft models, LAC117 has a strong inhibitory impact on tumor growth, enhancing its potential as a therapeutic agent against HCC [26].

5.3. *Indoles*

5.3.1. *3,3′-diindolylmethane*

3,3′-diindolylmethane (DIM), obtained from cruciferous plants, has demonstrated antineoplastic effects in different types of human malignancies. The involvement of MAPKs, particularly JNK and p38 MAPK, have been identified in the induction of apoptosis and their potential as targets for inhibiting proliferation and inducing death in liver cancer cells by DIM. The cleavage of caspase-3 produced by DIM relies on the initiation of phospho-p38 MAPK, indicating a possible mechanism for DIM-induced apoptosis. Elevating the cytosolic concentration of Ca^{2+} in a continuous manner might disrupt the delicate balance of Ca^{2+} regulation within the cell and initiate a series of reactions that ultimately lead to programmed cell death in tumor cells. Proliferating cell nuclear antigen (PCNA) (proliferation marker) was discovered to be suppressed in HCC cells as a result of DIM treatment. Concurrently, there was a reduction in cell growth and an elevation in the activation of p38 MAPK via phosphorylation. These findings indicate that the p38 MAPK pathway plays a role in the suppression of HCC cell proliferation by DIM, which aligns with previous studies conducted on different types of tumor cells. Administration of an inhibitor targeting p38 MAPK mitigated the inhibitory effect on cell proliferation induced by DIM in HCC cells, hence further substantiating the role of this pathway in the growth suppression of HCC cells by DIM. Extended increase in the concentration of Ca^{2+} within the cytoplasm might be harmful and initiate cell death.

Research has demonstrated that DIM-induced production of interferon-γ in breast cancer cells is facilitated by p38, which relies on cytosolic calcium signaling. Carvacrol, a different chemical, has similarly been demonstrated to induce apoptosis by the depolarization of mitochondria saturated with calcium. Following DIM therapy, there was a detected elevation in cytosolic calcium levels, indicating that DIM may enhance the sensitivity of HCC cells by disrupting the balance of cytosolic calcium.

The indoles found in cruciferous vegetables, such as indole-3-carbinol and its dimeric derivative 3,3′-diindolylmethane (DIM), have demonstrated potential as antitumor drugs. To do this, they disrupt many cellular signaling pathways and exert influence over the activity of transcription factors and non-coding RNAs. These acts improve their ability to hinder the spread of tumors and overcome resistance to therapy. Drug resistance poses a significant obstacle to the efficacy of cancer therapy with chemotherapeutics. This resistance can stem from several processes, including increased drug expulsion, DNA repair, mutation, or alteration of drug targets, epigenetic control, and factors within the tumor microenvironment. Indole compounds derived from natural sources have shown potential as antineoplastic agents. Vincristine and vinblastine, which are indole alkaloid drugs, have been proven to be effective therapies for tumor problems [27, 28].

5.4. *Isoflavones*

5.4.1. *Genistein*

Genistein is a flavonoid, a naturally occurring chemical included in soy. Flavonoids are recognized for their physiological effects and positive impact on health, specifically their association with reduced incidence of metastatic cancer as demonstrated in many population-based studies. HCC has anti-mutagenic characteristics and can cause apoptosis by blocking TPA-induced cell invasion and decreasing MMP-9 synthesis. MMP-9 is a protein that enhances the infiltration of cells and is upregulated by diverse stimulants. TPA is a substance that has been well researched for its capacity to stimulate the production of MMP-9 in HCC cells. The generation of MMP-9 caused by TPA is facilitated by the activation of many signaling pathways, including MAPK, IκB, and Akt. These pathways induce the activation of transcription factors NF-κB and AP-1, which are responsible for the synthesis of MMP-9. Gen achieved this by suppressing the MAPK/AP-1 and PI3K/AKT/NF-κB signaling pathways, resulting in the suppression of tumor migration and invasion in human hepatoma HepG2 cells. EGFR autocrine/paracrine pathways refer to the signaling pathways in which the EGFR protein interacts with itself or neighboring cells to regulate various cellular functions. EGFR exhibits significant upregulation in a wide range of human malignancies, including lung, colon, breast, head and neck, ovarian, bladder, and liver cancers. There is a strong correlation between this elevated expression and more advanced tumor stage, as well as a worse clinical prognosis.

EGFR initiates intracellular signaling cascades, including Ras/Raf/MEK/ERK and PI3K/Akt, which govern cellular processes such as cell proliferation, motility, and apoptosis. Gen demonstrates therapeutic efficacy as a pharmaceutical agent for the treatment of HCC by inhibiting the spread of cancer cells to distant anatomical locations.

Song et al. discovered that the combination of Taurine, Epigallocatechin gallate (EGCG), and Genistein (TEG) decreased the expression of AMPK and mTOR phosphorylation proteins in hepatic stellate cells (HSCs), hence impacting the AMPK-mTOR pathway. The medicines also decreased autophagy-related gene expression in LC3 and Beclin1. TEG intervention on liver tissue and HSCs in *in vivo* and *in vitro* tests is discussed in the highlighted section. HSC proliferation and hepatic autophagy were reduced by TEG. TEG inhibits the AMPK-mTOR pathway to protect the liver against autophagosomes. Inhibiting cell autophagy to convert HSCs from activated to quiescent (inactive) for liver fibrosis treatment is crucial to its advancement. HSC activation involves autophagy. TEG lowers autophagosomes, limits HSC proliferation, and heals liver tissue damage by blocking the AMPK-mTOR pathway, making it promising for HCC [29, 30].

5.4.2. *Deguelin*

Deguelin, a rotenoid compound belonging to the flavonoid group, is derived from botanical sources such as Lonchocarpus, Derris, and Tephrosia. Deguelin, a well-known compound with notable anticancer properties, has demonstrated its ability to inhibit the development of many forms of cancer, such as stomach malignancies like MGC-803 and MKN-45 cells, in laboratory settings. The anti-proliferative effects of this substance on cancer cells occur by influencing many signaling pathways, such as PI3K/Akt, NF-kB, Wnt, and EGFR. Deguelin specifically targets key molecules that play a significant role in the development and spread of cancer cells, including Bmi1, COX-2, galectin-1, and Hexokinase II. Moreover, it hinders the growth and spread of tumor cells by specifically targeting biological processes such as the formation of new blood vessels (angiogenesis), the formation of new lymphatic vessels (lymphangiogenesis), the focal adhesion kinase (FAK), the epithelial-mesenchymal transition (EMT), and the NIMA-related kinase 2 (NEK2). In addition to these, deguelin also demonstrates a wide range of biological activities, including the ability to halt the cell cycle, regulate autophagy, block the hedgehog pathway, and enhance differentiation in mutant NPM1 acute myeloid leukemia.

Studies on the effects of deguelin on the growth of several liver cancer cell lines, such as Hep3B, HepG2, and MHCC97-H, have been conducted to examine the drug's potential as an anticancer agent. Determining the function of angiogenesis in the development of HCC and evaluating the anti-angiogenic effects of deguelin are major goals of this study. Research has indicated that, in laboratory settings, deguelin suppresses the proliferation, migration, invasion, and creation of tubes in human umbilical vascular endothelial cells (HUVECs). Additionally, it lessens *in vivo* tumor vascularization. Deguelin efficiently inhibits HUVECs' VEGF receptor-mediated signaling and reduces HCC cells' autocrine VEGF synthesis. It reduces HGF-induced VEGF production by blocking the activation of the c-Met signaling pathway, which is initiated by HGF. Deguelin has demonstrated therapeutic effectiveness in patient-derived xenograft models of

HCC, primarily through the lowering of proangiogenic factors in cancer cells and the suppression of angiogenesis in vascular endothelial cells [31, 32].

5.5. *Polyphenols*

5.5.1. *Curcumin*

The polyphenol curcumin, which comes from the Curcuma longa plant, is presently being investigated as a possible novel anticancer medication in early clinical studies. However, the exact method via which curcumin prevents the growth of cancer is yet unknown. Numerous proposed cellular targets have been identified. However, none of these appear to be the primary goal.

Curcumin exhibited a dose-dependent influence on colony formation in RMS cell lines. A concentration of 20 μM led to a significant reduction of over 80% in all examined cell lines. However, the impact of 10-μM curcumin varied across various cell lines. Curcumin, an Indian spice, has been thoroughly researched for its anti-tumorigenic effects on rhabdomyosarcoma. It has been found to limit the growth and survival of cancer cells. Nevertheless, due to curcumin's inadequate absorption, quick degradation, and absence of specificity, it is not suited for clinical application. Consequently, scientists are investigating its non-specific reactivity in order to find possible targets for therapeutic intervention and drug creation.

EF24, a synthetic analog resembling curcumin, exhibits improved absorption into the body and has demonstrated the capacity to inhibit liver cancer growth and trigger programmed cell death in mice liver cancer cells. Curcumin therapy reduces the amount of bcl-2 protein and increases the amount of bax protein, causing toxicity in human hepatoma cells. EF24 causes cell cycle arrest at the G2/M phase in liver cancer cells by decreasing the amounts of cyclin B1 and cdc2. Additionally, curcumin therapy triggers the activation of the Chk1-mediated G2 checkpoint, leading to G2/M arrest and resistance to curcumin-induced cell death in cancer cells [33, 34].

5.5.2. *Fisetin*

One flavonoid that is common in strawberries, apples, persimmons, onions, and other fruits and vegetables is called fisetin, and it has drawn interest because it may be an anticancer agent. Fisetin's effectiveness as a cancer treatment has been demonstrated by both *in vitro* and *in vivo* research. The main mechanism of action of this compound is the suppression of the PI3K/Akt and mTOR signaling pathways. Fisetin inhibits many pathways' constituents, such as mLST8, PRAS40, Raptor, and RICTOR, which reduces the production of mTORC1 and mTORC2 complexes. Fisetin inhibits the proliferation of several cancer cell types and induces apoptosis as a result of its molecular action. It efficiently inhibits mTOR's downstream targets, including S6K1, eIF4E, and 4E-BP1. Furthermore, fisetin activates AMPK, diminishes Akt and mTOR phosphorylation, and lowers the expression of the regulatory (p85) and catalytic (p110) subunits of PI3K.

In rat models of HCC, specifically Aflatoxin-B1 (AFB1)-induced HCC, fisetin has demonstrated encouraging effects in tumor regression. This is accomplished by preventing ROS-induced proinflammatory factors from activating, which is essential for the advancement of HCC. The core of this signaling cascade is the dynamic interaction between phosphatase and tensin homolog deleted on chromosome 10 (PTEN) and 3-phosphoinositol kinase (PI3K). Fisetin's action causes 3-phosphoinositol-dependent kinase 1 (PDK1) to phosphorylate at Thr308, which activates protein kinase B (Akt). Through GSK3β phosphorylation at Ser 9 by p-Akt^thr308, this phosphorylation promotes the fast cell proliferation inside the neoplastic niche. According to the research findings, fisetin's suppression of proinflammatory pathways plays a role in the HCC's reversal. Furthermore, fisetin modifies a sequence of signals that activate Akt, a crucial regulator of cell development. PCNA immunohistochemical study revealed a decrease in actively dividing cells in the liver affected by HCC, suggesting that fisetin may be used as a treatment drug for HCC by inhibiting Akt signaling and reducing cell proliferation [35, 36].

5.5.3. *Resveratrol*

A naturally occurring polyphenol called resveratrol has demonstrated strong cytotoxic effects on cancer cells. Its diverse antitumor activity affects several important facets of cancer development. One of the main ways that resveratrol works is by preventing metastasis and angiogenesis, two processes that are necessary for the development and multiplication of cancer cells. As a result, it promotes the controlled processes of cellular death, autophagy and apoptosis, which kill cancer cells. Bax, NOXA, and PUMA are among the pro-apoptotic proteins in the p53 family that are molecularly activated by resveratrol. Cancer cells undergo apoptosis as a result of this activation, which eliminates them. Moreover, resveratrol increases the activation of AMPK and Sirt1, two important factors in the autophagic process. Resveratrol stimulates autophagy, which aids in the lysis of cancer cells.

Apart from its direct cytotoxic effects, resveratrol also efficiently prevents the spread of cancer cells by blocking many pathways linked to the disease's advancement. These include the Gli1 pathway, TGF-β1/Smads, Wnt/β-catenin, PI3K/Akt/NF-κB, and EMT, which are all involved in tumor development and metastasis. Resveratrol's capacity to prevent angiogenesis — the development of new blood vessels that provide nutrition to tumor cells — is another essential component of its activity. It accomplishes this by preventing VEGF from acting in a way that is dependent on HIF-α1.

Resveratrol treatment reduced the negative effects of FB1 on the levels of oxidative stress markers and liver enzymes in mice. Its capacity to lessen aflatoxin B1 and fluoride-induced oxidative damage has been demonstrated by earlier studies. However, in high concentrations, it can cause oxidative stress and may have dangerous side effects, depending on the dosage and duration of exposure. It decreased the high blood sialic acid levels brought on by FB1, which acts as a biomarker for FB1-induced liver damage. Resveratrol comes in two isomeric forms: trans- and cis-resveratrol. It has several health benefits, including modifying gene expression and protecting liver cells from oxidative damage.

Because it affects cell signaling and metabolism, resveratrol, a phenolic phytocompound found in peanuts and grapes, has been used medicinally to treat several conditions, including HCC. Throughout history, this material has been consumed in the form of wines and other delights due to its flavor and potential health benefits against specific illnesses. Numerous research investigations have shown that resveratrol has anticancer properties. It works by regulating many pathways. Research indicates that it suppresses oxidative stress and inflammation in the liver, initiates programmed cell death (apoptosis), and prevents the growth and division of cancer cells. It is thought that some enzymes and signaling molecules are activated, and others are suppressed to produce these effects. Resveratrol shows promise as a medicinal substance for the prevention and treatment of HCC in general. To fully understand its modes of action and potential therapeutic applications, more study is needed [37–39].

5.5.4. *Epigallocatechin gallate (EGCG)*

Green tea contains a significant catechin called epigallocatechin-3-gallate (EGCG), which has been shown to have a variety of biological benefits, particularly in the treatment and management of HCC. As an antioxidant, EGCG provides defence against oxidative stress and free radicals, which can harm cells. It has a major impact on the PI3K/AKT signaling pathway, which is essential for cancer cells to proliferate and migrate. Studies show that EGCG can efficiently reduce the mRNA expression of key players in this system, such as PI3K, AKT, and NF-κB.

Particularly noticeable is the influence of EGCG on the activation kinetics of AKT, where phosphorylation at critical sites (Ser473 and Thr308) is essential for controlling downstream effectors such as NF-κB. These chemicals, particularly in SMMC7721 cells, are essential for the behaviors of cells. EGCG acts on both sides of the AKT signaling axis, impacting downstream and upstream pathways such as the HIF-1α/VEGF axis and the thrombin-PAR1/PAR4-p42/p44 MAP. By inhibiting Bcl-2 family signaling or inducing apoptosis through the downregulation of COX-2 and Bcl-2, which activates caspase-9 and caspase-3, EGCG can prevent the development of HCC cells.

In addition, EGCG has anti-metastatic properties by inhibiting the activity of matrix metalloproteinases MMP-2 and MMP-9. This characteristic highlights its therapeutic promise in the management of HCC, since it specifically suppresses the PI3K/AKT signaling pathway to modify the cell cycle and cause death.

Subsequent investigation indicates that the p21wafl/Cipl/CDC25A axis is involved in EGCG's effect on liver cancer. In individuals with HCC, elevated CDC25A in liver cancer is associated with malignancy and worse prognoses. Research employing rat models of diethylnitrosamine (DEN)-induced HCC and human hepatoma cell lines shows that EGCG inhibits the development of HepG2 and Huh7 cells by raising p21wafl/Cipl and lowering CDC25A, particularly in HepG2 cells. *In vivo*, EGCG dramatically lowers tumor volume and raises the survival rate of HCC-affected mice. It increases the expression of p21wafl/Cipl mRNA and protein, while decreasing CDC25A mRNA and protein levels in liver tissues and serum γ glutamyl transpeptidase in rats treated with EGCG. Under similar circumstances, the effectiveness of EGCG is comparable to that of green tea extract, indicating a mechanism involving EGCG-induced downregulation of CDC25A and overexpression of p21wafl/Cipl. Research on how EGCG affected HCCLM6 cells revealed possible targets for HCC treatment. Four proteins were identified by proteomic analysis of EGCG-treated versus untreated cells as being related to cell growth and proliferation: FUBP1, HSPB1, CH60, and NPM. A DNA-binding protein called FUBP1 increases c-Myc in HCC, suggesting a potential role for metastasis. EGCG has the potential to inhibit the growth of HCCLM6 and HCC that involves FUBP1. In HCCLM6 cells, EGCG administration also raises NPM expression, which may prevent RNA synthesis and cell division. The complicated impact of EGCG in HCC intervention is demonstrated by the association between HSP60 and improved motility and invasiveness in human pharyngeal squamous carcinoma cells, as well as CH60, which is connected to tumor growth through immune response regulation.

5.5.5. *Quercetin*

Quercetin is a polyphenolic component included in several food sources including tea, onions, red grapes, and apples. Quercetin hinders the development of cancer by obstructing the signaling of mTOR, as well as the functioning of two other proteins, PI3K and Ras, which serve as regulators of mTOR. In addition, quercetin stimulates AMPK, a protein that is recognized for its ability to suppress mTOR signaling. Quercetin additionally enhances the production of TSC1, a protein that acts as a suppressor of mTOR signaling. Nevertheless, quercetin's effectiveness as a therapeutic cancer therapy is hindered by its limited ability to be absorbed and distributed in the body. To enhance its efficiency, it is necessary to develop novel formulations or chemically modify quercetin.

Hexokinase-2 (HK2) is a protein that is excessively produced in HCC, a kind of liver cancer. Quercetin, a type of flavonoid present in various fruits and vegetables, has demonstrated the capacity to impede the survival and growth of HCC cell lines Bel-7402 and SMMC-7721 at doses lower than 50 μM. At this dosage, quercetin additionally decreases cellular glucose absorption and lactate generation. The observed phenomenon is most likely caused by a reduction in the abundance of HK2 protein, which is typically regulated by the PI3K/AKT/mTOR pathway, a signaling network that plays a role in cellular proliferation and viability. Given that the STAT3 route may also regulate the overexpression of HK2 in HCC cell lines, it implies that both pathways may have a role in controlling this crucial enzyme. Quercetin has the ability to maintain the impact of proven chemotherapeutic drugs, potentially enabling a decrease in their doses. The challenges posed by Quercetin's limited water solubility, chemical instability, and low bioavailability can be addressed by utilizing innovative delivery technologies, thereby expediting its transition from laboratory research to clinical application [40, 41].

5.5.6. *Gallic acid*

The naturally occurring polyphenol gallic acid is obtained from plants and has gained notice for its anticancer properties. Using MTT and colony formation tests, a recent research investigated the effects of gallic acid on two liver cancer cell lines, HepG2 and SMMC-7721. The study found that the proliferation of these cancer cells was greatly suppressed by gallic acid, with the effectiveness of this suppression being dose-dependent and time-dependent. Gallic acid was discovered to cause apoptosis, or programmed cell death, in SMMC-7721 cells. Western blotting and flow cytometry were used in the investigation to explore the fundamental processes of this apoptotic process. The findings showed that in SMMC-7721 cells, gallic acid enhanced reactive oxygen species and activated caspase-3 and caspase-9. Its particular apoptotic effect in cancer cells in contrast to normal hepatocytes was further highlighted by the reduction of mitochondrial membrane potential and the elevation of pro-apoptotic Bcl-2-like protein 4 expression.

Additionally, the study found that gallic acid caused SMMC-7721 cells to undergo apoptosis via mitochondrial pathways, suggesting that it may be a promising new treatment for HCC. In addition to its direct anticancer actions, gallic acid has pro- and antioxidant qualities. Additional research examining its function in hepatocarcinogenesis *in vivo*, namely in rat models of HCC, has discovered that gallic acid displays a variety of bioactivities and enhances liver tissue structure. These include apoptotic, anti-inflammatory, antioxidant, and anticancer properties, which support its promise as a versatile therapeutic and control tool for liver cancer [42, 43].

5.6. *Other natural compounds*

5.6.1. *Tocotrienol*

Tocotrienols, natural compounds found in vegetable oils, wheat germ, barley, nuts, and various grains, represent a unique group within the vitamin E family. These compounds exist in four isoforms — alpha, beta, gamma, and delta, each distinguished by their potent antioxidant and anti-inflammatory properties. Unlike tocopherols, tocotrienols feature an unsaturated isoprenoid side chain, which enhances their tissue penetration, especially in organs with saturated fatty layers such as the brain and liver.

Studies have highlighted that tocotrienols, particularly gamma-tocotrienol, exhibit exceptional antioxidant and anti-inflammatory activities, outperforming alpha-tocopherol in combating chronic diseases. Tocotrienols exhibit diverse biological properties, including neuroprotection, anticancer effects, anti-inflammatory actions, and cholesterol-lowering capabilities. Upon supplementation, tocotrienols are detectable in plasma and accumulate in vital organs, although the precise plasma levels required for significant physiological impact remain unclear. In liver health, α-T3 and γ-T3 tocotrienols demonstrate hepatoprotective effects by inhibiting lipid peroxidation and oxidative damage. Moreover, γ-T3 and δ-T3 tocotrienols enhance the expression of enzymes like CYP450 and UGT1A1, as well as MDR-protein 1. The tocotrienol-rich fraction (TRF) from sources such as palm oil and rice bran oil further contributes to these protective effects. Additionally, α-T3, γ-T3, and δ-T3 tocotrienols boost hepatic antioxidant status, as evidenced by biodistribution studies.

In the context of HCC, tocotrienols modulate various cellular pathways, leading to anticarcinogenic effects. They enhance the expression of Prx4, Bax, caspase-8, and caspase-9, while suppressing Bcl-2, Bcl-xL, cyclin D1, Mcl-1, and VEGF. Tocotrienols, particularly δ-tocotrienol, have shown promise in inhibiting liver cancer progression in rat models, exhibiting selective distribution to tumor tissues. δ-Tocotrienol also acts as a potent proteasome inhibitor, triggering apoptosis in liver cancer cell lines by reducing the production of proteasomal subunits and TNF-α. Tocotrienols offer a potentially safer, more natural alternative to conventional pharmaceuticals in treating liver damage and liver cancer. They target specific molecular pathways, such as the Nrf2/Keap1 pathway, which may contribute to liver protection and cancer prevention. Given their enhanced antioxidant and biological properties compared to tocopherols, tocotrienols are emerging as promising agents in mitigating liver damage and preventing liver cancer. Their ability to counteract oxidative stress and liver toxicity positions them as potential molecular targets for liver health [44, 45].

5.6.2. *Timosaponin*

Timosaponin AIII, a cholesterol-derived steroidal saponin found in *Anemarrhena asphodeloides* Bge., exhibits various biological activities and plays a significant role in the modulation of several diseases. In the realm of cancer research, the impact of Timosaponin AIII on cancer cells involves complex signaling networks. It induces apoptosis in HCC cells through pathways involving Bcl-2, Bcl-xL, Mcl-1, XIAP, cIAP-1, and cIAP-2. Additionally, it triggers autophagy via mechanisms linked to LC3-II, AMPKα, and mTOR pathways. Specifically in HCC cells, Timosaponin AIII targets XIAP, a protein often overexpressed in cancerous cells, to promote apoptosis. It induces AMPKα/mTOR-dependent autophagy, leading to the suppression and lysosomal degradation of XIAP. This process underlines Timosaponin AIII's ability to selectively target cancer cells. Importantly, while demonstrating significant cytotoxic effects on human HCC cells, Timosaponin AIII does not inflict severe damage to liver tissues. This selective cytotoxicity underscores its potential as a therapeutic agent in treating HCC, offering a promising avenue for targeted cancer therapy with minimal collateral damage to healthy liver cells [46, 47].

5.6.3. *Phloretin*

Using Soluplus as a polymer matrix to formulate and characterize a phloretin amorphous solid dispersion. Phloretin's dissolution profile and oral bioavailability were enhanced by the solid dispersion, opening up the possibility of using it to treat metabolic disorders linked to non-alcoholic fatty liver disease (NAFLD) and related conditions. SEM, P-XRD, FT-IR, and TGADSC were among the analyses used to assess the formulation. In NAFLD mice, the oral bioavailability of the solid dispersion was studied, and it was discovered to have a protective effect against hepatic degenerative changes, lipid accumulation, and inflammation. Tumor necrosis factor-a and interleukin-6 levels in the liver were also lowered by the solid dispersion, and the serum lipid profile was also improved [48].

5.6.4. *Diosgenin*

Diosgenin is a steroid saponin present in several plants, including yam, a widely consumed vegetable globally and utilized as a medicinal substance in traditional Chinese medicine. The effectiveness of diosgenin in HCC cells was examined in Bel-7402, SMMC-7721, and HepG2 cells, with its impact varying according to the concentration used. It was discovered that administering therapy for a duration of 24 hours resulted in the arrest of the G2/M phase of the cell cycle, inhibition of cell growth, and induction of apoptosis. Diosgenin exhibited these effects through the inhibition of Akt phosphorylation, the upregulation of p21 and p27 expression, and the activation of caspase cascades-3, -8, and -9. Therefore, it has the potential to act as an anti-HCC drug [49].

The anticancer mechanisms of these compounds were studied using Glc/CNHphth-diosgenin (GND), a diosgenin derivative. Organic anion-transporting polypeptide 1B1 allowed GND to pass the plasma membrane and enter the ER, lysosome, and mitochondria. GND caused ER enlargement, mitochondrial damage, and autophagosome production, which kill cells. GND increased the expression of IRE-1α, a protein implicated in autophagy and apoptosis. GND caused autophagy to stimulate caspase-8-dependent apoptosis, since chloroquine slowed the emergence of cleaved poly (ADP-ribose) polymerase and inhibited caspase-8. These findings imply that diosgenyl saponin is a strong liver cancer drug that induces ER stress and mitochondria-mediated apoptosis. Diosgenin, the major steroidal saponin in fenugreek seeds, inhibits proinflammatory and pro-survival signaling pathways in tumor cells and induces death. Trillin and other diosgenyl saponins trigger apoptosis in cancer cells, suggesting they may interact with several targets and have a complicated mode of action. To study its mechanisms, a fluorescent trillin (GND) counterpart reached maximum brightness at 6 hours, demonstrating that temperature-related passive transport was responsible for cellular uptake. GND enters cells via OATPs, an essential membrane transporter superfamily. Inhibiting OATP1B1, a particular

OATP family member, decreased GND entry and apoptosis-related proteins [50].

Diosgenin suppressed HepG2 and SMMC-7721 HCC cell migration and invasion by upregulating DDX3 and down-regulating Cyclin D1, Notch-1, and β-catenin. It also inhibits STAT3, c-Src, JAK1, and JAK2 signaling pathways that promote cell growth and survival. Thus, Disogenin inactivates these proteins, slowing cell development. diosgenin maintains JNK/p38 MAPK phosphorylation. ASK1, a protein that initiates apoptosis in response to stress signals, activates in liver cancer cells and increases apoptosis in malignant cells. It may cure liver cancer by blocking signaling pathways and decreasing cell development. Researchers discovered that diosgenin suppressed liver cancer cell proliferation at dosage and time-dependent levels, with 50-μM and 75-μM doses showing considerable suppression at 72 hours. By inhibiting TAZ (transcriptional co-activator with PDZ binding motif) in liver cancer cells, it also reduced cell migration and invasion. These data imply that diosgenin may treat liver cancer [49–51].

5.6.5. *Silymarin*

Silymarin is a flavonolignan that is derived from the seeds of *Silybum marianum* (L.) Gaertn, often known as milk thistle. The primary constituents of silymarin are silibinin, isosilibinin, silicristin, and silidianin. Silymarin is a widely recognized herbal treatment for chronic liver problems that has been used for a long time around the world. Silibinin, the primary bioactive constituent of silymarin, has been extensively investigated for its hepatoprotective and anticancer properties, both in laboratory settings (*in vitro*) and in living organisms (*in vivo*). The primary challenges in the clinical utilization of silymarin encompass its inadequate solubility and bioavailability. Novel variations of silymarin, such as siliphos, have recently emerged as potential therapies for liver diseases. The newly developed synthetic compound incorporates lecithin, which greatly enhances the solubility and bioavailability of silymarin (70).

5.6.6. *Baicalin*

Isolated from *Scutellaria baicalensis* Georgi, it was demonstrated to be capable of protecting hepatocytes from the damaging effects of oxidative stress by upregulating the expression of liver fatty acid binding protein as well as the activity of intracellular SOD and GSH.

5.6.7. *Emodin*

Natural anthraquinone derivative emodin is derived from traditional Chinese medicines and is well-known for its antibacterial, anticancer, and anti-inflammatory effects. It has been discovered that combination therapy, which combines emodin with other medicinal agents, produces synergistic effects, lowers toxicity, and postpones the development of drug resistance. Emodin or its analogs in combination with other bioactive substances have demonstrated significant synergistic effects in the treatment of a number of diseases, such as cancer, inflammation, antimicrobial effects, disorders of the central nervous system, glucose and lipid metabolism, and infections [52].

One of *Polygonum multiflorum*'s (PM) main ingredients, emodin, affects many cell types in both harmful and protective ways. Emodin's effects and modes of action on hepatic cells are still unknown. Emodin induces apoptosis and substantially reduces the viability of L02 human hepatic cells in a time- and dose-dependent manner. In these cells, it also boosts autophagy. Without affecting the expression of PI3K, AKT, or mTOR, emodin dose-dependently reduces the expression of p-PI3K, p-AKT, and p-mTOR. Compared to emodin treatment alone, cotreatment with 3-methyladenine (3-MA) or rapamycin increases and decreases the apoptosis rate of L02 cells, respectively. Emodin induces autophagy by suppressing the PI3K-AKT-mTOR signaling pathway and demonstrates cytotoxicity in L02 cells by promoting apoptosis. After emodin treatment, autophagy might be protective (Table 2) [53].

6. Challenges and Considerations for Clinical Translation

Phytochemicals, typically present in traditional remedies, are thought to be efficacious in promoting general well-being and averting ailments like cancer. Scientists have conducted extensive research on these substances for many years with the aim of creating treatments for cancer. Before they may be extensively employed as chemotherapeutic medications, certain concerns must be resolved despite their considerable potential. The hurdles involved with these concerns include insufficient solubility, limited cell permeability, hepatic distribution, a narrow therapeutic range, and fast absorption by normal tissues. Phytochemicals have a substantial apparent volume of dispersion, leading to their accumulation in healthy organs. Moreover, the specific application of these chemicals has not yet been completely developed.

Due to factors including low solubility in water, poor bloodstream absorption, digestive tract instability, and difficulties penetrating cells, phytochemical distribution in the body is difficult to understand. Due to their size and hydrophobic nature, these chemicals have trouble navigating bodily barriers such as the mucosa, gastrointestinal tract, endothelium lining blood vessels, and blood-brain barrier. Furthermore, they are broken down by enzymes in the digestive tract. A workable approach would be to conjugate or encapsulate these chemicals with nanocarriers to increase their efficacy. Through this method, their solubility, velocity of absorption, and gastrointestinal stability can all be enhanced. While proliferating cells are the primary target of most cancer treatments, they can also affect rapidly proliferating cells in the body, such as those in the bone marrow, digestive tract, and hair follicles. These adverse effects may include alopecia, gastrointestinal issues, and compromised immune function. In order to tackle these concerns, scientists are investigating the application of nanotechnology for targeted delivery of cancer therapies to cancerous cells, while minimizing harm to healthy cells. Nevertheless, there are still obstacles to be surmounted in efficiently administering

Table 2: Efficacy of phytochemicals in liver cancer: *in vitro* and *in vivo* studies, molecular targets, and outcomes

Phytochemicals	*In Vitro* Cell Lines	*In-Vivo* Models	Molecular Target	Outcome	Ref.
Resveratrol		Fumonisin B1 induced hepatotoxicity in Bal B/c mice		Resveratrol has a protective effect against oxidative stress and liver damage caused by FB1. Total sialic acid levels in the serum can serve as a biomarker of FB1 toxicity and liver damage.	[38]
Gamma-tocotrienol	HepG2 liver cancer cell line		Peroxiredoxin-4 (Prx-4) protein	The study suggests that GTT might directly influence the expression dynamics of peroxiredoxin-4 to control proliferation in liver cancer.	[54]
Timosaponin AIII	Human hepatocellular carcinoma cell lines HepG2, PLC/PRF/5 and Hep3B	Xenograft model of female nude mice (s.c injection of MHCC97L)	Tumor proliferation marker — Ki67	the expression of Ki67 was significantly reduced in the TAIII-treated xenograft compared to a control group. Study revealed that TAIII was more toxic to carcinoma cell lines (cancer cells) than to normal hepatocytes (healthy liver cells). Hence, it targets tumor cells specifically.	[46]

Gallic acid	i. HepG2 and SMMC-7721 cell line		GA induces apoptosis in SMMC-7721 cells *in vitro* via mitochondrial-mediated pathways (↑ caspase, ↑ ROS, ↑ expression of BCL-2-like proteins)	GA shows potential effects for treating hepatocellular carcinoma (HCC) by inhibiting cell growth and inducing apoptosis *in vitro*.	[43]
		ii. N-nitrosodiethylamine NDEA (CAS no. 55-18-5) induced HCC in Wistar male rats	STAT3 signaling pathway	GA also has potential therapeutic effects on HCC in rats by regulating the signaling pathway may be a possible mechanism for its anti-liver cancer effect that may mitigate hepatic carcinogenesis.	[42]
Diosgenin	HepG2 liver cancer cells		TAZ (transcriptional co-activator with PDZ binding motif)	MTT assay demonstrated the suppression of cell growth in a dose and time-dependent manner.	[51]
EGCG	i. HepG2, SMMC7721 and SK-hep1 cells		Downstream signaling molecules include p-ERK, p-Akt, p-Stat-3, and p-GSK-3β proteins	EGCG inhibited HCC cell growth by affecting cell cycle and induced apoptosis via downregulation of PI3K/AKT signaling.	[55]

(*Continued*)

Table 2: (*Continued*)

Phytochemicals	*In Vitro* Cell Lines	*In-Vivo* Models	Molecular Target	Outcome	Ref.
		ii. DEN-induced Sprague Dawley (65 male rats) i.p. injected (20 mg/ml)	Upregulation of a protein called p21waf1/Cip1 and the downregulation of another protein called CDC25A.	EGCG was able to reduce the size of tumors and slow down their growth significantly. The study also found that a daily dose of 25 mg of EGCG was effective in prolonging the survival rates of rats with HCC.	[56]
Genistein	i. Human HCC cells (PLC/PRF5)		ERK-1/2 and AKT as key regulators	GE could be a promising treatment option for liver cancer, particularly for tumors that are driven by estrogen.	[29]
		Carbon tetrachloride-induced liver fibrosis rat model (male SD)	AMPK-mTOR pathway affects autophagy and anti-hepatic fibrosis	Combination therapy with TEG can protect the liver against autophagosomes by inhibiting the AMPK-mTOR pathway, which is an important mechanism for treating liver fibrosis by converting activated HSCs to a quiescent state and inhibiting cell autophagy.	[30]

Deguelin	Hep3B, HepG2, and MHCC97-H cells	PDX model by using three different orthotopic hepatocellular carcinomas which exhibit similar clinical characteristic in C57/BL/6 mice	Targeting HGF-c-Met and VEGF-VEGFR pathways in cancer cells. Also inhibits PI3K-Akt, IKK-IκBα-NF-κB and AMPK-mTOR-surviving pathways.	Deguelin may be a valuable addition to treatments available for hepatocellular carcinoma, and that further research is warranted to explore its potential clinical applications. Deguelin is a potent angiogenesis inhibitor and thus can be useful for the clinical application.	[32]

these therapies. Transporting bioactive phytochemicals as a chemotherapeutic drug presents numerous obstacles. These factors encompass inadequate solubility, reduced stability, restricted absorption in the gastrointestinal tract, limited bioavailability, extensive metabolism in the liver during the first pass, chemical degradation, quick elimination, and absence of selectivity.

The principal objectives of phytochemical-based clinical studies are to increase the susceptibility of cancer cells to conventional chemotherapy and radiation therapy, mitigate the severe side effects associated with regular cancer treatment, and detect any negative interactions with standard therapy. Numerous phytochemicals, including EGCG, lycopene, quercetin, resveratrol, green tea, berberine, curcumin, and sulforaphane, have been shown in preclinical research to have positive benefits. Though promising preclinical efficacy results have been obtained, the clinical trials examining berberine's complete potential as an anticancer drug remain narrowly focused. Owing to its substantial medical potential, curcumin, a naturally occurring chemical, has been the subject of much research. Turmeric, or curcumin, has been demonstrated to be incredibly successful in treating a wide range of ailments in various clinical studies. Unfortunately, curcumin's potential to provide health advantages is thought to be limited, mostly because of its low bioavailability.

This can be related to insufficient absorption, increased metabolic rate, and fast elimination from the body. After a comprehensive analysis of all the clinical trials, it was shown that while some studies have expressed concerns about the low bioavailability, others have demonstrated notable benefits in the treatment of chronic diseases at the standard levels of bioavailability. The Phase I clinical studies of Curcumin have shown that it is safe, well-tolerated, and non-toxic, even at high dosages. Nevertheless, it has exhibited suboptimal bioavailability in the human population. Notwithstanding this obstacle, clinical trials evaluating curcumin as an anticancer drug, either as a standalone treatment or in conjunction with other therapies, have shown effectiveness against different disease locations. Resveratrol exhibits restricted bioavailability and undergoes rapid metabolism, posing difficulties in sustaining therapeutic concentrations and impeding its practical application in cancer management.

7. Future Perspective

The current chemotherapy approach encounters significant challenges due to the deleterious side effects induced by chemotherapy and the development of drug resistance. Consequently, there is a rising apprehension regarding the efficacy and safety of existing chemotherapy treatments, prompting researchers to explore alternative remedies. Phytochemicals offer a promising approach in the quest for improved and safer therapies for breast cancer. These naturally occurring compounds, found in many plant-based foods including vegetables, spices, fruits, and grains, have been recognized for their exceptional compatibility with living organisms and their potent capacity to eradicate cancer cells through diverse methods. Moreover, the use of nanocarriers encapsulating phytochemicals, either alone or in conjunction with other phytotherapeutics or chemotherapeutics, has demonstrated promising outcomes in the treatment of liver cancer. The essay thoroughly explains the mechanisms underlying the anticancer properties of phytochemicals.

The combination of phytochemicals and chemotherapeutic medications using nanotechnology has great promise for producing substantial and diverse impacts in the future. Phytochemicals, derived from natural sources, have been utilized in traditional medicine for millennia, assisting in the preservation of well-being and the avoidance of diseases, including cancer. While research based on cell cultures and certain animal studies has shown the anticancer effects of various phytochemicals, clinical trials involving humans have shown varying and inconclusive outcomes. The discrepancy seen can be attributed to the limitations observed in administering significant doses of phytochemicals in human trials, as well as their restricted solubility in water, stability, bioavailability, and selectivity in targeting cancer cells and tumors. Moreover, these chemicals undergo significant breakdown and modification by enzymes in the gastrointestinal tract, liver, and other organs, leading to brief periods of circulation and low levels in the bloodstream.

Thus far, nanotechnology has become a crucial method in developing and producing nano-sized delivery systems for curcumin. These systems include solid dispersions, liposomes, conjugates, polymeric nanoparticles, peptide carriers, and micelles. Micelles have become more important as nanocarriers in the fields of medication delivery and cancer therapy. These polymeric micelles possess the capacity to enhance aqueous formulations of medications that exhibit poor solubility in water. In addition, they extend the duration of these medications in the body, improve their absorption by cells, and specifically target cancer locations by taking advantage of the improved permeability and retention effects. Nanotechnology encompasses the deliberate manipulation of materials on a scale typically less than 100 nm. Recently, there has been a significant surge in the utilization of nanotechnology to boost the transportation of phytochemicals to tumors or cancer cells, hence increasing the effectiveness of therapy. Various phytochemicals can be enclosed in nanoparticles that are both compatible with living organisms and capable of breaking down naturally. This encapsulation provides advantages such as enhanced absorption, safeguarding against enzymatic breakdown, improved stability, extended circulation, and targeted uptake by cancer cells or tumors. These benefits minimize toxicity by preventing premature interaction with the biological environment.

Plant-derived chemicals, including alkaloids, flavonoids, terpenoids, soluble polysaccharides, and phenolic acids, are utilized as reducing and stabilizing agents during the synthesis of metal nanoparticles. The innovative approach of using phytochemicals to facilitate nanoparticle production has great promise, as the botanical constituents act as both capping and reducing agents. Liposomes, nanoemulsions, micelles, solid lipid nanoparticles (SLNs), nanostructured lipid carriers (NLCs), and poly (lactide-co-glycolide) (PLGA) nanoparticles are examples of frequently used biocompatible and biodegradable nanoparticles. There are several ways to administer these nanoparticles: orally, intravenously, intraperitoneally, and transdermally. Polymeric nanoparticles (PNs) are a class of nanomaterials that have garnered interest because of their easily modifiable surface, uncomplicated production method, high compatibility with living cells, and little adverse effects. A frequently employed strategy for personalized cancer treatment delivery involves incorporating phytonutrients into pharmaceutical nanoparticles (PNs). Techniques for delivering nanodrugs based on lipids are thought to be particularly promising colloidal carriers of phytochemicals. Liposomes, SLNs, and NLCs are examples of lipid-based nanoparticles that may transfer hydrophobic and hydrophilic molecules efficiently by using an internal aqueous core or the phospholipid bilayer. Liposomes have a noticeably low degree of toxicity and exhibit biocompatibility and biodegradability. They provide a wide range of benefits, such as the ability to combine both water-loving and fat-loving drugs, create lipid regions, display flexibility, participate in multiple binding interactions, promote merging, allow for prolonged drug retention, have a large drug-carrying capacity, facilitate targeting to specific sites, and enable controlled release of drugs. In addition, liposomes provide extended therapeutic effects, decrease the probability of potential negative effects, and provide improved safeguarding for medications against physiological circumstances. Therefore, the inclusion of anticancer phytochemicals in liposomes is considered a more strategic option for overcoming the constraints of conventional chemotherapy in suppressing the development of cancer and substantially reducing adverse effects.

Niosomes are highly developed drug delivery devices that form nanoscale lamellar vesicles by combining a helper lipid that resembles cholesterol with a nonionic surfactant. In hydrophilic conditions, these nonionic surfactants require energy to form a stable bilayer vesicle, especially when there is physical agitation and heating. The hydrophilic heads of the bilayer structure are oriented toward the aqueous side, while the hydrophobic segments are positioned away from it. Surfactants with biocompatible, biodegradable, and nonimmunogenic qualities are used in the production of niosomes. Niosomes demonstrate similar characteristics to liposomes in both *in vivo* and *in vitro* settings, therefore extending the duration of the encapsulated phytochemical in the circulation, altering its distribution within organs, and enhancing its bioavailability. It has been demonstrated that niosomes are very useful for enhancing the stability and solubility of phytochemicals. These substances are primarily intended to make precise administration and regulated dispensing of these physiologically powerful substances easier.

Lipids, surfactants, water, and maybe co-surfactants are combined to generate lipid-based particles known as SLNs and NLCs. They are made up of a hydrophobic lipid core and a hydrophilic outer layer. Triglycerides, waxes, or fatty acids make up the inner core, which repels water, while phospholipids and surfactants often make up the outer layer, which has an attraction for water. It should be noted that the lipid cores of SLNs and NLCs are made of solid or semi-solid materials, as opposed to emulsions. The lipid core structure of SLNs is very well-organized, but the lipid cores of NLCs are less well-organized, which increases their ability to transfer phytochemicals.

Although a number of studies conducted on animals and in laboratories have suggested that nanoparticles may augment the anticancer qualities of phytochemicals, questions about their long-term toxicity, cost, safety, and possible adverse consequences still remain. As a result, a specialized area within the study of nanotechnology called nanotoxicology has developed to specifically tackle these challenges. Although oral administration is preferred, the majority of nano-encapsulated phytochemicals, especially those intended for tumor targeting, are largely supplied to animals through intravenous, subcutaneous, or intraperitoneal methods. The development of nano-delivery systems for orally administering phytochemicals has challenges due to concerns over gastrointestinal digestion and degradation. A burgeoning field of study focuses on improving the effectiveness and selectivity of directing phytochemical nanoparticles toward cancer cells or tumors. The goal is to enhance the anticancer potency of these compounds while reducing their toxicity and negative impact on healthy cells and tissues. Prospective clinical trials are necessary to evaluate the anticancer efficacy of phytochemical nanoparticles and

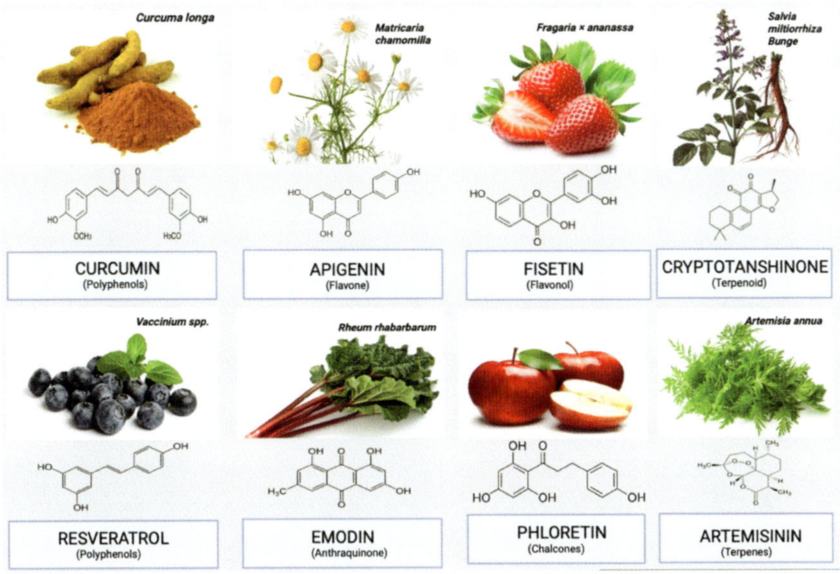

Figure 4: An overview of phytochemical sources

determine their toxicity and side effects in humans, after conducting cell and animal investigations.

8. Conclusion

In this chapter, we explored the substantial influence of phytochemicals as inhibitors of mTOR in relation to liver cancer. The diversity of these natural compounds, categorized into groups like flavones, diterpenes, indoles, isoflavones, and polyphenols, highlights the vast potential of phytomedicine in offering novel therapeutic avenues for this challenging disease.

Each category of phytochemicals exhibits distinct characteristics in regulating the mTOR pathway, indicating a potentially effective approach for liver cancer treatment that complements or enhances current therapies. This approach could potentially lead to more targeted, effective, and less toxic treatment modalities.

The potential of phytochemicals in liver cancer therapy is not just a theoretical prospect but a tangible pathway toward innovative treatments. The capacity of these natural chemicals to target cancer cell pathways like mTOR emphasizes the need for ongoing study to translate these results into clinical practice.

References

1. Xu T, Sun D, Chen Y, Ouyang L. Targeting mTOR for fighting diseases: a revisited review of mTOR inhibitors. *European Journal of Medicinal Chemistry* 2020;199:112391.
2. Patra S, Mishra SR, Behera BP, Mahapatra KK, Panigrahi DP, Bhol CS, et al. Autophagy-modulating phytochemicals in cancer therapeutics: current evidences and future perspectives. *Seminars in Cancer Biology* 2022.
3. Lian C, Huang Y, Hu P, Cao Y, Zhang Z, Feng F, et al. Nitidine chloride triggers autophagy and apoptosis of ovarian cancer cells through Akt/mTOR signaling pathway. *Current Pharmaceutical Design* 2023;29(19):1524.
4. Tan HK, Moad AIH, Tan ML. The mTOR signalling pathway in cancer and the potential mTOR inhibitory activities of natural phytochemicals. *Asian Pacific Journal of Cancer Prevention* 2014;15(16):6463–6475.
5. Zhao Y, Xiong X, Sun Y. DEPTOR, an mTOR inhibitor, is a physiological substrate of SCFβTrCP E3 ubiquitin ligase and regulates survival and autophagy. *Molecular Cell* 2011;44(2):304–316.
6. Mossmann D, Park S, Hall MN. mTOR signalling and cellular metabolism are mutual determinants in cancer. *Nature Reviews Cancer* 2018;18(12):744–757.
7. Asnaghi L, Bruno P, Priulla M, Nicolin AJ. mTOR: a protein kinase switching between life and death. *Pharmacological Research* 2004;50(6):545–549.
8. Jhanwar-Uniyal M, Wainwright JV, Mohan AL, Tobias ME, Murali R, Gandhi CD, et al. Diverse signaling mechanisms of mTOR complexes: mTORC1 and mTORC2 in forming a formidable relationship. *Advances in Biological Regulation* 2019;72:51–62.

9. Tian L-Y, Smit DJ, Jücker MJIJoMS. The role of PI3K/AKT/mTOR signaling in hepatocellular carcinoma metabolism. *International Journal of Molecular Sciences* 2023;24(3):2652.
10. Matter MS, Decaens T, Andersen JB, Thorgeirsson SS. Targeting the mTOR pathway in hepatocellular carcinoma: current state and future trends. *Journal of Hepatology* 2014;60(4):855–865.
11. Guichard C, Amaddeo G, Imbeaud S, Ladeiro Y, Pelletier L, Maad IB, et al. Integrated analysis of somatic mutations and focal copy-number changes identifies key genes and pathways in hepatocellular carcinoma. *Nature Genetics* 2012;44(6):694–698.
12. Szwed A, Kim E, Jacinto E. Regulation and metabolic functions of mTORC1 and mTORC2. *Physiological Reviews* 2021;101(3): 1371–1426.
13. Dibble CC, Cantley LC. Regulation of mTORC1 by PI3K signaling. *Trends in Cell Biology* 2015;25(9):545–555.
14. Tian T, Li X, Zhang JJIjoms. mTOR signaling in cancer and mTOR inhibitors in solid tumor targeting therapy. *International Journal of Molecular Sciences* 2019;20(3):755.
15. Hua H, Kong Q, Zhang H, Wang J, Luo T, Jiang YJ. Targeting mTOR for cancer therapy. *Molecules* 2019;12(1):1–19.
16. Gomez-Pinillos A, Ferrari AC. mTOR signaling pathway and mTOR inhibitors in cancer therapy. *Cell & Bioscience* 2012;26(3):483–505.
17. Zoncu R, Efeyan A, Sabatini DM. mTOR: from growth signal integration to cancer, diabetes and ageing. *Nature Reviews Molecular Cell Biology* 2011;12(1):21–35.
18. Dancey J. mTOR signaling and drug development in cancer. *Nature Reviews Clinical Oncology* 2010;7(4):209–219.
19. Chiang GG, Abraham RT. Targeting the mTOR signaling network in cancer. *Trends in Molecular Medicine* 2007;13(10):433–442.
20. Ersahin T, Tuncbag N, Cetin-Atalay R. The PI3K/AKT/mTOR interactive pathway. *Molecular BioSystems* 2015;11(7):1946–1954.
21. Yang J, Pi C, Wang G. Inhibition of PI3K/Akt/mTOR pathway by apigenin induces apoptosis and autophagy in hepatocellular carcinoma cells. *Biomedicine & Pharmacotherapy* 2018;103:699–707.

22. Tong X, Pelling J. Targeting the PI3K/Akt/mTOR axis by apigenin for cancer prevention. *Anti-Cancer Agents in Medicinal Chemistry* 2013; 13(7):971–978.
23. Pan F-f, Zheng Y-B, Shi C-J, Zhang F-W, Zhang J-F, Fu W-M. H19-Wnt/β-catenin regulatory axis mediates the suppressive effects of apigenin on tumor growth in hepatocellular carcinoma. *European Journal of Pharmacology* 2021;893:173810.
24. Chen W, Lu Y, Chen G, Huang S. Molecular evidence of cryptotanshinone for treatment and prevention of human cancer. *Anti-Cancer Agents in Medicinal Chemistry* 2013;13(7):979–987.
25. Kim J, Jung KH, Choi JG, Oh MS, Hong S-S. *Artemisiae iwayomogii* Herba inhibits growth, motility, and the PI3K/AKT/mTOR signaling pathway in hepatocellular carcinoma cells. *Planta Medica* 2020; 86(10):717–727.
26. Kim J, Jung KH, Yan HH, Cheon MJ, Kang S, Jin X, et al. *Artemisia capillaris* leaves inhibit cell proliferation and induce apoptosis in hepatocellular carcinoma. *BMC Complementary and Alternative Medicine* 2018;18(1):1–10.
27. Jiang Y, Fang Y, Ye Y, Xu X, Wang B, Gu J, et al. Anti-cancer effects of 3,3′-diindolylmethane on human hepatocellular carcinoma cells is enhanced by calcium ionophore: the role of cytosolic Ca^{2+} and p38 mapK. *Frontiers in Pharmacology* 2019;10:1167.
28. Biersack B. 3,3′-Diindolylmethane and its derivatives: nature-inspired strategies tackling drug resistant tumors by regulation of signal transduction, transcription factors and microRNAs. *Cancer Drug Resistance* 2020;3(4):867.
29. Wang S-D, Chen B-C, Kao S-T, Liu C-J, Yeh C-C. Genistein inhibits tumor invasion by suppressing multiple signal transduction pathways in human hepatocellular carcinoma cells. *BMC Complementary and Alternative Medicine* 2014;14(1):1–12.
30. Song P, Hu S, Li Y, Guan Z, He D, Huang Z, et al. Taurine, EGCG and Genistein regulate AMPK-mTOR pathway to inhibit hepatic stellate cells autophagy and alleviate liver fibrosis in rats. 2022.
31. Lin ZY, Yun QZ, Wu L, Zhang TW, Yao TZ. Pharmacological basis and new insights of deguelin concerning its anticancer effects. *Pharmacological Research* 2021;174:105935.

32. Li M, Yu X, Li W, Liu T, Deng G, Liu W, et al. Deguelin suppresses angiogenesis in human hepatocellular carcinoma by targeting HGF-c-Met pathway. *Oncotarget* 2018;9(1):152.
33. Beevers C, Zhou H, Huang S. Hitting the golden TORget: curcumin's effects on mTOR signaling. *Anticancer Agents in Medicinal Chemistry* 2013;13(7):988–994.
34. Sharma S, Tanwar A, Gupta DK. Curcumin: an adjuvant therapeutic remedy for liver cancer. *Hepatoma Research* 2016;22:23.
35. Syed D, Adhami V, Khan M, Mukhtar H. Inhibition of Akt/mTOR signaling by the dietary flavonoid fisetin. *Anti Cancer Agents in Medicinal Chemistry* 2013;13:995–1001.
36. Maurya BK, Trigun SK. Fisetin attenuates AKT associated growth promoting events in aflatoxinb1 induced hepatocellular carcinoma. *Anti-Cancer Agents in Medicinal Chemistry* 2018;18(13):1885–1891.
37. Sarfraz M, Arafat M, Zaidi SHH, Eltaib L, Siddique MI, Kamal M, et al. Resveratrol-laden nano-systems in the cancer environment: views and reviews. *Cancers* 2023;15(18):4499.
38. Yalçın R, Kart A, Özmen Ö, Zeybek E. Protective effects of resveratrol against fumonisin B1-induced liver toxicity in mice. *Arhiv za Higijenu Rada i Toksikologiju* 2023;74(2):115–119.
39. Bhattacharya S, Perris A, Jawed JJ, Hoda M. Therapeutic role of resveratrol against hepatocellular carcinoma: a review on its molecular mechanisms of action. *Pharmacological Research-Modern Chinese Medicine* 2023;6:100233.
40. Bruning A. Inhibition of mTOR signaling by quercetin in cancer treatment and prevention. *Anti-Cancer Agents in Medicinal Chemistry* 2013;13(7):1025–1031.
41. Maugeri A, Calderaro A, Patanè GT, Navarra M, Barreca D, Cirmi S, et al. Targets involved in the anti-cancer activity of quercetin in breast, colorectal and liver neoplasms. *International Journal of Molecular Sciences* 2023;24(3):2952.
42. Aglan HA, Ahmed HH, El-Toumy SA, Mahmoud NS. Gallic acid against hepatocellular carcinoma: an integrated scheme of the potential mechanisms of action from *in vivo* study. *Tumour Biology* 2017; 39(6):1010428317699127.

43. Sun G, Zhang S, Xie Y, Zhang Z, Zhao W. Gallic acid as a selective anticancer agent that induces apoptosis in SMMC-7721 human hepatocellular carcinoma cells. *Oncology Letters* 2016;11(1):150–158.
44. Ahsan H, Ahad A, Iqbal J, Siddiqui WA. Pharmacological potential of tocotrienols: a review. *Nutrition & Metabolism* 2014;11:1–22.
45. Abdullah A, Atia A. The role of tocotrienols in liver health and disease. *Current Topics in Pharmacology* 2018;22:135–142.
46. Wang N, Feng Y, Zhu M, Siu F-M, Ng K-M, Che C-M. A novel mechanism of XIAP degradation induced by timosaponin AIII in hepatocellular carcinoma. *Biochimica et biophysica acta* 2013;1833(12):2890–2899.
47. Han F-Y, Song X-Y, Chen J-J, Yao G-D, Song S-J. Timosaponin AIII: a novel potential anti-tumor compound from *Anemarrhena asphodeloides. Steroids* 2018;140:125–130.
48. Chhimwal J, Dhritlahre RK, Anand P, Patial V, Saneja A, Padwad YS. Amorphous solid dispersion augments the bioavailability of phloretin and its therapeutic efficacy via targeting mTOR/SREBP-1c axis in NAFLD mice. *Biomaterials Advances* 2023;154:213627.
49. Li Y, Wang X, Cheng S, Du J, Deng Z, Zhang Y, et al. Diosgenin induces G2/M cell cycle arrest and apoptosis in human hepatocellular carcinoma cells. *Oncology Reports* 2015;33(2):693–698.
50. Meng X, Dong H, Pan Y, Ma L, Liu C, Man S, et al. Diosgenyl saponin inducing endoplasmic reticulum stress and mitochondria-mediated apoptotic pathways in liver cancer cells. *Journal of Agricultural and Food Chemistry* 2019;67(41):11428–11435.
51. Chen Z, Xu J, Wu Y, Lei S, Liu H, Meng Q, et al. Diosgenin inhibited the expression of TAZ in hepatocellular carcinoma. *Biochemical and Biophysical Research Communications* 2018;503(3):1181–1185.
52. Hu Y, Yang L, Lai YJB. Recent findings regarding the synergistic effects of emodin and its analogs with other bioactive compounds: insights into new mechanisms. *Biomedicine & Pharmacotherapy* 2023;162:114585.
53. Zheng X-Y, Yang S-M, Zhang R, Wang S-M, Li G-B, Zhou S-W, et al. Emodin-induced autophagy against cell apoptosis through the PI3K/AKT/mTOR pathway in human hepatocytes. *Drug Design, Development and Therapy* 2019:3171–3180.
54. Sazli FAR, Jubri Z, Rahman MA, Karsani SA, Top AGM, Ngah WZW, et al. Gamma-tocotrienol treatment increased peroxiredoxin-4

expression in HepG2 liver cancer cell line. ***BMC Complementary and Alternative Medicine*** 2015;15:64.

55. Shen X, Zhang Y, Feng Y, Zhang L, Li J, Xie Y-A, et al. Epigallocatechin-3-gallate inhibits cell growth, induces apoptosis and causes S phase arrest in hepatocellular carcinoma by suppressing the AKT pathway. ***International Journal of Oncology*** 2014;44(3):791–796.
56. Tang Y, Cao J, Cai Z, An H, Li Y, Peng Y, et al. Epigallocatechin gallate induces chemopreventive effects on rats with diethylnitrosamine-induced liver cancer via inhibition of cell division cycle 25A. ***Molecular Medicine Reports*** 2020;22(5):3873–3885.

https://doi.org/10.1142/9789811293320_0008

Chapter 8

Therapeutic Role of Phytochemicals in Angiogenesis and Metastasis of Liver Cancer

Dr. Shweta Kumar*

**Research Associate III, Department of General Medicine, AIIMS Bhopal, India*

Table of Contents

---

*Corresponding author: ORCID: 0000-0003-4484-3184; E-mail address: drshwetakumar786@gmail.com

Abbreviations

HCC — Hepatocellular carcinoma
VEGF — Vascular endothelial growth factor
PDGF — Platelet-derived growth factors
Ang — Angiopoietins
FGF — Fibroblast growth factor
ECs — Endothelial cells
VEGFR — Vascular endothelial growth factor and its receptor
TGF-β — Transforming growth factor-β
PGF — Placental growth factor
TNF-α — Tumor necrosis factor-α
CSF-1 — Colony-stimulating factor-1
IL-8 — Interleukin-8
PGE2 — Prostaglandin E2
S1P — Sphingosine-1-phosphate
MMP — Matrix metalloproteinases
HIF-1α — Hypoxia-inducible factor-1α
RNAi — RNA interference
FDA — Food and Drug Administration
mAbs — Monoclonal antibodies
MAPK — Mitogen-activated protein kinase
mTOR — Mammalian target of rapamycin
PI3K — Phosphoinositide 3-kinases
PDGFR — Platelet-derived growth factor receptors
PlGF — Placental growth factor
EMA — Epithelial membrane antigen
PEM — Polymorphic epithelial mucin
MUC1-CT — Cytoplasmic tail of MUC1
ECD — Extracellular domain
TMD — Transmembrane domain
CT — Cytoplasmic tail
CTGF — Connective tissue growth factor
PDGF-β — Platelet-derived growth factor-β
MRP1 — Multidrug resistance protein 1

PHGDH — Phosphoglycerate dehydrogenase
CAMs — Chorioallantoic membrane
CTCs — Circulating tumor cells
NRP-1 — Neuropilin-1
PDA — Pancreatic ductal adenocarcinoma
NSCLC — Non-small-cell lung cancer

Abstract

One of the more common malignancies is liver cancer. Accelerated tumorigenesis is a result of metabolic imbalance. It is generally known that metabolic alterations maintain the growth, proliferating, and survival of tumors. Phytochemicals present in large quantities in plants possess numerous anticarcinogenic qualities as inhibiting tumor growth, angiogenesis, and metastasis, while also inducing apoptosis. Furthermore, they can regulate immune system functions and protect healthy cells from damage caused by free radicals. Most studies on the anticancer effects of phytochemicals used isolated substances. However, various research has shown that by combining them synergistically with chemically related or unrelated substances, anticancer efficacy and scope of action can be further increased. The prevention and resistance to development of liver cancer can be achieved by targeting metabolic dysregulation in organisms, which has significant ramifications to create innovative therapeutic strategies for the control and treatment of cancer. This chapter systematically illustrates the role of various phytochemicals in angiogenesis and metastasis in liver cancer.

1. Introduction

One of the more common malignancies is liver cancer. Liver cancer, also referred as hepatocellular carcinoma (HCC), is a malignancy that starts in the hepatic cells. It is a significant global health concern and is often associated with individuals dealing with chronic liver conditions such as cirrhosis resulting from hepatitis B or C infection, excessive alcohol consumption, or fatty liver diseases. Early stages may not present noticeable symptoms, making early detection challenging [1].

2. Treatment Modalities of Lung Cancer: Conventional and Current Strategies

Possible treatment modalities encompass surgical procedures, chemotherapy, radiation therapy, targeted therapy, and immunotherapy depending on the stage and overall health of the individual. However, these days, there is rise in resistance of tumors to several drugs. As a result, research efforts are expanding to find novel anticancer chemicals with high sensitivity to cancer cells. *In vitro* and preclinical studies conducted have demonstrated the potential of exogenous antioxidants to mitigate the damage caused by free radicals that is linked to the onset of cancer. Nevertheless, clinical studies are still limited and ongoing. Another naturally occurring process that regulates the creation of new blood vessels from existing ones is angiogenesis. It is now thought that most of the malignancies have the capacity for angiogenesis, and that angiogenesis is necessary for the growth, metastasis, and invasion of these tumors. Endothelial cells (ECs) secrete unique enzymes such as heparin and matrix metalloproteinase (MMP), which cause the extracellular matrix and basal lamina to be broken down during angiogenesis. The robust connections between the ECs get fragmented because of this process. ECs can be produced through this mechanism, which then organizes immigration and reproduction to construct new capillary tubes. Factors that promote angiogenesis are vascular endothelial growth factor (VEGF), platelet-derived growth factors (PDGF), fibroblast growth factor (FGF), epidermal growth factor (EGF), transforming growth factor-β (TGF-β), angiopoietins (Ang1 and Ang2), and cytokines like interleukin-1 (IL-1), tumor necrosis factor-α (TNF-α), colony-stimulating factor-1 (CSF-1), and. Various cell types, including smooth muscle cells, keratinocytes, platelets, macrophages stimulate the formation of these angiogenic mediators [2, 3].

The prevention and resistance to development of liver cancer can be achieved by targeting metabolic dysregulation in organisms, which has significant ramifications for the development of novel therapeutic approaches for the control and treatment of cancer. This chapter systematically illustrates the role of various phytochemicals in angiogenesis and metastasis in liver cancer. The regulation of angiogenesis involves maintaining an equilibrium between activating molecules such as cytokines and growth factors that stimulate ECs, and inhibitory agents that restrain these cells. Thus, inhibiting or preventing excessive angiogenesis is an effective strategy for HCC prevention.

3. Inflammatory Mediators in Antiangiogenic Therapy

Notably, VEGF and FGF have emerged as potential targets for antiangiogenic therapy. VEGF is a circulating glycoprotein which primarily operates through the VEGF receptor 2 (VEGFR2 or flk-1/kdr), a receptor tyrosine kinase (RTK) expressed by ECs. In cancer, hypoxia-induced by increased demand for nutrients and oxygen creates a situation where cancer cells release molecules such as growth factors, cytokines, anti-apoptotic factors, and hypoxia-inducible factor-1α (HIF-1α).

In contrast, the process of angiogenesis can be hindered by inhibitory proteins, which fall into two categories: direct and indirect angiogenesis inhibitors. The direct inhibitors act by suppressing ECs within developing blood vessels, while the indirect inhibitors inhibit either tumor cells or other stromal cells related to tumors. Integrin receptors, functioning via diverse intracellular signaling pathways, can exert a direct inhibitory impact. Certain molecules such as angiostatin, endostatin, arrestin, canstatin, and tumstatin, generated through the degradation of specific EC-matrix components, impede the proliferation and migration of vascular ECs against angiogenic signals. Moreover, inhibitors of angiogenesis include interferons, retinoic acid, interleukin-1 (IL-1), interleukin-12 (IL-12), tissue inhibitors of metalloproteinases, and multimerin 2.

Reiterating, the equilibrium between activators and inhibitors of angiogenesis is pivotal. Hypoxia, a key factor, disrupts this balance by upregulating HIF-1α, resulting in heightened expression of pro-angiogenic factors and diminished expression of angiogenesis inhibitors. As a result, all the molecules involved in these pathways could potentially be targeted for therapeutic interventions focused on inhibiting angiogenesis.

In the realm of pharmacological antiangiogenic agents, substantial advancement has been achieved since Folkman introduced the concept of angiogenesis inhibitors for cancer treatment. Promising antiangiogenic interventions include gene therapy, monoclonal antibodies (mAbs), chimeric antigen receptor T-cell (CAR-T) treatment, RNAs interference (RNAi) therapy-MicroRNAs (miRNAs)/small interfering RNAs (siRNAs), aptamers, small molecules, and chemotherapeutic agents. Several drugs inhibiting angiogenesis have been developed such as Sorafenib (inhibiting oral multi-kinase), Regorafenib (a multi-kinase suppressor of VEGFR1-3), Ramucirumab (an mAb), Bevacizumab (an anti-VEGF mAb), and Everolimus. However, these agents have shown limited effectiveness in tumor response and patient survival [2].

On the other hand, phytochemicals, which are natural compounds found in plants, have gained attention for their potential role in inhibiting angiogenesis and metastasis in liver cancer. Phytochemicals present in large quantities in plants possess numerous anticarcinogenic qualities such as inhibiting tumor growth, angiogenesis, and metastasis, while also inducing apoptosis. Furthermore, they can regulate immune system functions and protect healthy cells from damage caused by free radicals. Most studies on the anticancer effects of phytochemicals used isolated substances [4].

mAbs are designed to target crucial receptors such as vascular endothelial growth factor receptors (VEGFRs) and their associated signal transduction pathways. In contrast, small molecules aim at variety of molecules like mammalian target of rapamycin (mTOR), Raf (rapidly accelerated fibrosarcoma), mitogen-activated protein kinase

(MAPK), and phosphoinositide 3-kinases (PI3K). Medicinal herbs present promising attributes as multi-target agents, offering broader mechanisms, cost-effectiveness, and reduced toxicity for the development of novel anticancer drugs. Their focus on targeting the VEGF signaling pathway and RTKs in angiogenesis is particularly noteworthy. Currently, cancer treatment drugs comprise antiangiogenic small molecules and phytochemicals that function by inhibiting VEGF and the process of angiogenesis. Herbal anti-VEGF agents are deemed crucial targets for clinical applications in cancer treatment. A few of them have been validated, with their receptors and downstream signaling pathways now well-established [5, 6].

VEGF comprises of two identical parts of about 45 kDa [7]. There are other variants such as VEGF-B, VEGF-C, VEGF-D, VEGF-E (viral VEGF), VEGF-F (snake venom VEGF), and placental growth factor (PlGF), which share similarities with VEGF due to different splicing patterns [8]. VEGF-A and its receptors, VEGFR-1 (flt-1) and VEGFR-2 (KDR/flk-1 in mice), play a significant role in promoting oncogenic angiogenesis under hypoxic conditions. Additionally, among various VEGF isoforms, VEGF165 is widely recognized for its capacity to stimulate angiogenic sprouting and the formation of EC tubes, as evidenced by both *in vitro* and *in vivo* studies [9–15]. The crosstalk between signaling pathways, involving various angiogenic factors, cell surface receptors, and intracellular signaling components, is frequently intensified within the tumor microenvironment, promoting tumor growth, invasion, and metastasis. Genetic instability in cancer cells often results in mutations in oncogenes and tumor suppressor genes, leading to an increase in angiogenic factors. As tumors grow, hypoxia in the core triggers the upregulation of pro-angiogenic factors, including vascular endothelial growth factor receptors (VEGFR 1–3), and the stabilization of HIF-1α, playing a crucial role in angiogenesis. Therapeutic strategies targeting angiogenesis are primarily classified by their capacity to: (i) hinder the transcription and translation of specific angiogenic factors; (ii) functionally neutralize pro-angiogenic factors; and (iii) specifically bind to the extracellular domain of VEGF receptors, effectively blocking ligand-induced angiogenic activity. However, an intrinsic resistance to antiangiogenic drugs is commonly observed toward these drugs in most cancer patients [16–19].

3.1. *Membrane-bound mucin (MUC1)*

MUC1 (or episialin) is highly glycosylated protein and is found on the apical borders of glandular epithelial cells. In tumor cells, MUC1 has been reported to play a role in several types of cancer. It is found to be associated in the intrinsic apoptotic pathways. It has been reported that overexpression of MUC1 leads to decreased caspase-3 activation and, in many tumor cells, activates angiogenic factors, mainly VEGFs, through the activation of intracellular signaling pathways such as Ras/MAPK and JAK2/STAT3. It decreases its phosphorylation by attenuating activation of the phosphoinositide 3-kinase (PI3K)/AKT/mechanistic target of rapamycin (mTOR) [20]. Furthermore, the HIF-1α transcription factor has the capability to bind to the MUC1 promoter, leading to the upregulation of MUC1 expression [21]. This strengthens the movement and penetration of cancer cells to adjacent tissues [22].

Despite extensive research on angiogenesis-related pathways, many targeted agents have failed to achieve significant therapeutic outcomes. Understanding the association between abnormally elevated MUC1 expression and factors related to angiogenesis could provide valuable insights for the advancement of innovative therapeutic strategies for cancer patients [23].

4. Tumor Progression Through Metastasis

Metastasis is a complex process that involves cancer cells to spread from their original location to distant organs, and accounts for majority of cancer-related deaths. Despite its significance, metastasis remains poorly understood in the context of cancer pathogenesis. After establishing colonies at the primary site, tumor cells undergo a series of steps to invade surrounding tissues, enter the bloodstream or lymphatic system (intravasation), travel through the bloodstream at distant sites (extravasation), and grow there to establish new colonies [24] (Figure 1).

This multistep process can be broadly categorized into two main phases: physical transfer of cancer cells and colonization [25]. At the time of cancer diagnosis, 60–70% of patients already show evidence of metastasis. Importantly, no single molecular pathway is solely responsible for cancer metastasis; instead, complex signaling networks interact to facilitate tumor migration and invasion [26].

4.1. *Key molecular players in metastasis*

Several molecular factors have been implicated in cancer metastasis. Phosphoglycerate dehydrogenase (PHGDH) contributes to increased tumor cell metastasis, with its heterogeneity associated with cancer invasion [27]. Slit2, an inhibitor of metastasis in breast cancer,

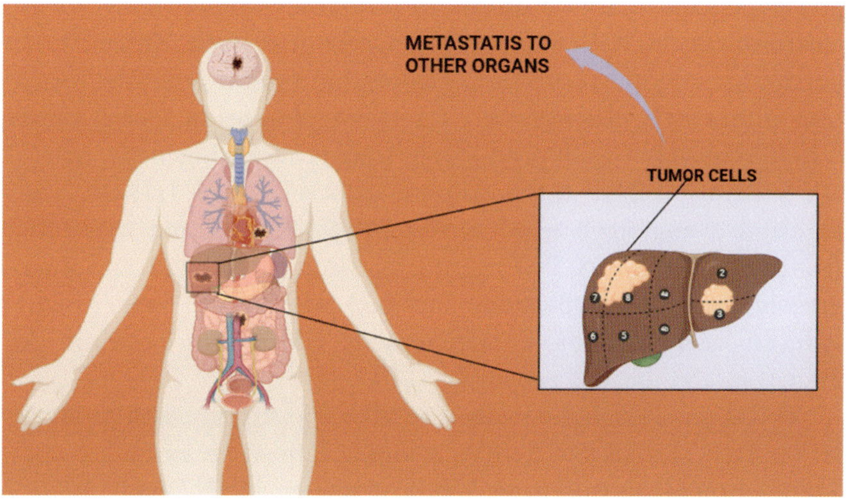

Figure 1: A diagram illustrating the process of tumor progression through metastasis. Following the growth of cancer cells at their initial location, they enter the bloodstream through a process called intravasation. Subsequently, they spread throughout the body, targeting specific locations. Upon reaching their destination, they exit blood vessels in a step called extravasation and form new colonies

promotes the spread of breast tumor cells by activating M1-like phagocytic and anti-fibrotic macrophages [28].

Efforts to combat metastasis have led to the development of anticancer agents with anti-metastatic activity. Ginsenoside Rh2, for instance, promotes the expression of miR-491, suppressing colon cancer cell metastasis [29]. Metformin, by inducing AMPK signaling and inhibiting mTOR expression, prevents invasion and metastasis of colorectal tumor cells. These studies underscore the intricate and interconnected nature of metastasis regulation, highlighting the complex interactions among molecular pathways [30]. The section below emphasizes the action of MUC1 in regulating tumor metastasis. Metastasis is a critical stage in the survival of tumor cells. Cancer cells can break free from the basement membrane, eat away at the surrounding matrix, target nearby tissues, and/or enter the bloodstream [16].

Cancer cells, adapting to thrive in hypoxic environments, induce pro-angiogenic factors' expression, promoting angiogenesis. In this environment, MUC1 raises pro-angiogenic gene levels. This elevation initiates new blood vessel formation within tumors and tube formation within ECs. Aberrant MUC1 overexpression in several cancer cells upregulates VEGF production, leading to angiogenesis. MUC1 also promotes PDGF-A expression in association with HIF-1α, a key regulator of angiogenesis. Moreover, MUC1-CD activates connective tissue growth factor (CTGF) gene expression (a metastasis and angiogenesis mediator) via β-catenin and p53 attachment. Thus, MUC1-induced factors promote angiogenesis and enhance cancer cell migratory and invasive properties [20].

It was revealed in the study that MUC1 overexpression promotes IGF-1-IGF-1R/AKT/VEGF signaling in human breast cancer cases. MUC1 expression stimulates VEGF synthesis via AKT and ERK1/2 signaling pathways, impacting diverse processes, including tumor growth, angiogenesis, and metastasis. The MUC1-mediated signaling cascade activates IGF-1R, a potent angiogenic factor, enhancing angiogenesis in cancer cells. Inhibition of MUC1 expression reduces IGF-1R phosphorylation, indicating a crucial role for MUC1 in tumor angiogenesis [20]. Neuropilin-1 (NRP-1) facilitates angiogenesis by acting as a co-receptor for the VEGF family. Overexpression of NRP-1 in various cancers correlates with disease progression and metastasis. Another study involving cells of pancreatic ductal adenocarcinoma (PDA), demonstrated an NRP1-dependent VEGFR signaling modulation by tumor-associated (TA) MUC1 [31].

5. Role of Phytochemicals in Angiogenesis and Metastasis of Liver Cancer

Researchers view plants as valuable resources for validating and creating novel pharmaceuticals. Since using plants to cure cancer has a long history, plants have historically been the main source of traditional medications that are useful in the treatment of cancer.

Research on isolating molecules from plants and other natural organisms confirmed that plants are important resources for synthesis inhibitors that have the potential to develop production of anticancer drugs, following the discovery of new proteins that had significant regulatory effects on the development of the tumor cell cycle. Several compounds with plant origin and with antiangiogenic properties have been identified. Multi-targeting antiangiogenic drugs have been developed to modulate several signaling pathways involved in angiogenesis simultaneously, exerting anticancer effects. (Figure 2 illustrates these multi-targeting drugs).

6. Conclusion

Antiangiogenic therapy for cancer has been recognized as a crucial treatment strategy for numerous cancer subtypes since its initial proposal in 1971. Angiogenesis in non-small-cell lung cancer (NSCLC) is associated with highly invasive and metastatic features of the illness, like other solid tumors. Antiangiogenic drugs are one of the promising treatment modalities that are now undergoing clinical testing. To address the known toxicities and disadvantages, additional research in this field is vitally needed. Exploring the potential of phytochemicals derived from our diets presents an intriguing and innovative method for preventing and treating HCC. These dietary compounds have

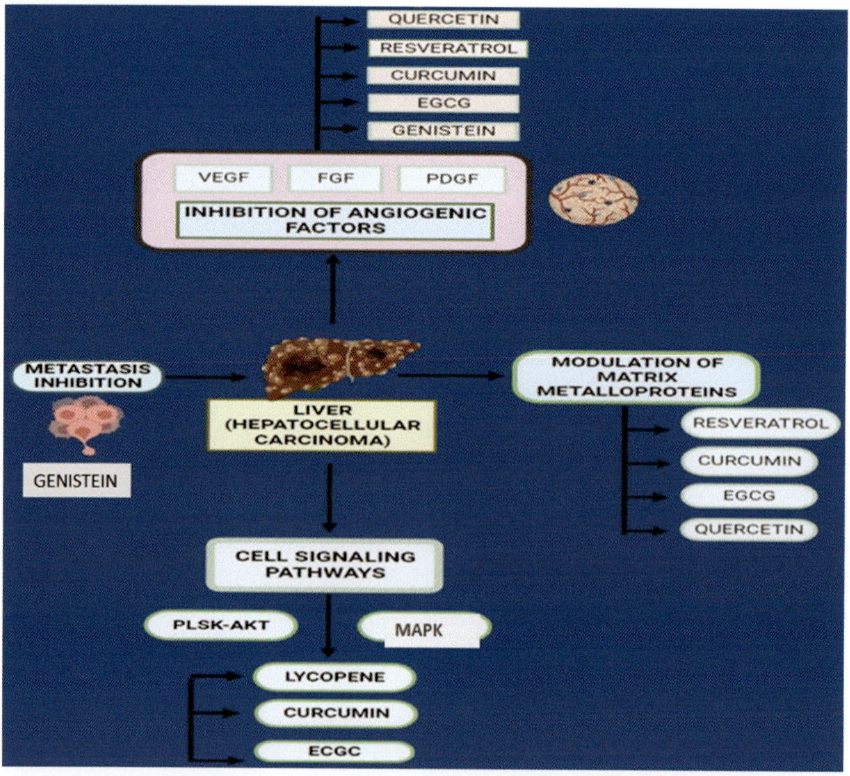

Figure 2: Schematic representation of phytochemicals targeting various steps of cancer progression; EGCG: epigallocatechin gallate; PI3K: phosphatidylinositol-3-kinase; VEGF: vascular endothelial growth factor; FGF: fibroblast growth factor; PDFG: platelet-derived growth factor

robust antioxidant and anti-inflammatory capabilities, essential for countering the oxidative stress and inflammation often associated with liver cancer. A multitude of phytochemicals have displayed significant potential as viable options for both preventing and treating HCC. However, various research has shown that by combining them synergistically with chemically related or unrelated substances, anticancer efficacy and scope of action can be further increased. The prevention and resistance to development of liver cancer can be achieved by targeting metabolic dysregulation in organisms, which

Table 1: Spectrum of potent phytochemicals exhibiting antiangiogenic and anti-metastatic action (*in vitro* and *in vivo*)

Name of Phytochemical	Source	Mechanism of Action	Reference(s)
Paclitaxel	*Taxus brevifolia*	Anti-VEGF action	Belotti et al. [32]
Podophyllotoxins	*Podophyllum peltatum*	Decreased expression of modulator proteins such as VEGFA, STAT-3, p-ERK, ERK1/2, and AKT-1	Nguyen et al. [33]
Vinblastine, Vinflunine	*Catharanthus roseus*	Block endothelial chemotaxis and proliferation also	Vacca et al. [34]
Curcumin	Turmeric	Suppression of vascular endothelial growth factor (VEGF), downregulation of angiogenic factors [fibroblast growth factors (FGF) and platelet-derived growth factors (PDGF)], anti-inflammatory properties, inhibition of matrix metalloproteinases (MMPs), regulation of microRNAs, and inhibition of cell signaling pathways	Varinska et al. [4] Arbiser et al. [35]
Epigallocatechin gallate (EGCG)	Green tea	Inhibition of VEGF, suppression of pro-angiogenic factors [basic fibroblast growth factor (bFGF) and matrix metalloproteinases (MMPs)], anti-inflammatory effects, suppression of endothelial cell proliferation and migration, suppression of invasion and metastasis, induction of apoptosis, regulation of cell signaling pathways (PI3K-AKT and MAPK pathways), and anti-oxidative properties	Bimonte et al. [36] Shirakami et al. [37]

(*Continued*)

Table 1: (*Continued*)

Name of Phytochemical	Source	Mechanism of Action	Reference(s)
Resveratrol	Red grapes and red wine	Inhibition of angiogenic factors (VEGF, FGF, and PDGF), anti-inflammatory effects, interference with endothelial cell function, modulation of matrix metalloproteinases (MMPs), cell signaling pathways (PI3K-AKT and MAPK pathways), and microRNA regulation	Varinska et al. [4] Bråkenhielm et al. [38]
Quercetin	Various fruits and vegetables	Inhibition of angiogenic factors (VEGF, FGF, and PDGF), antioxidant and anti-inflammatory properties, regulation of matrix metalloproteinases (MMPs), suppression of endothelial cell function, induction of apoptosis, cell signaling pathways, and microRNA regulation	Wu L et al., 2017 Gacche et al. [39]
Genistein	Isoflavones from Soy products	Antiangiogenic effects (VEGF) and metastasis inhibition	Kadioglu et al. [40] Kim et al., 2003
Lycopene	Tomatoes and red or pink fruits and vegetables	Antioxidant effects, anti-inflammatory effects, and regulation of cell signaling	Ranjan et al. [1]
Castanospermine	Indolizidine alkaloid isolated from the seeds of *Castanospermum australe*	Inhibit migration and invasion of endothelial cells (*in vitro*)	Pili et al. [41]
Sanguinarine	Benzophenanthridine alkaloid derived from rhizomes of the plant species *Sanguinaria canadensis*	VEGF-induced endothelial cell migration and sprouting *in vitro* and blood vessel formation *in vivo*	Llovet et al. [42]

Vinblastine	Alkaloid from *Catharanthus roseus*	Inhibit VEGF-mediated angiogenesis [human hepatocellular carcinoma-use of the chick embryo chorioallantoic membrane (CAM) assay]	Ribatti et al. [43] Nurcahyanti et al. [44]
Brucine	Indole alkaloid from Nuxvomica (*Strychnos nuxvomica)*	VEGF-mediated angiogenesis (cell lines)	Saraswati et al. [45]
Colchicine	Alkaloid from *Colchicum autumnale*	Antiangiogenic activity through direct apoptotic effect on endothelial cells	Stafford et al. [46] Baby et al. [47]
Benzyl isothiocyanate (BITC)	*Alliaria petiolata*, mustard plant, and papaya seeds	Downregulation of MMP-2/9 via PKC and MAPK signaling pathway, inhibition of STAT3 mediated HIF-1α/VEGF/Rho-GTPases, inhibition of PI3K/AKT/FOXO pathway	Ranjan et al. [1]
Luteolin	Celery, parsley, broccoli, onion leaves, carrots, peppers, cabbages, apple skins, and chrysanthemum flower	Suppress tumor growth by acting on cellular mechanisms such as apoptosis, angiogenesis, and migration	Haiaty et al. [48]
Retinoic acid	Carrots, sweet potatoes, spinach, kale, apricots, cantaloupe, mangoes, papayas, red and yellow bell peppers, liver (beef, chicken, or pork)	Metastasis was suppressed by preventing tumor cells from adhering to the vascular endothelium and subendothelium	Edward et al. [49]

has significant ramifications for the development of novel therapeutic approaches for the control and treatment of cancer. This chapter systematically illustrates the role of various phytochemicals in angiogenesis and metastasis in liver cancer.

References

1. Ranjan A, Ramachandran S, Gupta N, Kaushik I, Wright S, Srivastava S, et al. Role of phytochemicals in cancer prevention. *Int J Mol Sci.* 2019 Oct 9;20(20):4981.
2. Berretta M, Rinaldi L, Di Benedetto F, Lleshi A, De Re V, Facchini G, et al.. Angiogenesis inhibitors for the treatment of hepatocellular carcinoma. *Front Pharmacol.* 2016 Nov 9;7:428.
3. Morse MA, Sun W, Kim R, He AR, Abada PB, Mynderse M, et al. The role of angiogenesis in hepatocellular carcinoma. *Clin Cancer Res.* 2019 Feb 1;25(3):912–20.
4. Varinska L, Mirossay L, Mojzisova G, Mojzis J. Antiangogenic effect of selected phytochemicals. *Pharmazie.* 2010 Jan;65(1):57–63.
5. Kadioglu O, Seo EJ, Efferth T. Targeting angiogenesis by phytochemicals. *Med Aromat Plants [Internet].* 2012;2(5). [cited 2023 Oct 30]. Available from: https://www.omicsgroup.org/journals/targeting-angiogenesis-by-phytochemicals-2167-0412.1000134.php?aid=18338
6. Parveen A, Subedi L, Kim HW, Khan Z, Zahra Z, Farooqi MQ, et al. Phytochemicals targeting VEGF and VEGF-related multifactors as anticancer therapy. *J Clin Med.* 2019 Mar 12;8(3):350.
7. Azimi-Nezhad M. Vascular endothelial growth factor from embryonic status to cardiovascular pathology. *Rep Biochem Mol Biol.* 2014 Apr;2(2):59–69.
8. Robinson CJ, Stringer SE. The splice variants of vascular endothelial growth factor (VEGF) and their receptors. *J Cell Sci.* 2001 Mar;114(Pt 5):853–865.
9. Khodabakhsh F, Merikhian P, Eisavand MR, Farahmand L. Crosstalk between MUC1 and VEGF in angiogenesis and metastasis: a review highlighting roles of the MUC1 with an emphasis on metastatic and angiogenic signaling. *Cancer Cell Int.* 2021 Dec;21(1):200.

10. Shibuya M. Differential roles of vascular endothelial growth factor receptor-1 and receptor-2 in angiogenesis. *BMB Rep.* 2006 Sep 30; 39(5):469–478.
11. Holmes K, Roberts OL, Thomas AM, Cross MJ. Vascular endothelial growth factor receptor-2: structure, function, intracellular signalling and therapeutic inhibition. *Cell Signal.* 2007 Oct;19(10):2003–2012.
12. Roskoski R. Vascular endothelial growth factor (VEGF) signaling in tumor progression. *Crit Rev Oncol Hematol.* 2007 Jun;62(3): 179–213.
13. Shibuya M. Vascular Endothelial Growth Factor (VEGF) and its receptor (VEGFR) signaling in angiogenesis: a crucial target for anti- and pro-angiogenic therapies. *Gene & Cancer.* 2011 Dec 1;2(12):1097–1105.
14. Chen SH, Murphy D, Lassoued W, Thurston G, Feldman MD, Lee WMF. Activated STAT3 is a mediator and biomarker of VEGF endothelial activation. *Cancer Biol Ther.* 2008 Dec;7(12):1994–2003.
15. Neve A, Cantatore FP, Maruotti N, Corrado A, Ribatti D. Extracellular matrix modulates angiogenesis in physiological and pathological conditions. *BioMed Res Int.* 2014;2014:1–10.
16. Darvishi B, Majidzadeh-A K, Ghadirian R, Mosayebzadeh M, Farahmand L. Recruited bone marrow derived cells, local stromal cells and IL-17 at the front line of resistance development to anti-VEGF targeted therapies. *Life Sci.* 2019 Jan;217:34–40.
17. Tamamouna V, Pitsouli C. The hypoxia-inducible factor-1α in angiogenesis and cancer: insights from the drosophila model. Gene expression and regulation in mammalian cells: transcription toward the establishment of novel therapeutics. 2018 Feb 28:209.
18. Graziani G, Ruffini F, Tentori L, Scimeca M, Dorio AS, Atzori MG, et al. Antitumor activity of a novel anti-vascular endothelial growth factor receptor-1 monoclonal antibody that does not interfere with ligand binding. *Oncotarget.* 2016 Nov 8;7(45):72868–72885.
19. Marmé D. Tumor angiogenesis: a key target for cancer therapy. *Oncol Res Treat.* 2018;41(4):164.
20. Woo JK, Choi Y, Oh SH, Jeong JH, Choi DH, Seo HS, et al. Mucin 1 enhances the tumor angiogenic response by activation of the AKT signaling pathway. *Oncogene.* 2012 Apr 26;31(17):2187–2198.

21. Aubert S, Fauquette V, Hémon B, Lepoivre R, Briez N, Bernard D, et al. MUC1, a new hypoxia inducible factor target gene, is an actor in clear renal cell carcinoma tumor progression. *Cancer Res.* 2009 Jul 15;69(14):5707–5715.
22. Sahraei M, Roy LD, Curry JM, Teresa TL, Nath S, Besmer D, et al. MUC1 regulates PDGFA expression during pancreatic cancer progression. *Oncogene.* 2012 Nov 22;31(47):4935–4945.
23. Nath S, Mukherjee P. MUC1: a multifaceted oncoprotein with a key role in cancer progression. *Trends Mol Med.* 2014 Jun;20(6):332–342.
24. Fidler IJ. The pathogenesis of cancer metastasis: the "seed and soil" hypothesis revisited. *Nat Rev Cancer.* 2003 Jun;3(6):453–458.
25. Chaffer CL, Weinberg RA. A perspective on cancer cell metastasis. *Science.* 2011 Mar 25;331(6024):1559–1564.
26. Li J, Meng H, Bai Y, Wang K. Regulation of lncRNA and its role in cancer metastasis. *Oncol Res.* 2016 Apr 13;23(5):205–217.
27. Rossi M, Altea-Manzano P, Demicco M, Doglioni G, Bornes L, Fukano M, et al. PHGDH heterogeneity potentiates cancer cell dissemination and metastasis. *Nature.* 2022 May;605(7911):747–753.
28. Ahirwar DK, Charan M, Mishra S, Verma AK, Shilo K, Ramaswamy B, et al. Slit2 inhibits breast cancer metastasis by activating M1-like phagocytic and antifibrotic macrophages. *Cancer Res.* 2021 Oct 15; 81(20):5255–5267.
29. Wei W, Guo Q, Guo C, Cui X, Ma X, Shen X, et al. Ginsenoside Rh2 suppresses metastasis and growth of colon cancer via miR-491. Yuchi A, editor. *J Oncol.* 2021 Sep 24;2021:1–7.
30. Huang R, Li J, Fu Y, Deng Y. Downregulation of FEM1C enhances metastasis and proliferation in colorectal cancer. *Ann Transl Med.* 2021 Sep;9(17):1391.
31. Zhou Q, Lui VWY, Lau CPY, Cheng SH, Ng MHL, Cai Y, et al. Sustained antitumor activity by co-targeting mTOR and the microtubule with temsirolimus/vinblastine combination in hepatocellular carcinoma. *Biochem Pharmacol.* 2012 May 1;83(9):1146–1158.
32. Belotti D, Vergani V, Drudis T, Borsotti P, Pitelli MR, Viale G, et al. The microtubule-affecting drug paclitaxel has antiangiogenic activity. *Clin Cancer Res.* 1996 Nov;2(11):1843–1849.
33. Nguyen HT, Nguyen Thi QG, Nguyen Thi TH, Thi PH, Le-Nhat-Thuy G, Dang Thi TA, et al. Synthesis and biological activity, and

molecular modelling studies of potent cytotoxic podophyllotoxin-naphthoquinone compounds. *RSC Adv.* 12(34):22004–22019.

34. Vacca A, Iurlaro M, Ribatti D, Minischetti M, Nico B, Ria R, et al. Antiangiogenesis is produced by nontoxic doses of vinblastine. *Blood.* 1999 Dec 15;94(12):4143–4155.
35. Arbiser JL, Klauber N, Rohan R, van Leeuwen R, Huang MT, Fisher C, et al. Curcumin is an *in vivo* inhibitor of angiogenesis. *Mol Med.* 1998 Jun;4(6):376–383.
36. Bimonte S, Albino V, Piccirillo M, Nasto A, Molino C, Palaia R, et al. Epigallocatechin-3-gallate in the prevention and treatment of hepatocellular carcinoma: experimental findings and translational perspectives. *Drug Des Devel Ther.* 2019 Feb 12;13:611–621.
37. Shirakami Y, Shimizu M, Adachi S, Sakai H, Nakagawa T, Yasuda Y, et al. (-)-Epigallocatechin gallate suppresses the growth of human hepatocellular carcinoma cells by inhibiting activation of the vascular endothelial growth factor-vascular endothelial growth factor receptor axis. *Cancer Sci.* 2009 Oct;100(10):1957–1962.
38. Brâkenhielm E, Cao R, Cao Y. Suppression of angiogenesis, tumor growth, and wound healing by resveratrol, a natural compound in red wine and grapes. *FASEB J.* 2001 Aug;15(10):1798–1800.
39. Gacche RN, Shegokar HD, Gond DS, Yang Z, Jadhav AD. Evaluation of selected flavonoids as antiangiogenic, anticancer, and radical scavenging agents: an experimental and in silico analysis. *Cell Biochem Biophys.* 2011 Dec;61(3):651–663.
40. Kadioglu O, Seo EJ, Efferth T. Targeting angiogenesis by phytochemicals. *Med Aromat Plants.* 2013;2(5):1000134.
41. Pili R, Chang J, Partis RA, Mueller RA, Chrest FJ, Passaniti A. The α-glucosidase I inhibitor castanospermine alters endothelial cell glycosylation, prevents angiogenesis, and inhibits tumor growth. *Cancer Res.* 1995 Jul 1;55(13):2920–2926.
42. Llovet JM, Zucman-Rossi J, Pikarsky E, Sangro B, Schwartz M, Sherman M, et al. Hepatocellular carcinoma. *Nat Rev Dis Primers.* 2016 Apr 14;2(1):16018.
43. Ribatti D, Nico B, Mangieri D, Longo V, Sansonno D, Vacca A, et al. In vivo inhibition of human hepatocellular carcinoma related angiogenesis by vinblastine and rapamycin. *Histol Histopathol.* 2007 Mar;22(3):285–289.

44. Nurcahyanti ADR, Wink M. Cytotoxic potentiation of vinblastine and paclitaxel by L-canavanine in human cervical cancer and hepatocellular carcinoma cells. *Phytomedicine.* 2015 Dec;22(14):1232–1237.
45. Saraswati S, Agrawal SS. Brucine, an indole alkaloid from Strychnos nux-vomica attenuates VEGF-induced angiogenesis via inhibiting VEGFR2 signaling pathway *in vitro* and *in vivo. Cancer Lett.* 2013 May;332(1):83–93.
46. Stafford SJ, Schwimer J, Anthony CT, Thomson JL, Wang YZ, Woltering EA. Colchicine and 2-methoxyestradiol inhibit human angiogenesis. *J Surg Res.* 2005 May;125(1):104–108.
47. Baby J, Devan AR, Kumar AR, Gorantla JN, Nair B, Aishwarya TS, et al. Cogent role of flavonoids as key orchestrators of chemoprevention of hepatocellular carcinoma: a review. *J Food Biochem.* 2021 Jul;45(7):e13761.
48. Haiaty S, Rashidi M, Akbarzadeh M, Maroufi NF, Yousefi B, Nouri M. Targeting vasculogenic mimicry by phytochemicals: a potential opportunity for cancer therapy. *IUBMB Life.* 2020 May;72(5):825–841.
49. Edward M, Gold JA, Mackie RM. Retinoic acid-induced inhibition of metastatic melanoma cell lung colonization and adhesion to endothelium and subendothelial extracellular matrix. *Clin Exp Metast.* 1992; 10:61–67.

https://doi.org/10.1142/9789811293320_0009

Chapter 9

Cucurbitacin B: A Potential Therapeutic Agent Against Liver Cancer

A Amrutha Nisthul[1], US Aiswarya[2], MA Faisal[1] and VB Smitha[1,*]

[1]*Department of Biotechnology, University of Calicut, Thenhipalam, Kerala, India*
[2]*Rajiv Gandhi Centre for Biotechnology, Poojappura, Thiruvananthapuram, Kerala, India*

Table of Contents:

Abbreviations:

AD — Alzheimer's disease
Akt — Protein kinase B

*Corresponding author: Tel.: E-mail address: smithanishad@gmail.com

ALP — Alkaline phosphatase
APP — Amyloid precursor protein
ARE — Antioxidant response element
Bcl-xL — B-cell lymphoma-extra large
BL — Bilirubin
BTLA — B and T lymphocyte attenuator
CCL4 — Carbon tetrachloride
CDKN1A — Cyclin-dependent kinase inhibitor 1A
CDKN2A — Cyclin-dependent kinase inhibitor 2A
Chk — Checkpoint kinase
CIP2A — Cancerous inhibitor of PP2A
c-MET — c-Mesenchymal-epithelial transition factor
c-Myc — Cellular Myc
CTLA-4 — Cytotoxic T-lymphocyte-associated protein 4
CuB — Cucurbitacin B
DCLK1 — Doublecortin-like kinase 1
DNA — Deoxyribonucleic acid
EGF — Epidermal growth factor
EGFR — Epidermal growth factor receptor
ERK — Extracellular signal-regulated kinase
FDA — Food and Drug Administration
FoxO3a — Forkhead box protein O3A
Gal-SLNs — Galactosylated solid-lipid nanoparticle
GOT — Glutamate oxaloacetate transaminase
GPT — Glutamate pyruvate transaminase
GR — Glucocorticoid receptor
GR-NSCLC — Gefitinib-resistant non-small cell lung cancer
GSH — Reduced glutathione
GSSG — Oxidized glutathione
H1299 — Human non-small cell lung carcinoma
HBV — Hepatitis B virus
HCC — Hepatocellular carcinoma
HCV — Hepatitis C virus
HDAC — Histone deacetylase

Hes-1 — Hairy and enhancer of split 1
HGF — Hepatocyte growth factor
HIF-1 — Hypoxia-inducible factor-1
ICI — Immune checkpoint inhibitor
IGF — Insulin-like growth factor
IGF1R — Insulin-like growth factor 1 receptor
IGFBPrP1 — Anti-insulin-like growth factor binding protein-related protein
IL-17 — Interleukin-17
IL-23 — Interleukin-23
JAK — Janus kinase 2
JNK — c-Jun N-terminal kinase
K-RAS — Kirsten rat sarcoma viral oncogene homolog
LAG3 — Lymphocyte activation gene 3
LGR5 — Leucine-rich repeat-containing G-protein coupled receptor 5
MAPK/MEK1/2 — Mitogen-activated protein kinase 1/2
MMP-9 — Matrix metalloproteinase 9
mTOR — Mammalian target of rapamycin
NASH — Nonalcoholic steatohepatitis
NF-κB — Nuclear factor kappa B
NLRP3 — NOD-, LRR- and pyrin domain-containing protein 3
Nrf2 — Nuclear factor erythroid 2-related factor 2
NSLC — Non-small cell lung cancer
PD-1 — Programmed death-1
PI3K — Phosphoinositide 3-kinase
PKC — Protein kinase C
PLC — Phospholipase C
PP2A — Protein phosphatase 2A
PS1 — Human presenilin 1
RAF — Rapidly accelerated fibrosarcoma
RAS — Rat sarcoma virus
RB — Retinoblastoma
ROS — Reactive oxygen species

SGOT — Serum glutamate oxaloacetate transaminase
SGPT — Serum glutamate pyruvate transaminase
SIRT1 — Sirtuin 1
SOCS — Suppressor of cytokine signaling
STAT3 — Signal transducer and activator of transcription 3
SREBP — Sterol regulatory element-binding protein
TACE — Transcatheter arterial chemoembolization
TGFβ1 — Transforming growth factor beta 1
TIGIT — T-cell immunoreceptor with Ig and ITIM domains
TIM3 — T-cell immunoglobulin and mucin domain 3
TP53 — Tumor protein p53
TrkA — Tropomyosin receptor kinase A
VEGF — Vascular endothelial growth factor
γGT — γ-glutamyl transpeptidase

Abstract

Liver cancer is the third-leading cause of cancer death worldwide. Despite therapeutic interventions against liver cancer, survival rates are poor, and there is an urgent need to identify effective therapeutic regimens. Cucurbitacin B (CuB) is a triterpenoid widely distributed in a variety of plants, mainly isolated from plants in the Cucurbitaceae family. CuB has been found to have potent anticancer potential against cancers of different tissue origins. In this chapter, we discuss its characteristic anticancer potential against liver cancer.

Numerous preclinical studies have demonstrated the ability of CuB to inhibit the growth and proliferation of liver cancer cells both *in vitro* and *in vivo*. Mechanistically, CuB modulates multiple signaling pathways implicated in cell survival, apoptosis, and metastasis, such as MAPK, JAK/STAT, and PI3K/Akt/mTOR pathways. By targeting these pathways, CuB effectively inhibits tumor cell proliferation and induces apoptosis in liver cancer cells. Additionally, CuB has demonstrated the ability to inhibit angiogenesis, a crucial process for tumor growth and metastasis, through downregulation of vascular endothelial growth factor (VEGF) and other angiogenic factors. Furthermore, it possesses the potential to enhance the efficacy of existing anticancer drugs and sensitize liver cancer cells to chemotherapy when used in combination. Moreover, the hepatoprotective effect of CuB is also well documented.

In conclusion, CuB holds substantial promise as a potent therapeutic agent against liver cancer due to its multifaceted anticancer properties and favorable safety profile, and it is worth further clinical investigations to elucidate its therapeutic efficacy in patients.

1. Introduction

Liver cancer is one of the most lethal malignancies worldwide. It ranks third in cancer-related mortality, following lung cancer and colorectal cancer (GLOBOCAN 2020). It is more prevalent in sub-Saharan Africa and Southeast Asia than in Western countries [1]. Primary liver cancer originates in different types of cells in the liver. Hepatocellular carcinoma (HCC), derived from the major cell type in the liver, epithelial hepatocyte, is the most common type of primary liver cancer, accounting for approximately 90% of liver cancer cases [2]. Other types of liver cancers, such as intrahepatic cholangiocarcinoma (which starts in the bile ducts within the liver) and hepatoblastoma (a malignant liver cancer that primarily affects children), are much less common [3].

The major risk factor for HCC is chronic liver inflammation and liver cirrhosis, caused by infection with hepatitis viruses HBV and HCV, by chronic alcohol abuse, and rarely by hereditary diseases such as hemochromatosis. Exposure to aflatoxin-contaminated food and smoking exacerbate the situation. However, nonalcoholic steatohepatitis (NASH) associated with metabolic syndrome or diabetes mellitus has recently emerged as a major risk factor for liver cancer [4, 5].

The genetic alterations in HCC lead to disruption of the TP53 network, inactivation of cell cycle regulation by RB and constitutive activation of the Wnt and STAT signaling pathways [6, 7]. In addition, autocrine or paracrine signaling of growth factors and their receptors, such as HGF/c-MET and insulin-like factor IGF/IGF1R, are also implicated in the growth and survival of hepatocellular carcinoma by promoting proliferation and decreasing apoptotic cell death via MAPK and Akt signaling [8, 9].

Current treatment modalities for liver cancer encompass a range of approaches, including surgery, ablation therapy, chemotherapy, targeted therapy, radiation therapy, immunotherapy, and embolization therapy. Partial hepatectomy (surgery to remove part of the liver) and liver transplant are the major surgical procedures used to treat liver cancer [5]. However, these are applicable only to those who are in the early stages of liver cancer [10]. Ablation therapy is a technique used to remove small tumors, by employing very high or very low temperatures. Radiofrequency ablation and microwave ablation are done using a probe that generates heat and ablates the tumor. Cryoablation destroys the tumor by freezing it with a metal probe, and ethanol ablation uses concentrated percutaneous ethanol injection to damage the cancer cells. The major drawback of ablation therapy is that it can only be used for small tumors (no larger than 5 cm across), and it is not recommended for treating tumors near major blood vessels and bile ducts [11].

Embolization is another method used to treat liver cancer patients who cannot receive the curative therapies mentioned above. The process involves blocking artery in the liver by directly injecting substances to obstruct the blood supply to the tumor site. Among the two sources of blood supply to the liver, the portal vein and the hepatic artery [12, 13], it is the hepatic artery that supplies blood to the cancer cells [14]. This differential blood supply is exploited in intra-arterial therapies, where anticancer therapies can be specifically delivered to cancer cells without affecting normal hepatocytes [15]. Chemoembolization and radioembolization are the major types of trans-arterial approaches utilized in HCC. In chemoembolization, chemotherapeutic agents are injected into the feeding arteries of the tumor and are further combined with substances to block the arteries, reducing the blood supply to the tumor site. In radioembolization, a radioisotope such as Yttrium-90 (90Y) is delivered in microspheres into the blood vessels near the tumor site, where it emits small amounts of radiation to the tumor [16, 17].

The systemic therapies for HCC include sorafenib or lenvatinib in the first line and regorafenib, cabozantinib or ramucirumab in the second line, all of which fall under the molecular targeted therapy [18]. Unfortunately, cancer cells can develop resistance to systemic therapies [19] which necessitates the development of alternative therapy options for treating HCC. Advances in understanding the tumor microenvironment have led to the development of immunotherapy. Cancer cells escape detection and elimination by immune cells by regulating modulators of immune responses called immune checkpoints. The most studied immune receptors are PD-1, CTLA-4, LAG3, TIM3, TIGIT, and BTLA [20, 21]. Several immune checkpoint inhibitors (ICI) that target CTLA-4, PD-1, and its ligand PD-L1 have been tested to date. A combination of PD-1 inhibitor nivolumab and CTLA-4 inhibitor ipilimumab was approved by the FDA for patients with HCC who had been previously treated with sorafenib [22]. In recent years, a combination of ICI with molecular targeted therapy or locoregional treatments such as chemoembolization and radiofrequency ablation has emerged as a promising strategy for managing HCC [23–26].

2. Cucurbitacins: An Overview

Most of the chemotherapeutic drugs used for the treatment of HCC invoke chemoresistance and induce serious side effects [27]. In this context, compounds derived from nature, which in fact represent 60% of anticancer drugs used in clinics, are ideal candidates worth exploring for chemotherapeutic efficacy against liver cancer [28]. Curcumin, the principal polyphenolic curcuminoid obtained from the turmeric rhizome (*Curcuma longa*), has demonstrated effectiveness against HCC in both *in vitro* and *in vivo* models of hepatocarcinogenesis [29]. Additionally, resveratrol, a polyphenolic stilbenoid found in several plants, has exhibited chemopreventive and chemotherapeutic activities against liver cancer both *in vitro* and *in vivo* [30]. The chemopreventive and therapeutic effects of tea polyphenols against HCC have also been extensively researched [31]. Notably, the FDA has

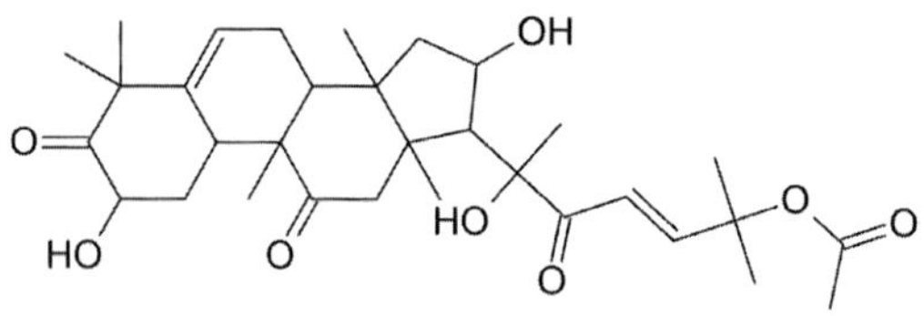

Figure 1: Chemical structure of cucurbitacin B

granted orphan drug designation to uttroside B, a saponin from *Solanum nigrum* Linn, for the treatment of HCC. The compound has shown activity 10 times greater than the standard drug sorafenib [32]. These developments create opportunities to identify new natural compounds for the efficient management of HCC.

Cucurbitacins are a group of highly oxidized tetracyclic triterpenoids, originally identified as the bitter principles of the Cucurbitaceae family [33] and later found to be present in plants of other families such as Begoniaceae, Cruciferae, Desfontainiaceae, Elaeocarpaceae, and Rubiaceae [34, 35]. They are derivatives of 19-(10→9-β)-abeo-5 alpha-lanostane with various oxygen substitutions at different positions and are classified into 12 main categories: cucurbitacins A to T [36, 37]. Cucurbitacin B ($C_{32}H_{46}O_8$), having a molecular weight of 558.702, is the most explored one for its effect in biological systems (Figure 1).

3. Cucurbitacin B: A Spectrum of Biological Actions

Cucurbitacin B (CuB) is reported to exhibit a repertoire of biological activities, including anti-inflammatory, neuroprotective, hepatoprotective, hypoglycemic, and anticancer effects, by regulating multiple signaling pathways [38]. Several studies have demonstrated the significant anti-inflammatory activity of CuB, attributed to the regulation of cytokines, chemokines, and multiple transcription factors (NF-κB, STAT3, and Nrf2) involved in inflammation, showcasing its potential for the prevention and treatment of a variety of inflammatory diseases [38]. It has been reported to inhibit the NLRP3 inflammasome and suppress gout arthritis in mice [39]. Another study by

Chu et al. demonstrated that CuB attenuates cerebral ischemia/reperfusion injury by inhibiting NLRP3 inflammasome-mediated inflammation and reducing oxidative stress [40]. A recent study by Reiszadeh-Jahromi demonstrated that CuB has prophylactic effect only for those with neuroinflammatory diseases like multiple sclerosis, via reduction in STAT3 activation, microgliosis, and regulation of the IL-23/IL-17 axis [41]. The neuroprotective effects of CuB can be attributed to its ability to modulate STAT/NF-κB anti-inflammatory signaling, Nrf2/ARE antioxidant signaling and also by targeting neuroreceptors and regulating neurotransmitter levels [38]. A recent study has shown the ability of CuB to induce neurogenesis and provide protection against memory impairment in APP/PS1 mice, by modulating the GR/PLC/PKC and TrkA/Ras/Raf/ERK signaling pathways [42]. Yet another study has demonstrated the neuroprotective effect of CuB in a murine Alzheimer's disease (AD) model. CuB protected neurons against intracerebroventricular streptozotocin neurotoxicity and decreased AD symptoms by modulating oxidative stress, inflammation, and neurotransmitter levels [43].

The hepatoprotective activity of CuB is well recognized, particularly in alleviating liver fibrosis. In 1999, the first study demonstrating the ability of CuB to prevent and treat hepatotoxicity induced by carbon tetrachloride (CCl4) was reported [44]. Since then, several studies have shown the ability of CuB to protect the liver from toxicity. The study by Mukerjee et al. [45] examined the hepatoprotective activity of the toluene fraction of *Citrullus colocynthis* root extract, the primary compound of which was CuB. The fraction reduced serum glutamate pyruvate transaminase (SGPT), serum glutamate oxaloacetate transaminase (SGOT), alkaline phosphatase (ALP), and total bilirubin (BL) in a rat model with CCl4-induced hepatotoxicity. Naggar et al. [46] substantiated this by showing that CuB treatment significantly reduced liver lesions in a rat model of CCl4-induced hepatotoxicity. Sallam et al. [47] further confirmed that CuB (at doses of 1 and 5 mg/kg) inhibits CCl4-induced liver fibrosis in mice. This inhibition was evident through reduced levels of hydroxyproline in liver tissues, decreased expression of collagen-1α, α-smooth muscle actin, and transforming growth factor β (TGF-β). Importantly, Signal

Transducer and Activator of Transcription 3 (STAT3) activity was inhibited upon CuB treatment. Similarly, Yang et al. [48] provided evidence that CuB (at doses of 1, 2, and 4 mg/kg) significantly attenuated the release of pro-inflammatory cytokines induced by concanavalin A in mice, thereby alleviating liver fibrosis. Its mechanism of action was primarily attributed to the inhibition of the sirtuin 1 (SIRT1)/anti-insulin-like growth factor binding protein-related protein (IGFBPrP1)/transforming growth factor beta 1 (TGFβ1) axis.

Moreover, Xiao et al. have demonstrated that CuB protects against cardiac hypertrophy by increasing autophagy level in cardiomyocytes via inhibition of Akt/mTOR/FoxO3a signal axis [49]. Furthermore, CuB has been reported to exhibit the ability to suppress hyperglycemia associated with a high-sugar diet and promote sleep pattern in *Drosophila melanogaster* [50]. CuB also induces browning of white adipocytes by inhibiting phospholipase D2, with the possibility of being a potential lead for new drugs to prevent obesity by promoting energy expenditure in adipocytes [51].

CuB has shown promising anticancer activity against malignancies of different tissue origins [52]. The antitumor activity of CuB is mainly achieved by inhibiting cell proliferation, inducing cell cycle arrest, autophagy, and/or cell apoptosis, and modulating cytoskeletal dynamics [38]. It has been reported to inhibit the progression of gastric cancer by suppressing STAT3, thereby reducing the expression of STAT3 target genes like c-Myc and Bcl-xL [53]. Alafnan et al. have demonstrated the ability of CuB to suppress the growth of prostate cancer cells by generating ROS and reducing the expression of key components in Notch signaling [54]. Additionally, Liu et al. [55] demonstrated that CuB suppresses the growth and invasion of gefitinib-resistant non-small cell lung cancer (GR-NSCLC) cells by inducing the lysosomal degradation of EGFR and downregulating the CIP2A/PP2A/Akt signaling axis. The therapeutic potential of CuB against non-small-cell lung cancer growth has been investigated both *in vitro* using NSCLC cell lines and *in vivo* in an H1299 tumor xenograft nude mouse model. Interestingly, CuB disrupted cellular redox status by depleting cellular GSH and protein thiol levels, as well as cellular GSH/GSSG ratios, through direct interaction with GSH [56].

Further, Tao et al. [57] demonstrated the significant antitumor activity of CuB against tongue squamous cell carcinoma cells by regulating the expression of the X-inactive specific transcript and microRNA 29b, which regulates the p53 protein. CuB has also been reported to inhibit DNA methyltransferase (DNMT) and histone deacetylase (HDAC) in H1299 cells, which might result in epigenetic modifications that lead to reactivation of key tumor suppressor genes such as CDKN1A and CDKN2A, as well as downregulation of oncogenes c-MYC and K-RAS along with the key tumor promoter gene, human telomerase reverse transcriptase. Remarkably, CuB significantly inhibited the tumor incidence and multiplicity in 4-(methylnitrosamino)-1-(3-pyridyl)-1-butanone (NNK)-induced lung tumorigenesis in A/J mice [58]. An *in vivo* study from our laboratory has provided evidence for the potent antimelanoma activity of CuB. The compound induced apoptotic mode of cell death in melanoma cells and effectively inhibited proliferative signals via inhibition of MEK1/2 and ERK 1/2 activation, demonstrating the role of CuB in regulating the MAPK proliferative signaling pathway [59]. In addition, CuB effectively inhibited the growth of colon cancer cells, both *in vitro* and *in vivo*. It achieved this inhibition by modulating the Notch signaling pathway, leading to a reduction in the expression of Notch 1–4 receptors, their ligands, and the downstream target Hes-1. Moreover, CuB significantly decreased the expression of cancer stem cell markers such as CD44, DCLK1, and LGR5 in the colon cancer cells, which was substantiated by a notable reduction in tumor xenograft growth in nude mice [60]. To summarize, this section highlights the multifaceted capability of CuB to modulate various biological activities and its prospects for therapeutic applications.

4. Anticancer Mechanism of Cucurbitacin B in Liver Cancer Cells

Many studies have explored the chemotherapeutic activity of CuB in the management of liver cancer, both *in vitro* and *in vivo*, which implicates the clinical utility of CuB in a clinical setting. Notably, Zhang et al. [61] identified that CuB induces S phase arrest followed by apoptotic cell death of HepG2 cells by inhibiting STAT3 activation and antiapoptotic B-cell lymphoma-2 (Bcl-2) expression. The therapeutic efficacy of the synergistic combination involving CuB and sorafenib, the first-line agent for the treatment of advanced hepatocellular carcinoma, was demonstrated by Wang et al. in a HepG2 xenograft mouse model [62], where the combination inhibited epidermal growth factor (EGF)-induced STAT3 activation. CuB was also found to sensitize CD133+ HepG2 cancer stem cells to sorafenib *in vitro* and *in vivo* by inhibiting the Janus kinase 2/signal transducers and activators of transcription-3 (JAK/STAT) signaling pathway, which leads to induction of cell cycle arrest at G2/M phase [63].

Overactivity of the STAT pathway is a common occurrence in HCC, often resulting from the hypermethylation of the SOCS1 promoter and the loss of heterozygosity (LOH) at 16p13, leading to the absence of the SOCS1 protein [64]. The JAK-STAT pathway, which plays a crucial role in transmitting growth and survival signals from cytokines, is inhibited in a feedback loop by SOCS1 [65]. In the absence of SOCS1, signals through the STAT pathway can become prolonged and more strongly promote resistance to apoptosis. The ability of CuB to inhibit JAK-STAT3 signaling has been proven beyond doubt [66]. Interestingly, computational docking analysis has illustrated that CuB interacts with the DNA-binding domain of STAT3 at several hydrophobic residues. Importantly, pull-down experiments have confirmed CuB as a direct inhibitor of STAT3 activity [53], further solidifying its potential as a promising therapeutic agent for managing HCC.

Zhou et al. [67] have shown that CuB effectively inhibits 12-O-tetradecanoylphorbol 13-acetate-induced migration and invasion of hepatoma cells through suppression of ERK1/2, p38, and Akt phosphorylation, and downregulation of MMP-9 expression. The efficacy of CuB against hepatocellular carcinoma can also be attributed to ROS-mediated DNA damage, apoptosis, and protective autophagy, as has been demonstrated in BEL-7402 cells. CuB increased γ-H2AX expression and phosphorylation of ATM/ATR and Chk1/Chk2 kinases, suggestive of DNA damage. CuB increased p-PTEN expression, which was inhibited by DNA damage inhibitors and N-acetyl-L-cysteine suggesting that activation of PTEN was mediated by DNA damage following ROS generation by CuB [68]. Moreover, Dat et al. [69] have shown that CuB inhibits hypoxia-inducible factor-1 (HIF-1) activation in Hep3B cells. HIF-1 is a heterodimeric DNA-binding protein that regulates the expression of several hypoxia-inducible target genes, such as VEGF, that promotes angiogenesis [70].

Interestingly, a recent study by Ji et al. [71] using AKT/c-Met-induced hepatocellular carcinogenesis in a genetically engineered mouse model has analyzed the therapeutic effect of CuB using metabolomics techniques. The results revealed that CuB substantially reduced the expression levels of activated Akt and phosphorylated mTOR in the liver lesions. Furthermore, CuB therapy resulted in a decrease in the protein expression of the *de novo* lipogenesis regulator SREBP1, downstream of the Akt/mTORC1 cascade, and effector lipogenic enzymes such as fatty acid synthase and acetyl CoA carboxylase. CuB administration also downregulated the critical proteins of glycolysis, such as hexokinase (HK) and pyruvate kinase M2, which were upregulated in AKT/c-Met group. The study provided evidence for CuB's ability to hinder tumor progression by regulating Akt-induced lipid, amino acid, and glucose metabolism in AKT-c-MET-induced HCC mouse models.

The efficacy of other cucurbitacins against hepatocellular carcinoma cells has also been reported. Cucurbitacins I and D have been found to modulate the JAK/STAT3, MAPK/ERK, and Akt/mTOR signaling pathways and induce cell cycle arrest and apoptosis in HepG2 cells [72, 73]. Furthermore, Liu et al. [74] demonstrated that CuE inhibited the proliferation, migration, and angiogenesis of Huh7 hepatoma cells by increasing JNK activation and suppressing ERK and p38 activation. CuE also significantly suppressed JAK2 and STAT3 phosphorylations, as well as STAT3 nuclear translocation, in Huh7 cells. CuE also exhibited synergism with sorafenib in inducing apoptosis in HCC cells by modulating JAK/STAT3, ERK/MAPK, and PI3K/Akt/mTOR signaling pathways [75].

In the 1970s and 1980s, China pioneered the development of cucurbitacin tablets, primarily consisting of cucurbitacins B and E, for adjuvant therapy in cases of chronic hepatitis and liver cancer. Clinical trials involving CuB tablets conducted in 13 Chinese hospitals revealed their effectiveness in alleviating common symptoms of chronic hepatitis and reducing SGPT and bilirubin levels while avoiding toxic side effects [38]. Furthermore, a study on transcatheter arterial chemoembolization (TACE) using cucurbitacin tablets in combination with thalidomide for the treatment of elderly patients with unresectable liver cancer demonstrated a short-term effectiveness rate of 89.4%. This approach also improved overall survival to 21.5 ± 2.8 months and progression-free survival to 17.4 ± 1.6 months, both of which were significantly higher than those in the control group [38].

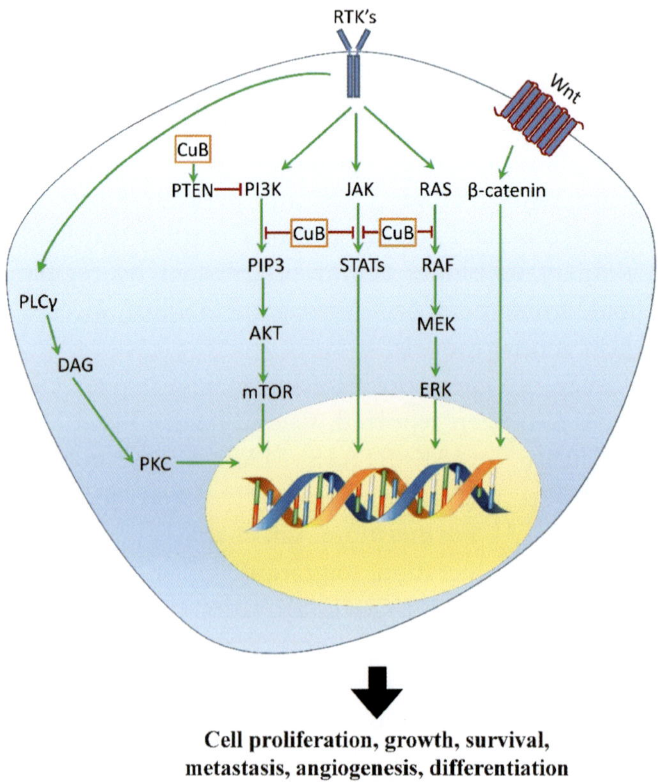

Figure 2: Molecular overview of oncogenic signaling pathways in HCC and molecules regulated by Cucurbitacin B, based on available data

5. Challenges in Clinical Applicability of Cucurbitacin B

The assessment of pharmacological properties related to the absorption, distribution, metabolism, and excretion (ADME) of a candidate drug is crucial for predicting its clinical effectiveness. While CuB has demonstrated potent anticancer properties against various cancer types, its bioavailability is relatively low. Hunsakunachai and colleagues [76] investigated the absolute oral bioavailability of CuB and reported it as 10% of the administered dose (2–4 mg/kg) in male Wistar rats. However, alternative strategies are being explored to increase the bioavailability of CuB, which in turn increases its therapeutic efficacy against cancer [77–80].

One such interesting study investigated the liver targetability of CuB using galactosylated solid-lipid nanoparticles (Gal-SLNs) as a drug delivery carrier. Hepatocytes possess asialoglycoprotein receptors that can recognize terminal β-D-galactose residues, and conjugating drug carriers with galactosylated residues can enhance liver targeting efficiency [81]. The encapsulation of CuB in Gal-SLNs significantly improved its cytotoxic activity in HepG2 cells compared to CuB solution. Furthermore, the tissue distribution experiments in mice (2 mg/kg) revealed that the liver targetability of CuB-Gal-SLNs was almost 2.5 times greater than that of CuB solution [82]. These findings highlight the potential of appropriate drug delivery systems to enhance CuB's bioavailability and tissue distribution for therapeutic applications.

Several studies have consistently indicated that CuB exhibits moderate cytotoxicity toward normal cells. Interestingly, an increasing body of recent research has highlighted that at lower doses, CuB appears to have minimal toxicity in normal cells and experimental animals [38]. In a study by Iwanski et al. [83], intraperitoneal administration of CuB at a lower dose (0.5 mg/kg) as well as a higher dose (1 mg/kg), three times per week for a period of 43 days, in a murine Panc-1 xenograft model, did not result in any significant weight loss in treated animals. Histopathological examinations revealed the absence of treatment-related toxicities such as liver fibrosis, expansion of red pulp, renal tubular damage, or glomerular congestion. Additionally, serum parameters, including glutamate oxaloacetate transaminase (GOT), glutamate pyruvate transaminase (GPT), γ-glutamyl transpeptidase (γGT), total bilirubin, creatinine, glucose levels (in the unstarved state), and cholesterol, were also in the normal range. However, assessment of bone marrow toxicity by colony-forming unit assay indicated that CuB, at both doses, reduced colony numbers. Interestingly, no significant difference in total blood count was observed for both doses. In a study by Kurman et al. [84], intraperitoneal administration of CuB at 1 mg/kg to the MB49 xenograft C57BL/6 mouse strain, administered three times per week for 3 weeks, did not cause significant weight loss in treated animals. Furthermore, histopathological analysis revealed that CuB showed no observable toxic effects on vital organs, such as the lung, liver, kidney, heart, and bladder.

Collectively, these reports show CuB may not pose significant toxicity concerns when administered to experimental cells and animals, provided that the dosage and duration of exposure are kept within reasonable limits. Table 1 presents the median lethal dose (LD50) of CuB in its pure form across various species. However, it is essential to note that there is a current lack of comprehensive and systematic toxicological investigations regarding CuB. Consequently, further in-depth research is warranted to delve into its toxicity and underlying mechanisms in the future.

Nonetheless, it has been demonstrated that CuB derivatives synthesized by Ge et al. [85] possess lower toxicity. Ge and colleagues found that the introduction of a phenylsulfonyl-substituted furoxan NO-releasing moiety to CuB (derivative 10b) could reduce toxicity against normal cells while maintaining anti-HCC activity.

Table 1: LD50 (mg/kg body weight) of cucurbitacin B in various species

Animal	LD50 (mg/kg)	Route of Administration	References
Mouse	1	intraperitoneal	[86]
	5	Oral	[87]
Cat	0.32	intravenous	[88]
Rabbit	0.5	intravenous	[89]

6. Conclusion

According to Cancer Global Statistics, liver cancer is ranked sixth in incidence and third in mortality worldwide. The use of phytomedicine in cancer management has gained significant attention in the past few decades. CuB, the most abundant and active member of cucurbitacins, has demonstrated potent activity against HCC. Various signaling pathways, including PI3K/Akt/mTOR, JAK/STAT, Wnt/β-catenin, and Ras/Raf/MAPK, play critical roles in HCC development and progression. Preclinical studies have shown that CuB effectively regulates these pathways, controlling cell proliferation, differentiation, apoptosis, invasion, and metastasis in HCC.

However, CuB has limitations as a chemotherapeutic agent, such as low bioavailability and moderate toxicity. TACE, the only globally recommended standard of care for intermediate-stage HCC, is used for patients who are not eligible for curative therapies like surgery or transplantation. This treatment strategy is designed to concentrate the effects of chemotherapeutic drugs on the tumor. In addition, the hypoxic stress due to reduced blood flow also contributes to tumor cell death. Administering CuB via chemoembolization can potentially overcome its limitations by enhancing drug delivery to the tumor, while minimizing toxicity to other normal tissues of the body. However, further studies in the clinical setting are needed to explore this promising approach. In conclusion, CuB, which targets major oncogenic signaling pathways in HCC, holds promise as a chemotherapeutic agent against this challenging cancer.

Conflict of Interest

The authors declare no conflict of interest.

References

1. Forner, A., M. Reig, and J. Bruix, Hepatocellular carcinoma. *Lancet*, 2018. **391**(10127): p. 1301–1314.
2. Chakraborty, E. and D. Sarkar, Emerging therapies for hepatocellular carcinoma (HCC). *Cancers (Basel)*, 2022. **14**(11).

3. Srivatanakul, P., H. Sriplung, and S. Deerasamee, Epidemiology of liver cancer: An overview. *Asian Pac J Cancer Prev*, 2004. **5**(2): p. 118–125.
4. Suresh, D., A.N. Srinivas, and D.P. Kumar, Etiology of hepatocellular carcinoma: Special focus on fatty liver disease. *Front Oncol*, 2020. **10**: p. 601710.
5. Llovet, J.M., et al., Hepatocellular carcinoma. *Nat Rev Dis Primers*, 2021. **7**(1): p. 6.
6. Midorikawa, Y., et al., Accumulation of molecular aberrations distinctive to hepatocellular carcinoma progression. *Cancer Res*, 2020. **80**(18): p. 3810–3819.
7. Kan, Z., et al., Whole-genome sequencing identifies recurrent mutations in hepatocellular carcinoma. *Genome Res*, 2013. **23**(9): p. 1422–1433.
8. Wang, H., et al., The function of the HGF/c-Met axis in hepatocellular carcinoma. *Front Cell Dev Biol*, 2020. **8**: p. 55.
9. Ngo, M.T., et al., The role of IGF/IGF-1R signaling in hepatocellular carcinomas: Stemness-related properties and drug resistance. *Int J Mol Sci*, 2021. **22**(4).
10. Anwanwan, D., et al., Challenges in liver cancer and possible treatment approaches. *Biochim Biophys Acta Rev Cancer*, 2020. **1873**(1): p. 188314.
11. Chu, K.F. and D.E. Dupuy, Thermal ablation of tumours: Biological mechanisms and advances in therapy. *Nat Rev Cancer*, 2014. **14**(3): p. 199–208.
12. Breedis, C. and G. Young, The blood supply of neoplasms in the liver. *Am J Pathol*, 1954. **30**(5): p. 969.
13. Eipel, C., K. Abshagen, and B. Vollmar, Regulation of hepatic blood flow: The hepatic arterial buffer response revisited. *World J Gastroenterol*, 2010. **16**(48): p. 6046.
14. Matsui, O., et al., Benign and malignant nodules in cirrhotic livers: Distinction based on blood supply. *Radiology*, 1991. **178**(2): p. 493–497.
15. Paul, S.B. and H. Sharma, Role of transcatheter intra-arterial therapies for hepatocellular carcinoma. *J Clin Exp Hepatol*, 2014. **4**: p. S112–S121.
16. Bozkurt, M.F., B.V. Salanci, and Ö. Uğur. Intra-arterial radionuclide therapies for liver tumors. in *Seminars in Nuclear Medicine*. 2016. Elsevier.

17. Kim, H.-C., Radioembolization for the treatment of hepatocellular carcinoma. *Clin Mol Hepatol*, 2017. **23**(2): p. 109.
18. Llovet, J.M., et al., Immunotherapies for hepatocellular carcinoma. *Nat Rev Clin Oncol*, 2022. **19**(3): p. 151–172.
19. Tang, W., et al., The mechanisms of sorafenib resistance in hepatocellular carcinoma: Theoretical basis and therapeutic aspects. *Signal Transduct Target Ther*, 2020. **5**(1): p. 87.
20. He, X. and C. Xu, Immune checkpoint signaling and cancer immunotherapy. *Cell Res*, 2020. **30**(8): p. 660–669.
21. Villarruel-Melquiades, F., et al., Current and novel approaches in the pharmacological treatment of hepatocellular carcinoma. *World J Gastroenterol*, 2023. **29**(17): p. 2571–2599.
22. Saung, M.T., et al., FDA approval summary: Nivolumab plus ipilimumab for the treatment of patients with hepatocellular carcinoma previously treated with Sorafenib. *Oncologist*, 2021. **26**(9): p. 797–806.
23. Duffy, A.G., et al., Tremelimumab in combination with ablation in patients with advanced hepatocellular carcinoma. *J Hepatol*, 2017. **66**(3): p. 545–551.
24. Kudo, M., Combination cancer immunotherapy with molecular targeted agents/anti-CTLA-4 antibody for hepatocellular carcinoma. *Liver Cancer*, 2019. **8**(1): p. 1–11.
25. Yoo, C., et al., Regorafenib plus nivolumab as first-line therapy for unresectable hepatocellular carcinoma (uHCC): Multicenter phase 2 trial (RENOBATE). *J Clin Oncol*, 2022. **40**(4_suppl): p. 415–415.
26. Leone, P., et al., The evolving role of immune checkpoint inhibitors in hepatocellular carcinoma treatment. *Vaccines (Basel)*, 2021. **9**(5).
27. Niu, M., et al., Advances of targeted therapy for hepatocellular carcinoma. *Front Oncol*, 2021. **11**: p. 719896.
28. Zheng, Y., et al., Recent progress in understanding the action of natural compounds at novel therapeutic drug targets for the treatment of liver cancer. *Front Oncol*, 2021. **11**: p. 795548.
29. Darvesh, A.S., B.B. Aggarwal, and A. Bishayee, Curcumin and liver cancer: A review. *Curr Pharm Biotechnol*, 2012. **13**(1): p. 218–228.
30. Bishayee, A., T. Politis, and A.S. Darvesh, Resveratrol in the chemoprevention and treatment of hepatocellular carcinoma. *Cancer Treat Rev*, 2010. **36**(1): p. 43–53.

31. Darvesh, A.S. and A. Bishayee, Chemopreventive and therapeutic potential of tea polyphenols in hepatocellular cancer. *Nutr Cancer*, 2013. **65**(3): p. 329–344.
32. Nath, L.R., et al., Evaluation of uttroside B, a saponin from Solanum nigrum Linn, as a promising chemotherapeutic agent against hepatocellular carcinoma. *Sci Rep*, 2016. **6**: p. 36318.
33. Enslin, P.R., Bitter principles of the cucurbitaceae. VI.† — the isolation and characterization of six new crystalline bitter principles. *J Sci Food Agric*, 1957. **8**(12): p. 673–678.
34. Miro, M., Cucurbitacins and their pharmacological effects. *Phytother Res*, 1995. **9**(3): p. 159–168.
35. Kaushik, U., V. Aeri, and S.R. Mir, Cucurbitacins — An insight into medicinal leads from nature. *Pharmacogn Rev*, 2015. **9**(17): p. 12–18.
36. Alghasham, A.A., Cucurbitacins — A promising target for cancer therapy. *Int J Health Sci (Qassim)*, 2013. 7(1): p. 77–89.
37. Chen, J.C., et al., Cucurbitacins and cucurbitane glycosides: Structures and biological activities. *Nat Prod Rep*, 2005. **22**(3): p. 386–399.
38. Dai, S., et al., Cucurbitacin B: A review of its pharmacology, toxicity, and pharmacokinetics. *Pharmacol Res*, 2023. **187**: p. 106587.
39. Xue, Y., et al., NLRP3 inflammasome inhibitor cucurbitacin B suppresses gout arthritis in mice. *J Mol Endocrinol*, 2021. **67**(2): p. 27–40.
40. Chu, X., et al., Cucurbitacin B alleviates cerebral ischemia/reperfusion injury by inhibiting NLRP3 inflammasome-mediated inflammation and reducing oxidative stress. *Biosci Biotechnol Biochem*, 2022. **86**(7): p. 846–854.
41. Reiszadeh-Jahromi, S., et al., Prophylactic effects of cucurbitacin B in the EAE model of multiple sclerosis by adjustment of STAT3/IL-23/IL-17 axis and improvement of neuropsychological symptoms. *Metab Brain Dis*, 2022. **37**(8): p. 2937–2953.
42. Li, J., et al., Cucurbitacin B induces neurogenesis in PC12 cells and protects memory in APP/PS1 mice. *J Cell Mol Med*, 2019. **23**(9): p. 6283–6294.
43. Liu, Z., M. Kumar, and A. Kabra, Cucurbitacin B exerts neuroprotection in a murine Alzheimer's disease model by modulating oxidative stress, inflammation, and neurotransmitter levels. *Front Biosci (Landmark Ed)*, 2022. **27**(2): p. 71.

44. Agil, A., et al., Isolation of ani-hepatotoxic principle form the juice of *Ecballium elaterium*. *Planta Med*, 1999. **65**(7): p. 673–675.
45. Mukerjee, A., Antihepatotoxic potential of *Citrullus colocynthis* root extract, fractions and isolated compounds. *J Exp Sci*, 2012. **3**(9).
46. El Naggar el, M.B., et al., Hepatoprotective and proapoptotic effect of *Ecballium elaterium* on CCl4-induced hepatotoxicity in rats. *Asian Pac J Trop Med*, 2015. **8**(7): p. 526–531.
47. Sallam, A.M., A. Esmat, and A.B. Abdel-Naim, Cucurbitacin-B attenuates CCl(4)-induced hepatic fibrosis in mice through inhibition of STAT-3. *Chem Biol Drug Des*, 2018. **91**(4): p. 933–941.
48. Yang, L., et al., SIRT1/IGFBPrP1/TGF beta1 axis involved in cucurbitacin B ameliorating concanavalin A-induced mice liver fibrosis. *Basic Clin Pharmacol Toxicol*, 2020. **127**(5): p. 371–379.
49. Xiao, Y., et al., Cucurbitacin B protects against pressure overload induced cardiac hypertrophy. *J Cell Biochem*, 2017. **118**(11): p. 3899–3910.
50. Sang, J., S. Dhakal, and Y. Lee, Cucurbitacin B suppresses hyperglycemia associated with a high sugar diet and promotes sleep in drosophila melanogaster. *Mol Cells*, 2021. **44**(2): p. 68–78.
51. Park, S.Y., et al., Cucurbitacin B-, E-, and I-induced browning of white adipocytes is promoted by the inhibition of phospholipase D2. *Int J Mol Sci*, 2022. **23**(23).
52. Tuli, H.S., et al., Cucurbitacins as potent chemo-preventive agents: Mechanistic insight and recent trends. *Biomolecules*, 2022. **13**(1).
53. Xu, J., et al., Cucurbitacin B inhibits gastric cancer progression by suppressing STAT3 activity. *Arch Biochem Biophys*, 2020. **684**: p. 108314.
54. Alafnan, A., et al., Cucurbitacin-B instigates intrinsic apoptosis and modulates notch signaling in androgen-dependent prostate cancer LNCaP cells. *Front Pharmacol*, 2023. **14**: p. 1206981.
55. Liu, P., et al., Cucurbitacin B induces the lysosomal degradation of EGFR and suppresses the CIP2A/PP2A/Akt signaling axis in gefitinib-resistant non-small cell lung cancer. *Molecules*, 2019. **24**(3).
56. Kausar, H., et al., Cucurbitacin B potently suppresses non-small-cell lung cancer growth: Identification of intracellular thiols as critical targets. *Cancer Lett*, 2013. **332**(1): p. 35–45.

57. Tao, B., et al., Cucurbitacin B inhibits cell proliferation by regulating X-inactive specific transcript expression in tongue cancer. *Front Oncol*, 2021. **11**: p. 651648.
58. Shukla, S., et al., Cucurbitacin B alters the expression of tumor-related genes by epigenetic modifications in NSCLC and inhibits NNK-induced lung tumorigenesis. *Cancer Prev Res (Phila)*, 2015. **8**(6): p. 552–562.
59. Aiswarya, S.U.D., et al., Cucurbitacin B, purified and characterized from the rhizome of *Corallocarpus epigaeus* exhibits anti-melanoma potential. *Front Oncol*, 2022. **12**: p. 903832.
60. Dandawate, P., et al., Cucurbitacin B and I inhibits colon cancer growth by targeting the notch signaling pathway. *Sci Rep*, 2020. **10**(1): p. 1290.
61. Zhang, M., et al., Targeted constitutive activation of signal transducer and activator of transcription 3 in human hepatocellular carcinoma cells by cucurbitacin B. *Cancer Chemother Pharmacol*, 2009. **63**(4): p. 635–642.
62. Wang, X., et al., Sorafenib and CuB exert synergistic antitumor effects against hepatocellular carcinoma cells via inhibition of STAT3 phosphorylation. *FEBS Open Bio*, 2021. **11**(1): p. 133–145.
63. Wang, X., et al., Cucurbitacin B exhibits antitumor effects on CD133+ HepG2 liver cancer stem cells by inhibiting JAK2/STAT3 signaling pathway. *Anticancer Drug*, 2021. **32**(5): p. 548–557.
64. Nishida, N., et al., Aberrant methylation of multiple tumor suppressor genes in aging liver, chronic hepatitis, and hepatocellular carcinoma. *Hepatology*, 2008. **47**(3): p. 908–918.
65. Liau, N.P.D., et al., The molecular basis of JAK/STAT inhibition by SOCS1. *Nat Commun*, 2018. **9**(1): p. 1558.
66. Fahmideh, H., et al., The role of natural products as inhibitors of JAK/STAT signaling pathways in glioblastoma treatment. *Oxid Med Cell Longev*, 2022. **2022**: p. 7838583.
67. Zhou, X., et al., Cucurbitacin B inhibits 12-O-tetradecanoylphorbol 13-acetate-induced invasion and migration of human hepatoma cells through inactivating mitogen-activated protein kinase and PI3K/Akt signal transduction pathways. *Hepatol Res*, 2012. **42**(4): p. 401–411.
68. Niu, Y., et al., PTEN activation by DNA damage induces protective autophagy in response to cucurbitacin B in hepatocellular carcinoma cells. *Oxid Med Cell Longev*, 2016. **2016**: p. 4313204.

69. Dat, N.T., et al., An isoaurone and other constituents from *Trichosanthes kirilowii* seeds inhibit hypoxia-inducible factor-1 and nuclear factor-κB. *J Nat Prod*, 2010. **73**(6): p. 1167–1169.
70. Jiang, B.H., et al., Dimerization, DNA binding, and transactivation properties of hypoxia-inducible factor 1. *J Biol Chem*, 1996. **271**(30): p. 17771–17778.
71. Ji, X., et al., Metabolomics profiling of AKT/c-Met-induced hepatocellular carcinogenesis and the inhibitory effect of Cucurbitacin B in mice. *Front Pharmacol*, 2022. **13**: p. 1009767.
72. Uremis, N., et al., Cucurbitacin I exhibits anticancer efficacy through induction of apoptosis and modulation of JAK/STAT3, MAPK/ERK, and AKT/mTOR signaling pathways in HepG2 cell line. *J Food Biochem*, 2022. **46**(10): p. e14333.
73. Mehdi Uremis, M., et al., Cucurbitacin D inhibits the proliferation of HepG2 cells and induces apoptosis by modulating JAK/STAT3, PI3K/Akt/mTOR and MAPK signaling pathways. *Curr Cancer Drug Targets*, 2022. **22**(11): p. 931–944.
74. Liu, Y., et al., Cucurbitacin E inhibits Huh7 hepatoma carcinoma cell proliferation and metastasis via suppressing MAPKs and JAK/STAT3 pathways. *Molecules*, 2020. **25**(3).
75. Uremis, M.M., N. Uremis, and Y. Turkoz, Cucurbitacin E shows synergistic effect with sorafenib by inducing apoptosis in hepatocellular carcinoma cells and regulates Jak/Stat3, ERK/MAPK, PI3K/Akt/mTOR signaling pathways. *Steroids*, 2023. **198**: p. 109261.
76. Hunsakunachai, N., et al., Pharmacokinetics of cucurbitacin B from *Trichosanthes cucumerina* L. in rats. *BMC Complement Altern Med*, 2019. **19**(1): p. 157.
77. Tang, L., et al., Modified mixed nanomicelles with collagen peptides enhanced oral absorption of cucurbitacin B: Preparation and evaluation. *Drug Deliv*, 2018. **25**(1): p. 862--871.
78. Lv, Q.Y., et al., Mucoadhesive buccal films containing phospholipid-bile salts-mixed micelles as an effective carrier for cucurbitacin B delivery. *Drug Deliv*, 2015. **22**(3): p. 351–358.
79. Cheng, L., et al., Improve bile duct-targeted drug delivery and therapeutic efficacy for cholangiocarcinoma by cucurbitacin B loaded phospholipid complex modified with berberine hydrochloride. *Int J Pharm*, 2015. **489**(1–2): p. 148–157.

80. Hu, H., et al., Preparation, characterization, cellular uptake and evaluation *in vivo* of solid lipid nanoparticles loaded with cucurbitacin B. *Drug Dev Ind Pharm*, 2013. **39**(5): p. 770–779.
81. Wu, J., M.H. Nantz, and M.A. Zern, Targeting hepatocytes for drug and gene delivery: Emerging novel approaches and applications. *Front Biosci*, 2002. 7: p. d717–d725.
82. Wang, W., et al., Galactosylated solid lipid nanoparticles with cucurbitacin B improves the liver targetability. *Drug Deliv*, 2010. **17**(3): p. 114–122.
83. Iwanski, G.B., et al., Cucurbitacin B, a novel in vivo potentiator of gemcitabine with low toxicity in the treatment of pancreatic cancer. *Br J Pharmacol*, 2010. **160**(4): p. 998–1007.
84. Kurman, Y., et al., Cucurbitacin B and cisplatin induce the cell death pathways in MB49 mouse bladder cancer model. *Exp Biol Med (Maywood)*, 2020. **245**(9): p. 805–814.
85. Ge, W., et al., Synthesis of cucurbitacin B derivatives as potential anti-hepatocellular carcinoma agents. *Molecules*, 2018. **23**(12).
86. David, A. and D. Vallance, Bitter principles of cucurbitaceae. *J Pharm Pharmacol*, 1955. 7(1): p. 295–296.
87. Le Men, J., et al., Relations entre la structure de quelques cucurbitacines leur toxicite et leuractivite laxative. *Chem Therapeut*, 1969. **6**: p. 459–465.
88. Garg, S., S.C. Kaul, and R. Wadhwa, Cucurbitacin B and cancer intervention: Chemistry, biology and mechanisms (Review). *Int J Oncol*, 2018. **52**(1): p. 19–37.
89. *WHO Monographs on Selected Medicinal Plants-Volume 4*. Vol. 4. 2009. World Health Organization.

https://doi.org/10.1142/9789811293320_0010

Chapter 10

Critical Role of Phytochemicals in Gut-Microbiota-Associated Liver Cancer

Sancharan Acharya and Chinnasamy Thirunavukkarasu*

Department of Biochemistry and Molecular Biology, Pondicherry University, Puducherry, India

Table of Contents:

Abbreviations:

AMPK — AMP-activated protein kinase
BAs — Bile acids

*Corresponding author: Tel.: +91 413 2654972; E-mail address: tchinnasamy@hotmail.com or tarasu.bbm@pondiuni.edu.in

CA — Cholic acid
CDCA — Chenodeoxycholic acid
CVD — Cardiovascular disease
DCA — Deoxycholic acid
FOS — Fructo-oligosaccharides
GABA — Gamma-aminobutyric acid
GI — Gastrointestinal
GMA — Gut-microbiome axis
GPCRs — G protein-coupled receptors
HCC — Hepatocellular carcinoma
HDAC — Histone deacetylase
LCA — Lithocholic acid
LPS — Lipopolysaccharides
MAMPs — Microbe-associated molecular patterns
MASLD — Metabolic dysfunction-associated steatotic liver disease
NADES — Natural deep eutectic solvents
ND — Neurological diseases
SCFAs — Short chain fatty acids
TGF-β — Transforming growth factor-β
TLR4 — toll-like receptor

Abstract

Every element of our body is influenced by the bacteria in our gut. The microbiome, a vast array of micro-organisms found in the human body, affects practically every bodily function. The microbiome is one environmental component that we are exposed to from the very beginning of our lives till the very end, and gene-environment interactions play a significant part in determining our susceptibility to various diseases including cancer. A growing body of research suggests a connection between the microbiome and cancer. The bacteria in our bodies may both raise the risk of carcinogenesis and treatment outcomes while also helping us prevent some malignancies. Changing the microbiome may be a novel strategy to treat and prevent many types of cancer. According to recent research, dietary phytochemicals like carotenoids, phenolics, and dietary fiber can change the human gut flora. The use of phytochemicals has regulatory effects on both pathogenic and non-pathogenic microorganisms. This shows that they may work in concert to reduce the risk of liver cancer and to improve gut health in people. The impact of phytochemicals on the gut microbiota in connection to liver cancer will be discussed in this chapter.

1. Introduction

"Death sits in the bowels"

— Hippocrates, 400 B.C. [1]

The onset of cancer is a long, multi-step process that is influenced by a number of variables. Some of the causes are food, smoking, drinking, and lack of physical activity, while others are outside of a person's direct control and include exposure to carcinogenic pollutants, chronic stress, radiation, and one's own microbiota [2]. Interactions between genes and the environment are important in the development of cancer. The predisposition to developing this fatal disease can be influenced by exposure to specific environmental variables. Our body's internal microbiota is one such environmental factor. Because our bodies contain such a wide diversity of microbes, we are frequently referred to as "superorganisms" [2]. Throughout an individual's life, the microbiota is susceptible to change due to environmental factors, while it generally remains stable in adults. Every aspect of how our bodies work is influenced by the microbiota, and changes to it can cause a number of problems. Father of modern medicine, the ancient Greek physician Hippocrates also talked about the role of gut microbiota in human health back in 400 B.C. Every anatomical compartment in the human body harbors its own population of microorganisms, including the tumor microenvironment. Up until recently, researchers paid little attention to the significance of the microbiota in cancer development. The advent of next-generation sequencing methods has made it extremely simple to research the epigenetic alterations and mutations that take place throughout the growth of cancers. International scientific groups are attempting to determine how microbiota and human health are related.

Plant's primary and secondary metabolisms produce phytochemicals, which are biologically active, non-nutritive plant substances. Dark chocolate, tea, seeds, nuts, whole grain products, legumes, and other natural functional foods all include phytochemicals, which have been linked to a lower risk of developing a number of chronic diseases [3]. There are tens of thousands of different types of phytochemicals, but only a small number of them have been recognized and extracted from plants. By selectively promoting the growth of some bacterial populations in the gut, known as "probiotics," phytochemicals improve the health of both human and animal bodies. These are endosymbionts that are associated with both human and animal gastrointestinal (GI) metabolism, which include Bifidobacterium, bacilli, lactic acid bacteria, and yeast [4]. Based on their metabolic origins, phytochemicals can be divided into several groups, including terpenoids (both carotenoid and non-carotenoid terpenoids), polyphenols, nitrogen-containing compounds, alkaloids, and organosulfur compounds [5]. The greatest group of these phytochemicals is made up of polyphenols. A growing body of research shows that phytochemicals can reduce inflammation, slow cancer cell growth, lower the production of carcinogens, control gene expression and hormone intracellular signaling, boost the immune system, reduce DNA damage, lessen oxidative cell death, and activate insulin receptors [6]. Due to their complicated chemical makeup and xenobiotic metabolism, phytochemicals have a very low bioavailability in comparison to micro- and macronutrients in the human body. Poor phytochemical absorption results in prolonged retention durations in the colon, where they may be useful by affecting the intestinal ecology [7]. Over the last 20 years, the impact of phytochemicals present in the diet on the GI microbial community has been shown, as have the basic mechanisms suggested for their therapeutic outcomes on and GI and extra-intestinal disorders.

2. Gut Microbiome

The human body is home to a vast variety of microorganisms, including bacteria, viruses, eukaryotes, and archaea. The term "human microbiota" refers to the collection of all microbes that are found on or in the human body, including the skin, placenta, lung, saliva, oral mucosa, seminal fluid, mammary glands, uterus, ovarian follicles, conjunctiva, biliary tract, and digestive tract. The collective genome of the microbiota is referred to as the "microbiome" [8]. More than 10^{14} bacteria are estimated to live in the GI tract. The microbiome contributes over one hundred times the amount of genetic material to the genome of humans [9]. According to a study by Sender et al. published in 2016, it is estimated that the overall count of bacteria within the body of an individual is around 3.9×10^{13}, with a cell-to-bacteria ratio of almost 1:1 [10]. The bulk of these microorganisms are digestive tract bacteria. "Gut microbiota" refers to the collection of bacteria, archaea, and eukarya found in the GI tract. Over the course of evolution, the microbiota and the host co-evolved, creating a relationship that is advantageous to both parties. Targeting the bacterial 16S ribosomal RNA (rRNA) gene and other high-throughput, low-cost sequencing methods have recently significantly improved our ability to scan the gut microbiota.

"Gut dysbiosis" is a condition where the host's microbial composition becomes out of balance compared to a healthy person. Inflammatory signaling pathways may be activated as a result, which may have an impact on the immune system as a whole rather than just the gut. Multiple sclerosis, inflammatory bowel disease, type I diabetes, and rheumatoid arthritis are only a few of the autoimmune and inflammatory diseases that have been related to gut microbial dysbiosis [11]. The method that researchers use to investigate the microbiome is metagenomics. Metagenomic research, however, is insufficient to establish whether a particular microbiome variation results in a disease state or is a direct cause of one. Finding out how the microbiota is related to a particular disease requires carefully controlled manipulation of the microbiota. The use of gnotobiotic mice models is therefore crucial for trials in this area of study. If their food is autoclaved and essential nutrients that the microbiota typically generates are delivered, laboratory mice can be bred and kept in specialized gnotobiotic facilities completely germ-free [12]. Even when given a high-fat diet, germ-free mice exhibit metabolic abnormalities, including hypoglycemia, decreased insulin and glycogen levels, and resistance to obesity. In studies, germ-free mice were contrasted with genetically similar controls who had a full but unidentified microbiota. Mice without germs consume more than controls, but they are leaner and contain around 35% less fat [13]. It can be claimed that these studies show that the gut bacteria improve the host's ability to collect calories. Germ-free mice have been used to demonstrate that the microbiota is also essential for controlling the immune system and inflammatory responses [14]. Mice lacking transforming growth factor-β1 exhibit inflammation and colon cancer, which can be avoided by maintaining them in a germ-free environment [15]. Interleukin-10 (IL-10), a potent immunosuppressive cytokine, causes colitis in mice and can be decreased by keeping the animals germ-free [16]. Additionally, given that these are known to be the characteristics of cancer, the functions played by the microbiota in cellular energetics, immunological response, and inflammation are highly important to cancer. As a result, numerous studies are shedding light on how the microbiome may make a host more vulnerable to a range of diseases, including cancer. The bacteria in the gut create bile acids (BAs), short chain fatty acids (SCFAs), and other important metabolites. BAs make up the majority of bile. Deoxycholic acid (DCA) and lithocholic acid (LCA) are the essential components of secondary BAs, while cholic acid (CA) and chenodeoxycholic acid (CDCA) make up the majority of primary BAs [17]. Taurine or glycine can be combined with BAs to produce conjugated-bile acids. Primary BAs are created by several liver enzymes, and then the gallbladder excretes them into the lumen of the intestine. The expression of bile salt hydrolase and 7-dehydroxylase by the gut microbiota significantly improves the generation of secondary BAs [18]. The majority of BAs in the colon initiate enterohepatic circulation upon return via the portal venous system to the liver. BAs can control energy metabolism and aid in lipid uptake. Additionally, via modulating a number of downstream signaling pathways, BAs play a crucial role in immunological regulation. SCFAs produced by the gut microbiota provide various health benefits, including the maintenance of mucosal integrity and reduction of inflammation via G protein-coupled receptors (GPCRs), for example, GPCR43, GPCR109A, and GPCR41 [19, 20]. Besides, SCFAs are carried inside the cells, where they impede the activity of histone deacetylase (HDAC) and cause histone hyperacetylation. HDAC inhibition can boost the making of transforming growth factor-β (TGF-β), colonic regulatory T cells, and IL-10, increasing cancer cell death [21]. Therefore, investigating the metabolites of the gut microbiota may provide vital insights into the etiology and management of a disease.

Human individuals differ greatly in terms of their microbiota at the levels of genus, species, and strain. This happens as a result of environmental factors, such as host genetics, nutrition, lifestyle, and health. A human being's microbiota changes during their lifespan as well as in reaction to their food, usage of chemotherapeutics, antibiotics, stress, and a number of other factors [11]. Human disease susceptibility is mostly caused by gene-environment interactions, while it is now thought that the microbiome plays a significant role as well. According to current knowledge, the majority of gut microorganisms belong to the taxonomic groups Firmicutes, Bacteroidetes, Proteobacteria, Actinobacteria, Verrucomicrobia, Fusobacteria, and Cyanobacteria, with Firmicutes and Bacteroidetes being the most common. Firmicutes and *Cytophaga-Flavobacterium-Bacteroides* account for the vast majority of beneficial bacteria in the gut microbiota of human [22].

3. Association of Gut Microbiome with Liver Cancer

Through the portal vein's vascular pathway, which transports intestinally derived materials to the liver and serves as the feedback loop of the liver for bile and immunoglobulins to the GI tract [23], the liver and microbiota communicate with one another. The gut mucosa and vascular barrier function as sites of contact between the gut and the liver by restricting systemic transmission of bacteria and toxins while permitting nutrients to travel through the circulation and access the liver. The bacteria that live in our digestive tracts are shielded from potential predators and receive a steady supply of nutrients from our diets, both of which are essential for their survival. In exchange, the microbiota supports the host in a number of ways, including energy harvesting [24], controlling host immunity [25], and maintaining the intestinal barrier, which prevents pathogenic organisms from infecting the epithelium [26]. As a source of energy for both the host and themselves, the symbiotic bacteria degrade glycans to create disaccharides and monosaccharides. As a result, our ability to absorb nutrients from our foods and derive the maximum energy from them is improved by our symbiotic association with these microorganisms.

Scientists showed that cirrhosis to early hepatocellular carcinoma (HCC) with cirrhosis led to an increase in fecal microbial diversity. Compared to cirrhosis, Actinobacteria were more common in early HCC. In contrast, 13 taxa, including Parabacteroides and Gemmiger, were more abundant in early HCC. Butyrate-producing genera were downregulated in early HCC relative to controls, but lipopolysaccharides (LPS)-producing genera were increased. LPS is a component of gram-negative bacteria's cell walls that activates toll-like receptor (TLR4) to cause inflammation. When intestinal permeability is increased, translocation of bacteria and LPS buildup result in overgrowth of bacteria in the intestine and alterations in the composition of gut microbiota. Additionally, a leaky gut makes it simpler for microbe-associated molecular patterns (MAMPs) and bacterial metabolites associated with dysbiotic microbiotas to translocate and reach the liver. In individuals having chronic liver disorders or cirrhosis, the degradation, detoxification, and clearance of LPS and other microbial metabolites are all impaired. The optimal 30 microbiological markers have been identified on a random forest model by fivefold cross-validation, and they yielded an area under the curve of 80.64% between 105 non-HCC and 75 early HCC samples. A significant susceptibility for early and also advanced HCC has been confirmed by gut microbial markers [27]. The microbiota that is connected to tumors, consists of Actinobacteria, Bacteroidetes,

Firmicutes, and Proteobacteria [28]. Additionally, it was found that *Ruminococcus gnavus* is a unique taxon for persons with HCC caused by viral hepatitis. Researchers have shown connections between the HCC stage, changes in the gut microbiota, and dysbiosis. According to Grat et al.'s prospectively matched analysis of 30 cirrhotic patients, patients with HCC had higher *Escherichia coli* counts in their feces. This analysis had a sensitivity of 66.7% and a specificity of 73.3% when predicting the presence of HCC based on *Escherichia coli* counts [29]. A similar sequencing tool has been utilized by Piero et al. to research 407 cases. The HCC group had a threefold rise in the family *Erysipelotrichaceae* and a fivefold decrease in the family *Leuconostocaceae* when compared to cirrhotic patients without HCC. Fusobacterium and Dorea, two *Lachnospiraceae* bacteria were found in significantly lower concentrations in HCC patients, whereas Odoribacter and Butyricimonas were shown to be more significantly enriched in HCC. The ratio of Bactericide to Prevotella increased in HCC [30]. Chen et al. created an obese mice model by feeding it a high-fat, high-sugar diet in order to assess the impact of the dietary supplement *Ganoderma lucidum* on the gut-liver axis [31]. Proopiomelanocortin, leptin, leptin receptor, and GABA neurons' expression levels were all shown to have changed, according to the scientists. They came to the conclusion that *G. lucidum* can treat metabolic syndrome via affecting the liver and intestines. Through long-distance pathways, gut dysbiosis can promote cancer. One example of it is the liver, which has no known microbiome. The gut microbiome may be involved in liver cancer through pro-inflammatory MAMPs and bacterial metabolites that enter the liver through the portal vein [32]. The direct exposure of several gut-microbiota constituents and metabolites to the liver is caused via this portal vein. Numerous studies have shown over the past ten years that the gut-liver axis plays a significant role in the course of liver disease from basic inflammation to fibrosis, cirrhosis, and cancer. Metabolic dysfunction-associated steatotic liver disease (MASLD) was demonstrated to occur in a mouse model following administration of a clinically isolated strain of *Klebsiella pneumoniae*. Additionally, MASLD in human patients has been linked to this bacterium,

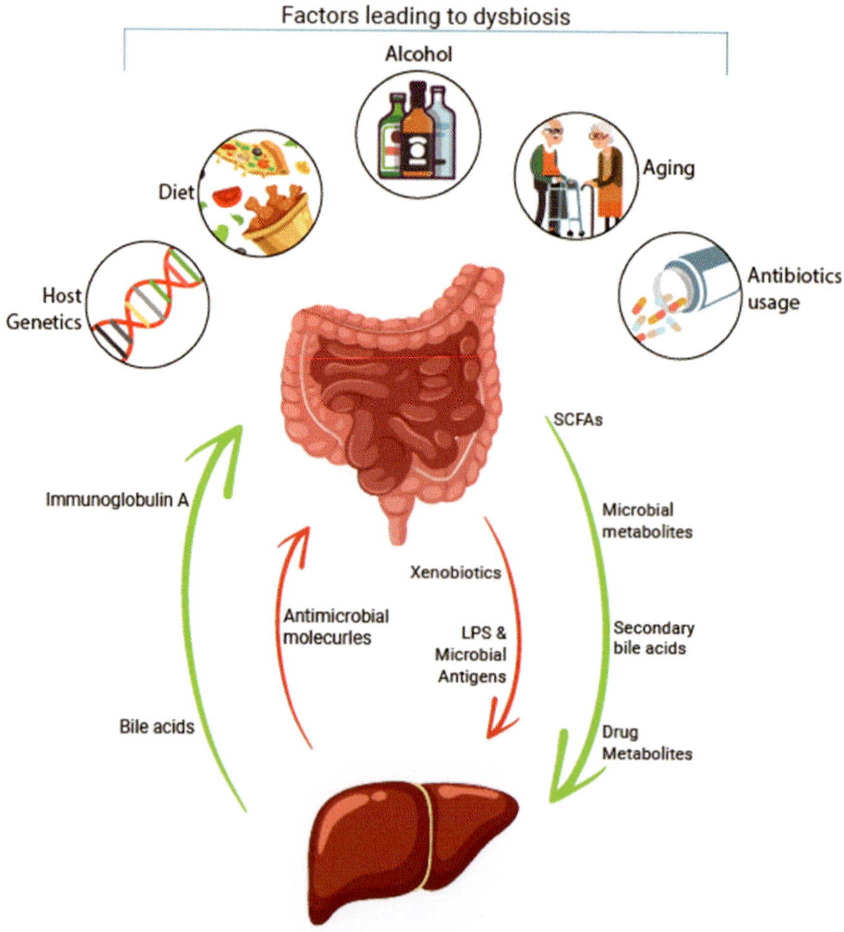

Figure 1: Gut-liver axis

according to reports. The gut microbiome of people with HCC is different from that of people with liver cirrhosis without HCC. In contrast to *Bifidobacterium*, *Bacteroides* and *Ruminococcaceae* were reported to be more prevalent in HCC patients [33]. Mice with a germ-free environment and antibiotics that are not absorbed reduce hepatic inflammation and slow the development of HCC.

4. What Are Phytochemicals

Plants produce phytochemicals, which are bioactive substances to serve as a form of defence. To date, over a thousand phytochemicals have been found, and they can be derived from a variety of foods such as vegetables, whole grains, nuts, fruits, and herbs. Among the key phytochemicals include saponins, polyphenols, carotenoids, phytosterols, dietary fibers, isoprenoids, and specific polysaccharides. These phytochemicals display antibacterial, antidiarrheal, anthelmintic, antiallergic, antispasmodic, and antiviral properties in addition to significant antioxidant activity [34]. Additionally, they support gap junction communication, boost immunity, regulate gene transcription, promote immunity, and offer defence against lung and prostate cancer [35]. Because of the increasing emphasis on translational research, functional foods now include more elements. Phytochemicals have a considerable impact on the development of functional foods and nutraceuticals after being derived from various sources. Different phytochemicals prefer different solvents and have varying heat tolerances. The solvent used influences the quality of the recovered phytochemical as well as its usage in the production of food and nutraceutical goods. The different types of solvents include green solvents [fatty acids/oils, ethanol, water, ionic liquids, acetic acid, carbon dioxide (CO_2), deep eutectic solvents, glycerol, natural deep eutectic solvents (NADES), etc.] and other solvents [36]. The use of inappropriate solvents and temperatures that vary can result in the loss of functional properties. Furthermore, the matrix within which the phytochemical is housed affects extraction efficiency. The effectiveness of phytochemical extraction processes and matrix-related variables such as pre-treatment, matrix type, structure, solid-liquid ratios, and particle size are all influenced by the matrix [37]. Phytochemicals need to be removed from source crops while maintaining their original structure and qualities if high-quality goods are to be produced. Therefore, choosing a proper phytochemical extraction technique is crucial.

5. Role of Phytochemicals in Gut-Microbiota Modulation

Plant-based functional foods' active ingredients are categorized into alkaloids, terpenoids, polyphenols or polysaccharides on the basis of the chemistry of natural products rather than nutrient metabolites. This division makes it easier to comprehend the precise components of a nutritious diet. By affecting the gut microbiota, bioactive substances lower the risk of numerous diseases, and this relationship between bioactive substances and gut microbiota is well-established. Modern medicine is also aware of how natural bioactive chemicals affect neurodegenerative diseases [38]. The impact of this mechanism on other

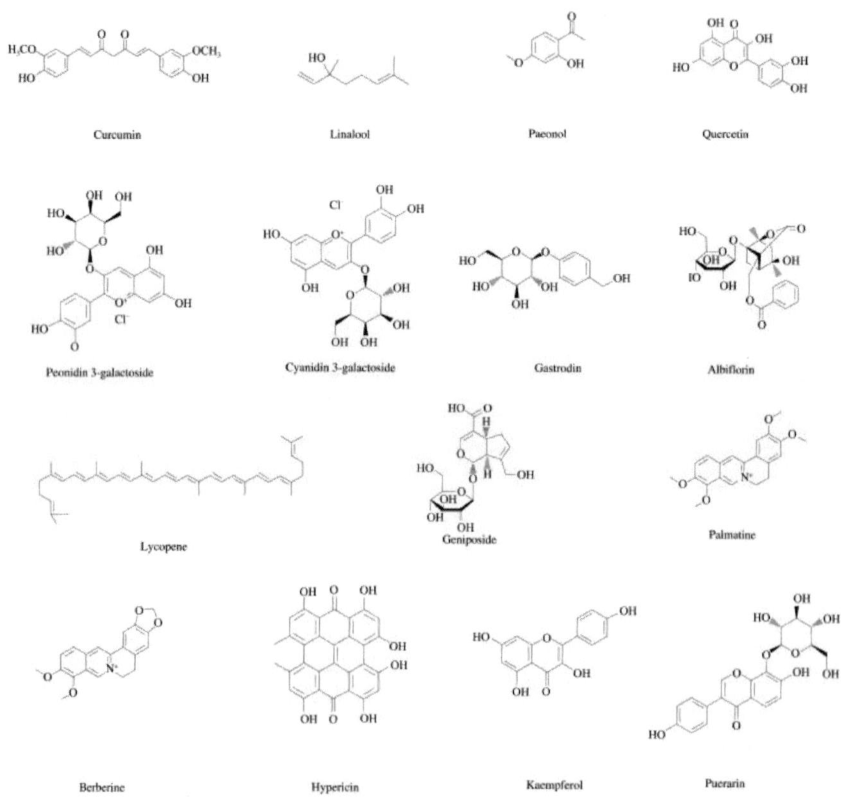

Figure 2: Structure of different phytochemicals related to gut microbiota

diseases or organs has been the subject of extensive inquiry. The immune system, the Vagus nerve, and microbial metabolites are the three main communication pathways by which bioactive substances communicate and influence human health in a bidirectional manner through the gut-microbiome axis (GMA) [39]. The fundamental mechanisms underlying the interaction of the phytochemicals with the GMA, however, have not undergone a thorough investigation.

Determining the connections between the phytochemicals and the GMA is essential for overcoming this restriction. Consumption of phytochemicals or functional meals obtained from whole plants affects the gut microbiota; these substances are then transformed into humoral and brain signals that are derived from the gut [40]. For instance, polyphenols defend against conditions like metabolic syndrome [41], the deterioration in cognitive function linked to neurological diseases (ND) [42], and cardiovascular disease (CVD) [43], all of which could be attributed to changes in the gut microbiota. Plant-based food is a significant alternative to allopathic medication because of its side effects and intolerance. Beyond the nutritional benefits, the regular ingestion of particular dietary components can modify the variety and function of the gut microbiota, which may have an impact on health. Phytochemicals can change the gut microflora composition by selectively enhancing the proliferation of specific microbial communities or inhibiting the expansion of other microbial communities present in the intestinal tract. Plants release these chemicals, which get accumulated in the cell sap compartments (body) and cell wall to support growth and survival. Because of their limited absorption, these substances have a limited bioavailability and a long duration retention in the colon, which benefits the gut microbial population. Feeding phytochemical-rich meals to humans and animals may alter gut flora, which may contribute to improved health and wellness. Dietary phytochemicals such as polyphenols, substances containing sulfur, polysaccharides, terpenoids, pigments, phytohaemagglutinins, and saponins have antiviral, antioxidant, anti-inflammatory, and cancer-prevention or therapeutic activities. These substances travel through the stomach, liver, small intestine, and colon after entering the body. In both the large intestine and small intestine, bacteria are critical for the digestion and absorption of dietary phytochemicals. The precise mechanisms by which dietary phytochemicals are ingested and processed in the human colon, however, are still largely unknown. Through metabolites, plant-based polysaccharides control the gut microbiota; they function as prebiotics, such as certain oligosaccharides that change the variety of the GI milieu [44]. The gut microbiota has access to substrates in the form of plant polysaccharides. By encouraging the gut's goblet cells to secrete mucus, they can aid in intestinal barrier repair by shielding the intestine from harm [45]. Polysaccharides regulate the gut microbiota to produce a more balanced composition by encouraging the development of probiotic bacteria and inhibiting the proliferation of harmful bacteria in terms of bacterial composition [46]. Additionally, polysaccharides have direct interactions with the epithelium, promote the production of mucin in the small intestine, and control cytokine secretions, hormones, and interleukins. These interactions make polysaccharides significant markers of the health of the intestinal immune system. Polysaccharides have a direct impact on gut metabolites and bacteria. Therefore, polysaccharides based on plants are crucial for preserving the balance of the gut microbiota.

Evidence demonstrates that flavonoids and their derivatives can alter microbiota composition to enhance host immune response and metabolism [47]. Flavonoids have both prebiotic and antimicrobial properties, according to the metabolic process [48]. During coculture with flavonoids, it was possible to demonstrate growth augmentation of *Lactobacillus*, Bifidobacterium, and *Enterococcus* species and suppression of *Bacteroides* and *Clostridium* species [49]. The technique of fluorescence in situ hybridization is being utilized to assess changes in the human gut microbiota. Flavonoid metabolism also involved the bacterial species *Clostridium orbiscindens* and *Eubacterium ramulus* [50, 51]. There are many flavonols in common diets, including quercetin and its glycoside derivatives [52]. The development of *Lactobacillus*, *Bacteroides galacturonics*, *Enterococcus caccae*, *Ruminococcus gauvreauii*, and *Escherichia coli* was shown to be dose-dependently inhibited by quercetin, but not by its glycoside derivatives [53]. Other flavonoids, which are frequently used in the food sector, also demonstrated antibacterial effects against food-borne pathogens. Based on the outcomes of mixed cultures containing the human microflora, it has been revealed that the metabolism of naringin (a flavanone) and rutin (a flavonol) is microbiota dependent [53]. The gut microbiota shows a significant influence on the metabolism of flavonoids and their related metabolites, which has a positive impact on health, according to all available evidence. During coincubation, raspberry anthocyanins (glycosides) were dramatically reduced in the presence of the live human microbiota [54]. The development of the gut microbiota, including that of *Staphylococcus aureus*, *Bifidobacterium sp.*, *Salmonella typhimurium*, and *Lactobacillus spp.*, was significantly influenced by anthocyanins from potato, black rice, and malvidin-3-glucoside during *in vitro* fermentation [55, 56]. It was also noted *in vivo* that anthocyanins and the gut bacteria have a reciprocal effect. Cyanidin-3-glucoside, a significant cyaniding derivative, is deglycosylated by the gut bacteria *Clostridium saccharogumia* and *Eubacterium ramulus* [56]. Anthocyanins, present in black raspberry, increased the development of *Lactobacillus sp.*, *Faecalibacterium prausnitzii*, and *Eubacterium rectale* in C57BL/6J mice while suppressing the growth of *Enterococcus sp.* and *Desulfovibrio sp.* [57]. Raspberry anthocyanins considerably changed the luminal abundances of Firmicutes (*Clostridium sp.*) and Bacteroidetes (*Barnesiella sp.*) [58]. In rats fed blackcurrant anthocyanins, *Prevotella*, *Bacteroides*, *Lactobacillus*, and *Porphyromonas* relative abundances greatly increased, but *Bifidobacterium and Clostridium* relative abundances dramatically decreased [59]. In the group with a high-fat diet, berry anthocyanins boosted the abundance of Gammaproteobacteria while inhibiting the pro-inflammatory bacteria *Bilophila wadsworthia*'s development [60]. *Eggerthella lenta, Bifidobacterium, and Enterococcus* were found in greater relative abundances at the genus level in the feces of individuals in human clinical trials who consumed red wine high in anthocyanins [61]. Gallotannins, Ellagitannins, complicated tannins, and condensed tannins are subcategories of tannins, which are polyphenolic chemicals [62]. Berry, walnut, plant seeds, and herbs all contain ellagitannins, hydrolyzable tannins. The colon microbiota gradually degraded ellagic acid to produce urolithin

B and urolithin A after ellagic acid was hydrolyzed from ellagagitannins [63]. The antioxidants urolithin C and urolithin D were also shown to be present in the intestines at considerably high amounts [64]. Evidently, the human lower GI tract is where urolithin metabolites are produced and tannins are metabolized, and both processes depend on the microbiota. Species from the genera *Prevotella, Ruminococcus, and Bacteroides* were found to be the predominant intestinal microbes in individuals who ingested urolithin-enriched walnut and pomegranate extracts, and the family *Coriobacteriaceae* has been linked to blood cholesterol levels and urolithin metabolites [65]. These findings have helped to identify specific microbes that are involved in the metabolism of ellagitannin. The genera *Clostridium, Bifidobacterium, Lactobacillus, and Bacteroides* may play a role in the formation of urolithins, according to other investigations [66, 67]. It was observed that *Clostridium and Bifidobacterium* were also associated with the metabolism of pomegranate ellagitannin in a bacteria species-dependent manner by evaluating the culture medium's optical density [68]. Another form of hydrolyzable tannin is gallotannin [69]. According to a human clinical study, gallotannins were metabolized by microbes and free gallic acid was released in the GI tract [70]. Tetraterpenoids called carotenoids are the colored pigments found in fruits and vegetables [71]. Carotenes (alpha, beta, and astaxanthin) and Xanthophylls (zeaxanthin, lutein) are two of the subgroups, and these substances have considerable antioxidant activity in maintaining human health [72, 73]. A plentiful oxycarotenoid found in some microalgae and marine life is astaxanthin. Phyla Proteobacteria and Bacteroidetes, genera *Parabacteroides, Bilophila, and Butyricimonas*, as well as species from *Akkermansia* and Verrucomicrobia, were all affected by dietary astaxanthin (50 mg/kg) in C57BL/6J mice [74]. On Balb/cA mice with *Helicobacter pylori* infection, astaxanthin (200 mg/kg body weight/day) decreased the bacterial count of the gram-negative pathogen *Helicobacter pylori* 119/95p and decreased stomach inflammation and the release of *Helicobacter pylori*-specific T-cell cytokines [75]. A study found that eating astaxanthin (0.04%, w/w) altered the phylum-level cecal microbiota in vivo by genotype and gender. Vegetables, whole grains, and fruits are examples of whole plant foods that are high in fiber. The composition of the gut microbiota of human is considerably altered by digestible fibers, one of the key bioactive components of whole-food dietary treatments [76]. A type of SCFA called butyrate is frequently generated by bacteria in the colon when dietary fibers are fermented. As a histone deacetylase inhibitor, GPCR activator, energy metabolite for ATP synthesis, antioxidant, anti-inflammatory, and brain health promoter, this fatty acid performs a number of critical biological functions [77]. Dietary fiber consumption was found to be substantially correlated with the abundances of particular gut microbes, including those of the bacterial phylum Actinobacteria, class Clostridia, and order Bifidobacteriales in human clinical trials [78]. In a randomized human clinical research, soluble maize fibers (21 grams/day) considerably changed the bacterial phyla Bacteroidetes and Firmicutes as well as the families *Porphyromonadaceae, Eubacteriaceae, Lachnospiraceae, and Ruminococcaceae* [79]. Consuming dietary fiber also stimulated metabolic pathways, such as those involved in the metabolism of amino acids, vitamins, nucleotides, and carbohydrates.

6. Effect of Phytochemicals on Liver Cancer Microbiome

Because of the gut-liver axis, which plays a significant role in HCC progression, gut microbiota is a key contributing component. However, the development of HCC may be prevented by altering the type and quantity of gut microbiota. This has a number of advantages, including a balanced and healthy gut flora, a significant reduction in intestinal inflammation, improved mucosal barrier functions, and a proven ability to effectively treat cirrhosis. Prebiotics are dietary components that promote the growth or activity of beneficial microorganisms. Prebiotics, probiotics, and synbiotics can all be used in concert with other strategies to manage gut flora overgrowth. As a result, galactans (galacto-oligosaccharides) and inulin-type fructans (such as fructo-oligosaccharides [FOS], inulin, and oligofructose) have attracted the most scientific focus. Inulin is a non-digestible polymer found in plants such as wheat, rye, barley, leeks, onions, chicory, and

Jerusalem artichokes. Inulin regulates the composition of the gut microbiota and hepatic fatty acid, preventing dysbiosis and its negative effects on host health [80]. Plants including chicory root, onions, leeks, garlic, Jerusalem artichokes, asparagus, and bananas are the main sources of FOS. According to recent research, FOS may contribute to resistance to the colonization of *Clostridium difficile.* According to several studies that link intestinal microflora with liver cancer, *Clostridium* cluster XIVa, cluster XI, or other bacteria that catalyze the conversion of primary to secondary BAs can be factors in the development of liver cancer [81]. Other oligosaccharides have lately attracted interest, including isomalto-oligosaccharides and soybean oligosaccharides. Prebiotic oligosaccharides can be found in a variety of fruits, vegetables, cereals, and legumes. Dietary fibers are categorized as either soluble (such as fructans, gums, and pectins) or insoluble (such as hemicellulose, cellulose, and lignin) depending on how soluble they are in water. Only soluble fibers have "prebiotic" properties that can impact host health and can be digested by gut microbiota [82]. Foods having high FOS and inulin, such as onions, mushrooms, lettuce, celery, garland chrysanthemum, beans, squash, garlic shoots, and carrots, had a substantial inverse relationship with liver cancer, demonstrating their anti-HCC benefits [83], according to a study examining the link between food groups and liver cancer risk. Consuming bran, cereal fiber, and wholegrain may help lower HCC, according to a cohort study encompassing 125455 participants [84]. In recent years, prebiotic benefits have been attributed to compounds other than non-digestible oligosaccharides, like plant polyphenols. These substances enter the colon where the colonic microbiota processes them, benefiting the host's health. They are made up of the lignins, flavonoids, and phenolic acids that are present in fruits, tea, nuts, vegetables, and wine. Due to immunomodulation activity, polyphenols can slow the progression of HCC [85]. Coffee consumption has been shown in numerous studies to decrease the occurrence of HCC because it contains phenolic compounds with anticarcinogenic properties [86]. Tea, in particular, has been shown to promote gut-microbiota equilibrium by reducing the development of dangerous bacteria. Ellagic acid, an antioxidant found predominantly in berries and nuts that is transformed by the microbiota in the colon into urolithins with anticancer effects [87]. Consuming dietary fiber and whole grains, especially cereal fiber, has been associated with a lower incidence of obesity and MASLD, both of which are known risk factors for HCC, according to prior research. In fact, it has been hypothesized that long-term whole-grain diet can lower the risk of HCC by enhancing gut integrity and altering gut-microbiota makeup [88]. In addition, a meta-analysis of 19 trials comprising 1,290,045 people (3912 of whom had HCC) revealed that every increase in vegetable consumption of 100 g/d results in an 8% reduction in the chance of developing HCC [89]. Additionally, the use of prebiotics has been investigated as a strategy to modify the function of the intestinal barrier by preserving the integrity of tight junction (TJ). Prebiotics have shown gut-microbiota compositional effects that could result in favorable adjustments to TJ protein expression and distribution. Prebiotics' modulation of the microbiota's impact on TJ is less well understood than the effects of probiotic administration. FOS, inulin, and galacto-oligosaccharide are three prebiotics that have been shown in numerous studies to have positive effects on intestinal TJs. In a recent study, T84 cells were employed as an intestinal epithelial cell model to evaluate the influence of FOS on AMP-activated protein kinase (AMPK) action and TJ formation in non-inflammatory and inflammatory conditions. The findings showed that FOS increased gut epithelial TJ assembly by activating AMPK. Additionally, additional research showed that prebiotic administration causes AMPK to be strongly activated [90, 91].

7. Therapeutic Strategies

By acting as prebiotics and enhancing numerous physiological processes that have been proven to depend on the healthy operation of the gut and its microbiota, phytochemicals produce a variety of advantageous bioactivities. Prebiotics have the power to alter the composition of organisms in the gut microbiome, which is the GI system's most usual habitat. It has been demonstrated that pure polyphenols and foods high in polyphenols, together with traditional diets, give health benefits through preserving the gut's beneficial bacteria [92]. Polyphenols are known to have chemo-preventive effects on HCC through regulating the immune system [93]. Since they have been found to have positive effects on the population of gut microbes and to reduce harmful bacteria, tea phenols may help to maintain great GI health. Tea polyphenols are a potent replacement for HCC chemotherapy in both prevention and treatment [94]. The increased generation of antibodies and lymphocytes are two additional effects of polysaccharides' immunomodulating capabilities, in addition to their promotion of antigenotoxic and anticancer activities [95]. Sclerotia of *Pleurotus tuber-regium* and sporoderm-broken germinating spores (SBGS) of Reishi both contain mushroom polysaccharides that have a considerable anticancer impact, particularly in preventing the regrowth or spread of malignant cells. In certain people, it lessens the harmful and adverse effects of radiation and

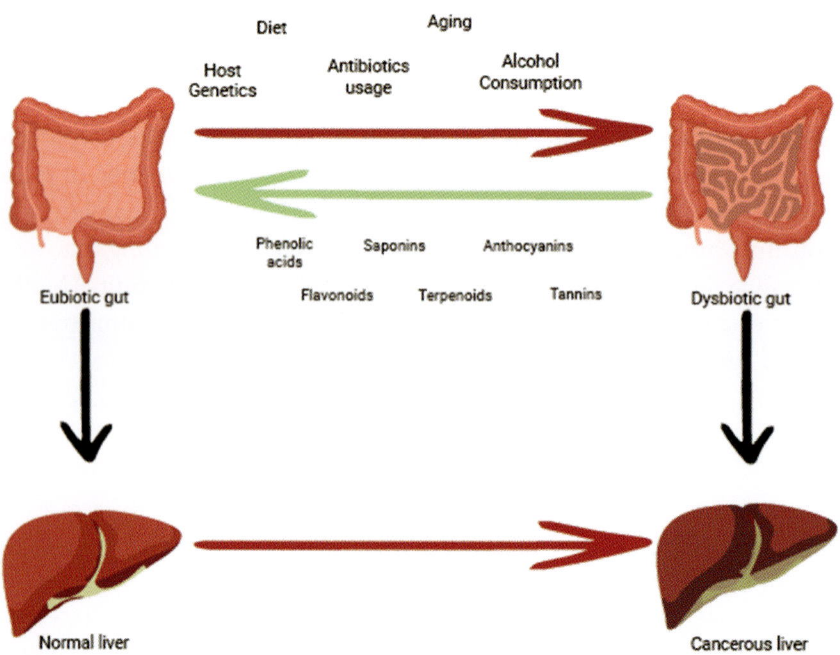

Figure 3: Connection between gut-microbiota, phytochemicals and liver cancer

chemotherapy [96]. Lactulose is one of the most frequent non-digestible oligosaccharides that is known to play a functional role in nature. Lactulose treatment has been shown to hasten liver regeneration in rats following hepatectomy, which may be because it lowers inflammation and oxidative stress. In patients with HCC who also have hepatocirrhosis and hypersplenism, lactulose administered orally after interventional therapy could balance out the imbalance of the antioxidant and oxidative systems, reduce liver damage, and improve antitumor immunity and prognosis [97].

8. Future of the Field

Gut microbiota is connected to nearly every aspect of human physiology, from basic food digestion and energy metabolism to memory and depression. The study of the microbiome has a very promising future. The relationship between cancer and the gut microbiota has already been accepted, despite the fact that the exact mechanisms by which these two interact are still largely unknown. Cancer treatment that involves gut microbiota modification may be effective. However, trying to change the composition of the tiny organisms in the gut might also have negative health effects because they are connected to other physiological processes. Critically conceived, creative research is necessary to fully comprehend how our gut microbiota and other physiological aspects are interconnected. Difficulties and hurdles still exist in research on the host-microbiota relationship, despite significant advancements. As the defining microbiota composition of "normal" or "healthy" gut has not yet been established, it is better not to use the term "disorder" rather abnormalities in the microbiome related to a specific disease or condition when compared to controls. There isn't a set criterion for treating with phytochemicals because the degree of "abnormality" in the gut-microbiota composition isn't exactly uniform. The majority of phytochemicals target chronic diseases; yet, because many chronic disease animal models improve gradually, the effects of phytochemical treatment may be limited. According to research, short-term interventions have only ephemeral effects on the core gut flora, whereas long-term normal diet has a higher impact [98]. Due to the cross-sectional nature of studies, variations in inclusion criteria, and difficulty to prove causation in the observed links, conducting comparative analyses of research findings is difficult. While whole genome sequencing allows us to investigate predicted metabolic patterns, more research is needed to clarify whether microbial functions and metabolites have increased or decreased. Highly distinct bacterial, archaeal, fungal, and viral compositions can be found in microbial communities. These microbes and their metabolites contribute to disease either alone or jointly. Consequently, it is difficult to pinpoint the specific factors that cause disease. Although it is still in its infancy and needs a lot of development, this field of cancer research holds out a lot of promise and has the potential to bring in a new era of cancer research.

References

1. G. Riscuta, "Probiotics and Cancer Prevention as a Part of the Healthy Microbiome," *J. Probiotics Health*, vol. 1, p. 3, Jan. 2013, doi: 10.4172/2329-8901.1000e103.
2. R. R. Dietert and J. M. Dietert, "The Human Superorganism: Microbes for Freedom vs. Fear," *Appl. Microbiol*, vol. 3, pp. 883–905, Jul. 2023, doi: 10.20944/preprints202307.0185.v1.
3. R. H. Liu, "Potential Synergy of Phytochemicals in Cancer Prevention: Mechanism of Action," *J. Nutr.*, vol. 134, no. 12, pp. 3479S–3485S, Dec. 2004, doi: 10.1093/jn/134.12.3479S.
4. L. Carrera-Quintanar, R. I. López Roa, S. Quintero-Fabián, M. A. Sánchez-Sánchez, B. Vizmanos, and D. Ortuño-Sahagún, "Phytochemicals that Influence Gut Microbiota as Prophylactics and for the Treatment of Obesity and Inflammatory Diseases," *Mediators Inflamm.*, vol. 2018, p. 9734845, Mar. 2018, doi: 10.1155/2018/9734845.
5. F. Rabizadeh, M. S. Mirian, R. Doosti, R. Kiani-Anbouhi, and E. Eftekhari, "Phytochemical Classification of Medicinal Plants Used in the Treatment of Kidney Disease Based on Traditional Persian Medicine," *Evid.-Based Complement. Altern. Med. ECAM*, vol. 2022, p. 8022599, Jul. 2022, doi: 10.1155/2022/8022599.

6. M. B. Ahmed, S. U. Islam, A. A. A. Alghamdi, M. Kamran, H. Ahsan, and Y. S. Lee, "Phytochemicals as Chemo-Preventive Agents and Signaling Molecule Modulators: Current Role in Cancer Therapeutics and Inflammation," *Int. J. Mol. Sci.*, vol. 23, no. 24, p. 15765, Dec. 2022, doi: 10.3390/ijms232415765.
7. S. Santhiravel et al., "The Impact of Plant Phytochemicals on the Gut Microbiota of Humans for a Balanced Life," *Int. J. Mol. Sci.*, vol. 23, no. 15, p. 8124, Jul. 2022, doi: 10.3390/ijms23158124.
8. S. L. Prescott, "History of Medicine: Origin of the Term Microbiome and Why It Matters," *Hum. Microbiome J.*, vol. 4, pp. 24–25, Jun. 2017, doi: 10.1016/j.humic.2017.05.004.
9. E. Thursby and N. Juge, "Introduction to the Human Gut Microbiota," *Biochem. J.*, vol. 474, no. 11, pp. 1823–1836, Jun. 2017, doi: 10.1042/BCJ20160510.
10. R. Sender, S. Fuchs, and R. Milo, "Are We Really Vastly Outnumbered? Revisiting the Ratio of Bacterial to Host Cells in Humans," *Cell*, vol. 164, no. 3, pp. 337–340, Jan. 2016, doi: 10.1016/j.cell.2016.01.013.
11. L. Jostins et al., "Host-Microbe Interactions Have Shaped the Genetic Architecture of Inflammatory Bowel Disease," *Nature*, vol. 491, no. 7422, pp. 119–124, Nov. 2012, doi: 10.1038/nature11582.
12. M. Al-Asmakh and F. Zadjali, "Use of Germ-Free Animal Models in Microbiota-Related Research," *J. Microbiol. Biotechnol.*, vol. 25, pp. 1583–1588, Jun. 2015, doi: 10.4014/jmb.1501.01039.
13. B.-N. Liu, X.-T. Liu, Z.-H. Liang, and J.-H. Wang, "Gut Microbiota in Obesity," *World J. Gastroenterol.*, vol. 27, no. 25, pp. 3837–3850, Jul. 2021, doi: 10.3748/wjg.v27.i25.3837.
14. N. Kamada, S.-U. Seo, G. Y. Chen, and G. Núñez, "Role of the Gut Microbiota in Immunity and Inflammatory Disease," *Nat. Rev. Immunol.*, vol. 13, no. 5, pp. 321–335, May 2013, doi: 10.1038/nri3430.
15. S. J. Engle et al., "Elimination of Colon Cancer in Germ-Free Transforming Growth Factor Beta 1-Deficient Mice," *Cancer Res.*, vol. 62, no. 22, pp. 6362–6366, Nov. 2002.
16. R. K. Sellon et al., "Resident Enteric Bacteria Are Necessary for Development of Spontaneous Colitis and Immune System Activation in Interleukin-10-Deficient Mice," *Infect. Immun.*, vol. 66, no. 11, pp. 5224–5231, Nov. 1998, doi: 10.1128/IAI.66.11.5224-5231.1998.

17. A. Di Ciaula et al., "Bile Acid Physiology," *Ann. Hepatol.*, vol. 16, no. Suppl. 1: s3–105, pp. s4–s14, Nov. 2017, doi: 10.5604/01.3001.0010.5493.
18. A. Wahlström, S. I. Sayin, H.-U. Marschall, and F. Bäckhed, "Intestinal Crosstalk between Bile Acids and Microbiota and Its Impact on Host Metabolism," *Cell Metab.*, vol. 24, no. 1, pp. 41–50, Jul. 2016, doi: 10.1016/j.cmet.2016.05.005.
19. K. M. Maslowski et al., "Regulation of Inflammatory Responses by Gut Microbiota and Chemoattractant Receptor GPR43," *Nature*, vol. 461, no. 7268, pp. 1282–1286, Oct. 2009, doi: 10.1038/nature08530.
20. P. M. Smith et al., "The Microbial Metabolites, Short-Chain Fatty Acids, Regulate Colonic Treg Cell Homeostasis," *Science*, vol. 341, no. 6145, pp. 569–573, Aug. 2013, doi: 10.1126/science.1241165.
21. P. Louis, G. L. Hold, and H. J. Flint, "The Gut Microbiota, Bacterial Metabolites and Colorectal Cancer," *Nat. Rev. Microbiol.*, vol. 12, no. 10, p. 10, Oct. 2014, doi: 10.1038/nrmicro3344.
22. S. M. Jandhyala, R. Talukdar, C. Subramanyam, H. Vuyyuru, M. Sasikala, and D. N. Reddy, "Role of the Normal Gut Microbiota," *World J. Gastroenterol. WJG*, vol. 21, no. 29, pp. 8787–8803, Aug. 2015, doi: 10.3748/wjg.v21.i29.8787.
23. A. Tripathi et al., "The Gut–Liver Axis and the Intersection with the Microbiome," *Nat. Rev. Gastroenterol. Hepatol.*, vol. 15, no. 7, p. 7, Jul. 2018, doi: 10.1038/s41575-018-0011-z.
24. G. den Besten, K. van Eunen, A. K. Groen, K. Venema, D.-J. Reijngoud, and B. M. Bakker, "The Role of Short-Chain Fatty Acids in the Interplay between Diet, Gut Microbiota, and Host Energy Metabolism," *J. Lipid Res.*, vol. 54, no. 9, pp. 2325–2340, Sep. 2013, doi: 10.1194/jlr.R036012.
25. T. Gensollen, S. S. Iyer, D. L. Kasper, and R. S. Blumberg, "How Colonization by Microbiota in Early Life Shapes the Immune System," *Science*, vol. 352, no. 6285, pp. 539–544, Apr. 2016, doi: 10.1126/science.aad9378.
26. S. R. Gill et al., "Metagenomic Analysis of the Human Distal Gut Microbiome," *Science*, vol. 312, no. 5778, pp. 1355–1359, Jun. 2006, doi: 10.1126/science.1124234.

27. Z. Ren et al., "Gut Microbiome Analysis as a Tool Towards Targeted Non-Invasive Biomarkers for Early Hepatocellular Carcinoma," *Gut*, vol. 68, no. 6, pp. 1014–1023, Jun. 2019, doi: 10.1136/gutjnl-2017-315084.
28. S. Komiyama, T. Yamada, N. Takemura, N. Kokudo, K. Hase, and Y. I. Kawamura, "Profiling of Tumour-Associated Microbiota in Human Hepatocellular Carcinoma," *Sci. Rep.*, vol. 11, no. 1, p. 1, May 2021, doi: 10.1038/s41598-021-89963-1.
29. J. Ni et al., "Analysis of the Relationship Between the Degree of Dysbiosis in Gut Microbiota and Prognosis at Different Stages of Primary Hepatocellular Carcinoma," *Front. Microbiol.*, vol. 10, Jun. 2019, Accessed: Aug. 10, 2023. [Online]. Available: https://www.frontiersin.org/articles/10.3389/fmicb.2019.01458
30. F. Piñero et al., "A Different Gut Microbiome Linked to Inflammation Found in Cirrhotic Patients with and without Hepatocellular Carcinoma," *Ann. Hepatol.*, vol. 18, no. 3, pp. 480–487, May 2019, doi: 10.1016/j.aohep.2018.10.003.
31. M. F. Ahmad et al., "*Ganoderma Lucidum*: Novel Insight into Hepatoprotective Potential with Mechanisms of Action," *Nutrients*, vol. 15, no. 8, p. 1874, Apr. 2023, doi: 10.3390/nu15081874.
32. A. Ochi et al., "MyD88 Inhibition Amplifies Dendritic Cell Capacity to Promote Pancreatic Carcinogenesis via Th2 Cells," *J. Exp. Med.*, vol. 209, no. 9, pp. 1671–1687, Aug. 2012, doi: 10.1084/jem.20111706.
33. J. Xu et al., "Clinical Aspects of Gut Microbiota in Hepatocellular Carcinoma Management," *Pathogens*, vol. 10, no. 7, p. 782, Jun. 2021, doi: 10.3390/pathogens10070782.
34. A. Kumar et al., "Major Phytochemicals: Recent Advances in Health Benefits and Extraction Method," *Molecules*, vol. 28, no. 2, p. 887, Jan. 2023, doi: 10.3390/molecules28020887.
35. M. A. Rahman et al., "Phytochemicals as a Complement to Cancer Chemotherapy: Pharmacological Modulation of the Autophagy-Apoptosis Pathway," *Front. Pharmacol.*, vol. 12, May 2021, Accessed: Oct. 06, 2023. [Online]. Available: https://www.frontiersin.org/articles/10.3389/fphar.2021.639628
36. E. Husanu et al., "Exploiting Deep Eutectic Solvents and Ionic Liquids for the Valorization of Chestnut Shell Waste," *ACS Sustain. Chem.*

Eng., vol. 8, no. 50, pp. 18386–18399, Dec. 2020, doi: 10.1021/acssuschemeng.0c04945.

37. E. Gil-Martín, T. Forbes-Hernández, A. Romero, D. Cianciosi, F. Giampieri, and M. Battino, "Influence of the Extraction Method on the Recovery of Bioactive Phenolic Compounds from Food Industry by-Products," *Food Chem.*, vol. 378, p. 131918, Jun. 2022, doi: 10.1016/j.foodchem.2021.131918.
38. R. H. Liu, "Health-Promoting Components of Fruits and Vegetables in the Diet," *Adv. Nutr.*, vol. 4, no. 3, pp. 384S–392S, May 2013, doi: 10.3945/an.112.003517.
39. D. O. Kennedy and E. L. Wightman, "Herbal Extracts and Phytochemicals: Plant Secondary Metabolites and the Enhancement of Human Brain function," *Adv. Nutr.*, vol. 2, no. 1, pp. 32–50, Jan. 2011, doi: 10.3945/an.110.000117.
40. W. C. Man, N. Xia, A. Daiber, and H. Li, "The Roles of Gut Microbiota and Circadian Rhythm in the Cardiovascular Protective Effects of Polyphenols," *Br. J. Pharmacol.*, vol. 177, no. 6, pp. 1278–1293, 2020, doi: 10.1111/bph.14850.
41. K. D. Crew et al., "Phase IB Randomized, Double-Blinded, Placebo-Controlled, Dose Escalation Study of Polyphenon E in Women with Hormone Receptor–Negative Breast Cancer," *Cancer Prev. Res. (Phila. Pa.)*, vol. 5, no. 9, pp. 1144–1154, Sep. 2012, doi: 10.1158/1940-6207.CAPR-12-0117.
42. M. J. Amiot, C. Riva, and A. Vinet, "Effects of Dietary Polyphenols on Metabolic Syndrome Features in Humans: A Systematic Review," *Obes. Rev.*, vol. 17, no. 7, pp. 573–586, 2016, doi: 10.1111/obr.12409.
43. D. Pantano, I. Luccarini, P. Nardiello, M. Servili, M. Stefani, and F. Casamenti, "Oleuropein Aglycone and Polyphenols from Olive Mill Waste Water Ameliorate Cognitive Deficits and Neuropathology," *Br. J. Clin. Pharmacol.*, vol. 83, no. 1, pp. 54–62, 2017, doi: 10.1111/bcp.12993.
44. L. ShuZhen et al., "Research Advance on Biological Activity and Structure-Activity Relationships of Bioactive Polysaccharide," *Food Res. Dev.*, vol. 38, no. 18, pp. 211–218, 2017.
45. C. Wu et al., "Effects of Dietary Radix Rehmanniae Preparata Polysaccharides on the Digestive Enzymes, Morphology, Microbial

Communities and Mucosal Barrier Function of the Intestine of *Luciobarbus Capito*," *Aquac. Res.*, vol. 51, no. 3, pp. 1026–1037, 2020, doi: 10.1111/are.14448.

46. N. Dong et al., "Astragalus Polysaccharides Attenuated Inflammation and Balanced the Gut Microflora in Mice Challenged with Salmonella Typhimurium," *Int. Immunopharmacol.*, vol. 74, p. 105681, Sep. 2019, doi: 10.1016/j.intimp.2019.105681.
47. G. D. Wu et al., "Linking Long-Term Dietary Patterns with Gut Microbial Enterotypes," *Science*, vol. 334, no. 6052, pp. 105–108, Oct. 2011, doi: 10.1126/science.1208344.
48. A. Braune and M. Blaut, "Bacterial Species Involved in the Conversion of Dietary Flavonoids in the Human Gut," *Gut Microbes*, vol. 7, no. 3, pp. 216–234, May 2016, doi: 10.1080/19490976.2016.1158395.
49. M. Hidalgo et al., "Metabolism of Anthocyanins by Human Gut Microflora and Their Influence on Gut Bacterial Growth," *J. Agric. Food Chem.*, vol. 60, no. 15, pp. 3882–3890, Apr. 2012, doi: 10.1021/jf3002153.
50. A. Braune, M. Gütschow, W. Engst, and M. Blaut, "Degradation of Quercetin and Luteolin by Eubacterium Ramulus," *Appl. Environ. Microbiol.*, vol. 67, no. 12, pp. 5558–5567, Dec. 2001, doi: 10.1128/AEM.67.12.5558-5567.2001.
51. L. Schoefer, R. Mohan, A. Schwiertz, A. Braune, and M. Blaut, "Anaerobic Degradation of Flavonoids by *Clostridium Orbiscindens*," *Appl. Environ. Microbiol.*, vol. 69, no. 10, pp. 5849–5854, Oct. 2003, doi: 10.1128/AEM.69.10.5849-5854.2003.
52. K. H. Miean and S. Mohamed, "Flavonoid (Myricetin, Quercetin, Kaempferol, Luteolin, and Apigenin) Content of Edible Tropical Plants," *J. Agric. Food Chem.*, vol. 49, no. 6, pp. 3106–3112, Jun. 2001, doi: 10.1021/jf000892m.
53. R. Yin et al., "Gut Microbiota, Dietary Phytochemicals and Benefits to Human Health," *Curr. Pharmacol. Rep.*, vol. 5, pp. 332–344, 2019, doi: 10.1007/s40495-019-00196-3.
54. R. González-Barrio, C. A. Edwards, and A. Crozier, "Colonic Catabolism of Ellagitannins, Ellagic Acid, and Raspberry Anthocyanins: *In Vivo* and *In Vitro* Studies," *Drug Metab. Dispos.*, vol. 39, no. 9, pp. 1680–1688, Sep. 2011, doi: 10.1124/dmd.111.039651.

55. Y. Zhu et al., "Metabolism and Prebiotics Activity of Anthocyanins from Black Rice (*Oryza Sativa* L.) *In Vitro*," *PLoS One*, vol. 13, no. 4, p. e0195754, Apr. 2018, doi: 10.1371/journal.pone.0195754.
56. H. Sun, P. Zhang, Y. Zhu, Q. Lou, and S. He, "Antioxidant and Prebiotic Activity of Five Peonidin-Based Anthocyanins Extracted from Purple Sweet Potato (*Ipomoea Batatas* (L.) Lam.)," *Sci. Rep.*, vol. 8, no. 1, p. 1, Mar. 2018, doi: 10.1038/s41598-018-23397-0.
57. L. Chen et al., "Chemoprevention of Colorectal Cancer by Black Raspberry Anthocyanins Involved the Modulation of Gut Microbiota and SFRP2 Demethylation," *Carcinogenesis*, vol. 39, no. 3, pp. 471–481, Mar. 2018, doi: 10.1093/carcin/bgy009.
58. J. Gu et al., "Dietary Black Raspberries Impact the Colonic Microbiome and Phytochemical Metabolites in Mice," *Mol. Nutr. Food Res.*, vol. 63, no. 8, p. 1800636, 2019, doi: 10.1002/mnfr.201800636.
59. G. Paturi, C. A. Butts, J. A. Monro, and D. Hedderley, "Effects of Blackcurrant and Dietary Fibers on Large Intestinal Health Biomarkers in Rats," *Plant Foods Hum. Nutr.*, vol. 73, no. 1, pp. 54–60, Mar. 2018, doi: 10.1007/s11130-018-0652-7.
60. S. Lee, K. I. Keirsey, R. Kirkland, Z. I. Grunewald, J. G. Fischer, and C. B. de La Serre, "Blueberry Supplementation Influences the Gut Microbiota, Inflammation, and Insulin Resistance in High-Fat-Diet–Fed Rats," *J. Nutr.*, vol. 148, no. 2, pp. 209–219, Feb. 2018, doi: 10.1093/jn/nxx027.
61. M. Boto-Ordóñez, M. Urpi-Sarda, M. I. Queipo-Ortuño, S. Tulipani, F. J. Tinahones, and C. Andres-Lacueva, "High Levels of Bifidobacteria are Associated with Increased Levels of Anthocyanin Microbial Metabolites: A Randomized Clinical Trial," *Food Funct.*, vol. 5, no. 8, pp. 1932–1938, Jul. 2014, doi: 10.1039/C4FO00029C.
62. K. Khanbabaee and T. van Ree, "Tannins: Classification and Definition," *Nat. Prod. Rep.*, vol. 18, no. 6, pp. 641–649, 2001, doi: 10.1039/B101061L.
63. J. M. Landete, "Ellagitannins, Ellagic Acid and their Derived Metabolites: A Review about Source, Metabolism, Functions and Health," *Food Res. Int.*, vol. 44, no. 5, pp. 1150–1160, Jun. 2011, doi: 10.1016/j.foodres.2011.04.027.

64. D. Bialonska, S. G. Kasimsetty, S. I. Khan, and D. Ferreira, "Urolithins, Intestinal Microbial Metabolites of Pomegranate Ellagitannins, Exhibit Potent Antioxidant Activity in a Cell-Based Assay," *J. Agric. Food Chem.*, vol. 57, no. 21, pp. 10181–10186, Nov. 2009, doi: 10.1021/jf9025794.
65. M. Romo-Vaquero et al., "Deciphering the Human Gut Microbiome of Urolithin Metabotypes: Association with Enterotypes and Potential Cardiometabolic Health Implications," *Mol. Nutr. Food Res.*, vol. 63, no. 4, p. 1800958, 2019, doi: 10.1002/mnfr.201800958.
66. R. García-Villalba, D. Beltrán, J. C. Espín, M. V. Selma, and F. A. Tomás-Barberán, "Time Course Production of Urolithins from Ellagic Acid by Human Gut Microbiota," *J. Agric. Food Chem.*, vol. 61, no. 37, pp. 8797–8806, Sep. 2013, doi: 10.1021/jf402498b.
67. D. Bialonska, P. Ramnani, S. G. Kasimsetty, K. R. Muntha, G. R. Gibson, and D. Ferreira, "The Influence of Pomegranate By-Product and Punicalagins on Selected Groups of Human Intestinal Microbiota," *Int. J. Food Microbiol.*, vol. 140, no. 2, pp. 175–182, Jun. 2010, doi: 10.1016/j.ijfoodmicro.2010.03.038.
68. D. Bialonska, S. G. Kasimsetty, K. K. Schrader, and D. Ferreira, "The Effect of Pomegranate (*Punica granatum* L.) Byproducts and Ellagitannins on the Growth of Human Gut Bacteria," *J. Agric. Food Chem.*, vol. 57, no. 18, pp. 8344–8349, Sep. 2009, doi: 10.1021/jf901931b.
69. K. Kawabata, Y. Yoshioka, and J. Terao, "Role of Intestinal Microbiota in the Bioavailability and Physiological Functions of Dietary Polyphenols," *Molecules*, vol. 24, no. 2, p. 2, Jan. 2019, doi: 10.3390/molecules24020370.
70. R. C. Barnes, K. A. Krenek, B. Meibohm, S. U. Mertens-Talcott, and S. T. Talcott, "Urinary Metabolites from Mango (*Mangifera indica* L. cv. Keitt) Galloyl Derivatives and *In Vitro* Hydrolysis of Gallotannins in Physiological Conditions," *Mol. Nutr. Food Res.*, vol. 60, no. 3, pp. 542–550, 2016, doi: 10.1002/mnfr.201500706.
71. J. Burns, P. D. Fraser, and P. M. Bramley, "Identification and Quantification of Carotenoids, Tocopherols and Chlorophylls in Commonly Consumed Fruits and Vegetables," *Phytochemistry*, vol. 62,

no. 6, pp. 939–947, Mar. 2003, doi: 10.1016/S0031-9422(02)00710-0.

72. E. Rinninella et al., "The Role of Diet, Micronutrients and the Gut Microbiota in Age-Related Macular Degeneration: New Perspectives from the Gut–Retina Axis," *Nutrients*, vol. 10, no. 11, p. 11, Nov. 2018, doi: 10.3390/nu10111677.
73. D. Magnuson et al., "Supplemental Microalgal Astaxanthin Produced Coordinated Changes in Intrinsic Antioxidant Systems of Layer Hens Exposed to Heat Stress," *Algal Res.*, vol. 33, pp. 84–90, Jul. 2018, doi: 10.1016/j.algal.2018.04.031.
74. H. Liu et al., "Astaxanthin Prevents Alcoholic Fatty Liver Disease by Modulating Mouse Gut Microbiota," *Nutrients*, vol. 10, no. 9, p. 9, Sep. 2018, doi: 10.3390/nu10091298.
75. M. Bennedsen, X. Wang, R. Willén, T. Wadström, and L. P. Andersen, "Treatment of H. Pylori Infected Mice with Antioxidant Astaxanthin Reduces Gastric Inflammation, Bacterial Load and Modulates Cytokine Release by Splenocytes," *Immunol. Lett.*, vol. 70, no. 3, pp. 185–189, Dec. 2000, doi: 10.1016/S0165-2478(99)00145-5.
76. K. M. Tuohy, L. Conterno, M. Gasperotti, and R. Viola, "Up-regulating the Human Intestinal Microbiome Using Whole Plant Foods, Polyphenols, and/or Fiber," *J. Agric. Food Chem.*, vol. 60, no. 36, pp. 8776–8782, Sep. 2012, doi: 10.1021/jf2053959.
77. M. W. Bourassa, I. Alim, S. J. Bultman, and R. R. Ratan, "Butyrate, Neuroepigenetics and the Gut Microbiome: Can a High Fiber Diet Improve Brain Health?," *Neurosci. Lett.*, vol. 625, pp. 56–63, Jun. 2016, doi: 10.1016/j.neulet.2016.02.009.
78. C. Dominianni et al., "Sex, Body Mass Index, and Dietary Fiber Intake Influence the Human Gut Microbiome," *PLoS One*, vol. 10, no. 4, p. e0124599, Apr. 2015, doi: 10.1371/journal.pone.0124599.
79. D. Holscher, J. G. Caporaso, S. Hooda, J. M. Brulc, G. C. Fahey, and K. S. Swanson, "Fiber Supplementation Influences Phylogenetic Structure and Functional Capacity of the Human Intestinal Microbiome: Follow-Up of a Randomized Controlled Trial," *Am. J. Clin. Nutr.*, vol. 101, no. 1, pp. 55–64, Jan. 2015, doi: 10.3945/ajcn.114.092064.
80. M. Albouery et al., "Soluble Fiber Inulin Consumption Limits Alterations of the Gut Microbiota and Hepatic Fatty Acid Metabolism

Caused by High-Fat Diet," *Nutrients*, vol. 13, no. 3, p. 1037, Mar. 2021, doi: 10.3390/nu13031037.

81. C. Ma et al., "Gut Microbiome-Mediated Bile Acid Metabolism Regulates Liver Cancer via NKT Cells," *Science*, vol. 360, no. 6391, p. eaan5931, May 2018, doi: 10.1126/science.aan5931.
82. K. Makki, E. C. Deehan, J. Walter, and F. Bäckhed, "The Impact of Dietary Fiber on Gut Microbiota in Host Health and Disease," *Cell Host Microbe*, vol. 23, no. 6, pp. 705–715, Jun. 2018, doi: 10.1016/j.chom.2018.05.012.
83. W. Zhang et al., "Vegetable Based Dietary Pattern and Liver Cancer Risk: Results from the Shanghai Women's and Men's Health Studies," *Cancer Sci.*, vol. 104, no. 10, pp. 1353–1361, Oct. 2013, doi: 10.1111/cas.12231.
84. W. Yang et al., "Association of Intake of Whole Grains and Dietary Fiber with Risk of Hepatocellular Carcinoma in US Adults," *JAMA Oncol.*, vol. 5, no. 6, pp. 879–886, Jun. 2019, doi: 10.1001/jamaoncol.2018.7159.
85. L. R. Ferguson and M. Philpott, "Cancer Prevention by Dietary Bioactive Components That Target the Immune Response," *Curr. Cancer Drug Targets*, vol. 7, no. 5, pp. 459–464, Aug. 2007, doi: 10.2174/156800907781386605.
86. S. K. Bøhn, R. Blomhoff, and I. Paur, "Coffee and Cancer Risk, Epidemiological Evidence, and Molecular Mechanisms," *Mol. Nutr. Food Res.*, vol. 58, no. 5, pp. 915–930, 2014, doi: 10.1002/mnfr.201300526.
87. M. Larrosa, A. González-Sarrías, M. T. García-Conesa, F. A. Tomás-Barberán, and J. C. Espín, "Urolithins, Ellagic Acid-Derived Metabolites Produced by Human Colonic Microflora, Exhibit Estrogenic and Antiestrogenic Activities," *J. Agric. Food Chem.*, vol. 54, no. 5, pp. 1611–1620, Mar. 2006, doi: 10.1021/jf0527403.
88. A. Costabile et al., "Whole-Grain Wheat Breakfast Cereal Has a Prebiotic Effect on the Human Gut Microbiota: A Double-Blind, Placebo-Controlled, Crossover Study," *Br. J. Nutr.*, vol. 99, no. 1, pp. 110–120, Jan. 2008, doi: 10.1017/S0007114507793923.
89. Y. Yang et al., "Increased Intake of Vegetables, But Not Fruit, Reduces Risk for Hepatocellular Carcinoma: A Meta-Analysis," *Gastroenterology*,

vol. 147, no. 5, pp. 1031–1042, Nov. 2014, doi: 10.1053/j.gastro.2014.08.005.

90. P. Wongkrasant et al., “A Prebiotic Fructo-Oligosaccharide Promotes Tight Junction Assembly in Intestinal Epithelial Cells via an AMPK-Dependent Pathway,” *Biomed. Pharmacother.*, vol. 129, p. 110415, Sep. 2020, doi: 10.1016/j.biopha.2020.110415.
91. J. Wang, S. Tian, H. Yu, J. Wang, and W. Zhu, “Response of Colonic Mucosa-Associated Microbiota Composition, Mucosal Immune Homeostasis, and Barrier Function to Early Life Galactooligosaccharides Intervention in Suckling Piglets,” *J. Agric. Food Chem.*, vol. 67, no. 2, pp. 578–588, Jan. 2019, doi: 10.1021/acs.jafc.8b05679.
92. U. Etxeberria, A. Fernández-Quintela, F. I. Milagro, L. Aguirre, J. A. Martínez, and M. P. Portillo, “Impact of Polyphenols and Polyphenol-Rich Dietary Sources on Gut Microbiota Composition,” *J. Agric. Food Chem.*, vol. 61, no. 40, pp. 9517–9533, Oct. 2013, doi: 10.1021/jf402506c.
93. D. S. Mandair, R. E. Rossi, M. Pericleous, T. Whyand, and M. Caplin, “The Impact of Diet and Nutrition in the Prevention and Progression of Hepatocellular Carcinoma,” *Expert Rev. Gastroenterol. Hepatol.*, vol. 8, no. 4, pp. 369–382, May 2014, doi: 10.1586/17474124.2014.894879.
94. H. C. Lee, A. M. Jenner, C. S. Low, and Y. K. Lee, “Effect of Tea Phenolics and Their Aromatic Fecal Bacterial Metabolites on Intestinal Microbiota,” *Res. Microbiol.*, vol. 157, no. 9, pp. 876–884, Nov. 2006, doi: 10.1016/j.resmic.2006.07.004.
95. H. S. Kim, S. Kacew, and B. M. Lee, “In Vitro Chemopreventive Effects of Plant Polysaccharides (*Aloe barbadensis* Miller, *Lentinus edodes, Ganoderma lucidum* and *Coriolus versicolor*),” *Carcinogenesis*, vol. 20, no. 8, pp. 1637–1640, Aug. 1999, doi: 10.1093/carcin/20.8.1637.
96. X. Bao, C. Liu, J. Fang, and X. Li, “Structural and Immunological Studies of a Major Polysaccharide from Spores of *Ganoderma lucidum* (Fr.) Karst,” *Carbohydr. Res.*, vol. 332, no. 1, pp. 67–74, May 2001, doi: 10.1016/S0008-6215(01)00075-1.
97. D.-W. Zong, C.-Y. Guo, H.-T. Cheng, H.-T. Hu, J.-C. Xiao, and H.-L. Li, “Influence of Lactulose on Interventional Therapy for HCC Patients

with Hepatocirrhosis and Hypersplenism," *Asian Pac. J. Trop. Med.*, vol. 9, no. 2, pp. 193–196, Feb. 2016, doi: 10.1016/j.apjtm.2016.01.011.

98. G. Ecklu-Mensah, J. Gilbert, and S. Devkota, "Dietary Selection Pressures and Their Impact on the Gut Microbiome," *Cell. Mol. Gastroenterol. Hepatol.*, vol. 13, no. 1, pp. 7–18, Jan. 2022, doi: 10.1016/j.jcmgh.2021.07.009.

https://doi.org/10.1142/9789811293320_0011

Chapter 11

Emerging Role of Plant-Derived Products in Immunotherapy: Plausible Exposition for HCC Treatment

Ayana R Kumar[1,2,#], SA Ajay[1,2,#], K Anusha[1,2,#], Bhagyalakshmi Nair[1,2], Aswathy R Devan[1,2], Gautam Sethi[3,*], and Lekshmi R Nath[1,*]

[1]*Department of Pharmacognosy, Amrita School of Pharmacy, Amrita Vishwa Vidyapeetham, AIMS Health Sciences Campus, Kochi-682 041, India*
[2]*Department of Pharmacology, Amrita School of Pharmacy, Amrita Vishwa Vidyapeetham, AIMS Health Sciences Campus, Kochi-682 041, India*
[3]*Department of Pharmacology, Yong Loo Lin School of Medicine, National University of Singapore, Singapore*
[#]*Equally contributed (first authors)*

Table of Contents:

*Corresponding authors: E-mail address: lekshmirnath@aims.amrita.edu; phcgs@nus.edu.sg

Abbreviations:

ACT — Adoptive cell therapy
AES — Adverse events
AFP — Alpha feto-protein
APC — Antigen-presenting cells
BCMA — B cell maturation antigen
CAR-T — Chimeric Antigen Receptor-T
CCl-19 — Chemokine CC motif ligand 19
CD — Cluster differentiation
CD133 — Cluster of differentiation 133
CDR — Complementary decision regions
CEA — Carcinoembryonic antigen
cGAS — Cyclic GMP-AMP synthase
CHOP — C/EBP homologous protein
CMV — Cucumber mosaic virus

CpG-ODN — Cytosine-phosphorothioate-guanine oligodeoxynucleotides
CRES — CAR-T cell-associated encephalopathy syndrome
CRS — Cytokine release syndrome
CT — Cryptotanshinon
CTL — Cytotoxic T lymphocytes
CTLA-4 — Cytotoxic T lymphocyte-associated protein-4
DC — Dendritic cells
DCR — Disease control rate
DNA — Deoxyribonucleic acid
DOR — Duration of response
EpCAM — Epithelial cellular adhesion molecule
GPC-3 — Glypican-3
HBV — Hepatitis B virus
HCC — Hepatocellular carcinoma
HCV — Hepatitis C virus
HDV — hepatitis D virus
HepG2 — Hepatoblastoma cell line
HVR1 — Hypervariable region
ICI — Immune checkpoint inhibitors
IFN — interferon
IgG — Immunoglobulin G
IKK — IκB kinase
IL — Interleukin
irAEs — Immune-related adverse reactions
LBP — *Lycium barbarum* polysaccharide
LNP-mRNA — Lipid nanoparticle mRNA
MAPK ERK — Mitogen-activated protein kinase family extracellular signal-regulated Protein kinase
MHC — Major histocompatibility complex
MMP-9 — Matrix metalloproteinase
mRNA — Messenger ribonucleic acid
MUC-1 — Mucin-1
NF — Nuclear factor
NFAT — Nuclear factor of activated T cells
NK — Natural killer cells

NKG-20 T cells — Natural killer group 2D
NSG — NOD-SCID-gamma mouse
ORR — Objective response rate
OS — Overall survival
PD-1 — Programmed cell death protein-1
PD-L1 — Programmed death ligand-1
PEG — Polyethylene glycol
PEG-IFN — PEGylated interferon
PI3K-Mtor — Protein kinase
RFS — Recurrence-free survival
ROBO-1 — Roundabout homolog-1
STAT3 — Signal transducer and activator of transcription 3
TCR — T cell receptor
TCR-T — T cell receptor-engineered T cells
TGF-β — Tumor growth factor
TIL — Tumor-infiltrating lymphocytes
TKI — Tyrosine kinase inhibitors
TME — Tumor microenvironment
Tregs — Regulatory T cells
TSA — Tumor-specific antigens
VEGF — Vascular endothelium growth factor
VEGFR — Vascular endothelium growth factor receptor
WT-1 — Wilms tumor-1

Abstract

Hepatocellular carcinoma (HCC) remains a major global healthcare challenge, with a predictable incidence of greater than 1 million cases by 2025. HCC is commonly detected at an advanced stage, and a limited range of treatment modalities are available, where oral multi-kinase inhibitor Sorafenib is considered a main systemic first-line treatment option. Nevertheless, the clinical utility of Sorafenib is limited because of its severe drug-related side effects and early emergence of drug resistance. Nowadays, immunotherapies including immune checkpoint inhibitors, adoptive cell therapy (CAR-T cells), therapeutic cancer vaccines, engineered cytokines, and so on have been used to tackle the advanced HCC. However, the activation of immune suppressive signals in the tumor milieu can hinder the success of cancer immunotherapy. More recently, plant-based products have been extended to comprise cancer immunotherapy agents. In this clinical setting, combining plant-based products with existing immunotherapies may improve the effectiveness of immunotherapies against HCC. In this book chapter, we have emphasized the possible role of plant-based products as an affordable, effective, more scalable, versatile, speedy, and safer repository of immune modulatory agents. In this chapter, we have also investigated the plausible combinatorial effect of plant-based products with established immunotherapies against HCC.

1. Introduction

HCC remains a major global healthcare challenge with a predictable incidence of more than 1 million annual cases by 2025 [1]. Over 70% of HCC cases are identified later in life, usually when treatment is no longer possible [2]. The primary risk factors for the development and the progression of HCC are chronic infection with hepatitis B virus (HBV), hepatitis C virus (HCV), hepatitis delta virus (HDV) and double or triple chronic infection with HBV and HCV, prolonged heavy alcohol consumption, liver cirrhosis, chronic ingestion of aflatoxin-contaminated foodstuffs, smoking, obesity, and type II diabetes [3]. Advanced-stage diagnosis and unavailability of curative treatment options result in a poor prognosis of HCC [4]. Tyrosine kinase inhibitor (TKI) Sorafenib is the first-line drug used for advanced HCC [5]. Lenvatinib, Regorafinib, and Cabozantinib are also used as second-line therapeutic options for HCC [6]. But, TKIs produce serious adverse effects like systemic hypertension, facial erythema, and so on [7]. Moreover, the clinical evidence suggests that the effectiveness of Sorafenib is hampered by drug resistance. The immune components present in the tumor microenvironment (TME) play a significant role in triggering Sorafenib resistance, and Sorafenib or any other approved TKIs do not address the immune evasion in the tumor milieu in the progression of HCC. The TME in the HCC is an ecosystem comprising a variety of immune cells that play an essential role in tumor initiation, progression, and distant metastasis [8]. Thus, targeting tumor-associating immune cells and proteins by the use of immunotherapies might be a promising approach to overcome the therapeutic obstacles in HCC [9].

1.1. *Immune evasion in hepatic tumor microenvironment*

Immunomodulation is co-regulated by the adaptive and innate immune around the TME, and the immunotherapies have been developed for activating the immune-mediated signaling pathways, for inhibit carcinogenesis [10]. Cancer cells attain evasion from immune surveillance by creating an immunosuppressive tumor microenvironment [11]. An immunosuppressive tumor microenvironment (TME) is achieved by the accumulation of inhibitory B cells, elevated levels of tolerogenic enzymes, increased levels of M2 polarized tumor-associated macrophages, increased levels of regulatory T cells, upregulate the expression of immune checkpoint receptors and their corresponding ligands on T cell and antigen-presenting cells (APC), respectively, and so on [10, 12]. The adaptive and innate immunities are suppressed in HCC patients due to the dysfunctional tumor-infiltrating lymphocytes (TIL) and natural killer cells (NK), and this will reduce the level of cytotoxic T cells in the tumor milieu and cause cancer progression [9]. In this context, targeting strategies by modulating the immune responses in the TME will help to hamper the immune evasion and produce more therapeutic effects with minimal side effects [13, 14].

2. Current Trends in Immunotherapy Against HCC

Immunotherapy is a well-established treatment modality, and it is identified as a "fifth pillar" of cancer therapy. Immunotherapy includes a wide range of treatment strategies comprising immune checkpoint inhibitors (ICIs), adoptive cell therapy, HCC vaccines, oncolytic virus therapies, and so on to inhibit HCC progression and metastasis [15].

2.1. *Immune checkpoint inhibitors (ICIs)*

The prime immunotherapeutic option against HCC is ICIs, which include monoclonal antibodies that can block the interactions of programmed cell death protein-1 (PD-1) or programmed death ligand-1 (PD-L1) and cytotoxic T lymphocyte-associated protein-4 (CTLA-4) present on the surface of activated T cells and APC. Studies also indicated that the combinations of ICIs are also beneficial for effective HCC therapy [16]. The treatment strategy with anti-PD-1-antibodies restricts the escape mechanism of T cells and retains the active T cells in the TME to combat cancer cells. The novelty of the sophisticated treatment modality is that, unlike conventional chemotherapy and molecular targeted therapy, these monoclonal antibodies can activate the body's immune system and produce natural anticancer immune responses against cancer cells. Anti-PD-L1-antibodies have similar actions to PD-1-antibodies. PD-L1 overexpression is a marker of tumor aggressiveness [17]. The CTLA-4 protein is over-expressed on regulatory T cells (Tregs) that are present in the tumor milieu, and it activates the signaling pathways that take place exclusively within lymph nodes. Thus, the CTLA-4 modifies the proliferation of activated lymphocytes. In contrast to PD-1, CTLA-4 is over-expressed on Tregs which can inactivate the actions of effector T cells *via* several mechanisms [18]. Inhibition of the immune checkpoints recovers the antitumor immune response. Nivolumab was the first ICI approved by the FDA in 2017 against advanced HCC [19]. Later on, another immune checkpoint inhibitor, Pembrolizumab, was approved in 2018 [20]. Nivolumab and Pembrolizumab are PD-L1 inhibitors that are reported to possess better tumor suppression in alone and also in combination with other ICIs and TKIs against HCC [21, 22]. Tremelimumab (CP-675,206) is a fully human IgG2 monoclonal antibody (mAb) that can restrict the interaction of CTLA-4 with the corresponding ligand [23, 24]. In 2020 National Medical Products Administration (NMPA) approved Camrelizumab as the second-line treatment for advanced HCC. A multicenter, phase-II clinical study (NCT02989922) was conducted in 2019 by Professor Qin Shukui in 220 patients with advanced stage of HCC. This clinical study revealed that the safety of Camrelizumab was similar to Pembrolizumab and

Nivolumab [25]. Tislelizumab is a humanized IgG4 anti-PD-1 monoclonal antibody independently developed in China [26]. It binds to PD-1 with great affinity and specificity and has high T cell activation. Tislelizumab monotherapy can produce a prolonged anti-tumor effect and patients showed good tolerance [27]. Durvalumab is an anti-PD-L1 type humanized monoclonal antibody that targets PD-L1. A phase-I-II clinical study was conducted on Durvalumab in the treatment of advanced HCC patients who failed to receive Sorafenib. [28] (Table 1).

2.2. *Dual therapies combining ICIs with anti-VEGF antibodies*

PD1/PD-L1 inhibitor with vascular endothelium growth factor (VEGF) inhibition has been developed as a new combination therapy for the treatment of advanced HCC. Atezolizumab-Bevacizumab combination in patients with untreated advanced HCC shows better safety and promising antitumor activity than Sorafenib, as the combination immunotherapy decreased the risk of death by 42%. This combinatorial approach also inhibits the VEGF-mediated immunosuppression and encourages T cell infiltration, and PD-L1 inhibition, and produces an anticancer immune response via T-effector cells [29]. A clinical study revealed that the combination of Atezolizumab (PD-L1 inhibitor) and Bevacizumab (anti-VEGF) enhances the anti-tumor immune response and also increases the survival rate with a tolerable safety profile [30]. The combination of Levatinib (multiple tyrosine kinase inhibitor of VEGFR1–3) with Pembrolizumab (anti-PD-L1 antibody) produced promising antitumor effect. [31]. Thus, the combination of VEGF inhibitors with ICIs can prevent the immunosuppressive TME and increase the antitumor immune response.

2.3. *Adoptive cell therapy*

Adoptive cell therapy (ACT) is currently used for treating patients with advanced HCC cases who are not responding to systematic therapies [32]. ACT is achieved by infusing autologous or allogenic immune cells to patients [33]. Various ACT therapies involve Chimeric Antigen Receptor (CAR)-NK, CAR-T, T cell receptor (TCR) therapy. Among these, CAR-T cell treatments have proven efficacy against HCC and are the most important ACT treatment currently in use [34]. ACT consists of a carrier CAR and an activated adjuvant cell. CAR cells have three domains which include extracellular structural domain, intracellular structural domain and transmembrane structural domain [35]. Antigen recognition and binding sites are present on extracellular domain whereas the trans-membrane and intracellular domain involves in activity enhancement and co-stimulation, respectively [32]. CAR-T cells are classified mainly into four classes, namely first, second, third, and fourth generation. First-generation CAR-T cells had an extracellular domain integrated with CD30 alone and possessed poor immunogenicity and proliferative capacity [36]. Second-generation CAR-T cells possess continuous proliferation due to the incorporation of co-stimulatory receptors [37]. Third-generation CAR-T cells provide longer protection and better antitumor efficacy due to the incorporation of two co-stimulatory signals [38]. In comparison to second- and third-generation CAR's, the fourth generation incorporates nuclear factor of activated T cells (NFAT). It attempts to control tumor mesenchyme by inhibiting the release of Treg cells and downregulating the immunosuppressive effects of cytokines like TGF-β and secreting cytokines like IL-12 and IL-18 [39].

2.3.1. *CAR-T therapy*

The term CAR-T refers to the genetic engineering methods of modifying T cells by inserting CARs into them using plasmids or viruses. The goal of the CAR-T cells is to stimulate the host defense system that the body naturally produces using T cells. The T cells can target particular tumor antigens with the help of chimeric molecules known as chimeric antigen receptors (CARs) [40]. Various preclinical and clinical studies have confirmed anticancer efficacy of CAR-T therapy, and US-FDA has approved six CAR-T therapies for treating different malignancies which include various lymphoma, acute B cell lymphocytic leukemia and multiple myeloma targeting B cell maturation antigen (BCMA) and CD19 [41]. Systemic toxicity associated with CAR-T therapy which includes neurotoxicity, cytokine release syndrome (CRS), CAR-T cell-associated encephalopathy syndrome (CRES) which limits its clinical translation [32]. The heterogenicity of solid tumors in liver cancer coupled with immunosuppressive microenvironment and lack of tumor-specific antigens (TSA) limits the utility of CAR-T cells against HCC [42]. Currently the tumor targets such as alpha feto-protein (AFP), cluster of differentiation 133 (CD133), glypican-3 (GPC-3), mucin-1 (MUC-1), carcinoembryonic antigen (CEA), and CD-147 are explored for their anticancer effects against HCC in preclinical and clinical studies [43].

GPC-3 is an oncofetal proteoglycan that plays a vital role in development and growth of the cell [44]. GPC-3 is highly expressed in the organs of an embryo and numerous studies reported that, expression of GPC-3 in adults may cause the development of various cancers, particularly in HCC [45]. An *in-vitro* study conducted by Gao et al. reports for the first time that GPC-3 targeted CAR-T treatment possesses potent antitumor effects against HCC, and the results were further confirmed by an *in-vivo* study which reported a direct correlation between antitumor effect of GPC-3 expression on HCC tumors [46]. Preliminary phase-I studies have reported the clinical safety and efficacy of CAR-GPC3 treatment [47]. Another *in-vivo* study utilizing patient-derived HCC model reports higher anticancer potency of CAR-GPC3 treatment with decreased expression of PD-L1, suggesting that CAR-GPC3 treatment on combination with ICI might produce a better anticancer potency against HCC [48]. CAR-GPC3 can produce high levels of cytokines which can enhance antitumor efficacy and accelerate CAR-T cell maturation. It can also leverage the immunomodulatory properties of cytokines to produce a dual antitumor effect [49]. A recent phase-I clinical study utilizing CAR-GPC3 T treatment secreting IL-7 and CCL19 cytokines reports better anticancer effects and complete tumor disappearance upon intratumor injection [50]. The study concludes that both CCL19 and IL-7 enhanced CAR-T cell survival and T cell infiltrate. Various preclinical and clinical studies are further exploring CAR-GPC3 T treatment incorporation of various chemokines.

AFP is another glycoprotein like GPC3 that is mainly expressed in fetus, and various HCC tumors have been identified to express AFP [51]. Few studies have explored the clinical applications of AFP-CAR-T treatment [33]. Preclinical studies involving *in-vivo* studies have reported the antitumor efficacy of AFP-CAR-T treatment against HCC [52, 53]. A phase-I clinical study on AFP-expressed HCC patients demonstrated the clinical safety of AFP-CAR-T treatment [54].

CD133 is a pentameric glycoprotein whose expression in solid tumors has been correlated to poor prognosis and tumor malignancy in HCC [55]. A phase-I clinical study conducted on CD133 expressed advanced HCC patients reports a 65.2% disease control rate and tumor shrinkage in few patients [56]. Another phase-II clinical study on advanced HCC patients demonstrated 12 months of median survival rate and 6.8 months of progression-free survival after CAR-CD133-T cell therapy [57].

2.3.2. *TCR-engineered T cell (TCR-T)*

T cells are immune cells present in the body naturally and have antitumor properties. All T cells express the T cell receptor which is a member of the immunoglobulin superfamily [58]. The major histocompatibility complex (MHC) can be specifically recognized by TCR-T cells, which are created by introducing the foreign TCR genes into T cells [59]. TCR-T cells can target both the intracellular and tumor-surface antigens as all tumor-derived proteins are susceptible to proteasomal processing and MHC presentation [60]. TCR strands consist of a constant region structural domain and a variable region structural domain [61]. There are three complementary decision regions (CDRs) in each structural domain. Through CDRs, TCRs with antigen specificity are built to control T cell development. TCRs form complexes with numerous CD3 dimers that have intracellular signaling capabilities because T cells lack intracellular signaling components [62]. The interaction of TCRs with MHC leads to the activation of T cells and produces antitumor immune response [63]. Currently AFP and virus-associated peptides are mainly targeted using TCR studies [64]. Multifunctional HBV-specific TCR-T cells are developed, and their safety and efficacy are evaluated in a phase-I clinical study (NCT02686372) [65]. Another phase-I study conducted on eight patients reported some adverse effects but concluded that HBV-specific TCR-T is well tolerated and safe [66].

AFP-specific TCR-T cells have been developed and studied against HCC. Various studies have reported that AFP-targeted TCR has low toxicity [67]. An *in-vivo* study has reported the anti-HCC effects of AFP158-specific TCR-T cells against HEPG2 cells in NSG mice model [68]. By using alanine scanning (X-scan) to screen specific clinical TCR candidates, any possibility of the chosen TCRs reacting negatively with the candidate proteins was removed. For the treatment of patients with HCC, preliminary clinical trials using this TCR-T cell have been started (NCT03971747) [54].

2.4. *Therapeutic cancer vaccines*

The therapeutic cancer vaccination is an immunotherapy that stimulates the patient's immune system to combat cancer by introducing tumor antigens in a variety of forms and overcome the tumor's immunosuppressive microenvironment [69]. DNA vaccines, dendritic cell vaccines, mRNA vaccines, peptide vaccines, and viral vector-based vaccines are the major therapeutic cancer vaccines used against HCC [70].

2.4.1. *Dendtritic cell vaccines*

Dendritic cells (DCs) are the strongest APCs in the human immune system. They are essential for both innate immunity activation and cytotoxic T lymphocyte (CTL)-mediated adaptive immunity induction [71]. Because of its expertise in presenting antigens to T cells, dendritic cells are essential for both triggering and controlling immune responses. They function as APCs to T cells. [72, 73]. As a result, the T cells produce an attack on the tumor with a specific immunological response.

A phase-I clinical study with a total of 18 participants analyzed the anticancer effects of AFP-primed DC vaccine and reported positive for immunogenicity with well-tolerated side effects (NCT01974661) [74]. Another phase-I study explored the safety and feasibility of autologous DC vaccine and reported that the treatment is well tolerated with a reduction in tumor markers in two patients upon vaccination [75]. A phase-II study reported the safety of HepG2 cell lysate-pulsed DC vaccine with a disease control rate of 28% [76]. Another phase-II study explored the safety and therapeutic efficacy of personalized DC vaccine pulsed with neoantigens combined with surgical resection and CTL infusion (NCT03067493). The study reports that the treatment was well tolerated with no tumor recurrence in 50% of study subjects for a period of 2 years [77]. The study also concludes that disease-free survival rates are higher for subjects who developed an immune reaction than for those who did not develop any, and the latter group is found to possess tumor recurrence [77]. Currently, clinical studies are exploring the therapeutic efficacy of combinatorial treatment with DC vaccine to produce a potent and well-tolerated treatment option.

2.4.2. *DNA vaccine*

DNA vaccine consist of tumor-specific antigen-encoded plasmids that are introduced into the patient's body and exhibit an immune response against cancer cells that exhibit the specific antigen corresponding to the vaccine [78]. The immunogenicity and safety of GPC-3 encoded DNA vaccine is analyzed in a phase-1 study (NCT01828762) [79]. The study reports that the vaccine exhibited a potent anticancer effect against HCC and is well tolerated in patients [79]. Another phase-1 study exploring the anticancer effect of HCV antigen-encoded DNA vaccine reported a modest anticancer effect, and the treatment is well tolerated [80]. Further studies are ongoing with the incorporation of various neoantigens and combinational therapy with ICI (NCT04251117) [81].

2.4.3. *Peptide vaccine*

Peptides can act as immune system antigens. Peptide-based vaccinations have a high specificity, which lowers the possibility of autoimmune reactions and off-target effects. Additionally, their production is rather simple, and safety assessments show generally favorable results [82]. GPC-3, AFP, Wilms tumor-1 (WT-1), round about homolog-1 (ROBO-1) are the most commonly targeted peptides for producing vaccines [83]. A phase-1 clinical study reported the safety and immunogenicity of the GPC-3 peptide vaccine [84]. The study also reports that the vaccine is well tolerated with a reduction in tumor biomarkers and produces a better overall survival rate [84]. Another phase-1 study explored the therapeutic efficacy of a combined vaccine which includes AFP, tumor-associated antigens, melanoma-associated gene A1, and human telomerase reverse transcriptase. The study reports no vaccine-specific adverse immune reaction occurred and the treatment was well tolerated [85]. There are several obstacles in the way of clinical translation of peptide-based vaccines, despite encouraging results. One obstacle is the considerable clonal heterogeneity of the tumor, which permits certain cancer cells lacking the target antigen to evade immune recognition. To maximize the overall anticancer effect, researchers advise combining peptide-based vaccinations with other immune-based therapies, such as immune checkpoint inhibitors [86]. More research is therefore required to address tumor heterogeneity, improve these vaccines, and create potent combination therapies.

2.4.4. *mRNA vaccines*

RNA tumor vaccines are prepared and injected into the body using translated protein template messenger RNA (mRNA). The protein synthesis machinery of human cells produces specific antigen proteins, which are then utilized to trigger the body's immune system to attack tumor cells [87]. AFP mRNA vaccine, neoantigen mRNA vaccine, and ICI mRNA vaccine are the major mRNA vaccines currently being investigated against HCC [88]. Studies reported that the LNP-mRNA vaccine targeting various tumor antigens exhibits antitumor effects against HCC [89]. Currently, two phase-1 trials are investigating the therapeutic efficacy of mRNA vaccine against HBV-related HCC (NCT05738447) (NCT05738447). As mRNA-based vaccination research for HCC is still in its infancy, more studies and clinical trials will be required to assess the vaccines' safety, effectiveness, and clinical usefulness in HCC patients.

2.5. *Role of engineered cytokines in the management of HCC*

Cytokines are essential elements of the immune system that are vital to the immune system's reaction against cancer. The use of cytokines in the treatment of cancer has a lot of attention in recent decades because of its promising therapeutic benefits [90]. Interleukin-2 (IL-2) is a pleiotropic and multifunctional cytokine that is essential for adaptive immune systems that play an essential role in T cell activation and function [91, 92]. The IFN-α is also used to treat HCC with diverse backgrounds. The effect of adjuvant IFN-α on postoperative recurrence varied between HBV-HCC and HCV-HCC cases [93]. Another meta-analysis examined the impact of adjuvant PEGylated interferon (PEG-IFN) therapy on patients' survival following curative treatment for hepatitis-related HCC. The adjuvant PEG-IFN therapy could enhance overall survival (OS) and recurrence-free survival (RFS) in patients with hepatitis-related HCC [94, 95] (Tables 1 and 2) (Figure 1).

3. Plausible Role of Plant-Based Products as an Immunotherapeutic Agent

Plant-based compounds are being progressively acknowledged as a potent complementary therapy for different cancers [114]. Several studies demonstrated that effective modulation of the tumor microenvironment (TME) using phytochemicals will help to increase the efficiency of immunotherapies against HCC. Nowadays plant-based natural products are used as combinational therapies of HCC with conventional chemotherapeutic agents [115]. Studies revealed that the combination of immunotherapy with plant-based products may

Table 1: Clinical trial results of immune checkpoint inhibitors in hepatocellular carcinoma

Treatment	Target	Trial Name	Phase	Sample Size	ORR (%)	DCR (%)	DOR (months)	Grade 3/4 AEs(%)	Result	Reference
Tremelim-umab	CTLA-4	NCT01008358	II	21	17.6	76.4	Not reported	Not reported	ICIs slightly alter the elevations of AT(alanine transaminase) levels with or without bilirubin.	[96]
Nivolumab	PD-1	NCT01658878	I/III	48	15	58	17	25	The report showed that Nivolumab had a feasible safety profile.	[97]
Durvalumab	PD-1	NCT01693562	I/II	40	10	32.5	Not reported	20	Recruitment is ongoing.	[98]
Camrelizumab	PD-1	NCT02989922	II	217	32	44.2	Not reported	22	Camrelizumab showed antitumor efficacy with tolerable toxicity.	[25]
Pembrolizumab	PD-1	NCT02702414	II	104	18	61	Not reported	24	The study reported that Pembrolizumab showed long-term effectiveness in patients who were previously treated with Sorafenib.	[99]
Tislelizumab	PD-1	NCT02407990	IA/B	50	12.2	51	Not reported	47.5	Teslelizumab was well tolerated, and anticancer activity was shown.	[100]

Combination of immune checkpoint inhibitors										
Durvalumab and Tremelimumab	PD-1 CTLA-4	NCT02519348	II	326	24	Not reported	Not reported	35.1	Report demonstrated that Durvalumab+ Tremelimumab combination gives the best risk-benefit profile.	[101]
Nivolumab and Ipilimumab	PD-1 CTLA-4	Checkmate 040, NCT01658878	I/II	148	39	41	17	37	Second-line Nivolumab+ Ipilimumab combination continued to show clinically significant responses and an advantage for long-term survival.	[102]
Combination with anti-VEGF and TKI										
Atezolizumab and bevacizumab	PD-1 VEGF	NCT03434379	III	336	26.7	73.6	Not reported	56.5	Bevacizumab plus Atezolizumab combination results in a longer progression-free survival than Atezolizumab alone.	[103]
Avelumab and Axitinib	PD-1 VEGF	NCT03289533	I	22	13.8	68.2	Not reported	Not reported	Patients with HCC who received treatment with Avelumab plus Axitinib reported a tolerable safety profile and antitumor efficacy.	[104]

(*Continued*)

Table 1: (*Continued*)

Treatment	Target	Trial Name	Phase	Sample Size	ORR (%)	DCR (%)	DOR (months)	Grade 3/4 AEs(%)	Result	Reference
Durvalumab–ramucirumab	PD-1 VEGF	NCT02572687	IB	28	11	69	Not reported	Not reported	Combination does not find any unexpected safety signal.	[105]
Pembrolizumab and Levantinib	PD-1 TKI	NCT03006926	IB	104	46	86	8.6	67	Pembrolizumab and Levantinib combination showed promising antitumor activity with acceptable safety profile.	[106]
Nivolumab and Cabozanitib	PD-1 TKI	NCT03299946	I	15	Not reported	Not reported	Not reported	67	These combinations were feasible and resulted in long-term survival.	[107]

ORR = objective response rate, DCR = disease control rate, DOR = duration of response, AES=adverse events

Table 2: Clinical study details of adoptive T cell therapies (CAR-T and TCR therapies)

Serial No	Treatment	Intervention	Phase	Clinical Trial No	Result	Reference
1	GPC3	CAR-T	1	NCT02395250	• Serum AFP and GPC-3 are reduced • The patients showed a 5-year disease-free survival • CTCs and image visible lesions are eliminated by CAR-T therapy	[108]
2	GPC3	CAR-T	1	NCT03884751	Result not published	
3	GPC3	CAR-T	1	NCT03146234	• Survival rate of 50.3% is reported for a duration of 6 months • The systemic adverse effects associated with CAR-T treatment were reversible	[47]
3	GPC3	CAR-T	1	NCT03980288	• The disease control rate is reported to be 50% • Median progression-free survival upto 4.2 months.	[109]
4	GPC3, RUNX-3	CAR-T	1	NCT03980288	• CT017 shows manageable safety profile and antitumor effects • Disease control rate of 50% and objective response rate of 16.7%	[110]
5	GPC3	CAR-T	1	NCT04951141	Ongoing	[111]

(*Continued*)

Table 2: (*Continued*)

Serial No	Treatment	Intervention	Phase	Clinical Trial No	Result	Reference
6	CD147	CAR-T	1	NCT03993743	Ongoing	[112]
7	HBV	TCR-T	1	NCT03899415	• Reduction in HBV DNA upon treatment • Treatment is safe and well tolerated	[66]
8	AFP	TCR-T	1	NCT04368182	Ongoing	[64]
9	AFP	TCR-T	1	NCT03132792	Result not published	[64]
10	HBV	TCR-T	1	NCT05417932	Safety and efficacy study ongoing	[113]

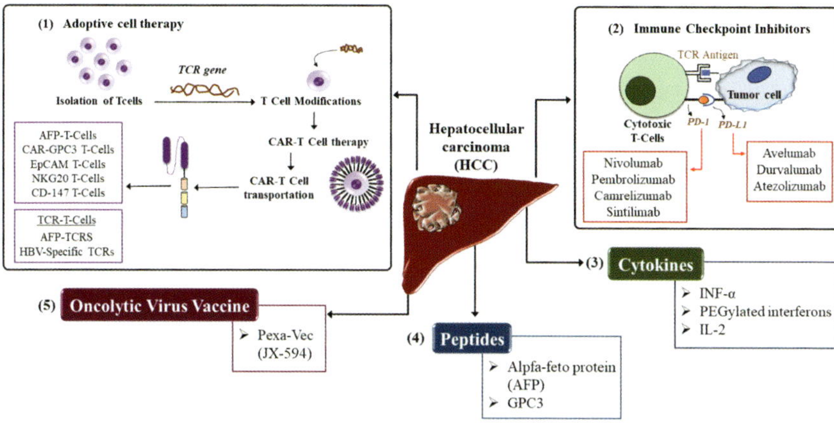

Figure 1: Current immunotherapies against hepatocellular carcinoma: Several immunotherapies such as immune checkpoint inhibitors (monoclonal antibodies of CTLA-4, PD-1 and PD-L1), adaptive cell therapy (CAR-T cells and TCR), therapeutic cancer vaccines (dendritic cell vaccines and peptide vaccine) and cytokines are used to tackle HCC

inhibit the development of cancer as well as also reduce the cancer progression through facilitating immune responses by modulating several signaling pathways [115, 116]. The combinatorial strategy of plant-derived natural products with immunotherapy persuades anticancer effects by restoring the immune recognition capacity of immune cells and causing antitumor immune response by regulating the immune function [117]. The studies also emphasized the importance of plant-derived products as a single treatment approach against HCC affordably and cost-effectively with minimal side effects [118]. More sophisticated techniques such as nanotechnology can be used to overcome the drawbacks of plant derived products to enhance their antitumor efficacy [115].

3.1. *Synergistic combination of plant-derived products with immunotherapies*

Icaritin is a prenylflavonoid isolated from the *Epimedium genus* plant, and it is widely used in traditional Chinese medicine as a tonic and energy-boosting agent [119]. The anticancer effect of Icaritin was studied in various cancers such as liver cancer, ovarian cancer, glioblastoma, and so on [120–122]. Two phase-3 clinical trials are also ongoing for the treatment of HCC (NCT03236636 and NCT03236649). Even though Icaritin is a promising antitumor agent, there have been limited studies on its immune checkpoint control activity. Mo et al. disclosed the possibility of Icaritin as an immune therapeutic agent against HCC. Icaritin abridged tumor cell proliferation and a combinatorial approach with anti-PD-1 monoclonal antibody elicits significant regulation on cancer cells. Additionally, Icaritin down-regulates the expression of PD-L1 by blocking/decreasing the complex formation of IκB kinase (IKK) and restricts the translocation of NF-κB p65, which acts as a promoter of PD-L1 [123]. Hence, Icaritin displays immune modulatory activities in HCC and can also normalize the expression of immune checkpoints in the TME and has great potential for synergistic treatment with ICI therapy.

Lycium barbarum polysaccharide (LBP) is isolated from the fruits of *Lycium barbarum* (wolfberry) [124]. Studies demonstrated that LBP in combination with cytokines such as CXCL10 can elicit an immune response against HCC. LBP endorses the release of Thl cytokines as well as helps to restore the balance of Thl/Th2. It also improves the production and function of dendritic cells (DCs) and increases the immune responses in the tumor-bearing bodies [125]. The combination of 10-hydroxycamptotenin and DC hepa-6 fusion vaccine can increase immune responses and prominently produce CTL cytotoxicity in HCC [126]. The report suggests that Vitamin C can increase the effectiveness of anti-PD-L1 antibodies in both *in-vitro* and *in-vivo*. The combination of Vitamin C with an anti-PD-L1 antibody can produce anti-angiogenesis effect via the normalization of the blood vessels that are present in the tumor milieu. This combination also improves the production and effectiveness of cytotoxic T cells in the TME via stimulating the cyclic GMP-AMP synthase (cGAS) and also increases the production of cGAMP. The activation of STING pathway of vascular endothelial cells will help to produce innate immune cells, which produce immune responses against cancer cells [127]. The immunosuppressant Cyclosporin A combined with Taxol upregulates the level of Caspase 9 and Caspase 3 in the TME, which facilitates the activation of PI3K-mTOR pathway and produces cancer cell apoptosis [128].

Cryptotanshinone (CT) known as Tanshinone C is a quinoid diterpene obtained from the roots of *Salvia miltiorrhiza* [48]. CT has clinical benefits for chronic diseases including Alzheimer's disease, blood and blood vessel-related disorders, and several cancers. Han Z et al. suggest that CT has an immune modulatory role in ICI therapy [129]. In preclinical settings, HCC-induced mice expressively reduce the cancer progression on CT and ICI combination. The combinational therapy of CT with anti-PD-L1 antibody significantly restricts tumor growth. The re-inoculation of the same tumor cells did not develop cancers; thus CT develops a long-term immunity around the tumor milieu. Additionally, the combined treatment of CT with ICI inhibitor against HCC amplified the secretion of tumor-infiltrating $CD8^+$ T cells and effector $CD8^+$ T cells from lymph nodes. Hence, CT is known as a potential synergetic phytoconstituent with ICI therapy for generating long-term tumor-specific immunity around TME [130].

3.2. *Plant-derived products: As a monotherapy against HCC*

Baicalein (5,6,7-trihydroxyflavone), a type of flavonoid, obtained from the roots of *Scutellaria baicalensis* and *Scutellaria lateriflora*. Baicalein and its conjugate Baicalin are established pharmacological agents having the role as an angiogenic agent, anti-inflammatory agent, antioxidant and hormone antagonist [118, 131, 132]. Several studies indicate that Baicalein and Baicalin possess anticancer action such as tumor cell apoptosis [30, 133]. Prominent evidences demonstrate that Baicalein and Baicalin have immune checkpoint inhibitory actions on TME. Baicalein and Baicalin can modulate the proliferation of HCC cells and immune suppression in the TME via downregulating the level of PD-LI expression on the surface of APCs. These phyto-molecules can also inhibit the STAT3 protein, subsequently inhibit the IFN-γ induced PD-L1 expression, and cause cytotoxic T cell-triggered cell death in HCC. Besides, Baicalein and Baicalin can inhibit the PD-1-expression via increasing the level of IL-2 secretion in the tumor milieu [134, 135]. Therefore, Baicalein and Baicalin can defeat the HCC development and progression through suppressing the expression of PD-L1/PD-1 and augmenting host immunity.

Fraxinellone is a natural terpenoid isolated from the root of *Raulinoa echinata* and has been recognized as a suitable candidate for cancer treatment. Xing et al. demonstrated that Fraxinellone can produce dose-dependent inhibition on PD-L1 expression in various cancers such as hepatic cancers, lung, cervical, and colon cancers. Fraxinellone can significantly downregulate the activation of STAT3 and the synthesis of HIF-1α protein through JAK/Src, mTOR/p70S6K/eIF4E, and MAPK signaling pathways. The signaling molecules such as STAT3 and HIF-1α are the transcription factors, that can increase the transcription of PD-L1. Thus the treatment with Fraxinellone can decrease the levels of PD-L1 on APC and reduce tumorigenesis. Moreover, Fraxinellone-triggered PD-L1 downregulation can reduce angiogenesis in endothelial cells by regulating VEGF and MMP-9 signaling [136].

Several phytoconstituents such as Terpenes and Saponins, also obligate immune modulatory action and regulate the immune system in the tumor milieu via restraining activities of immune cells and cytokine secretion in the TME [20]. Several terpenes can modulate immune checkpoints and PD-1/PD-L1 expression in cancer cells via molecular mechanisms. Triterpenoid saponins extracted from *Anemone flaccida Fr* remarkably induce the apoptosis of HCC cells [137]. Triterpenoid saponins can inhibit the expression and activity of PD1/PD-L1, p38 MAPK ERK1/2, STAT3, and JNK signaling pathways in the cancer cells; it can also alter the cancer cell metabolism and reduce the cancer development and progression and alter the metabolism of cancer. Moreover, it can produce immune modulatory actions in the TME by declining the level of regulatory T cells (Treg) and augmenting the level of cytotoxic T cells [138].

3.3. *Plant-derived vaccines mediated immunotherapies for HCC*

HBV and HCV infections are the global cause for the development of chronic hepatic diseases such as cirrhosis and HCC [139]. The development of plant-based vaccines against HBV and HCV-induced

HCC has much attention because it is an inexpensive, 'needle-free' vaccines that are stable at room temperature for long periods and are fundamentally safe and efficacious [140, 141]. Plant-derived HBV vaccine has been under development for two decades. Normally, transgenic plants were used for generating plant-derived vaccines. Numerous approaches have been employed for the development, processing, expansion and manufacturing of these vaccines for HBV infection from the plant varieties tomato, maize, lettuce and rice [142]. Recently studies revealed that maize germ wafers can express HBsAg as part of a prime-boost vaccination strategy. A primary dose of Recombivax was injected into mice, and an oral booster of HBsAg wafers was later given. Mice administrated with this vaccine regimen increase the level of mucosal IgA and long-term memory over 1-year after vaccination [143]. On the other hand, Pniewski et al. established micropropagation techniques for the development of transgenic lettuce lines, which can express uniform and high levels of HBsAg [144, 145].

The process of vaccine development for HCV infection has a lot of challenges, especially for the growth and development of virus in the tissue culture. In the beginning, tobacco mosaic virus (TMV) was considered as a vector to express potential neutralizing epitopes of HCV [146]. Cucumber mosaic virus (CMV) has also been used as an expression vector to generate HCV hypervariable region (HVR1) epitopes. The plant extracts comprising anti-HCV vaccine can increase the release of IFN-γ and cytokines from lymphocytes [147–149].

3.4. *Nano-based drug delivery strategies to improve the therapeutic benefits of plant-derived products in cancer immunotherapies*

The development of a nano-drug delivery system/nanotechnology can expand the clinical utility of phyto-molecules by improving their characteristics including drug solubility and drug stability, drug targeting properties, drug toxicity, and adverse effects. Paclitaxel-loaded nanoparticles combined with anti-CD-133 antibody can effectively target the tumor stem cells and produce apoptosis via inhibiting pro-apoptotic molecules such as CHOP and Caspase-12 [115]. Moreover, a combination of Paclitaxel with anti-human Stathmin 1 antibody restricts the proliferation of cancer cells, particularly in combination with synergism. Thus the combined treatment approaches produce more significant apoptosis in tumor cells than monotherapy [150].

Mannose (M)/CpG oligodeoxynucleotide (CpG-ODN)-conjugated liposomes encapsulated with tumor antigens (TA) particularly induces the production, maturation, and activation of DCs, and it achieves the immunotherapeutic effect via activating the effector cells, which destroys the cancer cells [115]. An innovative "core-shell" encapsulated with plant-based natural products such as Ursolic acid and Polyphenol conjugated with EpCAM-aptamer was studied against HCC. The natural products isolated from food-plant, Ursolic acid and Polyphenol had good antitumor activities and low toxicity. The combination of Ursolic acid and Polyphenol in a nano complex system elicits immune modulatory effects in the TME through activating the innate and acquired immunity. This dual-drug nanosystem can increase the secretion of IL-12, IFN-γ, and NK cells and significantly augment the tumor infiltration of $CD8^+$ T cells in the tumor milieu and produce synergistic effects against HCC [151]. (Table 3) (Figure 2)

4. Hurdles in the Clinical Translation of Plant-Derived Products

In recent years, plant-derived secondary metabolites such as flavonoids, terpenoids, alkaloids, and saponins are described as an excellent source of anticancer agents exhibiting low toxicity. Nevertheless, it has been recognized as a notable candidate for anticancer therapies, but they do not produce satisfactory clinical output. This may be for many reasons which include poor water solubility, low bioavailability, easy-to-develop drug resistance, low retention time in the body, poor targetability, etc. Therefore, monotherapy with phyto-molecule may not be capable to produce satisfactory efficacy against cancer progression [115]. The lack of understanding of the pharmacokinetic,

Table 3: Summary of the role of plant-derived products in cancer immunotherapy against HCC

Sl. No	Plant/Plant-derived Product	Effect on Immunotherapy	Mechanism of Action	References
Combination of plant-derived products with immunotherapies				
1	Icaritin	• Synergistic effect with anti-PD-1 antibody • Reduce PD-L1 expression	• Blocks the formation of IKK • Inhibit NF-κB translocation which promotes PD-L1 expression	[123]
2	*Lycium barbarum* polysaccharide (LBP)	• Synergistic effect with cytokine (CXCL10)	• Increase the release of Th1 cytokines • Restores balance of Thl/Th2 • Increase the production and function of dendritic cells (DCs)	[125]
3	10-hydroxycamptotenin	• Synergistic effect with DC hepa-6 fusion vaccine	• Produce CTL cytotoxicity	[126]
4	Vitamin C	• Synergistic effect with anti-PD-L1 antibody	• Produce anti-angiogenesis effect • Improves the production and effectiveness of cytotoxic T cells • Stimulating the cyclic GMP-AMP synthase (cGAS) • Increases the production of Cgamp • Activation of STING pathway	[127]
5	Taxol	• Synergism with Cyclosporin A	• Upregulate the level of Caspase 9 and Caspase 3 • Facilitate the activation of PI3K-mTOR	[128]
6	Cryptotanshinone (CT)	• Synergism with PD-L1 antibody	• Increase the secretion of tumor-infiltrating $CD8^+$ T cells and effector $CD8^+$ T cells from lymph nodes	[129, 130]

(Continued)

Table 3: (*Continued*)

Sl. No	Plant/Plant-derived Product	Effect on Immunotherapy	Mechanism of Action	References
Plant-derived products as monotherapy against HCC				
7	Baicalein and Baicalin	• Immune checkpoint inhibitory action	• Down regulating the level of PD-LI • Inhibit the STAT3 protein • Inhibit the IFN-γ • Increase the level of cytotoxic T cells • Increasing the level of IL-2 secretion	[134, 135]
8	Fraxinellone	• Immune checkpoint inhibitory action	• Inhibit PD-L1 expression • Downregulate the activation of STAT3 • Inhibit the synthesis of HIF-1α protein through JAK/Src, mTOR/p70S6K/eIF4E and MAPK signaling pathways	[136]
9	Triterpenoid saponins extracted from *Anemone flaccida Fr*	• Immune checkpoint inhibitory action	• Inhibit the expression and activity of PD1/PD-L1, p38 MAPK ERK1/2, STAT3 and JNK signaling pathways • Alter the cancer cell metabolism • Declining the level of regulatory T cells (Treg) • Increasing the level of cytotoxic T cells	[138]

Plant-derived products as anti-HCC vaccines				
10	Maize germ wafers	Anti-HBV vaccine	• Increase the expression of HBsAg • Increase the level of mucosal IgA	[143]
11	Lettuce	Anti-HBV vaccine	• Increase the expression of HBsAg	
12	Cucumber mosaic virus (CMV)	Anti-HCV vaccine	• Increase the release of IFN-γ and cytokines from lymphocytes	[147–149]
Nano-based drug delivery strategies to improve the therapeutic benefits of plant-derived products in cancer immunotherapies				
13	Paclitaxel-loaded nanoparticles	• Synergism with anti-CD-133 antibody • Synergism with stathmin 1 antibody	• Produce apoptosis via inhibiting pro-apoptotic molecules such as CHOP and Caspase-12	[115, 150]
14	Mannose (M)/CpG oligodeoxynucleotide (CpG-ODN)-conjugated liposomes encapsulated with tumor antigens	• Produce immune response in the TME	• Increase the production, maturation and activation of DCs • Activates the effector cells, which destroys the cancer cells	[115]
15	Ursolic acid and Polyphenol conjugated with EpCAM-aptamer	• synergistic treatment	• Increase the secretion of IL-12, IFN-γ, and NK • Augment the tumor infiltration of $CD8^+$ T cells in the tumor milieu	[151]

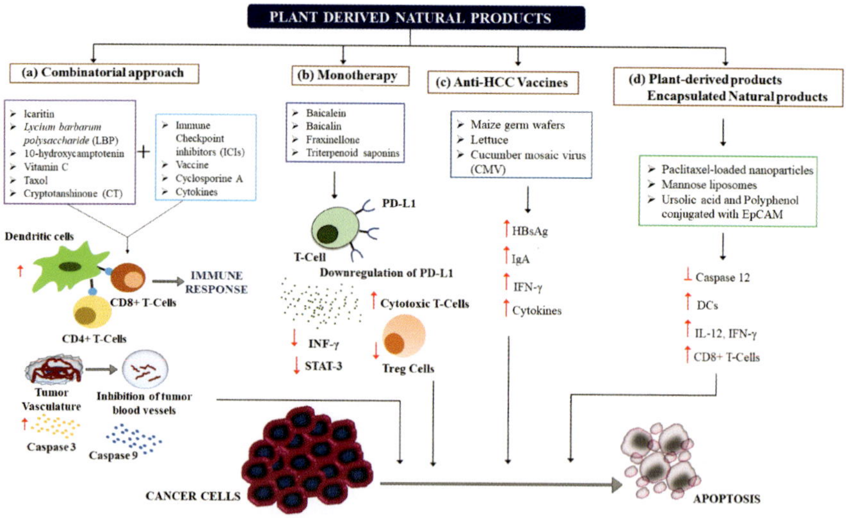

Figure 2: Role of plant-derived products as immunotherapeutic agents (a) as a combination of plant-derived with immunotherapies, (b) as a monotherapy, (c) as a cancer vaccine, and (d) as encapsulated nanoformulation

bio-distribution and pharmacodynamics profile also restricts its applications. This makes difficulties in predicting effectiveness and safety in the clinic difficult for phytoconstituents. The PK-PD challenges of phytochemicals complicate the determination of the potential interactions with other chemotherapeutic and immunotherapeutic agents that might influence the overall result of the cancer therapy [152].

The combinations of plant-based therapies along with conventional chemotherapies and immunotherapies show significant effects against cancers [153, 154]. The most favorable factor in the combinatorial approach is the dose reduction of each agent, which helps to reduce the side effects of cancer therapies as compared with a single treatment. Multiple drug combinations targeting various cancer pathways can also help to address tumor heterogeneity [155, 156].

The limitations of natural medicines can be improved by the use of nanotechnology. Nanoparticles can modulate the bioavailability, release kinetics, and targetability of phytomedicine [157, 158]. Targeted nanoparticle/nanoformulation-based delivery of plant-derived compounds has prominent benefits. Most plant-derived products have to be administered to patients with a large dosage, which may lead to the development of serious side effects. Hence, nanoparticle-based drug delivery systems should be designed for plant-derived products to overcome the limitations [159, 160]. The nanoformulations including liposomes, micelles, core-shell nanoparticles, and so on stand out due to the better therapeutic outcome for tumor-targeting, antitumor activities, dose reduction, immune-sensitization, stability, and safety.

5. Conclusion and Future Perspectives

In conclusion, the book chapter discusses the significant role of plant-derived products in cancer immunotherapy and the potential of phytochemicals as a possible alternative to combination therapy with immunotherapy to expand the therapeutic efficacy of existing immunotherapy with minimal side effects. Several phyto-molecules belonging to the category of flavonoids, terpenoids, saponins, and so on can elicit antitumor immune response through the downregulation of several immune pathways, and they can also modulate the function of immune cells in the tumor microenvironment. Moreover, plant derived products induce apoptosis, anti-angiogenic effect, and antitumor immune responses in HCC, and they also restrict the cancer progression and metastasis. The combination of plant-derived products with immunotherapy will help to improve the overall survival rate and control the off-targeted immune-related adverse reactions (irAEs). The incorporation of nanotechnology with plant derived products can improve the therapeutic effectiveness of phyto-molecules against cancer. In a nutshell, the potential of phytochemicals in combination with immunotherapy or as monotherapy should be authenticated in well-designed clinical settings for safety and efficacy. This may further help to develop an effective-versatile treatment modality against HCC.

References

1. Llovet JM, Kelley RK, Villanueva A, Singal AG, Pikarsky E, Roayaie S, Lencioni R, Koike K, Zucman-Rossi J, Finn RS. Hepatocellular carcinoma. *Nature Reviews. Disease Primers.* 2021;7(1):6.

2. Moawad AW, Szklaruk J, Lall C, Blair KJ, Kaseb AO, Kamath A, Rohren SA, Elsayes KM. Angiogenesis in hepatocellular carcinoma; pathophysiology, targeted therapy, and role of imaging. *Journal of Hepatocellular Carcinoma*. 2020 Apr 23;7:77–89.
3. Shen C, Jiang X, Li M, Luo Y. Hepatitis virus and hepatocellular carcinoma: Recent advances. *Cancers*. 2023 Jan 15;15(2):533.
4. McGlynn KA, Petrick JL, El-Serag HB. Epidemiology of hepatocellular carcinoma. *Hepatology*. 2021 Jan;73:4–13.
5. Schlachterman A, Craft Jr WW, Hilgenfeldt E, Mitra A, Cabrera R. Current and future treatments for hepatocellular carcinoma. *World Journal of Gastroenterology: WJG*. 2015 Jul 7;21(28):8478.
6. Chen R, Li Q, Xu S, Ye C, Tian T, Jiang Q, Shan J, Ruan J. Modulation of the tumour microenvironment in hepatocellular carcinoma by tyrosine kinase inhibitors: From modulation to combination therapy targeting the microenvironment. *Cancer Cell International*. 2022 Feb 11;22(1):73.
7. Jackson R, Psarelli EE, Berhane S, Khan H, Johnson PJ. Impact of viral status on survival in patients receiving sorafenib for advanced hepatocellular cancer: A meta-analysis of randomized phase III trials. *Journal of Clinical Oncology*. 2017 Feb 20;35(6):622–628.
8. Wei S, Wei F, Li M, Yang Y, Zhang J, Li C, Wang J. Target immune components to circumvent sorafenib resistance in hepatocellular carcinoma. *Biomedicine & Pharmacotherapy*. 2023 Jul 1;163:114798.
9. Chen C, Wang Z, Ding Y, Qin Y. Tumor microenvironment-mediated immune evasion in hepatocellular carcinoma. *Frontiers in Immunology*. 2023 Feb 10;14:1133308.
10. Sangro B, Sarobe P, Hervás-Stubbs S, Melero I. Advances in immunotherapy for hepatocellular carcinoma. *Nature Reviews Gastroenterology & Hepatology*. 2021 Aug;18(8):525–543.
11. Rabinovich GA, Gabrilovich D, Sotomayor EM. Immunosuppressive strategies that are mediated by tumor cells. *Annual Review of Immunology*. 2007 Apr 23;25:267–296.
12. Velcheti V, Schalper K. Basic overview of current immunotherapy approaches in cancer. *American Society of Clinical Oncology Educational Book*. 2016 Jan 1;36:298–308.

13. Devan AR, Kumar AR, Nair B, Anto NP, Muraleedharan A, Mathew B, Kim H, Nath LR. Insights into an immunotherapeutic approach to combat multidrug resistance in hepatocellular carcinoma. *Pharmaceuticals*. 2021 Jul 9;14(7):656.
14. Okusaka T, Ikeda M. Immunotherapy for hepatocellular carcinoma: Current status and future perspectives. *ESMO Open*. 2018 Jan 1;3: e000455.
15. Ghavimi S, Apfel T, Azimi H, Persaud A, Pyrsopoulos NT. Management and treatment of hepatocellular carcinoma with immunotherapy: A review of current and future options. *Journal of Clinical and Translational Hepatology*. 2020 Jun 6;8(2):168.
16. Foerster F, Gairing SJ, Ilyas SI, Galle PR. Emerging immunotherapy for HCC: A guide for hepatologists. *Hepatology*. 2022 Jun;75(6): 1604–1626.
17. van Doorn DJ, Takkenberg RB, Klümpen HJ. Immune checkpoint inhibitors in hepatocellular carcinoma: An overview. *Pharmaceuticals*. 2020 Dec 22;14(1):3.
18. Wing K, Onishi Y, Prieto-Martin P, Yamaguchi T, Miyara M, Fehervari Z, Nomura T, Sakaguchi S. CTLA-4 control over Foxp3+ regulatory T cell function. *Science*. 2008 Oct 10;322(5899):271–275.
19. Kumar AR, Devan AR, Nair B, Nath LR. Anti-VEGF mediated immunomodulatory role of phytochemicals: Scientific exposition for plausible HCC treatment. *Current Drug Targets*. 2021 Aug 1; 22(11):1288–1316.
20. Kumar R, De Mooij T, Peterson TE, Kaptzan T, Johnson AJ, Daniels DJ, Parney IF. Modulating glioma-mediated myeloid-derived suppressor cell development with sulforaphane. *PLoS One*. 2017 Jun 30;12(6):e0179012.
21. Li SQ, Yang Y, Ye LS. Angiogenesis and immune checkpoint dual blockade: Opportunities and challenges for hepatocellular carcinoma therapy. *World Journal of Gastroenterology*. 2022 Nov 11;28(42):6034.
22. Xu W, Liu K, Chen M, Sun JY, McCaughan GW, Lu XJ, Ji J. Immunotherapy for hepatocellular carcinoma: Recent advances and future perspectives. *Therapeutic Advances in Medical Oncology*. 2019 Jul;11:1758835919862692.

23. Sangro B, Gomez-Martin C, de la Mata M, Iñarrairaegui M, Garralda E, Barrera P, Riezu-Boj JI, Larrea E, Alfaro C, Sarobe P, Lasarte JJ. A clinical trial of CTLA-4 blockade with tremelimumab in patients with hepatocellular carcinoma and chronic hepatitis C. *Journal of Hepatology*. 2013 Jul 1;59(1):81–88.
24. El Dika I, Khalil DN, Abou-Alfa GK. Immune checkpoint inhibitors for hepatocellular carcinoma. *Cancer*. 2019 Oct 1;125(19):3312–3319.
25. Qin S, Ren Z, Meng Z, Chen Z, Chai X, Xiong J, Bai Y, Yang L, Zhu H, Fang W, Lin X. Camrelizumab in patients with previously treated advanced hepatocellular carcinoma: A multicentre, open-label, parallel-group, randomised, phase 2 trial. *The Lancet Oncology*. 2020 Apr 1; 21(4):571–580.
26. Lee A, Keam SJ. Tislelizumab: First approval. *Drugs*. 2020 Apr; 80(6):617–624.
27. Hu M, Yao W, Shen Q. Advances and challenges of immunocheckpoint inhibitors in the treatment of primary liver cancer. *Frontiers in Genetics*. 2022 Sep 30;13:1005658.
28. Wainberg ZA, Segal NH, Jaeger D, Lee KH, Marshall J, Antonia SJ, Butler M, Sanborn RE, Nemunaitis JJ, Carlson CA, Finn RS. Safety and clinical activity of durvalumab monotherapy in patients with hepatocellular carcinoma (HCC). *Journal of Clinical Oncology*. 2017; 35:4071–4071
29. Lee M, Ryoo BY, Hsu CH, Numata K, Stein S, Verret W, Hack S, Spahn J, Liu B, Abdullah H, He R. Randomised efficacy and safety results for atezolizumab (Atezo)+ bevacizumab (Bev) in patients (pts) with previously untreated, unresectable hepatocellular carcinoma (HCC). *Annals of Oncology*. 2019 Oct 1;30:v875.
30. Wang Z, Ma L, Su M, Zhou Y, Mao K, Li C, Peng G, Zhou C, Shen B, Dou J. Baicalin induces cellular senescence in human colon cancer cells via upregulation of DEPP and the activation of Ras/Raf/MEK/ERK signaling. *Cell Death & Disease*. 2018 Feb 13;9(2):217.
31. Taylor M, Dutcus CE, Schmidt E, Bagulho T, Li D, Shumaker R, Rasco D. A phase 1b trial of lenvatinib (LEN) plus pembrolizumab (PEM) in patients with selected solid tumors. *Annals of Oncology*. 2016 Oct 1;27:vi267.

32. Wu D, Li Y. Application of adoptive cell therapy in hepatocellular carcinoma. *Immunology.* 2023 Dec;170(4):453–469.
33. Fan J, Das JK, Xiong X, Chen H, Song J. Development of CAR-T cell persistence in adoptive immunotherapy of solid tumors. *Frontiers in Oncology.* 2021 Jan 6;10:574860.
34. Sermer D, Brentjens R. CAR T-cell therapy: Full speed ahead. *Hematological Oncology.* 2019 Jun;37:95–100.
35. Martinez M, Moon EK. CAR T cells for solid tumors: New strategies for finding, infiltrating, and surviving in the tumor microenvironment. *Frontiers in Immunology.* 2019 Feb 5;10:128.
36. Stoiber S, Cadilha BL, Benmebarek MR, Lesch S, Endres S, Kobold S. Limitations in the design of chimeric antigen receptors for cancer therapy. *Cells.* 2019 May 17;8(5):472.
37. Van Der Stegen SJ, Hamieh M, Sadelain M. The pharmacology of second-generation chimeric antigen receptors. *Nature Reviews Drug Discovery.* 2015 Jul;14(7):499–509.
38. Carpenito C, Milone MC, Hassan R, Simonet JC, Lakhal M, Suhoski MM, Varela-Rohena A, Haines KM, Heitjan DF, Albelda SM, Carroll RG. Control of large, established tumor xenografts with genetically retargeted human T cells containing CD28 and CD137 domains. *Proceedings of the National Academy of Sciences.* 2009 Mar 3; 106(9):3360–3365.
39. Chmielewski M, Hombach AA, Abken H. Of CARs and TRUCKs: Chimeric antigen receptor (CAR) T cells engineered with an inducible cytokine to modulate the tumor stroma. *Immunological Reviews.* 2014 Jan;257(1):83–90.
40. Mohanty R, Chowdhury CR, Arega S, Sen P, Ganguly P, Ganguly N. CAR T cell therapy: A new era for cancer treatment. *Oncology Reports.* 2019 Dec 1;42(6):2183–2195.
41. Liu Z, Liu X, Liang J, Liu Y, Hou X, Zhang M, Li Y, Jiang X. Immunotherapy for hepatocellular carcinoma: Current status and future prospects. *Frontiers in Immunology.* 2021 Oct 4;12:765101.
42. June CH, Sadelain M. Chimeric antigen receptor therapy. *New England Journal of Medicine.* 2018 Jul 5;379(1):64–73.

43. Qu C, Zhang H, Cao H, Tang L, Mo H, Liu F, Zhang L, Yi Z, Long L, Yan L, Wang Z. Tumor buster-where will the CAR-T cell therapy 'missile' go?. *Molecular Cancer.* 2022 Oct 19;21(1):201.
44. Nishida T, Kataoka H. Glypican 3-targeted therapy in hepatocellular carcinoma. *Cancers.* 2019 Sep 10;11(9):1339.
45. Yong CS, Dardalhon V, Devaud C, Taylor N, Darcy PK, Kershaw MH. CAR T-cell therapy of solid tumors. *Immunology and Cell Biology.* 2017 Apr;95(4):356–363.
46. Gao H, Li K, Tu H, Pan X, Jiang H, Shi B, Kong J, Wang H, Yang S, Gu J, Li Z. Development of T cells redirected to glypican-3 for the treatment of hepatocellular carcinoma. *Clinical Cancer Research.* 2014 Dec 15;20(24):6418–6428.
47. Shi D, Shi Y, Kaseb AO, Qi X, Zhang Y, Chi J, Lu Q, Gao H, Jiang H, Wang H, Yuan D. Chimeric antigen receptor-glypican-3 T-cell therapy for advanced hepatocellular carcinoma: Results of phase I trials. *Clinical Cancer Research.* 2020 Aug 1;26(15):3979–3989.
48. Jiang Z, Gao W, Huang L. Tanshinones, critical pharmacological components in Salvia miltiorrhiza. *Frontiers in Pharmacology.* 2019;10:202.
49. Bell M, Gottschalk S. Engineered cytokine signaling to improve CAR T-cell effector function. *Frontiers in Immunology.* 2021 Jun 4;12: 684642.
50. Pang, N., Shi, J., Qin, L. *et al.* IL-7 and CCL19-secreting CAR-T cell therapy for tumors with positive glypican-3 or mesothelin. *Journal of Hematology & Oncology.* 2021;14:118. https://doi.org/10.1186/s13045-021-01128-9
51. Luo P, Wu S, Yu Y, Ming X, Li S, Zuo X, Tu J. Current status and perspective biomarkers in AFP negative HCC: Towards screening for and diagnosing hepatocellular carcinoma at an earlier stage. *Pathology & Oncology Research.* 2020 Apr;26:599–603.
52. Sun L, Guo H, Jiang R, Lu L, Liu T, Zhang Z, He X. Artificial antigen-presenting cells expressing AFP158-166 peptide and interleukin-15 activate AFP-specific cytotoxic T lymphocytes. *Oncotarget.* 2016 Apr 4;7(14):17579.
53. Liu H, Xu Y, Xiang J, Long L, Green S, Yang Z, Zimdahl B, Lu J, Cheng N, Horan LH, Liu B. Targeting alpha-fetoprotein

(AFP)–MHC complex with CAR T-cell therapy for liver cancer. *Clinical Cancer Research*. 2017 Jan 15;23(2):478–488.

54. Luo X, Cui H, Cai L, Zhu W, Yang WC, Patrick M, Zhu S, Huang J, Yao X, Yao Y, He Y. Selection of a clinical Lead TCR targeting alpha-fetoprotein-positive liver cancer based on a balance of risk and benefit. *Frontiers in Immunology*. 2020 Apr 27;11:623.
55. Kohga K, Tatsumi T, Takehara T, Tsunematsu H, Shimizu S, Yamamoto M, Sasakawa A, Miyagi T, Hayashi N. Expression of CD133 confers malignant potential by regulating metalloproteinases in human hepatocellular carcinoma. *Journal of Hepatology*. 2010 Jun 1;52(6):872–879.
56. Wang Y, Chen M, Wu Z, Tong C, Dai H, Guo Y, Liu Y, Huang J, Lv H, Luo C, Feng KC. CD133-directed CAR T cells for advanced metastasis malignancies: A phase I trial. *Oncoimmunology*. 2018 Jul 3;7(7):e1440169.
57. Dai H, Tong C, Shi D, Chen M, Guo Y, Chen D, Han X, Wang H, Wang Y, Shen P. Efficacy and biomarker analysis of CD133-directed CAR T cells in advanced hepatocellular carcinoma: A single-arm, open-label, phase II trial. *Oncoimmunology*. 2020 Jan 1;9(1):1846926.
58. Nandi D, Pathak S, Verma T, Singh M, Chattopadhyay A, Thakur S, Raghavan A, Gokhroo A, Vijayamahantesh. T cell costimulation, checkpoint inhibitors and anti-tumor therapy. *Journal of Biosciences*. 2020 Dec;45:1–36.
59. Watanabe K, Nishikawa H. Engineering strategies for broad application of TCR-T-and CAR-T-cell therapies. *International Immunology*. 2021 Nov 1;33(11):551–562.
60. Shafer P, Kelly LM, Hoyos V. Cancer therapy with TCR-engineered T-cells: Current strategies, challenges, and prospects. *Frontiers in Immunology*. 2022 Mar 3;13:835762.
61. Pandey PR, Różycki B, Lipowsky R, Weikl TR. Structural variability and concerted motions of the T cell receptor–CD3 complex. *Elife*. 2021 Sep 7;10:e67195.
62. Kuhns MS, Badgandi HB. Piecing together the family portrait of TCR-CD 3 complexes. *Immunological Reviews*. 2012 Nov;250(1): 120–143.

63. Reinherz EL. αβ TCR-mediated recognition: Relevance to tumor-antigen discovery and cancer immunotherapy. *Cancer Immunology Research*. 2015 Apr 1;3(4):305–312.
64. Ozer M, Goksu SY, Akagunduz B, George A, Sahin I. Adoptive cell therapy in hepatocellular carcinoma: A review of clinical trials. *Cancers*. 2023 Mar 16;15(6):1808.
65. Qasim W, Brunetto M, Gehring AJ, Xue SA, Schurich A, Khakpoor A, Zhan H, Ciccorossi P, Gilmour K, Cavallone D, Moriconi F. Immunotherapy of HCC metastases with autologous T cell receptor redirected T cells, targeting HBsAg in a liver transplant patient. *Journal of Hepatology*. 2015 Feb 1;62(2):486–491.
66. Ozer F, Zhao J, Tan AT, Hu W, Wang SY, Jin J, Wu J, Li Y, Shi L, Fu JL, Yu S. Immunotherapy of HBV-related advanced hepatocellular carcinoma with short-term HBV-specific TCR expressed T cells: Results of dose escalation, phase I trial. *Hepatology International*. 2021 Dec;15:1402–1412.
67. Cai L, Caraballo Galva LD, Peng Y, Luo X, Zhu W, Yao Y, Ji Y, He Y. Preclinical studies of the off-target reactivity of AFP158-specific TCR engineered T cells. *Frontiers in Immunology*. 2020 Apr 27;11:607.
68. Zhu AX, Finn RS, Edeline J, Cattan S, Ogasawara S, Palmer D, Verslype C, Zagonel V, Fartoux L, Vogel A, Sarker D. Pembrolizumab in patients with advanced hepatocellular carcinoma previously treated with sorafenib (KEYNOTE-224): A non-randomised, open-label phase 2 trial. *The Lancet Oncology*. 2018 Jul 1;19(7):940–952.
69. Zhu S, Zhang T, Zheng L, Liu H, Song W, Liu D, Li Z, Pan CX. Combination strategies to maximize the benefits of cancer immunotherapy. *Journal of Hematology & Oncology*. 2021 Sep 27; 14(1):156.
70. Mandlik DS, Mandlik SK, Choudhary HB. Immunotherapy for hepatocellular carcinoma: Current status and future perspectives. *World Journal of Gastroenterology*. 2023 Feb 2;29(6):1054.
71. Jeng LB, Liao LY, Shih FY, Teng CF. Dendritic-cell-vaccine-based immunotherapy for hepatocellular carcinoma: Clinical trials and recent preclinical studies. *Cancers*. 2022 Sep 8;14(18):4380.
72. Wang Y, Xiang Y, Xin VW, Wang XW, Peng XC, Liu XQ, Wang D, Li N, Cheng JT, Lyv YN, Cui SZ. Dendritic cell biology and its role

in tumor immunotherapy. *Journal of Hematology & Oncology*. 2020 Dec;13(1):1–8.

73. Liu J, Fu M, Wang M, Wan D, Wei Y, Wei X. Cancer vaccines as promising immuno-therapeutics: Platforms and current progress. *Journal of Hematology & Oncology*. 2022 Mar 18;15(1):28.
74. Rizell M, Sternby Eilard M, Andersson M, Andersson B, Karlsson-Parra A, Suenaert P. Phase 1 trial with the cell-based immune primer ilixadencel, alone, and combined with sorafenib, in advanced hepatocellular carcinoma. *Frontiers in Oncology*. 2019 Jan 21;9:19.
75. Iwashita Y, Tahara K, Goto S, Sasaki A, Kai S, Seike M, Chen CL, Kawano K, Kitano S. A phase I study of autologous dendritic cell-based immunotherapy for patients with unresectable primary liver cancer. *Cancer Immunology, Immunotherapy*. 2003 Mar;52: 155–161.
76. Palmer DH, Midgley RS, Mirza N, Torr EE, Ahmed F, Steele JC, Steven NM, Kerr DJ, Young LS, Adams DH. A phase II study of adoptive immunotherapy using dendritic cells pulsed with tumor lysate in patients with hepatocellular carcinoma. *Hepatology*. 2009 Jan;49(1): 124–132.
77. Peng S, Chen S, Hu W, Mei J, Zeng X, Su T, Wang W, Chen Z, Xiao H, Zhou Q, Li B. Combination neoantigen-based dendritic cell vaccination and adoptive T-cell transfer induces antitumor responses against recurrence of hepatocellular carcinoma. *Cancer Immunology Research*. 2022 Jun 3;10(6):728–744.
78. Yang B, Jeang J, Yang A, Wu TC, Hung CF. DNA vaccine for cancer immunotherapy. *Human Vaccines & Immunotherapeutics*. 2014 Nov 2;10(11):3153–3164.
79. Hochnadel I, Kossatz-Boehlert U, Jedicke N, Lenzen H, Manns MP, Yevsa T. Cancer vaccines and immunotherapeutic approaches in hepatobiliary and pancreatic cancers. *Human Vaccines & Immunotherapeutics*. 2017 Dec 2;13(12):2931–2952.
80. Jacobson JM, Zahrieh D, Strand CA, Cruz-Correa M, Pungpapong S, Roberts LR, Mandrekar SJ, Rodriguez LM, Boyer J, Marrero I, Kraynyak KA. Phase I trial of a therapeutic DNA vaccine for preventing hepatocellular carcinoma from chronic hepatitis C virus (HCV) infection. *Cancer Prevention Research*. 2023 Mar 1;16(3):163–173.

81. Yarchoan M, Gane E, Marron TU, Rochestie S, Cooch N, Peters J, Csiki I, Perales-Puchalt A, Sardesai N. Personalized DNA neoantigen vaccine in combination with plasmid IL-12 and pembrolizumab for the treatment of patients with advanced hepatocellular carcinoma. *Journal of Clinical Oncology*. 2021;39:TPS2680.
82. Wang N, Qian R, Liu T, Wu T, Wang T. Nanoparticulate carriers used as vaccine adjuvant delivery systems. *Critical Reviews in Therapeutic Drug Carrier Systems*. 2019;36(5):449–484.
83. Charneau J, Suzuki T, Shimomura M, Fujinami N, Nakatsura T. Peptide-based vaccines for hepatocellular carcinoma: A review of recent advances. *Journal of Hepatocellular Carcinoma*. 2021 Sep 2; 8:1035–1054.
84. Sawada Y, Yoshikawa T, Nobuoka D, Shirakawa H, Kuronuma T, Motomura Y, Mizuno S, Ishii H, Nakachi K, Konishi M, Nakagohri T. Phase I trial of a glypican-3–derived peptide vaccine for advanced hepatocellular carcinoma: Immunologic evidence and potential for improving overall survival. *Clinical Cancer Research*. 2012 Jul 1;18(13):3686–3696.
85. Greten TF, Forner A, Korangy F, N'Kontchou G, Barget N, Ayuso C, Ormandy LA, Manns MP, Beaugrand M, Bruix J. A phase II open label trial evaluating safety and efficacy of a telomerase peptide vaccination in patients with advanced hepatocellular carcinoma. *BMC Cancer*. 2010 Dec;10:1–7.
86. Chen DS, Mellman I. Elements of cancer immunity and the cancer–immune set point. *Nature*. 2017 Jan 19;541(7637):321–330.
87. Vishweshwaraiah YL, Dokholyan NV. mRNA vaccines for cancer immunotherapy. *Frontiers in Immunology*. 2022 Dec 14;13:1029069.
88. Han R. The potential of mRNA vaccine in HCC treatment. *International Journal of Immunotherapy and Cancer Research*. 2023 Jul 11;9(1):8–12.
89. Sahin U, Derhovanessian E, Miller M, Kloke BP, Simon P, Löwer M, Bukur V, Tadmor AD, Luxemburger U, Schrörs B, Omokoko T. Personalized RNA mutanome vaccines mobilize poly-specific therapeutic immunity against cancer. *Nature*. 2017 Jul 13;547(7662): 222–226.

90. Waldmann TA. Cytokines in cancer immunotherapy. *Cold Spring Harbor Perspectives in Biology*. 2018 Dec 1;10(12):a028472.
91. Sun Y, Wu H, Chen G, Huang X, Shan Y, Shi H, Zhang Q, Zheng Y. Genetically engineered recombinant adenovirus expressing interleukin-2 for hepatocellular carcinoma therapy. *Molecular Medicine Reports*. 2018 Jan 1;17(1):300–306.
92. Bertelli R, Di Donato A, Cioni M, Grassi F, Ikehata M, Bonanni A, Rastaldi MP, Ghiggeri GM. LPS nephropathy in mice is ameliorated by IL-2 independently of regulatory T cells activity. *PLoS One*. 2014 Oct 24;9(10):e111285.
93. Zhang Z, Zhu Y, Xu D, Li TE, Li JH, Xiao ZT, Chen M, Yang X, Jia HL, Dong QZ, Qin LX. IFN-α facilitates the effect of sorafenib via shifting the M2-like polarization of TAM in hepatocellular carcinoma. *American Journal of Translational Research*. 2021;13(1):301.
94. Ren H, Huang Y. Effects of pegylated interferon-α based therapies on functional cure and the risk of hepatocellular carcinoma development in patients with chronic hepatitis B. *Journal of Viral Hepatitis*. 2019 Jul;26:5–31.
95. Sakisaka M, Haruta M, Komohara Y, Umemoto S, Matsumura K, Ikeda T, Takeya M, Inomata Y, Nishimura Y, Senju S. Therapy of primary and metastatic liver cancer by human iPS cell-derived myeloid cells producing interferon-β. *Journal of Hepato-Biliary-Pancreatic Sciences*. 2017 Feb;24(2):109–119.
96. Kim C, Zhu S, Kouros-Mehr H, Khaldoyanidi S, Zu S. Incidence of elevated aminotransferases with or without bilirubin elevation during treatment with immune checkpoint inhibitors: A retrospective study of patients from community oncology clinics in the United States. *Cureus*. 2022 Apr 11;14(4).
97. El-Khoueiry AB, Yau T, Kang YK, Kim TY, Santoro A, Sangro B, Melero I, Kudo M, Hou MM, Matilla A, Tovoli F. Nivolumab (NIVO) plus ipilimumab (IPI) combination therapy in patients (Pts) with advanced hepatocellular carcinoma (aHCC): Long-term results from CheckMate 040. *Journal of Clinical Oncology*. 2021;39.
98. Gilbert J, Le Tourneau C, Mehanna H, Fayette J, Goswami T, Emeribe U, Jarkowski III A, Melillo G, Siu LL. Phase II, randomized, open-label

study of durvalumab (MEDI4736) or tremelimumab monotherapy, or durvalumab+ tremelimumab, in patients with recurrent or metastatic (R/M) squamous cell carcinoma of the head and neck (SCCHN): CONDOR. *Journal for ImmunoTherapy of Cancer* 2015 Nov 1;3(2).

99. Kudo M, Finn RS, Edeline J, Cattan S, Ogasawara S, Palmer DH, Verslype C, Zagonel V, Fartoux L, Vogel A, Sarker D. Updated efficacy and safety of KEYNOTE-224: A phase II study of pembrolizumab in patients with advanced hepatocellular carcinoma previously treated with sorafenib. *European Journal of Cancer*. 2022 May 1;167:1–2.
100. Deva S, Lee JS, Lin CC, Yen CJ, Millward M, Chao Y, Keam B, Jameson M, Hou MM, Kang YK, Markman B. A phase Ia/Ib trial of tislelizumab, an anti-PD-1 antibody (ab), in patients (pts) with advanced solid tumors. *Annals of Oncology*. 2018 Dec 1;29:x24–x25.
101. Lim HY, Heo J, Kim TY, Tai WM, Kang YK, Lau G, Kudo M, Tak WY, Watras M, Ali SK, Negro A. Safety and efficacy of durvalumab plus bevacizumab in unresectable hepatocellular carcinoma: Results from the phase 2 study 22 (NCT02519348). *Journal of Clinical Oncology*. 2022;40:436–436.
102. Kudo M, Chen M, Chow PK, Kaseb AO, Lee HC, Yopp AC, Becker L, Hernandez Painter S, Kovic B, Lian Q, Ma N. Efficacy, safety and patient reported outcomes (PROs) from the phase III IMbrave050 trial of adjuvant atezolizumab (atezo)+ bevacizumab (bev) vs active surveillance in patients with hepatocellular carcinoma (HCC) at high risk of disease recurrence following resection or ablation. *Journal of Clinical Oncology*. 2023;41:4002–4002.
103. Breder VV, Vogel A, Merle P, Finn RS, Galle PR, Zhu AX, Cheng AL, Feng YH, Li D, Gaillard VE, Li L. IMbrave150: Exploratory efficacy and safety results of hepatocellular carcinoma (HCC) patients (pts) with main trunk and/or contralateral portal vein invasion (Vp4) treated with atezolizumab (atezo)+ bevacizumab (bev) versus sorafenib (sor) in a global Ph III study. *Journal of Clinical Oncology*. 2021;39:4073–4073.
104. Kudo M, Motomura K, Wada Y, Inaba Y, Sakamoto Y, Kurosaki M, Umeyama Y, Kamei Y, Yoshimitsu J, Fujii Y, Aizawa M. Avelumab in combination with axitinib as first-line treatment in patients with

advanced hepatocellular carcinoma: Results from the phase 1b VEGF liver 100 trial. *Liver Cancer*. 2021 Jun 8;10(3):249–259.

105. Lin CC, Golan T, Corral J, Moreno V, Chung HC, Wasserstrom H, Yang J, Mi G, Bang YJ. Phase 1 study of ramucirumab (R) plus durvalumab (D) in patients (pts) with locally advanced and unresectable or metastatic gastrointestinal or thoracic malignancies (NCT02572687); Phase 1a results. *Annals of Oncology*. 2016 Nov 1;27:viii1.
106. Nowicki TS, Hu-Lieskovan S, Ribas A. Mechanisms of resistance to PD-1 and PD-L1 blockade. *Cancer Journal (Sudbury, Mass.)*. 2018 Jan;24(1):47.
107. Yarchoan M, Zhu Q, Durham JN, Gross N, Charmsaz S, Leatherman JM, Zhang S, Popovic A, Weiss MJ, Philosophe B, Burkhart RA. Feasibility and efficacy of neoadjuvant cabozantinib and nivolumab in patients with borderline resectable or locally advanced hepatocellular carcinoma (HCC). *Journal of Clinical Oncology*. 2021;39:335–335.
108. Shi Y, Shi D, Chi J, Cui D, Tang X, Lin Y, Wang S, Li Z, Jin H, Zhai B. Combined local therapy and CAR-GPC3 T-cell therapy in advanced hepatocellular carcinoma: A proof-of-concept treatment strategy. *Cancer Communications*. 2023 Sep;43(9):1064.
109. Fang W, Fu Q, Zhao Q, Zheng YI, Liu L, Li Z, Dai X, Wang H, Zhu X, Zhao P, Lin M. Phase I trial of fourth-generation chimeric antigen receptor T-cells targeting glypican-3 for advanced hepatocellular carcinoma. *Journal of Clinical Oncology*. 2021;39:4088–4088.
110. Fu Q, Zheng Y, Fang W, Zhao Q, Zhao P, Liu L, Zhai Y, Tong Z, Zhang H, Lin M, Zhu X. RUNX-3-expressing CAR T cells targeting glypican-3 in patients with heavily pretreated advanced hepatocellular carcinoma: A phase I trial. *EClinicalMedicine*. 2023 Sep 1;63: 102175.
111. Ilyas FZ, Beane JD, Pawlik TM. The state of immunotherapy in hepatobiliary cancers. *Cells*. 2021 Aug 15;10(8):2096.
112. Roddy H, Meyer T, Roddie C. Novel cellular therapies for hepatocellular carcinoma. *Cancers*. 2022 Jan 20;14(3):504.
113. Yin SY, Yang NS, Lin TJ. Phytochemicals approach for developing cancer immunotherapeutics. *Frontiers in Pharmacology*. 2017 Jun 19;8:386.

114. Abou-Alfa GK, Yong WP, Chang SL, Fan J, Toh HC, Yau T, Choo S, Wang J, Kusuma N, Ma C, Qin S. Autologous cytotoxic T-cell receptor T cell therapy (SCG101) against hepatitis B surface antigen phase I/II trial for patients with advanced hepatitis B-related hepatocellular carcinoma. *Journal of Clinical Oncology*. 2023;41:TPS4181.
115. Wang Y, Li J, Xia L. Plant-derived natural products and combination therapy in liver cancer. *Frontiers in Oncology*. 2023 Feb 14;13:1116532.
116. Kamat AM, Tharakan ST, Sung B, Aggarwal BB. Curcumin potentiates the antitumor effects of Bacillus Calmette-Guerin against bladder cancer through the downregulation of NF-κB and upregulation of TRAIL receptors. *Cancer Research*. 2009 Dec 1;69(23):8958–8966.
117. Du N, Bai R, Cui J. Mechanism of tumor immune escape and treatment strategy. *Chinese Journal of Cancer Biotherapy*. 2019;6: 454–462.
118. Chen Y, Wang J, Hong DY, Chen L, Zhang YY, Xu YN, Pan D, Fu LY, Tao L, Luo H, Shen XC. Baicalein has protective effects on the 17β-estradiol-induced transformation of breast epithelial cells. *Oncotarget*. 2017 Feb 2;8(6):10470.
119. Sze SC, Tong Y, Ng TB, Cheng CL, Cheung HP. Herba Epimedii: Anti-oxidative properties and its medical implications. *Molecules*. 2010 Nov 3;15(11):7861–7870.
120. Zhao H, Guo Y, Li S, Han R, Ying J, Zhu H, Wang Y, Yin L, Han Y, Sun L, Wang Z. A novel anti-cancer agent Icaritin suppresses hepatocellular carcinoma initiation and malignant growth through the IL-6/Jak2/Stat3 pathway. *Oncotarget*. 2015 Oct 10;6(31):31927.
121. Chen X, Song L, Hou Y, Li F. Reactive oxygen species induced by icaritin promote DNA strand breaks and apoptosis in human cervical cancer cells. *Oncology Reports*. 2019 Feb 1;41(2):765–778.
122. Liu Y, Shi L, Liu Y, Li P, Jiang G, Gao X, Zhang Y, Jiang C, Zhu W, Han H, Ju F. Activation of PPARγ mediates icaritin-induced cell cycle arrest and apoptosis in glioblastoma multiforme. *Biomedicine & Pharmacotherapy*. 2018 Apr 1;100:358–366.
123. Mo D, Zhu H, Wang J, Hao H, Guo Y, Wang J, Han X, Zou L, Li Z, Yao H, Zhu J. Icaritin inhibits PD-L1 expression by targeting protein IκB kinase α. *European Journal of Immunology*. 2021 Apr;51(4): 978–988.

124. Zhou F, Jiang X, Wang T, Zhang B, Zhao H. *Lycium barbarum* polysaccharide (LBP): A novel prebiotics candidate for Bifidobacterium and Lactobacillus. *Frontiers in Microbiology*. 2018 May 18;9:1034.
125. Li Y, Wang X, Ma X, Liu C, Wu J, Sun C. Natural polysaccharides and their derivates: A promising natural adjuvant for tumor immunotherapy. *Frontiers in Pharmacology*. 2021 Apr 14;12:621813.
126. Song WG, Qu X, Li YL, Xu YP, Wu C, Qin QL. Anti-tumor effects of 10-hydroxycamptothecinc-treated DC-Hepa1-6 fusion vaccines. *Zhonghua gan Zang Bing za zhi Zhonghua Ganzangbing Zazhi Chinese Journal of Hepatology*. 2004 Jun 1;12(6):344–346.
127. Magrì A, Germano G, Lorenzato A, Lamba S, Chilà R, Montone M, Amodio V, Ceruti T, Sassi F, Arena S, Abrignani S. High-dose vitamin C enhances cancer immunotherapy. *Science Translational Medicine*. 2020 Feb 26;12(532):eaay8707.
128. Lin HL, Lui WY, Liu TY, Chi CW. Reversal of taxol resistance in hepatoma by cyclosporin A: Involvement of the PI-3 kinase-AKT 1 pathway. *British Journal of Cancer*. 2003 Mar;88(6):973–980.
129. Chen W, Lu Y, Chen G, Huang S. Molecular evidence of cryptotanshinone for treatment and prevention of human cancer. *Anti-Cancer Agents in Medicinal Chemistry (Formerly Current Medicinal Chemistry-Anti-Cancer Agents)*. 2013 Sep 1;13(7):979–987.
130. Han Z, Liu S, Lin H, Trivett AL, Hannifin S, Yang D, Oppenheim JJ. Inhibition of murine hepatoma tumor growth by cryptotanshinone involves TLR7-dependent activation of macrophages and induction of adaptive antitumor immune defenses. *Cancer Immunology, Immunotherapy*. 2019 Jul 1;68:1073–1085.
131. Lee SI, Kim SY, Park KR, Kim EC. Baicalein promotes angiogenesis and odontoblastic differentiation via the BMP and Wnt pathways in human dental pulp cells. *The American Journal of Chinese Medicine*. 2016 Oct 25;44(07):1457–1472.
132. Ren M, Zhao Y, He Z, Lin J, Xu C, Liu F, Hu R, Deng H, Wang Y. Baicalein inhibits inflammatory response and promotes osteogenic activity in periodontal ligament cells challenged with lipopolysaccharides. *BMC Complementary Medicine and Therapies*. 2021 Dec; 21(1):1–1.

133. Dou J, Wang Z, Ma L, Peng B, Mao K, Li C, Su M, Zhou C, Peng G. Baicalein and baicalin inhibit colon cancer using two distinct fashions of apoptosis and senescence. *Oncotarget*. 2018 Apr 4; 9(28):20089.
134. Ke M, Zhang Z, Xu B, Zhao S, Ding Y, Wu X, Wu R, Lv Y, Dong J. Baicalein and baicalin promote antitumor immunity by suppressing PD-L1 expression in hepatocellular carcinoma cells. *International Immunopharmacology*. 2019 Oct 1;75:105824.
135. Zhang Q, Yang C, Gao X, Dong J, Zhong C. Phytochemicals in regulating PD-1/PD-L1 and immune checkpoint blockade therapy. *Phytotherapy Research*. 2023 Dec 5.
136. Xing Y, Mi C, Wang Z, Zhang ZH, Li MY, Zuo HX, Wang JY, Jin X, Ma J. Fraxinellone has anticancer activity in vivo by inhibiting programmed cell death-ligand 1 expression by reducing hypoxia-inducible factor-1α and STAT3. *Pharmacological Research*. 2018 Sep 1;135: 166–180.
137. Han LT, Fang Y, Li MM, Yang HB, Huang F. The antitumor effects of triterpenoid saponins from the *Anemone flaccida* and the underlying mechanism. *Evidence-Based Complementary and Alternative Medicine*. 2013 Oct;2013:517931.
138. Han L, Yao S, Cao S, Mo G, Li J, Cao Y, Huang F. Triterpenoid saponins from anemone flaccida suppress tumor cell proliferation by regulating MAPK, PD1/PDL1, and STAT3 signaling pathways and altering cancer metabolism. *OncoTargets and Therapy*. 2019;12:10917.
139. Wong CH, Goh KL. Chronic hepatitis B infection and liver cancer. *Biomedical Imaging and Intervention Journal*. 2006 Jul;2(3).
140. Joung YH, Park SH, Moon KB, Jeon JH, Cho HS, Kim HS. The last ten years of advancements in plant-derived recombinant vaccines against hepatitis B. *International Journal of Molecular Sciences*. 2016 Oct 13;17(10):1715.
141. Hefferon K. Reconceptualizing cancer immunotherapy based on plant production systems. *Future science OA*. 2017 Jul 12;3(3):FSO217.
142. Thanavala Y, Mahoney M, Pal S, Scott A, Richter L, Natarajan N, Goodwin P, Arntzen CJ, Mason HS. Immunogenicity in humans of an edible vaccine for hepatitis B. *Proceedings of the National Academy of Sciences*. 2005 Mar 1;102(9):3378–3382.

143. Hayden CA, Fischer ME, Andrews BL, Chilton HC, Turner DD, Walker JH, Tizard IR, Howard JA. Oral delivery of wafers made from HBsAg-expressing maize germ induces long-term immunological systemic and mucosal responses. *Vaccine.* 2015 Jun 9;33(25): 2881–2886.
144. Pniewski T, Czyż M, Wyrwa K, Bociąg P, Krajewski P, Kapusta J. Micropropagation of transgenic lettuce containing HBsAg as a method of mass-scale production of standardised plant material for biofarming purposes. *Plant Cell Reports.* 2017 Jan;36:49–60.
145. Rahimian N, Miraei HR, Amiri A, Ebrahimi MS, Nahand JS, Tarrahimofrad H, Hamblin MR, Khan H, Mirzaei H. Plant-based vaccines and cancer therapy: Where are we now and where are we going?. *Pharmacological Research.* 2021 Jul 1;169:105655.
146. Nemchinov LG, Liang TJ, Rifaat MM, Mazyad HM, Hadidi A, Keith JM. Development of a plant-derived subunit vaccine candidate against hepatitis C virus. *Archives of Virology.* 2000 Dec;145:2557–2573.
147. Piazzolla G, Nuzzaci M, Tortorella C, Panella E, Natilla A, Boscia D, De Stradis A, Piazzolla P, Antonaci S. Immunogenic properties of a chimeric plant virus expressing a hepatitis C virus (HCV)-derived epitope: New prospects for an HCV vaccine. *Journal of Clinical Immunology.* 2005 Mar;25:142–152.
148. Nuzzaci M, Piazzolla G, Vitti A, Lapelosa M, Tortorella C, Stella I, Natilla A, Antonaci S, Piazzolla P. Cucumber mosaic virus as a presentation system for a double hepatitis C virus-derived epitope. *Archives of Virology.* 2007 May;152:915–928.
149. Su H, van Eerde A, Rimstad E, Bock R, Branza-Nichita N, Yakovlev IA, Clarke JL. Plant-made vaccines against viral diseases in humans and farm animals. *Frontiers in Plant Science.* 2023 Mar 28;14:1170815.
150. Wang S, Liu X, Yuan S, Chen W, Wang S, Xu N. Effects of monoclonal antibodies against human stathmin 1 combined paclitaxel on proliferation of human hepatocellular carcinoma cell lines. *The Chinese-German Journal of Clinical Oncology.* 2009 Oct;8:603–606.
151. Zhang B, Jiang J, Wu P, Zou J, Le J, Lin J, Li C, Luo B, Zhang Y, Huang R, Shao J. A smart dual-drug nanosystem based on co-assembly of plant and food-derived natural products for synergistic HCC immunotherapy. *Acta Pharmaceutica Sinica B.* 2021 Jan 1;11(1):246–257.

152. Mohapatra P, Singh P, Singh D, Sahoo S, Sahoo SK. Phytochemical based nanomedicine: A panacea for cancer treatment, present status and future prospective. *OpenNano*. 2022 Jul;7:100055.
153. Dong S, Guo X, Han F, He Z, Wang Y. Emerging role of natural products in cancer immunotherapy. *Acta Pharmaceutica Sinica B*. 2022 Mar 1;12(3):1163–1185.
154. Deng LJ, Qi M, Li N, Lei YH, Zhang DM, Chen JX. Natural products and their derivatives: Promising modulators of tumor immunotherapy. *Journal of Leucocyte Biology*. 2020 Aug;108(2):493–508.
155. Parhi P, Mohanty C, Sahoo SK. Nanotechnology-based combinational drug delivery: An emerging approach for cancer therapy. *Drug Discovery Today*. 2012 Sep 1;17(17–18):1044–1052.
156. Iqbal J, Abbasi BA, Mahmood T, Kanwal S, Ali B, Shah SA, Khalil AT. Plant-derived anticancer agents: A green anticancer approach. *Asian Pacific Journal of Tropical Biomedicine*. 2017 Dec 1; 7(12):1129–1150.
157. Kashyap D, Tuli HS, Yerer MB, Sharma A, Sak K, Srivastava S, Pandey A, Garg VK, Sethi G, Bishayee A. Natural product-based nanoformulations for cancer therapy: Opportunities and challenges. In *Seminars in Cancer Biology* 2021 Feb 1 (Vol. 69, pp. 5–23). Academic Press.
158. More MP, Pardeshi SR, Pardeshi CV, Sonawane GA, Shinde MN, Deshmukh PK, Naik JB, Kulkarni AD. Recent advances in phytochemical-based nano-formulation for drug-resistant Cancer. *Medicine in Drug Discovery*. 2021 Jun 1;10:100082.
159. Gautam S, Lohani P, Purohit SD, Ambawani S, Maan P. Potential of natural-product-based nano-formulations as chemopreventive agents. In *Natural Products and Nano-Formulations in Cancer Chemoprevention* 2023 Feb 27 (pp. 129–142). CRC Press.
160. Banik D, Patra P. Possibility of liver cancer treatment by nanoformulation of phenolic phytochemicals. *Current Nanomedicine (Formerly: Recent Patents on Nanomedicine)*. 2022 Jul 1;12(2):108–125.

https://doi.org/10.1142/9789811293320_0012

Chapter 12

Overview of the Clinical Significance of Phytomolecules in Liver Cancer

PR Roshni[1], Bilha Baby[1] and Shine Sadasivan[2]

[1]*Department of Pharmacy Practice, Amrita School of Pharmacy, Amrita Vishwa Vidyapeetham, Kochi-41, Kerala, India*

[2]*Professor and Head, Department of Gastroenterology, Amrita Institute of Medical Sciences, AIMS Health Sciences Campus, Kochi-41, Kerala, India*

Table of Contents:

*Corresponding author: E-mail address: roshnipr@aims.amrita.edu

Abbreviations:

HCC — Hepatocellular carcinoma
EGCG — Epigallocatechin gallate
PMA — Phorbol 12-myristate 13-acetate
DMBA — Dimethylbenz(a)anthracene
APG — Apigenin
uPA — Urokinase plasminogen activator
VEGF — Vascular epithelial growth factor

EGFR — Epithelial growth factor receptor
uPAR — Urokinase plasminogen activator receptor
ROS — Reactive oxygen species
PDGFR — Platelet-derived growth factor receptor
AFP — Alpha-fetoprotein
TCM — Traditional Chinese medicine
Hep G2 — Human hepatoma
GO — Gene Ontology
KEGG — Kyoto encyclopedia of genes and genomes
PI3K-AKt — Phosphoinositide-3-kinase–protein kinase B/AK strain transforming
CSC — Colorectal cancer stem cell
CRLM — Colorectal liver metastases
FOLFOX — Folinic acid, fluorouracil, oxaliplatin
ALDH — Aldehyde dehydrogenase
5–FU — 5–Fluorouracil
SRT 501 — Micronized resveratrol

Abstract

This chapter provides a concise insight into the pivotal role of phytomolecules in managing liver cancer, highlighting their clinical significance. Liver cancer, a major global health concern, often presents challenges in treatment, prompting exploration into alternative therapeutic options. Phytomolecules, derived from plants, have gained attention due to their diverse biological activities and potential therapeutic effects in liver cancer. This overview discusses the various types of phytomolecules, including flavonoids, polyphenols, alkaloids, and terpenoids, elucidating their mechanisms of action in combating liver cancer. Emphasizing their antioxidant, anti-inflammatory, and apoptotic properties, this abstract sheds light on how phytomolecules intervene in key pathways implicated in liver cancer progression. Additionally, it explores the clinical studies and trials evaluating the efficacy and safety of phytomolecules as adjunctive or standalone therapies in liver cancer management. The challenges, such as bioavailability and standardization, associated with utilizing phytomolecules in clinical settings are also addressed. Understanding the clinical relevance of phytomolecules in liver cancer holds promise for future therapeutic advancements and personalized treatment strategies, potentially improving patient outcomes and quality of life.

1. Introduction

Hepatocellular carcinoma (HCC), the most common kind of liver cancer, poses a substantial threat to global health. It is the fourth most prevalent cause of cancer-related deaths globally, with an unjustifiably high incidence in places such as Asia and Africa. Despite considerable advancements in the field of medicine, liver cancer remains notoriously difficult to treat, primarily due to its late-stage diagnosis, belligerent nature, and the limited effectiveness of available therapeutic options.

1.1. *Liver cancer: A global health challenge*

This malignancy brings significant worldwide insinuations and disproportionately marks certain regions, making it a captivating topic for study and intervention. The incidence of liver cancer displays considerable geographic variation, with a particularly high prevalence in areas such as Asia and Africa [1]. This geographical variance can be attributed to differing distributions of risk factors, including hepatitis B and C infections, aflatoxin exposure, and lifestyle-related habits like excessive alcohol consumption. Chronic inflammation, fibrosis, and cellular damage within the liver contribute to the alteration of healthy hepatocytes into cancerous cells. Surgical options are often limited due to the liver's indispensable functions, and systemic therapies may not be as effective as in other cancers [2]. Access to healthcare, vaccination, and early detection services can be restricted in underserved populations, exacerbating the problem.

There are drawbacks to several liver cancer therapy options; surgical options, such as resection and transplantation, can possibly cure the disease but are only suitable for select patients due to factors such as tumor size, liver function, and overall health. Systemic treatments, such as chemotherapy and targeted therapies, show inadequate effectiveness in advanced hepatocellular carcinoma (HCC) and often yield modest survival benefits while being associated with significant side effects, highlighting the necessity for innovative approaches [3].

The prognosis for people with liver cancer appears to be miserable due to its late diagnosis and few available treatments. Liver cancer poses a unique challenge due to its silent progression until advanced stages, making early diagnosis difficult. By the time symptoms are evident or are spotted, the disease is often well-advanced, reducing the efficacy of available treatments. Surgical resection, liver transplantation, and local ablation techniques are options for early-stage patients, but the majority of patients are diagnosed at an advanced stage where curative therapies are no longer feasible [4].

1.2. *Need for alternative approaches*

Alternative treatment options for liver cancer must be explored due to a number of significant variables. First, conventional treatments such as surgery, chemotherapy, and radiation therapy have limited efficacy, especially in the advanced stages of the disease [5]. Early detection remains a significant challenge, highlighting the importance of interventions at earlier disease stages. Additionally, the adverse side effects of standard treatments which include Sorafenib, as seen in chemotherapy, can negatively impact patient's quality of life, imposing alternative methods that minimize these drawbacks. Alternative therapies are vital for a wider range of people since many patients are not good candidates for surgical procedures due to elements such as tumor size, liver function, and general health. Surgical options are often limited due to the liver's essential functions, and systemic therapies may not be as effective as in other cancers. Furthermore, given the global load of liver cancer and the diverse patient profiles, tailored alternative treatments can offer personalized care and address this pressing public health task effectively [6].

2. Phytomolecules: Nature's Treasure/Nature's Pharmacopoeia

Plant-derived bioactive second-generation metabolites identified as phytomolecules include polyphenols, alkaloids, terpenoids, glycosides, tannins, flavonoids, organosulfur compounds, saponins, monoterpenes, sesquiterpenes, and capsinoids [7]. Phytomolecules play a dynamic role in the treatment of liver cancer due to their extensive range of biochemical properties and the ability to target different components of cancer growth. These naturally occurring compounds, found in an array of plants, have been documented for their capacity to hamper with the initiation, promotion, and progression of liver cancer.

Due to the downsides of standard liver cancer pharmaceuticals, experts have begun looking into alternative treatment options. Phytomolecules, natural compounds found in plants, have garnered attention for their potential role in cancer treatment. Organic compounds found in plants called phytomolecules have drawn attention for possible applications in the treatment of cancer.

These compounds, often rich in antioxidants, polyphenols, alkaloids, and other bioactive constituents, have demonstrated promising anticancer properties in various studies. Their potential in liver cancer treatment is particularly appealing due to their relatively low toxicity compared to traditional chemotherapy agents [8].

Numerous biological properties of phytomolecules can be used in the battle against cancer. These comprise anti-inflammatory, antioxidant, antiproliferative, pro-apoptotic, and anti-angiogenic effects [9]. They mainly work by targeting specific receptors, intruding disease pathways, and disrupting pathogenic life cycles. Besides, some phytomolecules have shown the ability to modify the immune system, which plays a key role in cancer surveillance and control [10].

3. Anticancer Properties of Phytomolecules Against Hepatocellular Carcinoma

In the context of modern medicine, a rising trend exist in the use of phytomolecules to cure cancer is extremely significant [11]. It has been proven that chemotherapy medications made from plants and their derivatives are useful for both cancer prevention and treatment agents [12]. Chemotherapeutic medicines are nevertheless routinely used despite their renowned cytotoxic effects because of their affordability and reliability. Within this framework, the importance of using phytomolecules sourced from natural sources becomes evident in mitigating the conventional toxicities of chemotherapy treatments and other synthetic pharmaceuticals [13]. Vinca alkaloid and its derivatives have long been used to treat a variety of malignancies, both on their own and in conjunction with other therapeutic agents [12]. Following the discovery of the anticancer properties of vinblastine, vinca alkaloids, and other phytomolecules by 1950s, there has been a growing trend in investigating the antitumor potential of more plant-based anticancer medications [13]. The curative antitumor effects of saffron and its constituents, primarily come from *Crocus sativa*, *Syzygium aromaticum*, also referred to as cloves, and *Beta vulgaris*, lavender essential oils, are some of the established examples of phytomolecules used in cancer treatment [14]. Curcumin (Figure 1) has been shown in several studies to have antitumor activity against several cancer cell lines, including liver cancer, lung cancer, brain tumors, prostate cancer, head and neck squamous cell carcinoma, and breast cancer [15].

Despite of all the benefits listed above, curcumin's low water solubility, which leads to poor oral bioavailability and low chemical stability, limits its applicability [16]. The polyphenol obtained from green tea called epigallocatechin-3-gallate (EGCG) has been discovered to show anticancer effects. Green tea's primary ingredient, EGCG (Figure 2),

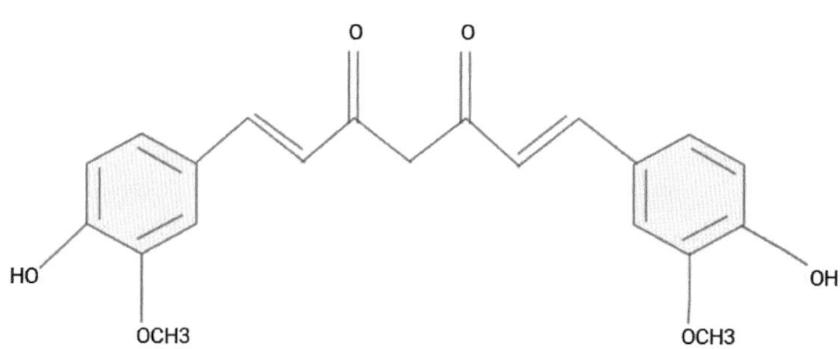

Figure 1: Molecular structure of curcumin

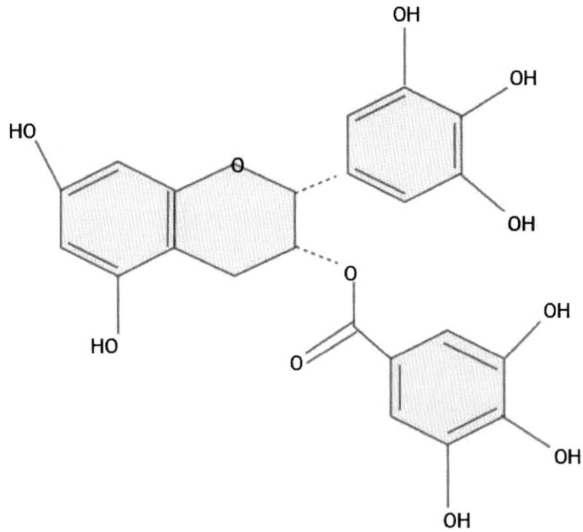

Figure 2: Molecular structure of EGCG

has antiproliferative, anti-inflammatory, antimutagenic, and antioxidative properties [17].

Research implemented both *in vivo* and *in vitro* advocates that EGCG may potently induce apoptosis and prevent proliferation in a variety of cancer types and can strongly engender apoptosis and inhibit growth in several types of cancers, including liver, colon, breast, kidney and brain cancers as well as leukemia [18]. When combined with medications used in clinical settings, resveratrol, a naturally occurring stilbene and non-flavonoid polyphenol found in grapes, apples and blueberries, can make cancer cells more liable to common chemotherapy treatments [19]. The dried fruit of milk thistle plant, *Silybum marianum*, is a frequent source of silymarin (Figure 3), belonging to a family of flavonoids that includes silybin, isosilybin, silychristin, silydianin, and taxifolin.

Silymarin is a chemopreventive agent *in vivo* against a range of carcinogens/tumor promoters, including UV radiation, phorbol 12-myristate 13-acetate (PMA), 7,12-dimethylbenz(a)anthracene (DMBA), and others, with regard to numerous investigations [20]. Quercetin (Figure 4), yet another bioactive flavonoid found in citrus

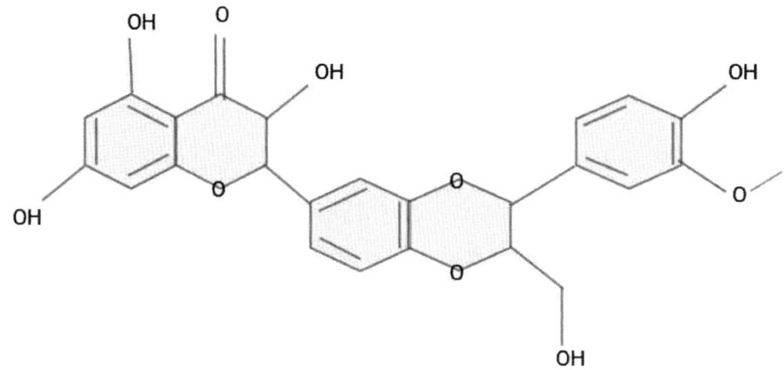

Figure 3: Molecular structure of silymarin

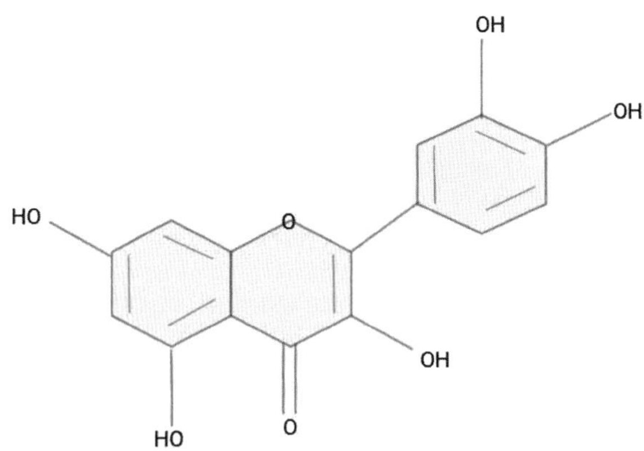

Figure 4: Molecular structure of quercetin

fruits, onions, grapes, and berries, directly induces apoptosis in tumor cells, hence impeding the progress of many human malignancies [21].

It is widely recognized that genistein makes up the greater part of isoflavone. The chemopreventive and therapeutic properties of genistein have been well studied. Genistein found in soymilk, barley meal, broccoli, and clover seeds modulates genes associated with apoptosis and cell cycle leading to pleiotropic effects. Furthermore, it has been proposed that it could suppress antioxidant events and angiogenesis via its molecular targets [22]. Another bioactive alkaloid present in many different plants, berberine, may also be used therapeutically in accordance with the growing need to control cancer by attenuating several cell signaling pathways [23]. Because of its low intrinsic toxicity and unique effects on cancer versus normal cells when compared to other structurally comparable flavonoids, apigenin (APG) has gained popularity as a medication in the present years. One important factor contributing to potential cancer-prevention benefits of apigenin is its powerful anti-inflammatory and antioxidant properties [24]. Gingerol, extracted from ginger, has drawn significant interest as a possible cancer treatment agent given that it serves as a natural scavenger of many chemical carcinogens that we are regularly exposed to such as aflatoxin B1 exo-8,9-epoxide, glycidamide, styrene oxide, vinyl carbamate epoxide, β-propiolactone, ethylene oxide, propylene oxide, 2-cyanoethylene oxide, and chloroethylene oxide [25]. Piperine, an alkaloid obtained from black pepper, is widely known for its chemopreventive properties by inhibiting cell alteration, angiogenesis, and so on [26].

4. Mechanism of Action by Which Phytomolecules Act Against Liver Cancer Cells

At various cellular levels, the phytochemicals have demonstrated a variety of distinct mechanisms of action. The majority of them have evolved into diverse sources of antioxidants which thereby target on several signaling pathways connected to factors for redox-mediated transcription. Additionally, they directly adjust the immune system, endocrine system and inflammation-related enzymes. Several of them demonstrated direct impact on the DNA breakage and repair processes [27]. Targeting certain cancer cells can prevent tumor growth, progression, and metastasis without having an adverse effect on health. Several anticancer drugs with various modes of action have been isolated from plant sources, including *Taxus brevifolia, Betula alba, Erythroxylum previllei, Curcuma longa, Catharanthus roseus, Cephalotaxus* species and many more in addition to the chemically developed anticancer medications [28]. Since ancient times, Asian medicine has used the low molecular weight polyphenol chemical curcumin [1,7-bis(4-hydroxy-3-methoxyphenyl)-1,6-heptadiene-3,5-dione], also known as diferuloylmethane, isolated from the plant *Curcuma longa Linn* [29]. Curcumin possesses certain anticancer potential, particularly both in terms of chemoprevention and therapy which is widely investigated [30]. Curcumin's anticancer action is due to its ability to modulate numerous biochemical and signaling pathways, which allows it to cause apoptosis and prevent tumor proliferation and invasion. A common transcription factor known as nuclear factor (NF)-B controls a large number of genes involved in the control of growth, inflammation, cancer, and apoptosis. Numerous cancer cells experience an attenuation of chemotherapy-induced apoptosis when NF-B is constitutively activated. In a similar vein, STAT3 is a key mediator of carcinogenesis. Constitutively active STAT3 has been linked to the generation of anti-apoptotic resistance, most likely via Bcl-xL and cyclin D1 expression. The expression of genes that control apoptosis, angiogenesis, promote proliferation, and invasion play a part in its role in carcinogenesis. In addition to its effects on the STAT3 and NF-B pathways, curcumin has been demonstrated to stop the cell cycle, reduce cell proliferation and promote apoptosis by modulating other transcription factors, including Erg-1, p53, AP-1, beta-catenin, Hif-1, Notch-1, and PPAR-α [31]. Additionally, it has been hypothesized that in CL-5 xenograft tumors, curcumin triggers apoptosis and promotes the down-regulation of Akt, EGFR, cMET, and cyclin D1 [32]. Housekeeping genes that are known to play a role in cell differentiation, tumor angiogenesis, and metastasis, including urokinase plasminogen activator (uPA), vascular epithelial growth factors (VEGF), epithelial growth factor receptor (EGFR), and urokinase plasminogen activator receptor (uPAR), have been linked to Sp-1. More specifically, curcumin has been proposed to lessen liver damage brought on by a variety of reasons and to function as an anticancer agent in cases of liver cancer [33]. The broad combination of curcumin can inhibit a variety of crucial metabolic processes in tumor cells and activate cell death pathways through several molecular triggers, hence improving the efficacy of eliminating tumors. Due to its potent antioxidant qualities, curcumin has a cytoprotective effect on healthy cells as a whole. It has been claimed to exert adjuvant effects when used in conjunction with several kinds of chemotherapeutic medications [34]. Curcumin exerts anticancer effect in liver cancer by specifically targeting on STAT 3 region. Being a STAT 3 inhibitor, curcumin acts by blocking STAT3 from being phosphorylated, reducing the creation of STAT3 dimers, or interfering with their ability to bind with DNA sequences, it prevents HCC cells from proliferating, surviving, and differentiating (Figure 5) [35].

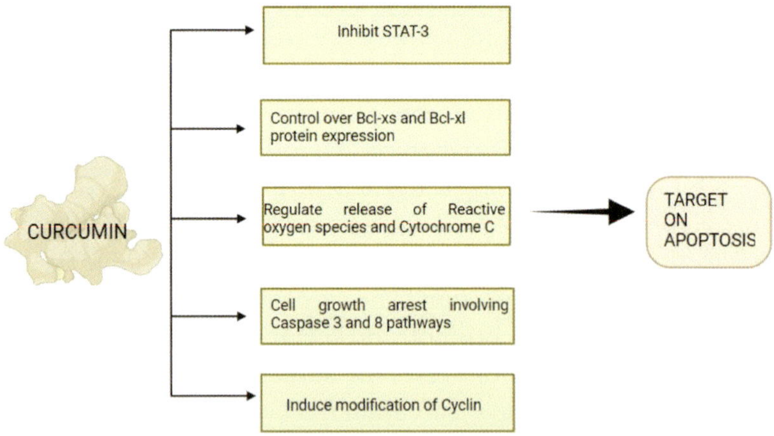

Figure 5: Anticancer mechanism of action by Curcumin. The major target where curcumin acts is STAT-3 pathway, caspase-3 and caspase-8, regulating the release of reactive oxygen species and cytochrome C finally ending up at apoptosis of the cancer cells.

By preventing STAT3 phosphorylation and nuclear translocation brought on by IL-6, the STAT3 small-molecule inhibitor LLL12 helps HCC cells proliferate less efficiently and undergo apoptosis [36]. The anticancer activities of curcumin have been linked to transcription factors including NF-B, beta-catenin, AP-1, and STAT-3, as well as protein kinases and growth factors such as MAPK, JAK, VEGF, AKT, PKA, ERK, and Bcl-2, according to research [37]. The primary three methods by which curcumin causes liver cancer cells to apoptosis were as follows: (1) control proteins involved in apoptosis, such as Bcl-xs and Bcl-xL; (2) Regulate the release of ROS and cytochrome C; and (3) causing cycle arrest by involving caspase-3 and caspase-8 pathways and by modifying the cyclin. In particular, the mitochondrial DNA of liver cancer cells is exposed to damage by the action of curcumin [38]. In HepG2 liver cancer tissues, curcumin can drastically lower COX-2 and VEGF production as well as tumor development and angiogenesis. The development of capillaries and associated heterogeneous networks might be prevented by curcumin. Neovascularization could therefore be partially inhibited [37]. Epigallocatechin-3-gallate [(2R,3R)-5,7-dihydroxy-2-(3,4,5-trihydroxyphenyl)chroman-3-yl]3,4,5-trihydroxy-benzoate is another phytomolecule which provide significant contribution with high anticancer effect. There exist several mechanisms by which this phytomolecule acts to show anticancer properties [39]. EGCG suppresses angiogenesis by downregulating VEGF and increasing cytotoxic T-lymphocyte infiltration [40]. By a similar mechanism, EGCG also provides angiogenesis and inhibition of tumor growth in colon cancer [41]. The protein tyrosine kinase activity of the EGF receptor, and platelet-derived growth factor receptor (PDGFR), 4 which have been recognized as a contributing factor in the proliferation of cancer cells, is additionally blocked by EGCG in addition to VEGF signaling [42]. In xenograft models, oral EGCG treatment suppresses the development of prostate cancer cells by upregulating apoptosis [43]. Anticancer treatment might focus on preventing tumor cells from migrating and invading healthy tissue. In order to prevent invasion and metastasis in hypopharyngeal cancer cells, EGCG inhibits hepatocyte growth factor (HGF)-induced matrix metalloproteinase (MMP)-9 and activation of urokinase-type plasminogen activator (uPA) (Figure 6) [44].

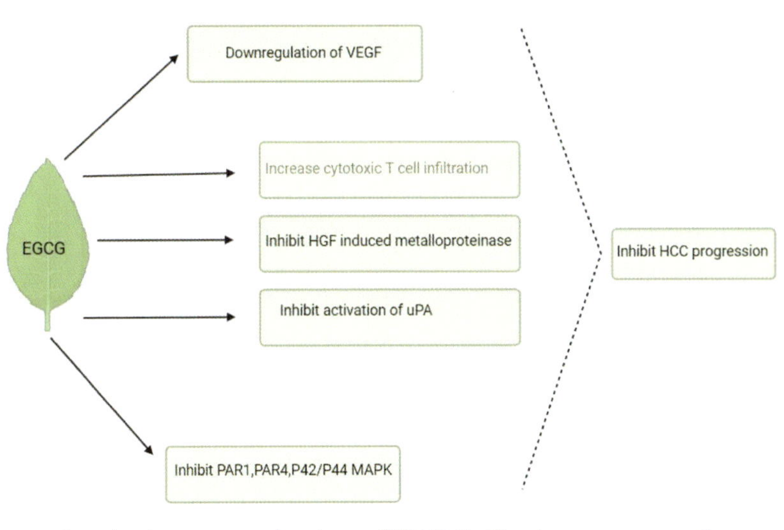

Figure 6: Anticancer mechanism of EGCG. Tea leaves are a major source for EGCG. By the action it targets to downregulate VEGF, increase infiltration of cytotoxic T cell infiltration, inhibit activation of uPA and so on thereby focusing to reduce the progression of hepatocellular carcinoma.

Through the modification of pharmacokinetics, the use of EGCG as an adjuvant may improve the curative properties of anticancer medications. The increased expression of P-glycoprotein causes multidrug resistance, which can be efficiently managed by ECGC [45]. Through alteration of P-glycoprotein function, EGCG causes vinblastine-induced drug-resistant cell death and doxorubicin-induced multidrug-resistant carcinoma cell death [46]. On the other hand, EGCG could interact directly with anticancer medications, which would negatively regulate their anticancer effects [47]. By changing the activity of MMPs, notably gelatinase A (MMP2) and gelatinase B (MMP9), EGCG has been found to limit cell invasion and metastasis development in a dose-dependent way [48]. The HCC progression-related PAR1, PAR4, and p42/p44 MAPKs all proved inhibited by EGCG [49]. The dose-dependent inhibition of cell proliferation by EGCG suggests that p53 is not the only component driving the inhibitory impact of EGCG on HCC growth [50]. Resveratrol has pharmacological properties that make it an effective treatment for a variety of liver conditions, including liver steatosis, fatty hepatitis, liver fibrosis, and liver cancer [51].

The capacity of HepG2 and Hep3B liver cancer cells to migrate and invade when exposed to phorbo-12-myristate 13-acetate (PMA) could be declined by resveratrol. Resveratrol lowered the activity of MMP-2 and MMP-9 while increasing the protein expression of TIMP-2 in Hep3B cells, with upregulating TIMP-1 protein expression and downregulating MMP-9 activity in HepG2 cells (Figure 7) [52].

A similar mechanism is also exhibited by silymarin. Silymarin hinders the recruitment of mast cells, which are implicated in invasion and angiogenesis, and subsequently reduced the expression of MMP-2 and MMP-9 (Figure 8) [53].

Silymarin modulates the state of the antioxidant defense system to prevent N-nitrosodiethylamine-induced hepatic carcinoma [54]. Additionally, silymarin treatment in the other trial significantly reduced the levels of carcinoembrional antigen (CEA), alpha-fetoprotein (AFP), malondialdehyde (MDA)-DNA adduct formation, and liver enzyme activity. Hence, a potential chemotherapeutic additive for the management of liver cancer could be silymarin [55]. Gingerol,

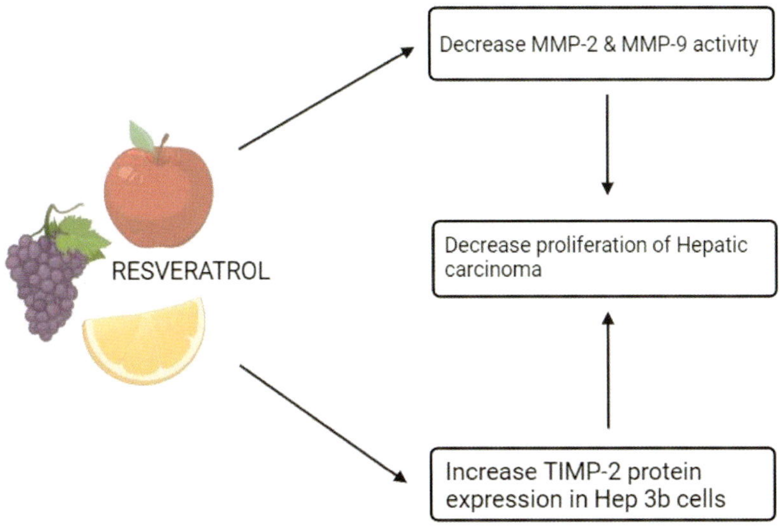

Figure 7: Anticancer mechanism of resveratrol. Fruits such as grapes, apples, and citrus are a major source for Resveratrol. It acts to reduce MMP-2 and MMP-9 activity, stimulating expression of TIMP-2 protein in Hep 3b cells, thereby reducing proliferation and growth of hepatic carcinomatous cells

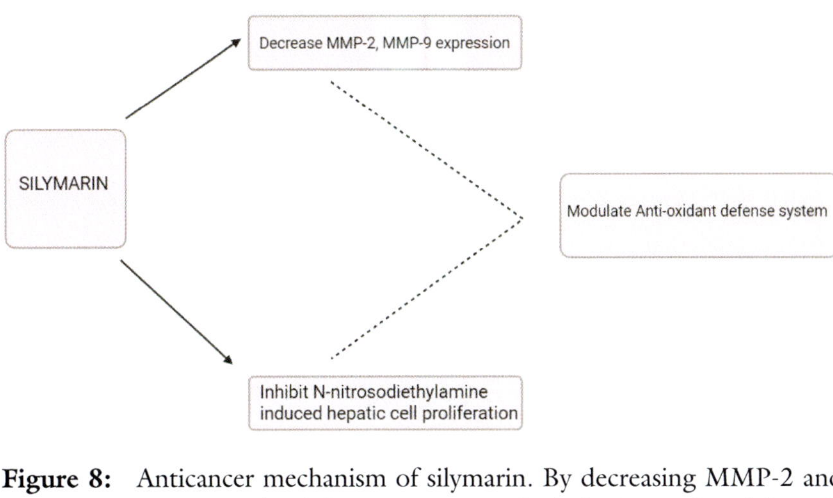

Figure 8: Anticancer mechanism of silymarin. By decreasing MMP-2 and MMP-9 expression and inhibiting N-nitrosodiethylamine-induced hepatic cell proliferation, Silymarin acts to modulate antioxidant defense system

derived from ginger, exerts antitumor activity in liver cells by targeting with good binding efficiency on PI3K and Akt. Gingerol and its derived compounds actively add to the reduction of HepG2 cell proliferation, enhance the progression of apoptosis in HepG2 cells, and upregulate the activity of Bax/Bcl-2 while downregulating the expression of p-Akt and Akt (Figure 9) [56].

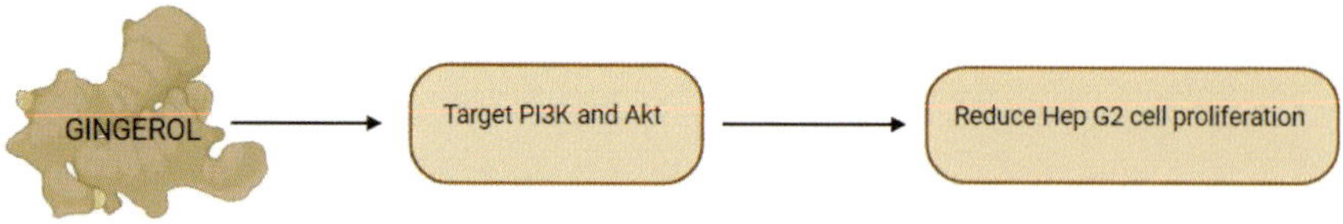

Figure 9: Anticancer mechanism of gingerol. PI3K and Akt inhibition are the major mechanism by which gingerol act to reduce Hep G2 cell proliferation

In hepatocellular carcinoma, Quercetin (3′,4′,5,7-tetrahydroxyflavonol) controls processes such as angiogenesis, fibrosis, migration, apoptosis, and inflammation. Additionally, it has a role in cell cycle arrest, cyclin synthesis inhibition, CDK inhibition, metabolic activity inhibition, cell death inhibition, and survival signal inhibition (Figure 10). Inhibiting the growth of hepatocellular carcinoma and

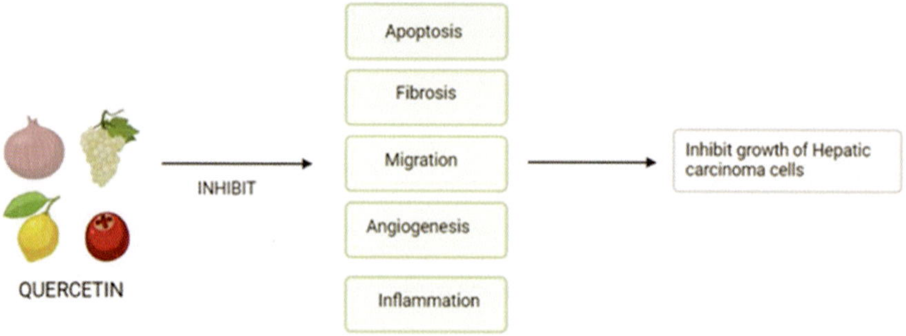

Figure 10: Anticancer mechanism of quercetin. This phytomolecule acts to reduce inflammation, apoptosis, fibrosis, migration, and angiogenesis, resulting in inhibition of growth of hepatic carcinoma cells

reducing the elements of the tumor microenvironment are other benefits associated with quercetin [57].

5. Challenges and Limitations

Undoubtedly, evaluating the difficulties and constraints of phytomolecules in the treatment of liver cancer is essential for an equitable evaluation of their therapeutic significance. The significant challenges and limitations in exploiting phytomolecules for liver cancer treatment are:

5.1. *Bioavailability*

Phytomolecules often have meager bioavailability, meaning that the body may not effectively absorb and utilize these compounds. This restriction can reduce their success in treating liver cancer. Policies to enhance bioavailability, such as nanoformulations or specific delivery systems, are still under examination [58].

5.2. *Standardization*

The lack of standardized formulations and dosage regimens for phytomolecules poses a weighty challenge. Variability in the quality and potency of natural products can lead to unreliable therapeutic outcomes and makes it difficult for clinicians to propose these compounds with confidence [59].

5.3. *Drug interactions*

Phytomolecules can interact with other medications a patient may be taking, potentially leading to adverse effects or reduced efficacy. This is particularly important in liver cancer, as many patients receive multiple medications, including chemotherapy drugs [59].

5.4. *Limited clinical evidence*

While there is growing interest in phytomolecules, clinical evidence supporting their efficacy in liver cancer treatment remains somewhat limited. Large-scale, long-term clinical trials are needed to establish their effectiveness definitively.

5.5. *Heterogeneity of liver cancer*

Liver cancer is a heterogeneous disease with various subtypes and genetic mutations. Phytomolecules may not be equally effective against all these subtypes, and identifying the most appropriate compounds for each patient's unique profile remains a challenge [60].

5.6. *Adverse effects*

Like any treatment, phytomolecules can have side effects. These side effects can vary depending on the specific compound and dosage used. Ensuring patient safety and managing these side effects can be challenging [61].

5.7. *Regulatory and safety concerns*

There is often limited oversight and regulation of phytomolecule products, which can lead to safety concerns and the risk of contamination. Ensuring product safety and efficacy is a challenge, and regulation in this area varies from country to country.

5.8. *Resistance and tolerance*

Over time, cancer cells can develop resistance or tolerance to phytomolecules, much like they do with traditional chemotherapy drugs. Development of resistance to phytomolecules in cancer treatment is a complicated problem involving genetic, molecular, and environmental factors. Understanding and overcoming resistance mechanisms is an unending challenge.

5.9. *Patient compliance*

Patients may find it tough to stick to intricate and occasionally stringent phytomolecule regimens, especially when coupled with standard treatment. Noncompliance to these medications may be due to complexity of regimen, side effects, lifestyle they need to follow and big financial burdens as these products are not covered by insurance.

5.10. *Cost and accessibility*

Some patients may lack easy access to superior phytomolecule supplements or products since they might be expensive to purchase, especially in areas with poor incomes.

5.11. *Lack of long-term data*

Long-term data on the safety and effectiveness of phytomolecule treatments for liver cancer are often lacking. This gap makes it challenging to make informed decisions regarding their use as long-term therapies.

It is important to note that while these challenges and limitations exist, phytomolecules also offer several advantages, including their potential as complementary or alternative treatments with fewer side effects. Researchers continue to investigate and address these issues to unlock the full therapeutic potential of phytomolecules in liver cancer treatment.

6. Drug Interactions and Side Effects

When using phytomolecules in the treatment of liver cancer, it is important to be aware of potential drug interactions and side effects. Phytomolecules, though considered natural compounds, can interact with other medications and produce side effects. Here are some drug interactions and side effects to consider:

6.1. *Drug interactions*

1. **Cytochrome P450 (CYP) interactions:** Phytomolecules can influence the activity of various cytochrome P450 enzymes, which play a crucial role in drug metabolism. This can lead to altered blood levels and efficacy of concurrently administered pharmaceuticals. For example, compounds like St. John's Wort may induce CYP3A4, potentially affecting the metabolism of certain chemotherapy drugs [62].
2. **Anticoagulants:** Phytomolecules such as ginkgo biloba and garlic can have anticoagulant properties. When combined with blood-thinning medications (e.g., warfarin), they may increase the risk of bleeding.
3. **Immunosuppressive drugs:** Phytomolecules with immunomodulatory effects, such as echinacea or astragalus, may interfere with immunosuppressive drugs used after liver transplantation, potentially reducing their efficacy.
4. **Anti-hypertensive medications:** Certain phytomolecules like hawthorn or coenzyme Q10 might interact with medications used to lower blood pressure, potentially leading to hypotension.
5. **Antidiabetic medications:** Phytomolecules like bitter melon and fenugreek may affect blood sugar levels. This interaction can be problematic for individuals taking antidiabetic medications.
6. **Herb-drug interactions:** Various herbs and phytomolecules can interact with medications. For example, Ginkgo supplements have been associated with increased bleeding risk, particularly when taken with anticoagulant medications like warfarin. It can interfere with blood clotting and lead to excessive bleeding [63].

6.2. *Common side effects of phytomolecules*

1. **Gastrointestinal disturbances:** Many phytomolecules, such as curcumin or green tea extracts, can cause digestive issues such as

nausea, diarrhea, abdominal discomfort, gas and bloating, indigestion, and heartburn.

2. **Allergic reactions:** Allergic reactions to phytomolecules are possible. Symptoms can range from rashes, itching, swelling, and breathing difficulties to severe anaphylactic reactions.
3. **Liver toxicity:** Liver toxicity related to phytomolecules or herbs is relatively rare but can be severe when it occurs. The mechanisms of liver toxicity can vary and may involve the production of toxic metabolites or the direct impact of certain compounds on liver function. Some herbs and phytomolecules, like kava and comfrey, have been associated with liver damage in rare cases.
4. **Hormonal effects:** Some phytomolecules may have hormonal activity. These effects may be attributed to the presence of phytoestrogens, adaptogens, or other bioactive compounds in certain plants or herbs. The hormonal effects of phytomolecules can vary depending on the specific compound, dose, and individual factors. For example, soy-derived compounds can affect estrogen levels. This may be of concern in certain liver cancer cases.
5. **Blood pressure changes:** Phytomolecules can affect the cardiovascular system and blood vessels. Phytomolecules like licorice root can influence blood pressure, leading to hypertension or hypotension in some individuals.
6. **Interference with blood clotting:** Certain phytomolecules can have antiplatelet or anticoagulant effects, potentially leading to bleeding issues. Example: Allicin present in garlic.
7. **Neurological effects:** Some herbal supplements, such as kava, have been associated with neurological symptoms such as headache, dizziness, changes in mood, tremors dystonia.

It is imperative to consult with a healthcare provider, preferably one experienced in integrative or complementary medicine, when considering the use of phytomolecules in the treatment of liver cancer. A healthcare professional can assess the individual patient's medical history, current medications, and tailor a treatment plan that minimizes drug interactions and side effects while maximizing potential benefits. Regular monitoring and open communication are key to ensuring safe and effective treatment.

7. Chemoprevention

Chemoprevention, a vital strategy in the battle against cancer, involves the use of specific agents to inhibit or delay the development of cancer. Phytomolecules, derived from plant sources, have emerged as promising candidates for chemoprevention due to their natural origin and potential to counteract cancer-promoting processes. These compounds, such as curcumin from turmeric or green tea catechins, are well-documented for their anti-inflammatory, antioxidant, and antiproliferative properties. Chemopreventive phytomolecules exert their effects at various stages of carcinogenesis, from preventing DNA damage to inhibiting the growth of cancer cells. They are particularly attractive due to their relatively low toxicity compared to conventional chemopreventive drugs, making them appealing for long-term use in high-risk populations or as complementary strategies alongside conventional therapies [64].

Studies focusing on the chemopreventive properties of phytomolecules have provided valuable insights into their mechanisms of action. For instance, curcumin has been shown to suppress inflammation-related signaling pathways, making it a potent agent against inflammation-associated liver cancer. Green tea catechins have demonstrated the ability to inhibit the progression of liver cancer by modulating cell cycle regulation and inducing apoptosis in cancer cells. The versatility of phytomolecules in targeting various molecular pathways implicated in carcinogenesis underscores their potential as effective and safe chemopreventive agents. However, while these findings are promising, further research is needed to establish optimal dosages, long-term safety, and efficacy in different populations to fully harness the chemopreventive potential of phytomolecules in liver cancer and beyond.

7.1. *Chemo sensitization*

Chemo sensitization refers to the process by which specific compounds or agents, such as phytomolecules, are used to enhance the sensitivity of cancer cells to conventional treatments like chemotherapy. In the context of liver cancer, this approach can be particularly valuable, given the resistance that liver cancer cells may develop against chemotherapy drugs. Phytomolecules have demonstrated the ability to sensitize liver cancer cells to these treatments through various mechanisms [65].

One crucial way in which phytomolecules can enhance chemosensitivity is by modulating drug efflux pumps. Many chemotherapy drugs are pumped out of cancer cells by proteins like P-glycoprotein, reducing their effectiveness. Certain phytomolecules, such as curcumin and quercetin, have been shown to inhibit these efflux pumps, allowing chemotherapy drugs to accumulate within the cancer cells, thereby increasing their cytotoxic effects. Additionally, phytomolecules possess the ability to interfere with cancer cell survival pathways, making the cells more vulnerable to the cytotoxic effects of chemotherapy. For example, compounds like resveratrol can inhibit the activation of survival proteins, such as NF-κB and Bcl-2, making liver cancer cells more susceptible to chemotherapy-induced cell death [66].

Furthermore, some phytomolecules have demonstrated the ability to reduce the production of pro-survival and anti-apoptotic molecules while increasing the expression of pro-apoptotic proteins within liver cancer cells. The overall result is an increased likelihood of chemotherapy drugs inducing apoptosis in these sensitized cancer cells. The combination of chemotherapy with phytomolecules that enhance chemosensitivity holds promise for improving the treatment outcomes for liver cancer patients, potentially reducing drug resistance and enhancing the overall effectiveness of chemotherapy regimens.

7.2. *Chemotherapy strategies*

Phytomolecules serve as promising adjuncts to chemotherapy in the treatment of liver cancer by augmenting the therapeutic outcomes. These natural compounds, found in various plant sources, offer several advantages in combination with chemotherapy. They can enhance the sensitivity of liver cancer cells to chemotherapy drugs, reducing the chances of drug resistance and improving the overall efficacy of treatment. Moreover, phytomolecules often exhibit antioxidant and anti-inflammatory properties, which can help mitigate the side effects associated with chemotherapy, such as oxidative stress and inflammation. Integrating phytomolecules as adjuncts to chemotherapy represents a comprehensive approach that seeks to maximize the benefits of conventional cancer treatment while minimizing its drawbacks, ultimately improving the overall quality of care for liver cancer patients [67].

7.3. *The role in enhancing the effectiveness of chemotherapy drugs*

Phytomolecules play a pivotal role in enhancing the effectiveness of chemotherapy drugs in the treatment of liver cancer through various mechanisms. These natural compounds, such as curcumin and green tea catechins, can sensitize liver cancer cells to chemotherapy by inhibiting drug efflux pumps, preventing the expulsion of chemotherapy drugs from the cells. Additionally, phytomolecules possess anti-inflammatory and antioxidant properties, reducing the harmful side effects associated with chemotherapy and supporting overall treatment tolerance. They can also influence cancer cell survival pathways, making the cells more susceptible to the cytotoxic effects of chemotherapy, ultimately increasing the likelihood of apoptosis and tumor regression. The combination of phytomolecules with chemotherapy represents a promising strategy to improve treatment outcomes, potentially overcoming drug resistance and offering a comprehensive approach to liver cancer therapy [68].

8. Real-World Application of Phytomolecules in Liver Cancer Treatment — Case Studies

In Phase I/II trials, researchers investigated the safety and efficacy of curcumin in patients with advanced hepatocellular carcinoma (HCC), a common type of liver cancer. The study showed that curcumin was well-tolerated, and some patients experienced stable disease. Some studies have explored the potential benefits of combining curcumin with conventional chemotherapy for liver cancer treatment [69].

Silymarin is a flavonoid complex derived from the milk thistle plant and its supplementation was associated with improved liver function and a reduction in certain liver enzymes. Silymarin may be considered as a complementary therapy to support liver health, mitigate chemotherapy-related liver damage, or help manage certain symptoms [70].

Numerous preclinical studies have shown that green tea polyphenols, especially EGCG, have the potential to inhibit the growth of liver tumors in animal models. Some research suggests that regular consumption of green tea or green tea extracts may reduce the risk of liver cancer, especially in high-risk populations such as individuals with chronic liver diseases (e.g., hepatitis B or C) or those with cirrhosis [71].

8.1. *Clinical studies*

Su et al. [72] explored gingerol's potential mechanism for treating liver cancer using network pharmacology and molecular docking technology and conducted *in vitro* experiments of human liver cancer cell HepG2 to verify important signaling pathways. They obtained potential targets of gingerol derivatives (6-gingerol, 8-gingerol and 10-gingerol) from PubChem and SwissTarget Prediction websites and collected related targets for liver cancer with the help of GeneCards and performed Gene Ontology (GO) and Kyoto Encyclopedia of Genes and Genomes (KEGG) enrichment analysis on key targets using the DAVID data platform and combined with Cytoscape 3.7.1 software to construct a component–target–signal pathway interaction map to study its mechanism of action. Subsequently, the components and key proteins were molecularly docked through Autodock Vina software. Finally, the important signal pathways were verified by HepG2 cell *in vitro* experiments. Bioinformatics analysis found that GO obtained 20 important functional items including cancer cell proliferation, protein kinase activity, phosphotransferase activity, and kinase activity; KEGG enrichment analysis yielded a total of 20 key signal pathways including the PI3K–Akt signaling pathway. The results of molecular docking show that the binding energy of gingerol derivatives has good binding activity with PI3K and Akt. The results of network pharmacology and experimental validation suggest that gingerol derivatives and compound gingerol can act against liver cancer by acting on the PI3K-Akt signaling pathway.

James et al. [73] investigated the potential of curcumin, a diet-derived agent, in enhancing the effectiveness of chemotherapy in colorectal cancer stem cell (CSC) models using patient-derived colorectal liver metastases (CRLM). The findings demonstrated that both curcumin alone and in combination with FOLFOX chemotherapy notably decreased spheroid number and reduced the population of cells displaying high aldehyde dehydrogenase activity (ALDH(high)/CD133(-)) in CSC models derived from patients. Moreover, the addition of curcumin to oxaliplatin/5-FU intensified antiproliferative and pro-apoptotic effects in a subset of patient-derived explants while diminishing the expression of stem cell-associated markers ALDH and CD133. The subsequent Phase I dose escalation study involving 12 patients with CRLM revealed that curcumin, at doses up to 2 grams daily, was safe and well-tolerated as an adjunct to FOLFOX chemotherapy, suggesting its potential to offer added benefit in specific patient subsets as a chemotherapy adjunct.

Siegel et al. [74] conducted a Phase I study in patients with advanced hepatocellular carcinoma (HCC) and compromised hepatic function. They were administered silybin phosphatidylcholine (Siliphos) to determine the maximum tolerated dose per day. The trial, conducted in a single institution, enrolled three participants across four planned cohorts escalating from 2 to 12 g per day in divided doses over 12 weeks. All three patients completed the 2 g per day regimen, leading to increased serum concentrations of silibinin and its metabolite silibinin glucuronide within 1 to 3 weeks. Despite observing progression in liver function abnormalities and the tumor marker α-fetoprotein in all patients, the third participant showed some improvement in liver function abnormalities and inflammatory biomarkers after day 56. However, unfortunately, all three participants succumbed within 23 to 69 days of enrollment, likely due to hepatic failure, although the possibility of the deaths being linked to the study drug could not be conclusively ruled out. The study could not establish the maximum tolerated dose, suggesting that patients in this severely ill population might not have benefited from an intervention aimed at improving liver function tests in the short term.

Howells et al. [75] did extensive preclinical investigations of cancer chemopreventive potential of resveratrol, a phytochemical compound. However, its limited systemic availability due to rapid metabolism poses a challenge for its efficacy in preventing malignancies in distant organs. Micronization has been proposed to enhance resveratrol's absorption, thereby improving its availability in the body. In this pilot study, SRT501, a micronized form of resveratrol, was administered at a dosage of 5.0 g daily for 14 days to patients with colorectal cancer and hepatic metastases scheduled for hepatectomy. The study aimed to evaluate the safety, pharmacokinetics, and pharmacodynamics of this formulation. SRT501 was well-tolerated, exhibiting significantly higher mean plasma resveratrol levels (1,942 ± 1,422 ng/mL) after a single dose compared to nonmicronized resveratrol at equivalent doses, surpassing them by 3.6-fold. Notably, hepatic tissue following SRT501 administration showed detectable levels of resveratrol (up to 2,287 ng/g), and there was a marked 39% increase in cleaved caspase-3, indicating heightened apoptosis in malignant hepatic tissue compared to placebo-treated patients. These promising findings suggest that SRT501 merits further clinical investigation to delineate its potential clinical application in cancer therapy.

9. Safety and Challenges

The safety profile of phytomolecules in the context of liver cancer treatment is generally favorable. These natural compounds are often associated with low toxicity, making them suitable for long-term use. While they offer numerous benefits, including anti-inflammatory and antioxidant properties, they can also produce side effects.

Careful monitoring of liver function is crucial, as some phytomolecules have been linked to rare cases of hepatotoxicity. Toxic effects are especially of concern for phytomolecules with narrow therapeutic index. Potential interactions with other medications should be considered, especially when used alongside chemotherapy or cancer-related drugs. Patients should be vigilant for allergic reactions, albeit rare, and consult healthcare professionals for guidance on individualized treatment plans. The quality and purity of phytomolecule products must be ensured to reduce safety concerns. In summary, phytomolecules offer a safe and valuable adjunct to liver cancer treatment, but their usage should be managed under the supervision of healthcare providers.

9.1. *Future directions*

Emerging trends in the field of phytomolecules and liver cancer treatment include a growing emphasis on personalized medicine, where treatment approaches are tailored to the individual patient's genetic and molecular profile. Additionally, there is a focus on nanotechnology, which aims to enhance the delivery and bioavailability of phytomolecules through the use of nanocarriers. Combinatorial approaches, using multiple phytomolecules in synergy with each other or conventional therapies, are gaining attention for their potential to improve therapeutic outcomes. Advances in bioinformatics and data analytics are aiding in the discovery of phytomolecules with anti-liver cancer properties and their mechanisms of action. Lastly, the development of standardized natural extracts and eco-friendly cultivation practices ensures the quality and sustainability of phytomolecule sources for liver cancer treatment.

10. Conclusion

Traditional medical practices such as Ayurveda, traditional Chinese medicine (TCM) and various indigenous traditions rely on phytomolecules. But scientific validation and sufficient quality control measures are necessary for collaborating phytomolecules with modern medicine. To merge phytomolecules into liver cancer treatment allows a personalized and holistic approach. By targeting key pathways and mechanisms, phytomolecules offer an exciting avenue for further research and therapeutic development. Additional research is also needed regarding the impact of phytomolecules in liver cancer and its cytotoxic effects on target cancer cells. Large-scale, well-controlled clinical trials are needed to validate their efficacies, adverse effects and safety before the use in treatment of hepatocellular carcinoma and in clinical practice.

Conflict of Interest

The authors declare no conflict of interest.

References

1. Sung H, Ferlay J, Siegel RL, Laversanne M, Soerjomataram I, Jemal A, et al. Global cancer statistics 2020: GLOBOCAN estimates of incidence and mortality worldwide for 36 cancers in 185 countries. *CA Cancer J Clin*, 2021.71(3):p. 209–249.
2. Bruix J, Reig M, Sherman M. Evidence-based diagnosis, staging, and treatment of patients with hepatocellular carcinoma. *Gastroenterology*, 2016.150(4):p. 835–853.
3. Llovet JM, Bruix J. Novel advancements in the management of hepatocellular carcinoma in 2008. *J Hepatol*, 2008.48(Suppl 1):p. S20–S37.
4. Smith J, Johnson A. Challenges of conventional liver cancer treatments. *Liver Oncol.* 2022.5(2):p. 123–135.
5. Brown R, Davis S. Early detection challenges in liver cancer. *Cancer Res*, 2021.30(4):p. 341–355.
6. Pandey KB, Rizvi SI. Plant polyphenols as dietary antioxidants in human health and disease. *Oxid Med Cell Longev*, 2009.2(5):p. 270–278.

7. Shukla S, Meena AK. *In vitro* and *in vivo* anticancer activity of a novel formulation of lycopene and quercetin. *J Cancer Res Ther*, 2017.13(1): p. 49–54.
8. Sahu SC, et al. Anticancer properties of phytochemicals present in medicinal plants of North America. *Int J Exp Bot*, 2013.54(392): p. 2923–2938.
9. Abotaleb M, Samuel SM, Varghese E, Varghese S, Kubatka P, Liskova A, et al. Flavonoids in cancer and apoptosis. *Cancers*, 2019.11(1): p. 28.
10. Mirza Z, Karim S. Structure-based profiling of potential phytomolecules with AKT1 a key cancer drug target. *Mol Basel Switz*, 2023.28(6): p. 2597.
11. Ali R, Mirza Z, Ashraf GMD, Kamal MA, Ansari SA, Damanhouri GA, et al. New anticancer agents: recent developments in tumor therapy. *Anticancer Res*, 2012.32(7):p. 2999–3005.
12. Das AP, Agarwal SM. Recent advances in the area of plant-based anti-cancer drug discovery using computational approaches. *Mol Divers*, 2023.21:p. 1–25.
13. Kaplan A. The nanocomposites designs of phytomolecules from medicinal and aromatic plants: promising anticancer-antiviral applications. *Beni-Suef Univ J Basic Appl Sci*, 2022.11(1):p. 17.
14. Anand P, Sundaram C, Jhurani S, Kunnumakkara AB, Aggarwal BB. Curcumin and cancer: an "old-age" disease with an "age-old" solution. *Cancer Lett*, 2008.267(1):p. 133–164.
15. Discovery of a new function of curcumin which enhances its anticancer therapeutic potency | Scientific Reports [Internet]. [cited 2023 Oct 22]. Available from: https://www.nature.com/articles/
16. Lecumberri E, Dupertuis YM, Miralbell R, Pichard C. Green tea polyphenol epigallocatechin-3-gallate (EGCG) as adjuvant in cancer therapy. *Clin Nutr Edinb Scotl*, 2013.32(6):p. 894–903.
17. Yang CS, Wang X, Lu G, Picinich SC. Cancer prevention by tea: animal studies, molecular mechanisms and human relevance. *Nat Rev Cancer*, 2009.9(6):p. 429–439.
18. The Role of Resveratrol in Cancer Therapy-PMC [Internet]. [cited 2023 Oct 22]. Available from: https://www.ncbi.nlm.nih.gov/pmc/articles/PMC5751192/

19. Agarwal R, Agarwal C, Ichikawa H, Singh RP, Aggarwal BB. Anticancer potential of silymarin: from bench to bed side. ***Anticancer Res***, 2006. 26(6B):p. 4457–4498.
20. Rauf A, Imran M, Khan IA, Ur-Rehman M, Gilani SA, Mehmood Z, et al. Anticancer potential of quercetin: a comprehensive review. *Phytother Res PTR*, 2018.32(11):p. 2109–2130.
21. Lee JY, Kim HS, Song YS. Genistein as a potential anticancer agent against ovarian cancer. ***J Tradit Complement Med***, 2012.2(2):p. 96–104.
22. Almatroodi SA, Alsahli MA, Rahmani AH. Berberine: an important emphasis on its anticancer effects through modulation of various cell signaling pathways. *Mol Basel Switz*, 2022.27(18):p. 5889.
23. Rahmani AH, Alsahli MA, Almatroudi A, Almogbel MA, Khan AA, Anwar S, et al. The potential role of Apigenin in cancer prevention and treatment. *Mol Basel Switz*, 2022.27(18):p. 6051.
24. Furlan V, Bren U. Protective effects of [6]-gingerol against chemical carcinogens: mechanistic insights. ***Int J Mol Sci***, 2020.21(3):p. 695.
25. Rather RA, Bhagat M. Cancer chemoprevention and piperine: molecular mechanisms and therapeutic opportunities. ***Front Cell Dev Biol***, 2018. p. 6–10.
26. Tripathi YB, Tripathi P, Arjmandi BH. Nutraceuticals and cancer management. ***Front Biosci J Virtual Libr***, 2005.1(10):p. 1607–1618.
27. Tomeh MA, Hadianamrei R, Zhao X. A review of curcumin and its derivatives as anticancer agents. ***Int J Mol Sci***, 2019.20(5):p. 1033.
28. Shahriari M, Kesharwani P, Johnston TP, Sahebkar A. Anticancer potential of curcumin-cyclodextrin complexes and their pharmacokinetic properties. ***Int J Pharm***, 2023.631:p. 122474.
29. Unlu A, Nayir E, Kalenderoglu MD, Kirca O, Ozdogan M. Curcumin (turmeric) and cancer. Available from: https://www.ncbi.nim.nih.gov/pubmed/17044766.
30. Davie JR, He S, Li L, Sekhavat A, Espino P, Drobic B, et al. Nuclear organization and chromatin dynamics--Sp1, Sp3 and histone deacetylases. *Adv Enzyme Regul*, 2008.48:p. 189–208.
31. Lee JY, Lee YM, Chang GC, Yu SL, Hsieh WY, Chen JJW, et al. Curcumin induces EGFR degradation in lung adenocarcinoma and

modulates p38 activation in intestine: the versatile adjuvant for gefitinib therapy. *PLoS One*, 2011.6(8):p.e23756.

32. Kim HJ, Park SY, Park OJ, Kim YM. Curcumin suppresses migration and proliferation of Hep3B hepatocarcinoma cells through inhibition of the Wnt signaling pathway. *Mol Med Rep*, 2013.8(1):p. 282–286.
33. Heger M, van Golen RF, Broekgaarden M, Michel MC. The molecular basis for the pharmacokinetics and pharmacodynamics of curcumin and its metabolites in relation to cancer. *Pharmacol Rev*, 2014.66(1): 222–307.
34. Jung KH, Yoo W, Stevenson HL, Deshpande D, Shen H, Gagea M, et al. Multifunctional effects of a small-molecule STAT3 inhibitor on NASH and hepatocellular carcinoma in mice. *Clin Cancer Res*, 2017.23(18):p. 5537–5546.
35. Zuo M, Li C, Lin J, Javle M. LLL12, a novel small inhibitor targeting STAT3 for hepatocellular carcinoma therapy. *Oncotarget*, 2015.6(13): p. 10940–10949.
36. Feng T, Wei Y, Lee RJ, Zhao L. Liposomal curcumin and its application in cancer. *Int J Nanomed*, 2017.12:p. 6027–6044.
37. Fan H, Tian W, Ma X. Curcumin induces apoptosis of HepG2 cells via inhibiting fatty acid synthase. *Target Oncol*, 2014.9(3):279–286.
38. National Library of Medicine. Anticancer effects and molecular mechanisms of epigallocatechin-3-gallate-PMC [Internet]. [cited 2023 Oct 22]. Available from: https://www.ncbi.nlm.nih.gov/pmc/articles/PMC5481703/
39. Mantena SK, Roy AM, Katiyar SK. Retracted: epigallocatechin-3-gallate inhibits photocarcinogenesis through inhibition of angiogenic factors and activation of CD^{8+} T Cells in tumors. *Photochem Photobiol*, 2005.81(5):p. 1174–1179.
40. Shimizu M, Shirakami Y, Sakai H, Yasuda Y, Kubota M, Adachi S, et al. (-)-Epigallocatechin gallate inhibits growth and activation of the VEGF/VEGFR axis in human colorectal cancer cells. *Chem Biol Interact*, 2010.185(3):p. 247–252.
41. Liang YC, Lin-shiau SY, Chen CF, Lin JK. Suppression of extracellular signals and cell proliferation through EGF receptor binding by (-)-epigallocatechin gallate in human A431 epidermoid carcinoma cells. *J Cell Biochem*, 1997.67(1):p. 55–65.

42. Khan N, Bharali DJ, Adhami VM, Siddiqui IA, Cui H, Shabana SM, et al. Oral administration of naturally occurring chitosan-based nanoformulated green tea polyphenol EGCG effectively inhibits prostate cancer cell growth in a xenograft model. *Carcinogenesis*, 2014.35(2):p. 415–423.
43. Lim YC, Park HY, Hwang HS, Kang SU, Pyun JH, Lee MH, et al. (–)-Epigallocatechin-3-gallate (EGCG) inhibits HGF-induced invasion and metastasis in hypopharyngeal carcinoma cells. *Cancer Lett*, 2008. 271(1):p. 140–152.
44. Jodoin J, Demeule M, Beliveau R. Inhibition of the multidrug resistance P-glycoprotein activity by green tea polyphenols. *Biochim Biophys Acta*, 2002.1542(1–3):p. 149–159.
45. Qian F, Wei D, Zhang Q, Yang S. Modulation of P-glycoprotein function and reversal of multidrug resistance by (–)-epigallocatechin gallate in human cancer cells. *Biomed Pharmacother*, 2005.59(3):p. 64–69.
46. Ge J, Tan BX, Chen Y, Yang L, Peng XC, Li HZ, et al. Interaction of green tea polyphenol epigallocatechin-3-gallate with sunitinib: potential risk of diminished sunitinib bioavailability. *J Mol Med Berl Ger*, 2011. 89(6):p. 595–602.
47. Lee SI, Kim HJ, Boo YC. Effect of green tea and (–)-epigallocatechin gallate on ethanol-induced toxicity in HepG2 cells. *Phytother Res PTR*, 2008.22(5):p. 669–674.
48. Kaufmann R, Henklein P, Henklein P, Settmacher U. Green tea polyphenol epigallocatechin-3-gallate inhibits thrombin-induced hepatocellular carcinoma cell invasion and p42/p44-MAPKinase activation. *Oncol Rep*, 2009.21(5):p. 1261–1267.
49. Bimonte S, Albino V, Piccirillo M, Nasto A, Molino C, Palaia R, et al. Epigallocatechin-3-gallate in the prevention and treatment of hepatocellular carcinoma: experimental findings and translational perspectives. *Drug Des Devel Ther*, 2019.13:p. 611–621.
50. Chupradit S, Bokov D, Zamanian MY, Heidari M, Hakimizadeh E. Hepatoprotective and therapeutic effects of resveratrol: a focus on anti-inflammatory and antioxidative activities. *Fundam Clin Pharmacol*, 2022.36(3):p. 468–485.
51. Weng CJ, Wu CF, Huang HW, Wu CH, Ho CT, Yen GC. Evaluation of anti-invasion effect of resveratrol and related methoxy analogues

on human hepatocarcinoma cells. *J Agric Food Chem*, 2010.58(5): p. 2886–2894.

52. Feher J, Lengyel G. Silymarin in the prevention and treatment of liver diseases and primary liver cancer. *Curr Pharm Biotechnol*, 2012.13(1):p. 210–217.
53. Ramakrishnan G, Lo Muzio L, Elinos-Báez CM, Jagan S, Augustine TA, Kamaraj S, et al. Silymarin inhibited proliferation and induced apoptosis in hepatic cancer cells. *Cell Prolif*, 2009.42(2):p. 229–240.
54. Ramakrishnan G, Augustine TA, Jagan S, Vinodhkumar R, Devaki T. Effect of silymarin on N-nitrosodiethylamine induced hepatocarcinogenesis in rats. *Exp Oncol*, 2007.1:p. 39–44.
55. Su M, Wang X, Cao G, Sun L, Ho RJY, Han Y, et al. Prediction of the potential mechanism of compound gingerol against liver cancer based on network pharmacology and experimental verification. *J Pharm Pharmacol*, 2022.74(6):p. 869–886.
56. Sethi G, Rath P, Chauhan A, Ranjan A, Choudhary R, Ramniwas S, et al. Apoptotic mechanisms of quercetin in liver cancer: recent trends and advancements. *Pharmaceutics*, 2023.15(2):p. 712.
57. Manach C, Scalbert A, Morand C, Rémésy C, Jiménez L. Polyphenols: food sources and bioavailability. *Am J Clin Nutr*, 2004.79(5):p. 727–747.
58. Gonçalves RV, Novaes RD, Sarandy MM, Júnior JV. Phytomolecules in the treatment of obesity: pharmacological, nutraceutical, and chemical aspects. *Eur J Nutr*, 2019.58(5):p. 1623–1637.
59. Huang SM, Lesko LJ. Drug interactions and the evolution of new regulations for clinical development. *J Clin Pharmacol*, 2007.47(5): p. 499–501.
60. Russo M, Spagnuolo C, Tedesco I, Bilotto S, Russo GL. The flavonoid quercetin in disease prevention and therapy: facts and fancies. *Biochem Pharmacol*, 2012.83(1):p. 6–15.
61. Zanger UM, Schwab M. Cytochrome P450 enzymes in drug metabolism: regulation of gene expression, enzyme activities, and impact of genetic variation. *Pharmacol Ther*, 2013.138(1):p. 103–141.
62. Bush TM, Rayburn KS, Holloway SW, Sanchez CA, Thomas JD. Adverse interactions between herbal and dietary substances and prescription medications: a clinical survey. *Altern Ther Health Med*, 2007.13(2): p. 30–35.

63. Surh YJ. Cancer chemoprevention with dietary phytochemicals. *Nat Rev Cancer*, 2003.3(10):p. 768–780.
64. Darvishi B, Manoochehri M, Kamalinia G, Fallah M, Saedi T. Chemosensitization effect of thymoquinone in cancer cells. *Drug Discov Today*, 2015.20(11):p. 1312–1322.
65. Shukla Y, Singh R. Resveratrol and cellular mechanisms of cancer prevention. *Ann N Y Acad Sci*, 2011.1:p. 1–8.
66. Aggarwal BB, Shishodia S. Molecular targets of dietary agents for prevention and therapy of cancer. *Biochem Pharmacol*, 2006.71(10): p. 1397–1421.
67. El-Tanbouly DM, Wadie W, Mady EA, Kassab AE, Khattab MM. Antimetastatic and anti-angiogenic properties of the combination of *Nigella sativa*, *Linum usitatissimum*, and *Papaver somniferum* ethanolic extracts. *Oncol Lett*, 2020.20(5):p. 286.
68. Kanai M, Otsuka Y, Otsuka K, Sato M, Nishimura T, Mori Y, et al. A phase I study investigating the safety and pharmacokinetics of highly bioavailable curcumin (Theracurmin) in cancer patients. *Cancer Chemother Pharmacol*, 2013.71(6):p. 1521–1530.
69. Abenavoli L, Capasso R, Milic N, Capasso F. Milk thistle in liver diseases: past, present, future. *Phytother Res*, 2010.24(10):p. 1423–1432.
70. Zhang LH, Huang YH, Zhao L. Phytomedicine polyphenol epigallocatechin-3-gallate: a systematic review of its anticancer properties and clinical use in liver cancer. *Food Chem*, 2015.5(1):p. 36–43.
71. Cao H, Wang C, Chen X, Hou Y, Xiang Z, Shen X. Protective role of green tea on hepatocellular carcinoma in clinical studies and animal models. *Chin Med J*, 2009.122(19):p. 2301–2305.
72. Su M, Wang X, Cao G, Sun L, Ho RJY, Han Y, et al. Prediction of the potential mechanism of compound gingerol against liver cancer based on network pharmacology and experimental verification. *J Pharm Pharmacol*, 2022.74:p. 869–886.
73. James MI, Iwuji C, Irving G, Karmokar A, Higgins JA, Griffin-Teal N, et al. Curcumin inhibits cancer stem cell phenotypes in ex vivo models of colorectal liver metastases, and is clinically safe and tolerable in combination with FOLFOX chemotherapy. *Cancer Lett*, 2015.364(2): p. 135–141.

74. Siegel AB, Narayan R, Rodrigues R, Goyal A, Jacobson JS, Kelly K, et al. A phase I dose-finding study of silybin phosphatidylcholine (Milk Thistle) in patients with advanced hepatocellular carcinoma. *Integr Cancer Ther*, 2014.13(1):p. 46–53.
75. Howells LM, Berry DP, Elliott PJ, Jacobson EW, Hoffmann E, Hegarty B, et al. Phase I randomised double-blind pilot study of micronized resveratrol (SRT501) in patients with hepatic metastases-safety, pharmacokinetics and pharmacodynamics. *Cancer Prev Res*, 2011.4(9): p. 1419–1425.

https://doi.org/10.1142/9789811293320_0013

Chapter 13

Phytochemicals in Liver Cancer-Translational Limitations and Strategies

Akhila S[1,*] and Remya K[2]

[1]*KVM College of Pharmacy, Cherthala, Alappuzha (Dist.), Kerala, India*
[2]*Alshifa College of Pharmacy, Perinthalmanna, Malappuram (Dist.), Kerala, India*

Table of Contents:

*Corresponding author: E-mail address: akhilamadathil84@gmail.com

Abbreviations:

HCC — Hepatocellular carcinoma
WHO — World Health Organization
WCRF — World Cancer Research Fund
LC — Liver cancer
RBC — Red blood corpuscles
DNA — Deoxyribonucleic acid
NF-κB — Nuclear factor kappa-light-chain-enhancer of activated B cells
IκB-α — IkappaB kinase
Bfl-1/A1 — Bcl-2 related gene in fetal liver
Bcl-xL — B-cell lymphoma-extra large
TNF-α — Tumor necrosis factor-alpha
Bcl-2 — B-cell lymphoma 2
P-gp — P-glycoprotein
HepG2 — Hepatoblastoma cell line
AST — Aspartate transaminase
ALT — Alanine transaminase
ALP — Alkaline phosphatase
EGC — Epigallocatechin
ROS — Reactive oxygen species
MAKPK — Mitogen activation protein kinase
Kip1/p27 — Cyclin-dependent kinase inhibitor 1B
MDR — Multiple drug resistance
pk — Pharmacokinetic

Abstract

Liver cancer (LC), particularly hepatocellular carcinoma (HCC), represents a significant world health burden because of its aggressive nature and limited options for therapy. With the growing interest in complementary and alternative medicine, phytochemicals have emerged as potential candidates for the treatment and prevention of liver carcinoma. Phytochemicals, derived from various plant sources, have several therapeutic properties, including anti-proliferative, anti-inflammatory, and anti-angiogenic properties, which can target the complex molecular pathways involved in liver carcinogenesis. Despite promising preclinical data demonstrating the efficacy of phytochemicals in inhibiting LC progression, their translation into clinical applications has encountered numerous challenges. One of the major limitations lies in the complexity of phytochemical action, which often involves multiple targets and intricate mechanisms. Moreover, the bioavailability, stability, and metabolism of phytochemicals pose significant hurdles in achieving consistent therapeutic outcomes. In addition, the lack of standardized protocols for phytochemical extraction, formulation, and dosage regimens has hindered their integration into conventional treatment approaches. To overcome these translational limitations, various strategies have been proposed. These include the invention of newer drug delivery methods to enhance the stability and bioavailability of phytochemicals, the identification of specific biomarkers to predict patient responsiveness, and the establishment of rigorous clinical trials to validate the safety and efficacy of phytochemical-based therapies. Furthermore, integrating phytochemicals with conventional treatments, such as chemotherapy and radiotherapy, holds promise for synergistic effects and improved therapeutic outcomes. In conclusion, while phytochemicals offer a potential avenue for the management of LC, their successful translation into clinical practice necessitates a comprehensive understanding of their pharmacokinetics, pharmacodynamics, and synergistic interactions with existing therapies. Addressing the challenges associated with standardization bioavailability and clinical validation is crucial for realizing the full therapeutic potential of phytochemicals in the context of LC treatment.

Graphical Abstract

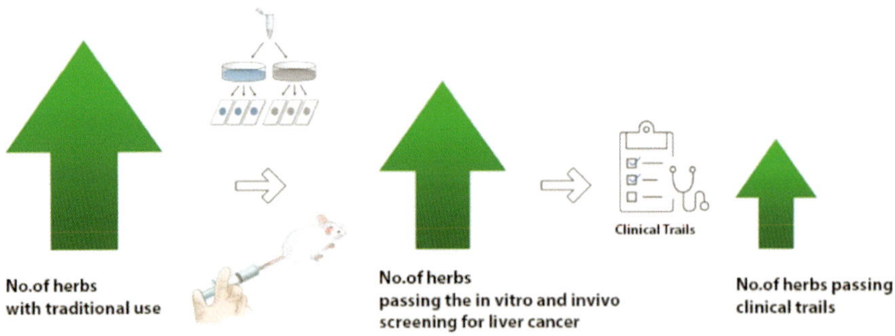

1. Introduction

1.1. *Cancer*

According to the World Health Organization, the term "cancer" refers to a broad category of diseases that can start and impact virtually any organ or tissue in the body when aberrant cells proliferate out of control. They may grow, and their growth crosses the usual boundaries and can affect the neighboring parts of the body [1]. Cancer is the second leading cause of death globally. According to the American Cancer Society's recent data, it is anticipated that there will be 1,958,310 new cancer cases and 609,820 cancer deaths in the US in 2023. Prostate, lung, stomach, liver, and colorectal cancers are the most common types of cancer in men, whereas colorectal, breast, colorectal, thyroid, cervical, and lung cancers are the most commonly found among women [1, 2]. According to World Cancer Research Fund International (WCRF), around 18 million cancer cases were reported worldwide in 2020. Based on the above report, 8.8 million cases were reported in women and 9.3 million cases were in men [3].

Cancer of the liver and intrahepatic bile ducts is the sixth primary cause of mortality from cancer in the US. It is the second most fatal cancer after pancreatic ductal adenocarcinoma [4–6]. There are two types of liver cancer (LC). They are primary and secondary LCs.

Although the original LC originates in the liver, metastases of the disease and the development of the most prevalent cases — colorectal, breast, pancreatic, ovarian, and lung cancers — cause secondary LC to start in other organs of the body and move to the liver. Hepatocellular carcinoma, cholangiocarcinoma, and sarcoma are examples of primary liver tumors that account for approximately 6% of the global cancer burden. Although primary LC originates in the hepatic cells, secondary LC starts in other body organs and then moves and spreads to the liver. The most common types of cancer include breast, colorectal, lung, ovarian, and pancreatic cancers. Primary LCs include cholangio carcinoma, sarcoma, and hepatocellular carcinoma, which account for approximately 6% of the total global cancer [7]. Hepatocellular carcinoma (HCC) is an aggressive disease that is often diagnosed in patients with chronic liver disease and cirrhosis. In contrast to the declining death rates seen for all other common cancers, mortality from HCC is increasing [6]. Hence, understanding from the basic level and thorough research on the known facts may bring out new targets to hit and new pathways to pierce down.

The liver is the most imperative and huge organ, weighing between 1 and 2.3 kg. This comprises a large portion of the right hypochondria region, part of the epigastric tract, and extends to the left at the top of the abdominal wall. To fit the diaphragm's underside, the liver's upper and lower surfaces should be smooth and perfectly shaped. Four lobes, called right, left, caudate, and quadral, constitute the liver. Liver lobe functional units are called lobules. They are hexagonal and are formed by hepatocytes, which are arranged as columns and radiate from the central vein. Sinusoids are channels that receive blood from the hepatic artery and portal vein. These blood samples were mixed and passed through the sinusoid of liver cells. Hepatic macrophages, called Kupffer cells, help to line the sinusoids and digest and destroy the remnants of RBCs and other foreign particles that enter the liver via the bloodstream [8]. Hepatocytes are highly specialized and metabolically active epithelial cells that, while they are responsible for the uptake of nutrients and detoxification of xenobiotics, are also responsible for the production of a huge amount of proteins, lipids, and bile acids [9]. Due to its diversified functions, the liver is exposed to various bacterial products entering through the portal vein, thus generating huge amounts of free radicals, leading to DNA damage and further liver cell death [10]. Intrahepatic cholangiocarcinoma and hepatocellular carcinoma are two types of primary LC with increasing mortality rates worldwide. Hepatocellular carcinoma leads to most primary LCs [11]. The dominant risk factors for hepatic cancer include chronic hepatitis C infection, hepatitis B infection, hyperglycemia, liver cirrhosis, oxidative stress, smoking, alcoholism, iron deposition, genetic alterations, and non-alcoholic liver disorders. The reasons behind cancer may vary from region to region. Of all the above factors, in most high-risk areas, the major risk factor is hepatitis B infection [12]. Hepatitis C virus-associated cirrhosis is the most prevalent etiological factor in Europe and the United States [13]. Hepatic cancer cells produce tubercular, clustered, and compact growth patterns within cancer cell

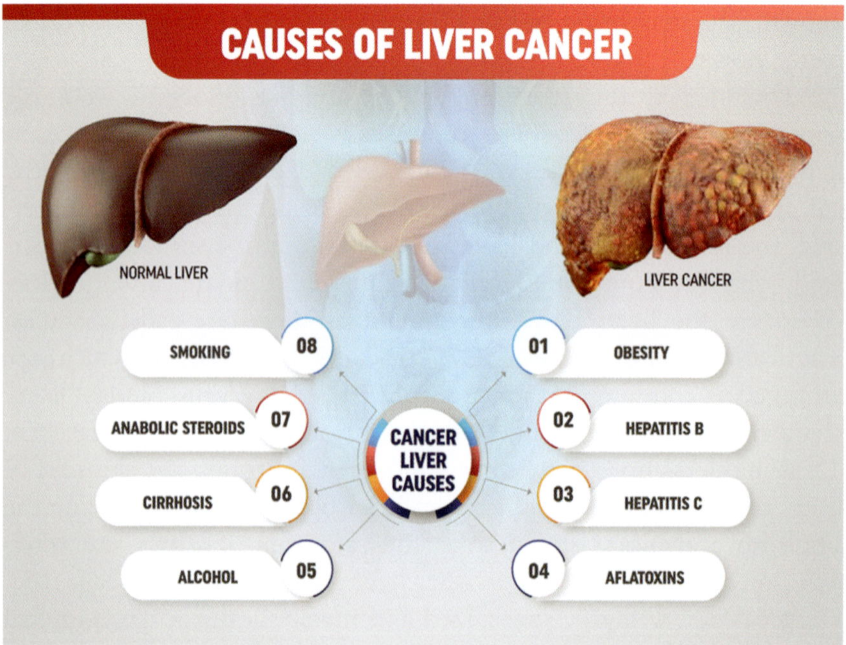

Figure 1: Causes of liver cancer

lines. Furthermore, liver cell architecture is completely lost with the crowding of high nuclear to cytoplasmic ratio [14]. In addition, it will cause physiological changes in the whole biological system, affecting the cell cycle phase, inflammation in cells and tissues, damage of the immune system, and changes in angiogenesis [7, 15].

1.2. *Cancer treatment*

The general treatment strategy for cancer includes surgical removal and radiation treatment followed by systematic chemotherapy for maintenance. However, related to these treatment methods, there are so many disadvantages. New approaches have also been utilized, such as stem cell therapies and anti-angiogenic and immune-mediated therapies, but they also cannot control the mortality rate [16–18]. In addition, these therapies have many side effects and disadvantages [19–21]. Hence, the search for newer cost-effective molecules devoid of disadvantages is relevant in the field of drug research.

The field of natural medicine can provide a finer solution to this problem as it has a reservoir of plant-derived molecules. Natural compounds are usually derived from various natural resources such as animals, plants, microorganisms, and minerals. Major potential compounds can be obtained from the plant source, and phytoconstituents include both primary and secondary metabolites of plants [22, 23]. The role of secondary metabolites in plants varies. They provide protection for plants from external agents such as insects, fungal infections, other microorganism attack, the generation of free radicals, and ionizing radiations. Hence, such produced compounds with structural diversity, upon ingestion by human beings, can benefit from protective effects by various mechanisms. There is no doubt that phytochemicals work in a complex and multidimensional manner through a variety of processes to prevent cancer [15].

Particularly in the case of cancer drugs, approximately 50% of approved drugs from 1940 to 2014 originated or are related to natural products. At times, it acts as a drug precursor, a template for synthetic modifications, or a model for the preparation of newer molecules known as pharmacological probes [24]. The major advantage of herbal drugs is that they act by regulating molecular pathways or by various mechanisms. The actions exerted by phytochemicals are very complex, and they act on different molecular targets and signal transduction pathways. Also, it acts at different stages, namely, tumor initiation, promotion, and progression stage, by increasing antioxidant status, downstreaming the activator proteins, carcinogen of cell cycle arrest and apoptosis, and regulating the immune system. Some typical phytochemical examples include vinca alkaloids, taxol analogs, and podophyllotoxin analogs [25, 26].

2. Phytochemicals for Clinical Use

Phytochemicals studied extensively for cancer treatment of the liver and in clinical use are vinca alkaloids and their derivatives, taxanes, podophyllotoxin and its derivatives, and camptothecin and its derivatives [24]. Vinca alkaloids are obtained from the whole plant of *Catharanthus roseus*, belonging to the Apocynaceae family. These alkaloids exhibit anticancer effects primarily by binding to β tubulin. This inhibits the polymerization and assembly of microtubules, which causes metaphase arrest and cell death. Synthetic analogs developed from these alkaloids, such as vinorelbine and vindesin, are also clinically effective [24, 27]. Taxanes are polyterpenoid compounds obtained from the bark of *Taxus* species belonging to the Taxaceae family. They exert an anticancer effect by stabilizing microtubules, which leads to cell cycle arrest. Semisynthetic derivatives of taxane, such as docetaxel and cabazitaxel, prove to be clinically effective [28, 29]. Podophyllotoxin is a lignan obtained from the roots and rhizomes of *Podophyllum peltatum*, *P. emodi* of the family Beriberidaceae. It reversibly binds to tubulin and prevents polymerization, which leads to metaphase arrest and cell death. Its derivatives, teneposide and etoposide, exert cytotoxicity by inhibiting topoisomerase II enzyme [30, 31]. Camptothecin is an alkaloid obtained from the bark and stem of *Camptotheca acuminata* of the family Nyssaceae. It acts by inhibiting topoisomerase I and prevents DNA relegation, leading to cell death. Its semisynthetic derivatives, including Irinotecan and topotecan, also exert antitumor activity [32, 33].

3. Phytochemicals in Clinical Trials and Limitations

Phytochemicals used in clinical trials include resveratrol, berberine, curcumin, epigallocatechin and lycopene, silibinin, and Tanshinone IIA [15, 24, 26, 34]. The respective major sources of these phytochemicals are tabulated in Table 1.

Resveratrol is a stilbenoid compound obtained from *Polygonum cuspidatum* of the family Polygonacxeae [35]. Resveratrol inhibits the fundamental activation of NF-κB through abolishing IκB-α kinase activation, which in turn downregulates certain pro-proliferation and anti-apoptotic gene products such as Bfl-1/A1, Bcl-xL, TNF-α receptor-associated factor 2, and Bcl-2. This causes apoptosis in

Table 1: Phytoconstituents and their major sources

Plant species	Chemical constituent
Polygonum cuspidatum 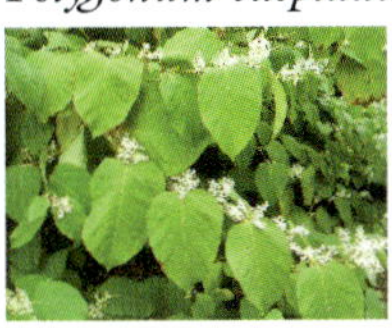	Resveratrol 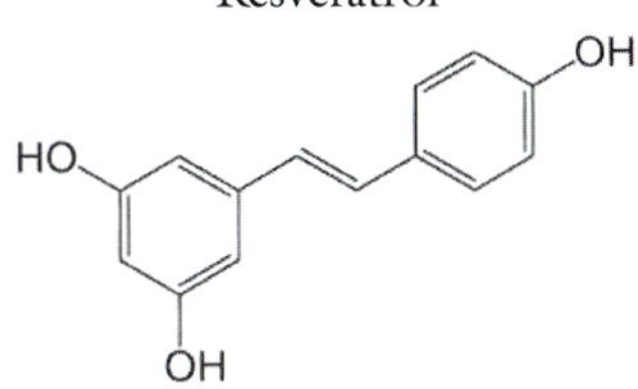
Berberis aristate 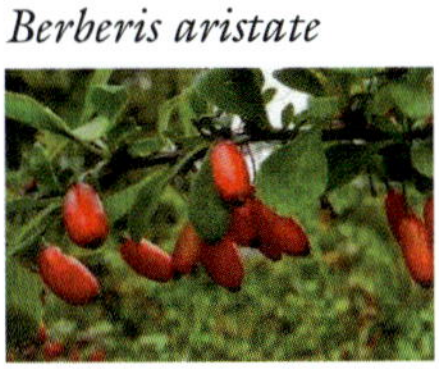	Berberine 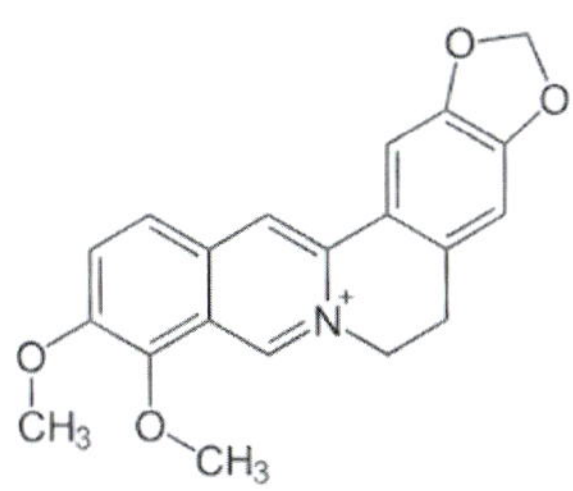
Curcuma longa 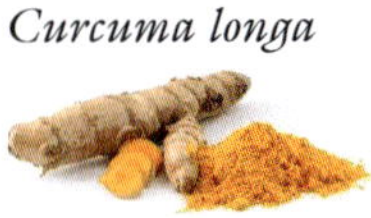	Curcumin 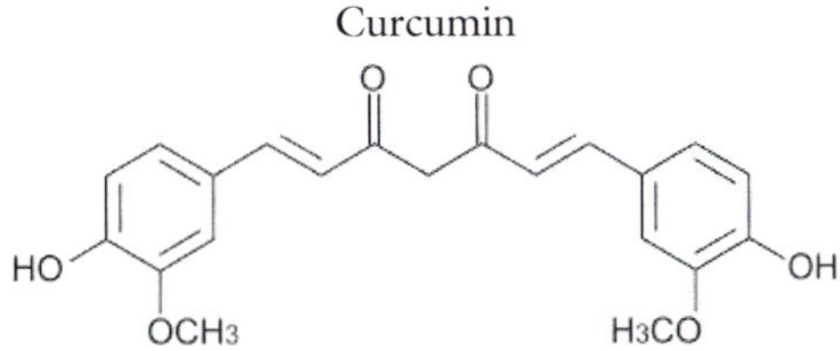

(*Continued*)

Table 1: (*Continued*)

Plant species	Chemical constituent
Camellia sinensis 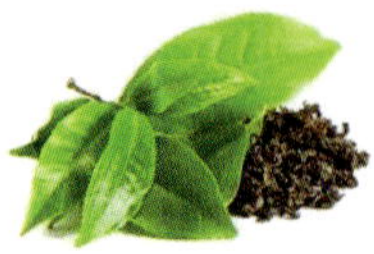	Epigallocatechin 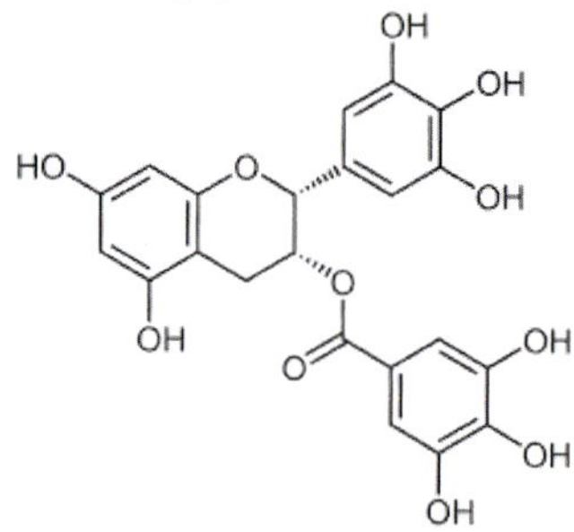
Solanum lycopersicum 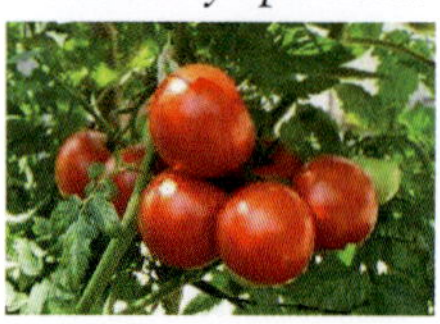	Lycopene 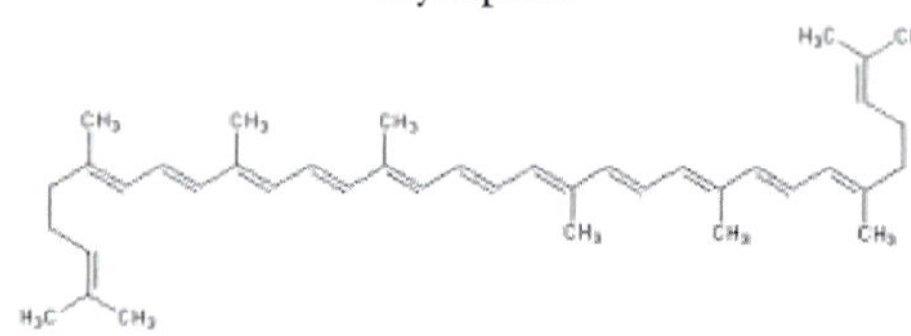
Silybum marianum 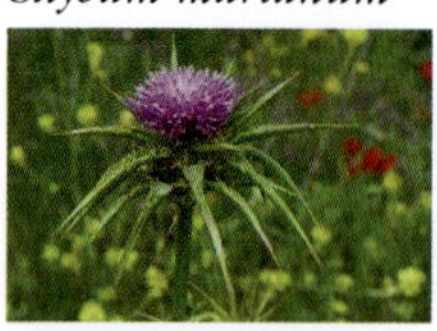	Silibinin 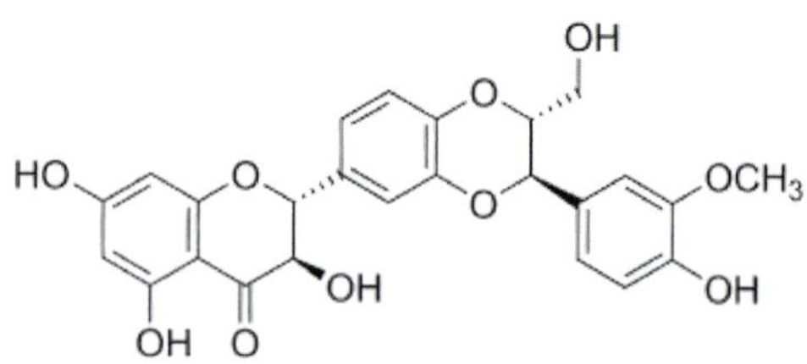
Salvia miltiorrhiza 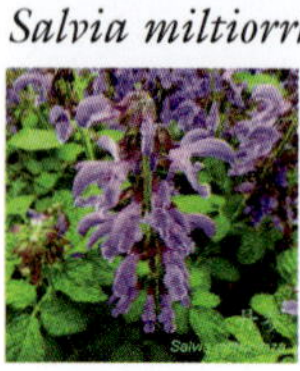	Tanshinone II A 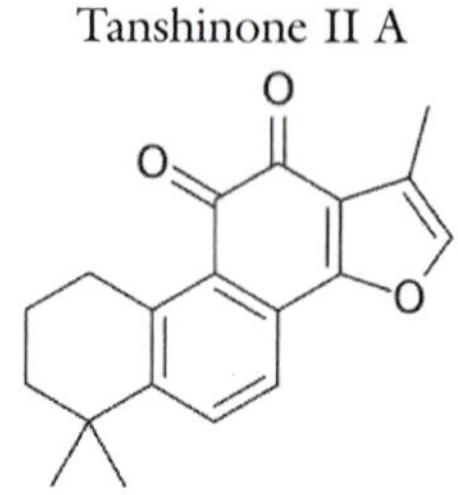

human multiple myeloma cells and prevents them from proliferation. The great acceptance of resveratrol with promising pharmacological activity has challenges regarding clinical trials. The primary obstacle to the therapeutic application of resveratrol seems to be its rapid metabolism, which results in a low level of *in vivo* bioavailability [36, 37].

Berberine is primarily obtained from the roots of *Berberis vulgaris and B. aristata* of the family Beriberidaceae [38]. Berberine was found to inhibit angiogenesis and cell proliferation by modulating cell apoptosis, cell cycle, tumor environment, and cell autophagy [39–41]. Although it has wide and effective anticancer activity, its slow absorption, efflux from intestinal cells by P-gp, and comprehensive metabolism by intestinal and hepatic cells render it difficult to use *in vivo* and in clinical use [42].

Curcumin is a colored pigment isolated from the rhizomes of *Curcuma longa* of the family Zingiberaceae [43]. Curcumin demonstrates a distinct anticancer mechanism primarily through triggering apoptosis and preventing tumor growth and invasion by suppressing numerous cellular signaling pathways [44]. Curcumin has high antioxidant and anti-inflammatory properties that can help control the development of human HepG2 cells and can be best opted for the prevention of oxidative stress-related hepatic disorders by lowering AST, ALT, ALP, and bilirubin levels [45]. Curcumin's limited stability, bioavailability, quick bodily clearance, and hydrophobicity make it impractical for use in clinical settings as an anticancer treatment [46, 47].

Epigallocatechin (EGC) is a catechin obtained from *Camellia sinensis* of the family Theaceae [48]. EGC inhibits tumorigenesis, carcinogen activity, angiogenesis, and cell proliferation, and induces cellular damage and death. These effects of epigallocatechins are associated with the inhibition of NF-κB, regulation of ROS production, upregulation of mitogen activation protein kinase (MAKPK) activation, and regulation of epigenomic change. Structure–activity relationship analysis revealed that esterification of gallic acid can help to increase activity significantly. Molecular dynamics assay studies also provided key ideas for pharmacophore modeling of derivatives. EGC possesses poor bioavailability and poor stability, representing a limitation for its use in human populations [49–52].

Lycopene is a natural red pigment obtained from *Solanum lycopersicum* of the family Solanaceae [53]. It scavenges free radicals such as singlet oxygen and thus guards against oxidative damage to DNA.

Consequently, lycopene stops normal cells from turning into cancerous cells. In addition, it suppresses apoptosis induction, cell division, the prevention of cell cycle progression, and the regulation of many signal transduction pathways through the modification of cell cycle regulation. As with most phytopharmaceuticals, lycopene also faces biopharmaceutical challenges in clinical trials [54–57].

Silibinin is a polyphenolic compound obtained from the seeds of *Silybum marianum* of the Asteraceae family. By inducing the Kip1/p27 messaging pathway and by inhibiting cycling D1, D3, and E as well as cyclin-dependent kinase, silibinin suppresses various hepatocellular tumors. Cytotoxicity caused by silibin can also result in apoptosis by activating various pathways. Commercial health supplements of silibinin are available in the market under various trade names. However, the real fact is that plasma concentration usually will not attain optimum therapeutic level due to its poor metabolism and after oral intake. Hence, the therapeutic use of this chemopreventive agent usually fails [58–62].

Tanshinone II A is a diterpenoid isolated from the roots and rhizomes of *Salvia miltiorrhiza* of the family Lamiaceae. Tan IIA exhibits a protective effect on various tumor cells. It usually acts by regulating the cell cycle, inhibiting cell diffusion, inducing apoptosis and differentiation, inhibiting tumor aggression and diversion, inhibiting angiogenesis and reversing tumor MDR, and so on. Cancer-related clinical studies in China have suggested the potential benefit of tanshinone for cancer patients. The use of tanshinone is usually limited due to its poor water solubility. Hence, bioavailability is a matter of concern for natural tanshinones [63–67].

Hence, the list of phytochemicals with promising *in vitro* and *in vivo* phytochemicals is thousands, but the compounds that are leading to clinical studies are only 1/10th. Those compounds that undergo preclinical and clinical studies mostly fail because of various factors [26, 68]. Limitations of herbs and limitations of herbs in clinical studies that prevent phytoconstituents from reaching clinical use are called clinical translational hurdles, and they must be discussed, studied, and researched to identify clinically effective molecules with promising hepato-protective actions.

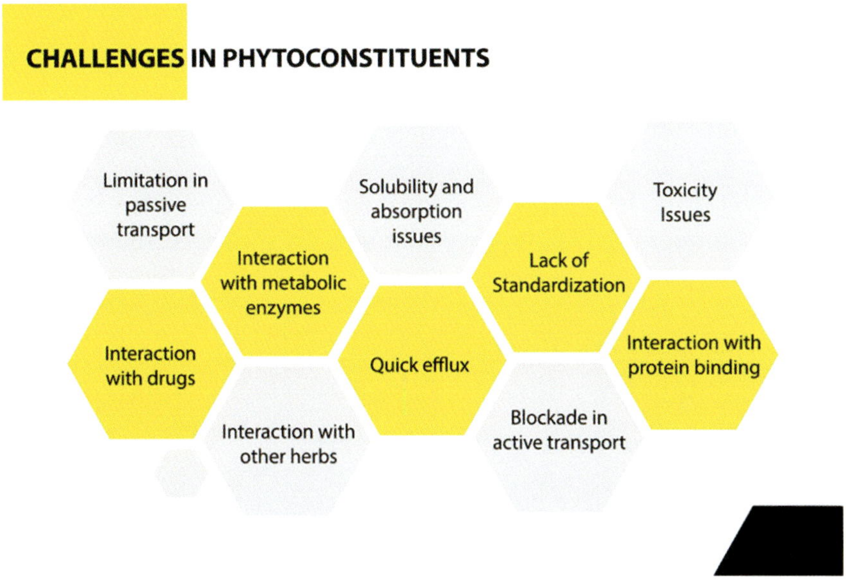

Figure 2: Challenges in phytoconstituents

4. Translational Hurdles [26]

From the studied phytoconstituents, the major factors that limit the phytoconstituents are

1. Solubility
2. Pharmacokinetic (pk) parameters
3. Pharmacodynamics factors
4. Safety
5. Shortcomings and limitations of *in vitro* studies
6. Limitations in *the in vivo* models
7. Statistical limitation
8. Lack of standardization techniques

4.1. *Solubility*

As mentioned earlier, even if phytoconstituents have excellent therapeutic properties, many of these compounds have poor solubility in water, or they will not be stable in water. This solubility issue brings notable risks of poor bioavailability, high-dose requirement, and adverse side effects. This limits the development of phytochemicals in the pharmaceutical industry, thereby restricting the comprehensive utilization of these plant resources [69, 70].

Newer drug delivery designs and chemical modifications are common techniques used to improve solubility, but these techniques may not work for all constituents. The development of biocompatible solvents such as natural deep eutectic solvents as delivery vehicles is another method to combat the solubility issue [71].

4.2. *Pharmacokinetic (pk) parameters*

Most herbal drugs have hundreds of bioactive molecules or mixtures of constituents. This complicates the standardization of herbal drugs. In addition, to evaluate the clinical significance of herbal drugs, the pharmacokinetic parameters of each constituent are significant. Orally ingested drugs have to undergo the same route as that of food and hence have to face the same challenges. pH, transporters, and enzymes Bioactive constituents succeeded *in vitro* models, and *in vivo* models sometimes get rejected in clinical trials because of poor absorption or poor distribution profile, metabolic issues with enzymes such as cytochrome P450, or quick excretion or poor excretion, leading to safety issues [72–76].

Some critical issues related to pharmacokinetics can be resolved by designing newer dosage forms using novel delivery systems and by targeting the drugs to the exact body part.

4.3. *Pharmacodynamics factors*

When applying pharmacodynamics for clinical study of herbal drugs, drugs fall into any of these three categories. (i) Herbal drugs whose efficacy is demonstrated — the active principles are familiar and their doses established; (ii) Herbal drugs whose efficacy is probable, which is not clearly demonstrated — the active agents can be utilized to standardize them; and (iii) Herbal drugs with uncertain efficacies, but have a long history of traditional usage — these drugs can be utilized for treating common disorders, but exactly as used in the traditional practice. This is a challenge for designing clinical trials of herbal drugs. While performing the studies, the dose to be used, the dosage route, and the willingness of the subjects make the study more challenging [68, 77].

Nowadays, *in silico* methods developed will help to an extent to predict the pharmacodynamics and pharmacokinetic parameters of drugs. This can help in solving the challenges faced by researchers in designing clinical trials. In addition, an exact understanding of the pharmacokinetics and pharmacodynamics of each constituent will help to prevent herb–drug interactions and to determine the correct dosage and frequency [68, 77, 78].

4.4. *Safety*

The use of herbal medicine is increasing day by day, and the incidence of toxicity and adverse effects is also increasing. Hence, studies and regulatory policies are needed to study each herbal drug. People also need to be educated about considering that all-natural drugs are safer as they are directly obtained from nature. The reality is that the terminologies "safety" and "natural" are not the same. Sometimes, interactions occurring between herbal medicines and drugs may be clinically insignificant, but this can become serious or relevant due to a variety of patient-related factors, such as the presence of multiple or other diseases or genetic predispositions in the patients. The studies should be designed as conventional drugs to monitor the dosage of drugs, half-life, and clearance rate, and on herb–drug interactions to ensure the safety of phytoconstituents [79–83].

4.5. *Shortcomings of the in vitro models*

Most of the *in vitro* models cease to give consistent results as they cannot replicate the conditions of cells in an organism. For example, isolated and cultured primary cells do not show the same properties as the corresponding cell type in an organism. This limits the *in vitro* data to predict the clinical value of a drug or even the *in vivo* behavior of a particular drug [84, 85]. Hence, the data obtained from these models mostly fail to be extrapolated to clinical trials and use.

4.6. *Limitations of the in vivo models*

In animal models, the extremely complex process of human carcinogenesis, physiology, and progression cannot often be mimicked. Hence, the results obtained for herbal drugs or phytoconstituents in safety and pharmacological studies with animals fail to be translated to human trials [86, 87]. Physiological differences and variations between mice and humans, especially in the homology of molecular targets, may be the major limitations in the translation of *in vivo* data to clinical trials [88].

4.7. *Statistical limitations*

Statistics are an important factor in upholding the integrity of clinical trials. The involvement of statistics is in every step of a trial, starting from design and protocol development, in the observation of data, the way of conducting an ongoing trial, management of data, analysis of data, and the reporting of trial results. The principal challenges in designing, monitoring, conducting, and analyzing preclinical studies are data variability and bias in the interpretation of data [89, 90]. Small studies are more vulnerable to the effects of missing data. A small change or the inclusion or exclusion of a single data point can alter the results and conclusions of a study [91].

4.8. *Lack of standardization techniques*

Lack of standardization in herbal medicine usually results in fluctuation of pharmacological effects and hence limits clinical use. There is a major possibility of change in the quality of herbal drugs due to variations in geographical conditions, climatic conditions, or time of collection, harvesting method, and storage conditions [92–94].

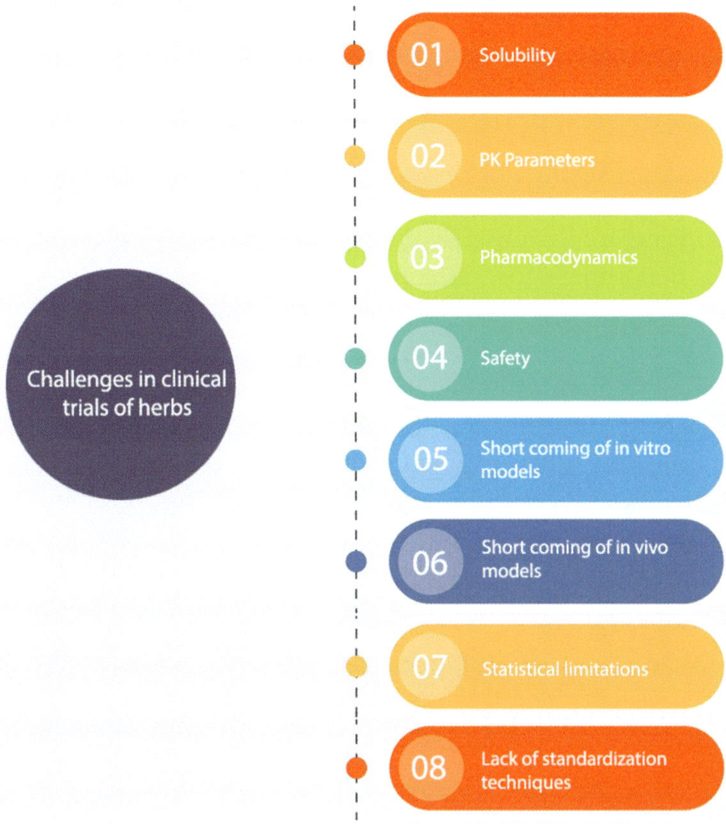
Challenges in clinical trials of herbs
01 Solubility
02 PK Parameters
03 Pharmacodynamics
04 Safety
05 Short coming of in vitro models
06 Short coming of in vivo models
07 Statistical limitations
08 Lack of standardization techniques

Figure 3: Challenges in Clinical Trials of Herbs

To attain reproducible therapeutic efficacy, the standardization of herbal drugs should be mandatory.

The hurdles of herbs in the clinical study are depicted in Figure 3.

5. Strategies to Use for Overcoming the Translational Hurdles

Different approaches are needed to overcome the clinical translational hurdles of phytoconstituents because each constituent has different limitations. In understanding and grouping these limitations, some strategies are pointed out by Sayed *et al.*, which include

a) Formulation-based approaches: Approaches, such as planning novel drug delivery systems for phytoconstituents, help to overcome major pharmacokinetic and pharmacodynamic hurdles associated with the constituents [95].
b) Prodrug and analog method: It can be used for phytoconstituents that have poor oral bioavailability due to rapid metabolism. Prodrugs are designed by linking carriers, using spacers, or utilizing dendrimers for sustained release. Moreover, they enhance cytocompatibility and reduce toxicity [95–98].
c) Concomitant administration of permeation enhancers and efflux inhibitors: Permeation enhancers can be used to increase the bioavailability of phytoconstituents by enhancing cell permeation without much emphasis on solubility. Efflux inhibitors also help to enhance bioavailability and can be studied using *in vitro* assays which help to obtain the data of drugs on its absorptivity and bioavailability in the preclinical stage itself [95, 99, 100].

6. Conclusion and Remarks

Although the role of phytochemicals in LC management shows promise, further research is necessary for successful clinical translation and to determine the optimal dosing regimens for effective clinical application. Integrating phytochemicals into comprehensive treatment strategies by utilizing advanced *in silico* modeling strategies has the potential to improve clinical translational rates and enhance the overall efficacy of conventional therapeutic approaches. Encouraging further investment in well-designed clinical trials, fostering interdisciplinary collaborations, establishing standardized protocols for quality control and streamlining regulatory pathways are essential steps to bridge the gap between preclinical research and human trials of phytochemicals in LC management.

Conflict of Interest

The authors declare no conflict of interest.

References

1. Siegel RL, Miller KD, Wagle NS, Jemal A. Cancer statistics. *Cancer Journal for Clinicians* 2023; 73(1): 17–48. https://doi.org/10.3322/caac.21763. PMID: 36633525.
2. https://www.wcrf.org/cancer-trends/worldwide-cancer-data/
3. Chew SA, Moscato S, George S, Azimi B, Danti S. Liver cancer: current and future trends using biomaterials. *Cancers* 2019; 11(12): 2026. https://doi.org/10.3390/cancers11122026
4. Zhang Y, Vaccarella S, Morgan E, Li M, Etxeberria J, Chokunonga E, Manraj SS, Kamate B, Omonisi A, Bray F. Global variations in lung cancer incidence by histological subtype in 2020: a population-based study. *The Lancet Oncology* 2023 Oct 11. https://doi.org/10.1016/S1470-2045(23)00444-8. Epub ahead of print. PMID: 37837979.
5. Manne A, Mulekar MS, Escobar DE, Prodduturvar P, Fahmawi Y, Henderson P, et al. Compliance with the American Association for the Study of Liver Diseases (AASLD) guidelines and its impact on overall survival in patients with hepatocellular carcinoma. *Journal of Clinical Oncology (Internet)* 2020 May 20 (cited 2023 Oct 25); 38(15 suppl): e16609. https://doi.org/10.4103/jcrt.jcrt_1861_20.
6. Mohammadian M, Mahadavifar N, Hafshejani MA, Salehiniya H. Liver cancer in the world: epidemiology, incidence, mortality and risk factors. *World Cancer Research Journal* 2018; 5(2): e1082.
7. Mishra NTP, Mohapatra L, Hussain Z. Herbal drugs against hepatic cancer: new possibilities as an alternative therapy. *Annals of RSCB* 2021; 25(6): 7708–7722.
8. Waugh A. *Ross and Wilson Anatomy and Physiology in Health and Illness, International Edition*. 12th edition. Edinburgh; New York: Elsevier Health-UK; 2014.
9. Schulze RJ, Schott MB, Casey CA, Tuma PL, McNiven MA. The cell biology of the hepatocyte: a membrane tracking machine. *Journal of Cell Biology* 2019; 218(7): 2096–2112.
10. Ramakrishna G, Rastogi A, Trehanpati N, Sen B, Khosla R, Sarin SK. From cirrhosis to hepatocellular carcinoma: new molecular insights on inflammation and cellular senescence. *Liver Cancer* 2013; 2(3–4): 367–383.

11. Hashem BE. Epidemiology of viral hepatitis and hepatocellular carcinoma. *Gastroenterology* 2012; 142(6): 1264–1273.
12. El-Serg HB, Rudolph KL. Hepatocellular carcinoma: epidemiology and molecular carcinogenesis. *Gastroenterology* 2007; 132(7): 2557–2576.
13. Hashem BE. Hepatocellular carcinoma: recent trends in the United States. *Gastroenterology* 2004; 127(5 suppl 1): S27–S34.
14. Erik SK, Purva G, Amit GS. The changing landscape of hepatocellular carcinoma: etiology, genetics and therapy. *The American Journal of Pathology* 2014; 184(3): 574–583.
15. Dave A, Parande F, Park EJ, Pezzuto JM. Phytochemicals and cancer chemoprevention. *Journal of Cancer Metastasis and Treatment* 2020; 6: 46. http://dx.doi.org/10.20517/2394-4722.2020.106
16. Saha D, Maity T, Jana M, Suprodip M. Cancer treatment strategy-an overview. *Asian Journal of Pharmacy and Technology* 2011; 1(2): 28–33.
17. Debela DT, Muzazu SG, Heraro KD, Ndalama MT, Mesele BW, Haile DC, Kitui SK, Manyazewal T. New approaches and procedures for cancer treatment: current perspectives. *SAGE Open Medicine* 2021 Aug 12; 9: 20503121211034366. https://doi.org/10.1177/20503121211034366. PMID: 34408877; PMCID: PMC8366192.
18. Atice Y, Nezehat PB, Seçil KT, Ozerk D, Fatma DÖD, Bengi U, Sibel AO. Treatment strategies in cancer from past to present. In: Grumezescu AM (eds.), *Drug Targeting and Stimuli Sensitive Drug Delivery Systems.* William Andrew Publishing; 2018, 1–37, ISBN 9780128136898.
19. Chakraborty S, Rahman T. The difficulties in cancer treatment. *E Cancer Medical Science* 2012 Nov 14; 6: ed16. https://doi.org/10.3332/ecancer.2012.ed16. PMID: 24883085; PMCID: PMC4024849.
20. Devlin EJ, Denson LA, Whitford HS. Cancer treatment side effects: a meta-analysis of the relationship between response expectancies and experience. *Journal of Pain and Symptom Management* 2017; 54(2): 245–258.
21. Van den Boogaard WMC, Komninos DSJ, Vermeij WP. Chemotherapy side-effects: not all DNA damage is equal. *Cancers* 2022; 14(3): 627. https://doi.org/10.3390/cancers14030627

22. Ranjan A, Ramachandran S, Gupta N, Kaushik I, Wright S, Srivastava S, Das H, Srivastava S, Prasad S, Srivastava SK. Role of phytochemicals in cancer prevention. ***International Journal of Molecular Sciences*** 2019 Oct 9; 20(20): 4981. https://doi.org/10.3390/ijms20204981. PMID: 31600949; PMCID: PMC6834187.
23. George BP, Blassan P, Chandran R, Abrahamse H. Role of phytochemicals in cancer chemoprevention: insights. ***Antioxidants*** 2021; 10(9): 1455. https://doi.org/10.3390/antiox10091455
24. Choudhari AS, Mandave PC, Deshpande M, Ranjekar P, Prakash O. Phytochemicals in cancer treatment: from preclinical studies to clinical practice. ***Frontiers in Pharmacology*** 2020 Jan 28; 10: 1614. https://doi.org/10.3389/fphar.2019.01614. Erratum in: Front Pharmacol. 2020 Feb 28; 11: 175. PMID: 32116665; PMCID: PMC7025531.
25. Devan AR, Nair B, Nath LR. Translational phytomedicines against cancer: promise and hurdles. ***Advanced Pharmaceutical Bulletin*** 2023 Mar; 13(2): 210–215. https://doi.org/10.34172/apb.2023.023. Epub 2022 Apr 28. PMID: 37342376; PMCID: PMC10278225.
26. Rodriguez S, Skeet K, Mehmetoglu-Gurbuz T, Goldfarb M, Karri S, Rocha J, Shahinian M, Yazadi A, Poudel S, Subramani R. Phytochemicals as an alternative or integrative option, in conjunction with conventional treatments for hepatocellular carcinoma. ***Cancers (Basel)*** 2021 Nov 17; 13(22): 5753. https://doi.org/10.3390/cancers13225753. PMID: 34830907; PMCID: PMC8616323.
27. ***LiverTox: Clinical and Research Information on Drug-Induced Liver Injury [Internet]***, Bethesda, MD: National Institute of Diabetes and Digestive and Kidney Diseases, 2012. Vinca Alkaloids. [Updated 2020 Sep 12]. Available from: https://www.ncbi.nlm.nih.gov/books/NBK547989
28. Yuan JH, Zhang RP, Zhang RG, Guo LX, Wang XW, Luo D, Xie Y, Xie H. Growth-inhibiting effects of taxol on human liver cancer ***in vitro*** and in nude mice. ***World Journal of Gastroenterology*** 2000 Apr; 6(2): 210–215. https://doi.org/10.3748/wjg.v6.i2.210. PMID: 11819558; PMCID: PMC4723486.
29. Okano J, Nagahara T, Matsumoto K, Murawaki Y. The growth inhibition of liver cancer cells by paclitaxel and the involvement of extracellular signal-regulated kinase and apoptosis. ***Oncology Reports*** 2007 May; 17(5): 1195–200. PMID: 17390065.

30. Fan HY, Zhu ZL, Xian HC, Wang HF, Chen BJ, Tang YJ, Tang YL, Liang XH. Insight into the molecular mechanism of podophyllotoxin derivatives as anticancer drugs. *Frontiers in Cell and Developmental Biology* 2021 Aug 10; 9: 709075. https://doi.org/10.3389/fcell.2021.709075. PMID: 34447752; PMCID: PMC8383743.
31. Sara M, Karolina J, Halina E, Javad SSR, Daniela C, Basem A, et al. Podophyllotoxin and its derivatives: potential anticancer agents of natural origin in cancer chemotherapy. *Biomedicine & Pharmacotherapy* 2023; 158: 114145. https://doi.org/10.1016/j.biopha.2022.114145.
32. Xiao L, Yu E, Yue H, Li Q. Enhanced liver targeting of camptothecin via conjugation with deoxycholic acid. *Molecules* 2019 Mar 26; 24(6): 1179. https://doi.org/10.3390/molecules24061179. PMID: 30917485; PMCID: PMC6472190.
33. Liu YQ, Li WQ, Morris-Natschke SL, Qian K, Yang L, Zhu GX, Wu XB, Chen AL, Zhang SY, Nan X, Lee KH. Perspectives on biologically active camptothecin derivatives. *Medicinal Research Reviews* 2015 Jul; 35(4): 753–789. https://doi.org/10.1002/med.21342. Epub 2015 Mar 21. PMID: 25808858; PMCID: PMC4465867.
34. Kumar G, Virmani T, Sharma A, Pathak K. Codelivery of phytochemicals with conventional anticancer drugs in form of nanocarriers. *Pharmaceutics* 2023 Mar 9; 15(3): 889. https://doi.org/10.3390/pharmaceutics15030889. PMID: 36986748; PMCID: PMC10055866.
35. Ko JH, Sethi G, Um JY, Shanmugam MK, Arfuso F, Kumar AP, Bishayee A, Ahn KS. The role of resveratrol in cancer therapy. *International Journal of Molecular Sciences* 2017 Dec 1; 18(12): 2589. https://doi.org/10.3390/ijms18122589. PMID: 29194365; PMCID: PMC5751192.
36. Singh CK, Ndiaye MA, Ahmad N. Resveratrol and cancer: challenges for clinical translation. *Biochimica et Biophysica Acta* 2015; 1852(6): 1178–1185. ISSN 0925-4439, https://doi.org/10.1016/j.bbadis.2014.11.004.
37. Boxu R, Marabeth XK, Cuiliu L, Zhaowu M, Muthu KS, Lingwen D et al. Resveratrol for cancer therapy: challenges and future perspectives. *Cancer Letters* 2021; 515: 63–72. ISSN 0304-3835. https://doi.org/10.1016/j.canlet.2021.05.001.

38. Rauf A, Abu-Izneid T, Khalil AA, Imran M, Shah ZA, Emran TB, et al. Berberine as a potential anticancer agent: a comprehensive review. *Molecules* 2021 Dec 4; 26(23): 7368. https://doi.org/10.3390/molecules26237368. PMID: 34885950; PMCID: PMC8658774.
39. Wang Y, Liu Y, Du X, Ma H, Yao J. The anti-cancer mechanisms of berberine: a review. *Cancer Management and Research* 2020 Jan 30; 12: 695–702. https://doi.org/10.2147/CMAR.S242329. PMID: 32099466; PMCID: PMC6996556.
40. Xu J, Long Y, Ni L, Yuan X, Yu N, Wu R, et al. Anticancer effect of berberine based on experimental animal models of various cancers: a systematic review and meta-analysis. *BMC Cancer* 2019; 19: 589. https://doi.org/10.1186/s12885-019-5791-1.
41. Almatroodi SA, Alsahli MA, Rahmani AH. Berberine: an important emphasis on its anticancer effects through modulation of various cell signaling pathways. *Molecules* 2022; 27(18): 5889. https://doi.org/10.3390/molecules27185889
42. Habtemariam S. Recent advances in berberine inspired anticancer approaches: from drug combination to novel formulation technology and derivatization. *Molecules* 2020; 25(6): 1426. https://doi.org/10.3390/molecules25061426.
43. Wilken R, Veena MS, Wang MB, Srivatsan ES. Curcumin: a review of anti-cancer properties and therapeutic activity in head and neck squamous cell carcinoma. *Molecular Cancer* 2011 Feb 7; 10: 12. https://doi.org/10.1186/1476-4598-10-12. PMID: 21299897; PMCID: PMC3055228.
44. Tomeh MA, Hadianamrei R, Zhao X. A Review of curcumin and its derivatives as anticancer agents. *International Journal of Molecular Sciences* 2019 Feb 27; 20(5): 1033. https://doi.org/10.3390/ijms20051033. PMID: 30818786; PMCID: PMC6429287
45. Gull N, Arshad F, Naikoo GA, Hussan IU, Pedram MZ, Ahmad A, et al. Recent advances in anticancer activity of novel plant extracts and compounds from *Curcuma longa* in hepatocellular carcinoma. *Journal of Gastrointestinal Cancer* 2022; 54: 368–390. https://doi.org/10.1007/s12029-022-00809-z.

46. Perrone D, Ardito F, Giannatempo G, Dioguardi M, Troiano G, Lo Russo, Lo Muzio L. Biological and therapeutic activities, and anti-cancer properties of curcumin. *Experimental and Therapeutic Medicine* 2015; 10: 1615–1623. https://doi.org/10.3892/etm.2015.2749.
47. Zoi V, Galani V, Lianos GD, Voulgaris S, Kyritsis AP, Alexiou GA. The role of curcumin in cancer treatment. *Biomedicines* 2021; 9(9): 1086. https://doi.org/10.3390/biomedicines9091086.
48. Min KJ, Kwon TK. Anticancer effects and molecular mechanisms of epigallocatechin-3-gallate. *Integrative Medicine Research* 2014 Mar; 3(1): 16–24. https://doi.org/10.1016/j.imr.2013.12.001. Epub 2013 Dec 9. PMID: 28664074; PMCID: PMC5481703.
49. Almatroodi SA, Almatroudi A, Khan AA, Alhumaydhi FA, Alsahli MA, Rahmani AH. Potential therapeutic targets of epigallocatechin gallate (EGCG), the most abundant catechin in green tea, and its role in the therapy of various types of cancer. *Molecules* 2020; 25(14): 3146. https://doi.org/10.3390/molecules25143146
50. Du GJ, Zhang Z, Wen XD, Yu C, Calway T, Yuan CS, Wang CZ. Epigallocatechin gallate (EGCG) is the most effective cancer chemo-preventive polyphenol in green tea. *Nutrients* 2012 Nov 8; 4(11): 1679–1691. https://doi.org/10.3390/nu4111679. PMID: 23201840; PMCID: PMC3509513.
51. Bimonte S, Cascella M, Barbieri A, Arra C, Cuomo A. Current shreds of evidence on the anticancer role of EGCG in triple negative breast cancer: an update of the current state of knowledge. *Infectious Agents and Cancer* 2020; 15(1): 2. https://doi.org/10.1186/s13027-020-0270-5.
52. Ren YG, Hua-Bin L, Zhong-Quan S, Harold C. Absorption, metabolism, anti-cancer effect and molecular targets of epigallocatechin gallate (EGCG): an updated review. *Critical Reviews in Food Science and Nutrition* 2018; 58(6): 924–941. https://doi.org/10.1080/10408398.2016.1231168.
53. Shanbhag VK. Lycopene in cancer therapy. *Journal of Pharmacy and Bioallied Sciences* 2016 Apr-Jun; 8(2): 170–171. https://doi.org/10.4103/0975-7406.171740. PMID: 27134472; PMCID: PMC4832910.

54. Wang JQ, Wang SS, Chu P, Ma X, Tang ZY. Investigating into the anti-cancer potential of lycopene: molecular targets. *Biomedicine & Pharmacotherapy* 2021; 138: 11546. ISSN 0753-3322, https://doi.org/10.1016/j.biopha.2021.111546.
55. Bhuvaneswari V, Nagini S. Lycopene: a review of its potential as an anticancer agent. *Current Medicinal Chemistry-Anti-Cancer Agents* 2005; 5(6): 627–635. https://dx.doi.org/10.2174/156801105774574667
56. Puah BP, Jalil J, Attiq A, Kamisah Y. New insights into molecular mechanism behind anti-cancer activities of lycopene. *Molecules* 2021; 26(13): 3888. https://doi.org/10.3390/molecules26133888.
57. Mekuria AN, Tura AK, Hagos B, Sisay M, Abdela J, Mishore KM, et al. Anti-Cancer Effects of lycopene in animal models of hepatocellular carcinoma: a systematic review and meta-analysis. *Frontiers in Pharmacology* 2020; 11: 1306. https://doi.org/10.3389/fphar.2020.01306. https://www.frontiersin.org/articles/10.3389/fphar.2020.01306
58. Bijak MS. A major bioactive component of milk thistle (*Silybum marianum* L. Gaernt.)-chemistry, bioavailability, and metabolism. *Molecules* 2017 Nov 10; 22(11): 1942. https://doi.org/10.3390/molecules22111942. PMID: 29125572; PMCID: PMC6150307.
59. Deep G, Agarwal R. Antimetastatic efficacy of silibinin: molecular mechanisms and therapeutic potential against cancer. *Cancer and Metastasis Reviews* 2010 Sep; 29(3): 447–463. https://doi.org/10.1007/s10555-010-9237-0. PMID: 20714788; PMCID: PMC3928361.
60. Mahdi MAB, Massoud MAB, Sepide G. Overview of silibinin anti-tumor effects. *Journal of Herbal Medicine* 2020; 23: 100375. https://doi.org/10.1016/j.hermed.2020.100375.
61. Zou H, Zhu XX, Zhang GB, Ma Y, Wu Y, Huang DS. Silibinin: an old drug for hematological disorders. *Oncotarget* 2017 Jul 11; 8(51): 89307–89314. https://doi.org/10.18632/oncotarget.19153. PMID: 29179521; PMCID: PMC5687691.
62. Tuli HS, Mittal S, Aggarwal D, Parashar G, Parashar NC, Upadhyay SK, et al. Path of Silibinin from diet to medicine: a dietary polyphenolic flavonoid having potential anti-cancer therapeutic significance.

Seminars in Cancer Biology 2021; 73: 196–218. https://doi.org/10.1016/j.semcancer.2020.09.014.

63. Fang ZY, Zhang M, Liu JN, Zhao X, Zhang YQ, Fang L. Tanshinone IIA: a review of its anticancer effects. *Frontiers in Pharmacology* 2021 Jan 14; 11: 611087. https://doi.org/10.3389/fphar.2020.611087. PMID: 33597880; PMCID: PMC7883641.
64. Cao YF, Wang SF, Li X, Zhang Y-L, Qiao Y-J. The anticancer mechanism investigation of tanshinone IIA by pharmacological clustering in protein network. *BMC Systems Biology* 2018; 12: 90. https://doi.org/10.1186/s12918-018-0606-6
65. Wu W, Zhang Y, Tang S, Ye M, Lu J, Jiang C. Anticancer potential of *Salvia miltiorrhiza* and its tanshinones: an efficacy perspective. *Botanics: Targets and Therapy* 2016; 6: 45–58. https://doi.org/10.2147/BTAT.S68097
66. Naz I, Merarchi M, Ramchandani S, Khan MR, Malik MN, Sarwar S, et al. An overview of the anti-cancer actions of Tanshinones, derived from *Salvia miltiorrhiza* (Danshen). *Exploration of Targeted Anti-tumor Therapy* 2020; 1: 153–170. https://doi.org/10.37349/etat.2020.00010
67. Zhang Y, Jiang P, Ye M, Kim S-H, Jiang C, Lü J. Tanshinones: sources, pharmacokinetics and anti-cancer activities. *International Journal of Molecular Sciences* 2012; 13(10): 13621–13666. https://doi.org/10.3390/ijms131013621
68. Parveen A, Parveen B, Parveen R, Ahmad S. Challenges and guidelines for clinical trial of herbal drugs. *Journal of Pharmacy and Bioallied Sciences* 2015 Oct-Dec; 7(4): 329–333. https://doi.org/10.4103/0975-7406.168035. PMID: 26681895; PMCID: PMC4678978.
69. Mohapatra D, Agrawal AK, Sahu AN. Exploring the potential of solid dispersion for improving solubility, dissolution & bioavailability of herbal extracts, enriched fractions, and bioactives. *Journal of Microencapsulation* 2021 Nov-Dec; 38(7–8): 594–612. https://doi.org/10.1080/02652048.2021.1963342. Epub 2021 Aug 17. PMID: 34338596.
70. Alaouna M, Penny C, Hull R, Molefi T, Chauke-Malinga N, Khanyile R, Makgoka M, Bida M, Dlamini Z. Overcoming the challenges of phytochemicals in triple negative breast cancer therapy: the path

forward. *Plants* 2023; 12(12): 2350. https://doi.org/10.3390/plants12122350

71. Jun C, Jiarui C, Huimin W, Luyao C, Fuliang C, Erzheng S. Solubility improvement of phytochemicals using (natural) deep eutectic solvents and their bioactivity evaluation. *Journal of Molecular Liquids* 2020; 318: 113997. https://doi.org/10.1016/j.molliq.2020.113997.
72. Mehta P, Shah R, Lohidasan S, Mahadik KR. Pharmacokinetic profile of phytoconstituent(s) isolated from medicinal plants-A comprehensive review. *Journal of Traditional and Complementary Medicine* 2015 Jan 28; 5(4): 207–227. https://doi.org/10.1016/j.jtcme.2014.11.041. PMID: 26587392; PMCID: PMC4624361.
73. Jia WW, Lu C, Lin G, Ge GB. Pharmacokinetics of herbal medicines and herb-drug interactions. *Frontiers in Pharmacology* 2022; 13. https://doi.org/10.3389/fphar.2022.1107777
74. Rein MJ, Renouf M, Cruz-Hernandez C, Actis-Goretta L, Thakkar SK, da Silva Pinto M. Bioavailability of bioactive food compounds: a challenging journey to bioefficacy. *British Journal of Clinical Pharmacology* 2013 Mar; 75(3): 588–602. https://doi.org/10.1111/j.1365-2125.2012.04425.x. PMID: 22897361; PMCID: PMC3575927.
75. Patra JK, Das G, Fraceto LF, Campos EVR, Rodriguez-Torres MDP, Acosta-Torres LS, et al. Nano based drug delivery systems: recent developments and future prospects. *Journal of Nanobiotechnology* 2018; 16(1): 71. https://doi.org/10.1186/s12951-018-0392-8
76. Durán-Iturbide NA, Díaz-Eufracio BI, Medina-Franco JL. *In silico* ADME/Tox profiling of natural products: a focus on BIOFACQUIM. *ACS Omega* 2020; 5(26): 16076–16084. https://doi.org/10.1021/acsomega.0c01581.
77. Husain GM, Khan MA, Urooj MK. Pharmacodynamic evaluation: herbal medicine. In: Hock F, Gralinski M (eds.), *Drug Discovery and Evaluation: Methods in Clinical Pharmacology*. Cham: Springer; 2017. https://doi.org/10.1007/978-3-319-56637-5_52-1
78. Sharma V, Madaan R, Bala R, Goyal A, Sindhu RK. Pharmacodynamic and pharmacokinetic interactions of herbs with prescribed drugs: a review. *Plant Archives* 2021; 21: 185–198. https://doi.org/10.51470/PLANTARCHIVES.2021.v21.S1.033.

79. Ekor M. The growing use of herbal medicines: issues relating to adverse reactions and challenges in monitoring safety. *Frontiers in Pharmacology* 2014 Jan 10; 4: 177. https://doi.org/10.3389/fphar.2013.00177. PMID: 24454289; PMCID: PMC3887317.
80. Neergheen-Bhujun VS. Underestimating the toxicological challenges associated with the use of herbal medicinal products in developing countries. *BioMed Research International* 2013; 2013: 804086, 9. https://doi.org/10.1155/2013/804086.
81. Bhat MDA, Malik R. Challenges in monitoring the safety of herbal medicines-an appraisal. *Journal of Pharmacovigilance and Drug Research* 2022; 3(4): 3. https://www.jpadr.com/index.php/jpadr/article/view/104.
82. Saikat S, Raja C, Biplab D. Challenges and opportunities in the advancement of herbal medicine: India's position and role in a global context. *Journal of Herbal Medicine* 2011; 1(3): 67–75. https://doi.org/10.1016/j.hermed.2011.11.001.
83. Zhou X, Li C-G, Chang D, Bensoussan A. Current status and major challenges to the safety and efficacy presented by Chinese herbal medicine. *Medicines* 2019; 6(1): 14. https://doi.org/10.3390/medicines6010014
84. Ghallab A, Bolt HM. *In vitro* systems: current limitations and future perspectives. *Archives of Toxicology* 2014; 88: 2085–2087. https://doi.org/10.1007/s00204-014-1404-6
85. Graudejus O, Ponce Wong RD, Varghese N, Wagner S, Morrison B. Bridging the gap between in vivo and *in vitro* research: reproducing *in vitro* the mechanical and electrical environment of cells in vivo. *Conference Abstract: MEA Meeting 2018 | 11th International Meeting on Substrate Integrated Microelectrode Arrays*, 2019. https://doi.org/10.3389/conf.fncel.2018.38.00069.
86. Mak IW, Evaniew N, Ghert M. Lost in translation: animal models and clinical trials in cancer treatment. *American Journal of Translational Research* 2014 Jan 15; 6(2): 114–118. PMID: 24489990; PMCID: PMC3902221.
87. Schleich N, Danhier F, Préat V. Iron oxide-loaded nanotheranostics: major obstacles to in vivo studies and clinical translation. *Journal of*

Controlled Release 2015 Jan 28; 198: 35–54. https://doi.org/10.1016/j.jconrel.2014.11.024. Epub 2014 Dec 4. PMID: 25481448.

88. Moran CJ, Ramesh A, Brama PAJ, Obyrne JM, Obrien FJ, Levingstone TJ. The benefits and limitations of animal models for translational research in cartilage repair. *Journal of Experimental Orthopaedics* 2016; 3: 1. https://doi.org/10.1186/s40634-015-0037-x
89. Herbert P, Xiaofei W. Statistical aspect of translational and correlative studies in clinical trials. *Chinese Clinical Oncology* 2016; 5(1): 11. https://doi.org/10.3978/j.issn.2304-3865.2014.07.04
90. Evans SR. Common statistical concerns in clinical trials. *Journal of Experimental Stroke & Translational Medicine* 2010 Feb 9; 3(1): 1–7. https://doi.org/10.6030/1939-067x-3.1.1. PMID: 21423790; PMCID: PMC3059317.
91. Yu D. Translational research: current status, challenges and future strategies. *American Journal of Translational Research* 2011; 3(5): 422–433. Epub 2011 Sep 12. PMID: 22046484; PMCID: PMC3204888.
92. Buț MG, Jîtcă G, Imre S, Vari CE, Ősz BE, Jîtcă C-M, Tero-Vescan A. The lack of standardization and pharmacological effect limits the potential clinical usefulness of phytosterols in benign prostatic hyperplasia. *Plants* 2023; 12(8): 1722. https://doi.org/10.3390/plants12081722.
93. Sachan AK, Vishnoi G, Kumar R. Need of standardization of herbal medicines in Modern era. *International Journal of Phytomedicine* 2016; 8: 300. https://doi.org/10.5138/09750185.1847.
94. Panossian A. Challenges in phytotherapy research. *Frontiers in Pharmacology* 2023; 14: 1199516. https://doi.org/10.3389/fphar.2023.1199516.
95. Sayed N, Khurana A, Godugu C. Pharmaceutical perspective on the translational hurdles of phytoconstituents and strategies to overcome. *Journal of Drug Delivery Science and Technology* 2019; 53: 101201. https://doi.org/10.1016/j.jddst.2019.101201.
96. Jornada DH, Fernandes GF, Chiba DE, Melo TRF, Santos JT, Chung MC. The prodrug approach: a successful tool for improving drug solubility. *Molecules* 2015; 21(1): 42.

97. Chen X, Zaro JL, Shen WC. Fusion protein linkers: property, design and functionality. *Advanced Drug Delivery Reviews* 2013; 65(10): 1357–1369.
98. Santos SS, Ferreira EI, Giarolla J. Dendrimer prodrugs. *Molecules* 2016; 21(6): 686.
99. Wadhwa S, Singhal S, Rawal S. Bioavailability enhancement by piperine: a review. *Asian Journal of Biomedical and Pharmaceutical Sciences* 2014; 4(36): 1–8.
100. Wei Y, Zhou S, Hao T, Zhang J, Gao Y, Qian S. Further enhanced dissolution and oral bioavailability of docetaxel by coamorphization with a natural P-gp inhibitor myricetin. *European Journal of Pharmaceutical Sciences* 2019; 129: 21–30.

https://doi.org/10.1142/9789811293320_0014

Chapter 14

Clinical Trials Using Phytochemicals in Liver Cancer Treatment: How Far is the Research?

Chameli Ratan[1] and Uday Kumar R[1,*]

[1]*Amrita School of Pharmacy, Amrita Vishwa Vidyapeetham, AIMS Health Science Campus, Kochi, Kerala, India*

Table of Contents:

List of Abbreviations:

HCC — Hepatocellular carcinoma
HBV — Hepatitis B virus

---

*Corresponding author: Tel.: 9686873535; E-mail address: udaykumarr@pharmacy.aims.amrita.edu

HCV — Hepatitis C virus
NAFLD — Non-alcoholic fatty liver disease
ROS — Reactive oxygen radicals
MARCH-1 — Membrane-associated RING-CH-1
HK2 — Hexokinase 2
MTA1 — Metastasis-associated protein 1
HDC1 — Histone deacetylase 1
PTEN — Phosphatase and tensin homolog
mTOR — Mammalian target of rapamycin
NF-κb — Nuclear factor kappa B
DAPI — 4′,6-diamidino-2-phenylindole
TNFα — Tumor necrosis factor alpha
IKκB — Inhibitor of kappa B kinase
pNF-κB — Phosphorylated nuclear factor kappa B
pIKκB — Phosphorylated inhibitor of kappa B kinase
PARP — Poly (ADP-ribose) polymerases
MLKL — Mixed lineage kinase domain-like pseudokinase
RIPK1 — Receptor-interacting serine/threonine-protein kinase 1
HNF-4α — Hepatocyte nuclear factor 4α
HIF-1α — Hypoxia-inducible factor 1 alpha
PKM1/PKM2 — Pyruvate kinase expression
EGFR — Endothelial growth factor receptor
AMPK — AMP-activated protein kinase
TF — Tatariside F
TGF-β — Transforming growth factor-β
SMAD2 — Mothers against decapentaplegic homolog 2
PJ-1 — Pulicaria jaubertii 1
JLGTE — Jujube leaf green tea extract
ERK — Extracellular signal-regulated kinase
GA — Gambogic acid
EGCG — Epigallocatechin-3-gallate
MAPK — Mitogen-activated protein kinase
FADD — Fas-associated protein with death domain
PF — Poncirus fructus
MMP-2/MMP-9 — Matrix metallopeptidase
AFP — Alpha-fetoprotein

ARE — Antioxidant response elements
UA — Ursolic acid
PPD — Protopanaxadiol
EMT — Epithelial-mesenchymal transition
BJO — Brucea javanica oil
BE-BJO — Brusatol-enriched BJO
BF-BJO — Brusatol-free BJO
TAE — Transarterial embolization
TACE — Transarterial chemoembolization
NK cells — Natural killer cells
GM-CSF — Granulocyte macrophage colony-stimulating factor
TTP — Time-to-progression
OS — Overall survival
CBR — Clinical benefit rate
VEGF — Vascular endothelial growth factor

Abstract

Hepatocellular carcinoma (HCC) poses significant clinical challenges worldwide due to its high incidence and limited treatment options, particularly in advanced stages. In recent years, there has been growing interest in exploring the potential of phytochemicals as adjunctive therapies for the prevention and management of HCC. Phytochemicals encompass a diverse array of compounds, including polyphenols, flavonoids, alkaloids, and terpenoids, each exhibiting distinct bioactive properties. Through various mechanisms, such as antioxidant, anti-inflammatory, and pro-apoptotic activities, phytochemicals have demonstrated efficacy in impeding carcinogenesis, inhibiting tumor proliferation, and suppressing metastasis in preclinical models. Despite promising preclinical and clinical evidence, challenges such as bioavailability limitations and standardization issues remain, necessitating further research and development efforts. The exploration of phytochemicals in HCC management represents a promising avenue for advancing therapeutic options, and warrants continued investigation to harness their full potential in combating HCC. This chapter mainly includes the phytochemicals — curcumin, resveratrol, epigallocatechin gallate (EGCG), quercetin, and silymarin. These compounds exhibit multifaceted anti-cancer effects by targeting signaling pathways implicated in HCC pathogenesis, including cell cycle regulation, apoptosis induction, and angiogenesis inhibition.

1. Introduction

Cancer ranks as the second most prevalent cause of death globally. As per data from the International Agency for Research on Cancer (GLOBOCAN 2020), liver cancer holds the sixth position in terms of most frequently diagnosed type of cancer and ranks as the second most prevalent cause of death [1]. Liver cancer encompasses various subtypes, including hepatocellular carcinoma (HCC), intrahepatic cholangiocarcinoma, and hepatoblastoma, with HCC being the most common, accounting for 75%–85% of all liver cancer cases [2, 3]. Unfortunately, the survival rate for HCC remains low at 8.37% over a 5-year period because of lack of efficient therapeutic alternatives [4]. The primary cause of death in HCC patients is the spread of cancerous cells to distant parts of the body [5]. Risk factors for HCC include hepatitis B (HBV) and hepatitis C virus (HCV) infections [6, 7], as well as chronic liver conditions such as non-alcoholic fatty liver disease (NAFLD) [8], fibrosis [9], or cirrhosis [10].

Currently, treatment options for HCC are restricted within the context of surgical interventions. Early-stage HCC is typically managed through liver ablation, surgical resection, or liver transplantation. However, it is important to note that each of these approaches comes with its own set of challenges and limitations [11]. The systemic drug treatments available for HCC are quite limited. Typically, kinase inhibitors such as lenvatinib and sorafenib are the primary therapies prescribed to individuals with inoperable HCC [12, 13]. Nevertheless, it is important to note that these medications are not curative in nature. They are administered with the goal of either managing the progression of cancer to make surgery possible or extending the patient's life expectancy, often by just a couple of months [14]. Moreover, it is a widely acknowledged reality that with the passage of time, patients develop resistance to these drugs, resulting in a limited duration of efficacy [15–17]. Furthermore, these treatments result in indiscriminate tissue damage and adverse effects, including alopecia, a decrease in red blood cell count, gastrointestinal tract infections, and immunosuppression. At present, medical approaches for HCC are limited, and even those available treatments lack high efficacy.

Regrettably, the most recent therapies and medications for HCC are plagued by numerous difficulties and constraints, which pose significant barriers to patients seeking treatments that could extend their lives. Given the evident need for alternative HCC treatment approaches, it is wise to explore the potential of plant-based solutions. Herbal medicines are still widely utilized worldwide; however, their recognition within the healthcare and scientific communities' lags because of the dearth of conclusive scientific data [18]. It is imperative to conduct further research on these compounds to connect the existing disparity between laboratory research and clinical practicality. This is especially crucial because plants contain a wealth of secondary metabolites with considerable potential previously demonstrated as chemotherapeutic or chemopreventive agents for a variety of chronic conditions, metabolic, including cardiovascular, neurodegenerative, and neoplastic diseases [19–21]. Many phytochemicals lack a strong scientific basis required to progress confidently into advanced research phases, primarily due to insufficient study. Despite the challenges associated with successful clinical translation, numerous phytochemicals have contributed significantly to advancements in the realm of cancer therapy, with a focus on HCC [18]. Plants have a rich history of being harnessed for their medicinal properties, primarily due to the valuable phytochemicals they contain [18]. Phytochemicals have demonstrated their effectiveness in reducing the primary characteristics of cancer, including proliferation, migration, and invasion. They can induce apoptosis to regulate the metastasis of HCC by targeting crucial molecular markers involved in these mechanisms [18]. In this chapter, our focus will be on exploring the impact of phytochemicals with diverse structures, including phenols, whole plant extracts, alkaloids, and lipids, on HCC.

1.1. *Phenols*

Phenols constitute a significant portion of secondary metabolites produced by plants, and they are characterized by aromatic compounds containing one or more hydroxyl groups. Phenols can be further classified into specific compound groups, such as stilbenes, flavonoids, xanthones, and catechins [22–24].

i. **Stilbenes: Resveratrol**, a natural stilbene found in grapes, peanuts, and pines, is known for its beneficial effects, such as antioxidative, anti-inflammatory, and cytoprotective properties (Figure 1). Resveratrol derivatives have demonstrated their ability to induce cell cycle arrest, increase intracellular ROS, and enhance caspase-3 activity in HepG2 cells, making them cytotoxic at a concentration of 21 μM [25, 26]. Additionally, resveratrol hinders the proliferation, migration, and invasion of HCC by downregulating MARCH1, an E3 ubiquitin ligase frequently overexpressed in HCC [27]. In animal trials, oral resveratrol therapy at 100 mg/kg for a 14-day period normalized antioxidant enzyme levels, such as glutathione peroxidase and catalase, typically decreased in HCC [28]. Resveratrol also inhibited hexokinase 2 (HK2) expression, an enzyme associated with anaerobic cell growth, and when

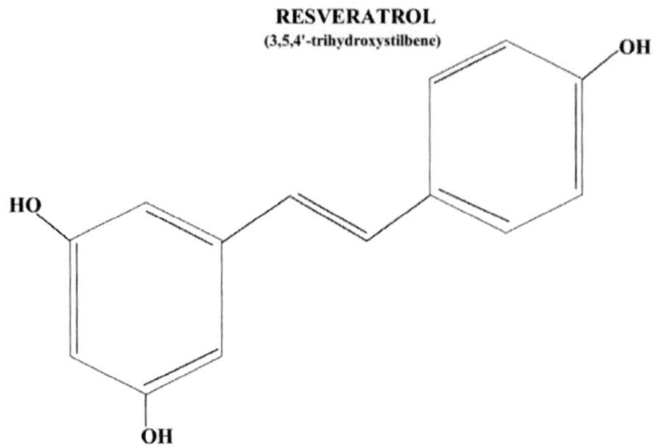

Figure 1: The figure represents the chemical structure of resveratrol

combined with sorafenib, it synergistically inhibited HCC cell growth [29]. In animal models, resveratrol displayed anticancer properties by increasing apoptosis, and in HCC mouse models, it inhibited tumor growth by reducing $CD8^{+}CD122^{+}$ regulatory T cells (Tregs) and increasing IFN-expressing $CD8^{+}$ T cells [30]. These effects were further enhanced when resveratrol was precisely delivered to the cancer site, such as through nanoparticle delivery systems [31]. Studies showed that nanoparticle and cationic liposome-based delivery systems significantly reduced liver nodules, indicating their potential in improving the anticancer effects of resveratrol [32]. **Pterostilbene**, another naturally occurring stilbenoid compound closely related to resveratrol but with greater bioavailability due to its two methoxy groups, has gained attention for its potential in cancer treatment. It exhibits inhibitory effects on various cellular processes involved in metastasis, acting through both programmed cell death (apoptosis) dependent and independent mechanisms [33]. Furthermore, it proficiently hampers the proliferation of HCC cells, exemplified by the SMMC-7721 cell line [34], by diminishing the expression of the metastasis-associated protein 1 (MTA1) and histone deacetylase 1 (HDC1) complex. This disruption of the complex amplifies the activation of the tumor suppressor PTEN within tumors, ultimately fostering apoptosis in HCC. In the prospective scenario, pterostilbene has the potential to function as an adjunctive treatment to decrease the incidence of metastasis in HCC [34, 35].

ii. **Flavonoids:** Flavonoids are commonly found in grains, wines, teas, fruits, and vegetables, and are known for their anti-inflammatory, antioxidant, antibacterial, and antiviral properties. Notably, some flavonoids have demonstrated promise as potential anti-cancer agents. **Quercetin** is a flavonoid primarily present in fruits and vegetables, such as grapes, onion, berries, apples, and broccoli, and in beverages such as red wine and tea. Its benefits include regulating ROS-mediated protein kinase C signaling, acting as an antioxidant to prevent oxidative damage, and inducing apoptosis in cancer cells [36, 37]. In HepG2 cells, quercetin increases the expression of p53 and Bax [38, 39]. Moreover, in SMMC-7721 and Bel-7402 cells, quercetin inhibits glycolysis by reducing HK-2 levels, a key glycolytic enzyme overexpressed in HCC. This glycolytic inhibition is associated with reduced phosphorylated mTOR and Akt levels [40–42]. Quercetin also represses the AKT/mTOR pathways in a dose-dependent manner. When administered to HCC xenograft tumors in mice, quercetin effectively inhibits tumor growth, by reducing HK-2 expression [40].

Citrus bergamia, also known as bergamot, is a tree native to the Italian Calabria region, and its juice is rich in flavonoids, including eriocitrin, neoeriocitrin, naringin, and neohesperidin. These individual flavonoids have demonstrated anticancer effects on HCC cell lines [43]. A study conducted by Ferlazzo et al. revealed that the combined administration of these flavonoids, as found in bergamot juice, led to anticancer effects. When HepG2 cells were treated with 10% bergamot juice, their proliferation rate decreased, and pro-apoptotic effects were induced. Bergamot juice caused cell cycle arrest in the G2 phase, with increased expression of p53 and p21 proteins [44]. Exposure to the flavonoids in bergamot juice additionally resulted in elevated expression

QUERCETIN

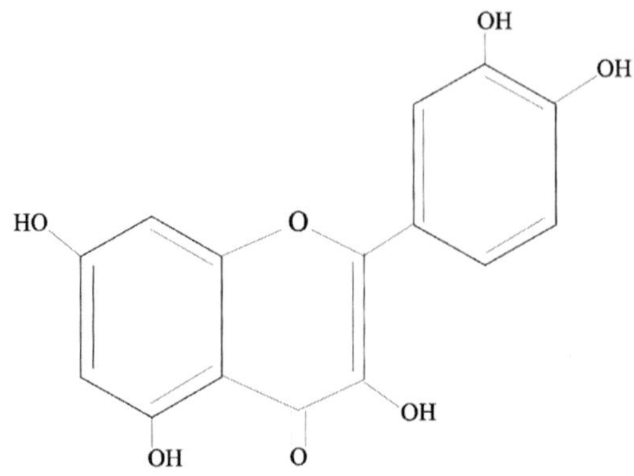

Figure 2: The figure represents the chemical structure of quercetin

of apoptosis-related genes and a decline in anti-apoptotic genes. Notably, the translocation of NF-kB to the nucleus was diminished, indicating that flavonoids from bergamot juice might trigger both the mitochondrial intrinsic and Fas-mediated extrinsic apoptotic pathways [44]. Another flavonoid, **fisetin**, is found in various fruits and vegetables, including grapes, persimmons, strawberries, onions, cucumber, and apples [45]. Fisetin triggers cell death through two methods: necroptosis and apoptosis. In the case of apoptosis, increased numbers of apoptotic cells were observed through DAPI staining, which revealed condensed chromatin, a characteristic of cells undergoing apoptosis. Morphological changes such as cell shrinkage, membrane blebbing, nuclear condensation, and apoptotic bodies confirmed the occurrence of apoptosis in HCC cells. Annexin V/PI staining further validated apoptosis, with its initiation linked to elevated TNFα expression and reduced NF-κB [46]. Fisetin led to alterations in the expression of various proteins, including the increase of IKκB and TNFα and the decrease of NF-κB, pIKκB, and pNF-κB. It also reduced Bcl2 levels while elevating Bax, caspase-3, and PARP levels in HepG2 cells. Moreover, fisetin triggered an increase in the expression of proteins associated with necroptosis, such as MLKL, pRIPK1, pRIPK3, RIPK3, and RIPK1, indicating cell death through necroptosis [46]. **Oroxylin A** is a promising flavonoid derived from the root of *Scutellariae radix*, a mint-like plant used in traditional Chinese medicine for centuries [47]. It has shown potential as a novel therapeutic modality for HCC. Research indicated that Oroxylin A enhanced the activation of HNF-4α in both SMMC-7721 and HepG2 cell lines. HNF-4α is involved in hepatocyte differentiation and positively influences HIF-1α. Additionally, Oroxylin A further elevated the PKM1/PKM2 ratio, subsequently activating HNF-4α and prompting differentiation in HepG2 and SMMC-7721 cells, with concentrations of 8 and 20 μM, respectively. This differentiation mechanism curbs unbridled proliferation and facilitates the transition into functional, non-malignant liver cells [48–50]. **Genistein**, an isoflavonoid found in soybeans, has demonstrated its preventive potential on Bel 7402 cells. It suppresses tumor cell proliferation and prompts cell cycle cessation in the G2/M and G0/G1 stages at a concentration of 10 μg/mL. In male BALB/c nude mice xenografted with Bel 7402 cells, intraperitoneal genistein treatment (50 mg/kg once a day for 15 days) reduced invasion, indicating its ability to inhibit metastasis *in vivo* [51]. Genistein also works effectively in combination with the EGFR inhibitor gefitinib in the Hep3B liver tumor cell line. In a chemical induction model of HCC in C57BL/6 mice, those fed with genistein through their diet (80 mg/kg/day for 5 months) showed a significant decrease in the incidence of HCC as opposed to those on regular chow [52]. Genistein increases phospho-AMPK levels in total liver tissue extracts and Hep3B cells, while also promoting apoptosis and suppressing pro-inflammatory responses, contributing to hepatic injury prevention [53]. **Tatariside F** (TF), a flavonoid found in the roots of *Fagopyrum tataricum* (tartary buckwheat), has demonstrated selective cytotoxicity to HCC cells in both *in vivo* and *in vitro* experiments. When HCC cells were exposed to TF (at 10 mg/kg), it significantly upregulated p53 and Bax, while downregulating Bcl-2. This effect was further enhanced when TF was combined with the chemotherapy drug cyclophosphamide. In HCC cells injected into mice, TF inhibited tumor growth and weight significantly, with even stronger effects when used alongside cyclophosphamide [54]. **Glabridin**, an isoflavone extracted from licorice roots, is not only used as a natural cosmetic and sweetener but also shows promise in combating cancer. In experiments with Huh-7 and HepG2 cell lines, glabridin (at 20 μM) was found to inhibit TGF-β and SMAD2 signaling pathways, impacting SMAD2 expression. Importantly, it did not affect the viability of normal liver cells (L02) when given at 10 and 20 μM [55]. In animal trials, the administration of glabridin in a xenograft model illustrated the inhibition of tumor formation. Mice with SK-Hep-1 xenografts, when administered with intraperitoneal glabridin for 28 days at 10 mg/kg, showed significantly reduced tumor volume compared to untreated control mice. These findings suggest that glabridin holds potential as a chemopreventive agent against HCC metastasis [56]. ***Pulicariajaubertii***, an aromatic plant native to Africa, Europe, and Asia, has demonstrated remarkable cancer-suppressing properties in HCC cells and human lung cells, even outperforming sorafenib, the primary drug for hepatic carcinoma treatment. Among the glycosides isolated from this plant, Pulicariajaubertii 1 (PJ-1) stood out for its ability to competitively suppress mutated K-Ras/B-Raf protein expression, specifically in HepG2 tumor cells without harming healthy liver cells. PJ-1 induced cellular toxicity in HepG2 cells at a dose of 1.5 mg/mL but had no adverse effects on normal hepatocytes. Additionally, PJ-1 activated p53 protein and reduced the expression levels of TGF-beta and IL-8 in HCC cells. These findings highlight PJ-1's potential as a targeted and safe therapy against HCC [57]. **Jujube leaf green tea extract (JLGTE)** demonstrated anti-proliferative effects on HepG2 cells at a concentration of 10 μg/mL. Significantly, it had no effect on the normal hepatocyte LO2 cell line, despite receiving the identical dose of 10 μg/mL. JLGTE showcased pro-apoptotic properties through the activation of AMP-activated protein kinase (AMPK)[58].

iii. **Xanthones: *Garcinia mangostana***, the mangosteen fruit, yields two unique xanthone compounds: mangostanaxanthone V and VI. Both xanthones have shown significant inhibitory effects on the proliferation of HepG2 cells. Mangostanaxanthone V halts' cells in the G0/G1 phase of the cell cycle, whereas mangostanaxanthone VI influences the G2/M phases. [59]. Alpha-mangostin, an additional bioactive xanthone from mangosteen, sensitizes HepG2 cells to anoikis, a programmed cell death process important in preventing metastasis. This is accomplished by activating mechanisms that promote apoptosis and suppressing proteins that inhibit apoptosis. Alpha-mangostin also reduces cell re-adhesion and migration, hindering molecules from participating in ERK and AKT signaling pathways [60]. Importantly, it exhibits minimal cytotoxicity to normal human osteogenic cells at various doses [61]. Gambogic acid (GA), isolated from gamboge resin, has anticancer effects [62]. It induces necrosis and reduced proliferation in SMMC-7721 cells and inhibits telomerase activity [63]. GA also triggers apoptosis through oxidative damage in HepG2 cells and blocks TrxR1 activity, leading to oxidative stress and programmed cell death in SMMC-7721 HCC cells [64]. These findings suggest the potential of these compounds as effective anticancer agents, especially in treating HCC.

iv. **Catechins: Green tea leaves (*Camellia sinensis*)** harbor numerous components with possible applications in cancer treatment. Epigallocatechin-3-gallate (EGCG), a polyphenol green tea extract, exhibits potential anti-neoplastic properties. It has been demonstrated that EGCG can hinder the multiplication of HCC cells in various cell lines, including SMMC-7721, SK-Hep1, Hep3B, HCC-LM3, HepG2, and Huh-7, by impeding the primary estrogen receptor, ERα36, which is prevalent in HCC cells [65]. EGCG markedly inhibits expansion and boosts apoptosis-inducing effects in HCC cells exhibiting elevated levels of ERα36 when exposed to concentrations of 30 or 60 μg/mL. This inhibitory effect is dose-dependent, and downstream effects include anti-proliferative actions by inhibiting the MAPK/ERK and PI3K/Akt pathways, as well as pro-apoptotic effects through caspase-3 activation and the ERα36-EGFR-Her-2 feedback loop. These findings suggest EGCG's potential in combating HCC [65]. Studies also showed that EGCG can disrupt HIF1α protein buildup in HepG2 cells when administered with 80 μg/mL by modifying the ERK1/2 and PI3K/Akt signaling pathways. Additionally, EGCG induces programmed cell death in HCC cells by lowering mitochondrial membrane potential and obstructing multiplication through G0/G1 cell cycle arrest. In Hep3B cells, EGCG activates caspase-3 and caspase-9 at a dose of 10 μg/mL [66–69]. Notably, EGCG was found to counteract a "poor prognosis" gene signature associated with HCC risk in cirrhotic liver tissue, indicating its potential to mitigate HCC development. In animal studies, intragastric EGCG treatment significantly reduced tumor volume and increased survival rates in DEN-induced HCC rats when administered at a dose of 25 mg/kg. Using the tea variety *Camellia sinensis* cv. CFT-1, high in EGCG, in male Wistar rats with HCC reduced hepatic nodules in size, number, and incidence [70–72]. EGCG has been observed to modify the gene expression profile of HCC cells in the presence of a simulated tumor microenvironment [73]. Remarkably, it opposes the effects of miR483-3p, a microRNA correlated with diminished survival and escalated progression of HCC in mouse models [74]. Combining EGCG with the EP1-selective antagonist ONO-8711 was more effective in inhibiting HepG2 cell viability and migration than EGCG alone when administered at various doses [75]. These investigations elucidate the mechanisms underlying EGCG's suppression of HCC growth.

1.2. *Whole plant extracts*

Whole plant extracts, obtained from plants, can encompass a multitude of phytochemicals, highlighting their potential as promising candidates for future cancer treatments. This is because these extracts contain a wide array of natural compounds and molecules, which may work synergistically to combat cancer cells, making them an attractive avenue for further research and development in the field of cancer therapy. ***Trametes robiniophila*** (Huaier) is a traditional Chinese medicinal mushroom with a history spanning over a millennium. Commonly, it is prepared as liquid extracts or granules. Its key component, proteoglycan, comprises of polysaccharides, water, and amino acids. Huaier displays powerful anti-HCC effects [76]. In an experiment conducted on HepG2 HCC cells, Huaier granules, administered at 15 mg/mL, exhibited decreased cell proliferation and migration. Importantly, this treatment did not harm normal human hepatocyte cells (L-02), indicating its specificity for HCC cells [77]. In a randomized controlled clinical trial, patients who had undergone liver resection for HCC and ingested a water-based extract of *Trametes robiniophila* (20 g in 100 mL of water, thrice daily for 96 weeks) exhibited markedly decreased rates of cancer recurrence and metastasis, coupled with enhanced survival rates [78]. Asian flatsedge, scientifically termed ***Cyperus amuricus***, is a grass indigenous to Europe, Russia, Japan, Korea, and China. It holds a longstanding presence in traditional oriental medicine. Research has shown that a methyl alcohol extract of the whole *C. amuricus* plant has cell-damaging effects on Hep3B cells at concentrations of 100–200 μg/mL. This cytotoxicity appears to result from an apoptotic mechanism, as indicated by observed morphological changes following 24-hour treatment [79]. The Hep3B cell treatment resulted in the suppression of cyclins and CDKs, inducing a halt in the cell cycle progression specifically at the sub-G1 phase. Moreover, it is suggested that *C. amuricus* triggers the splitting of procaspase-8 by FADD into its active form, caspase-8. Consequently, this triggers the division of Bid into tBid and its relocation to the mitochondria, fostering communication between intrinsic and extrinsic apoptotic pathways. The stepwise activation of cleaved caspases-3, -6, -7, -8, -9, and cleaved PARP, alongside other apoptosis-related proteins, additionally reinforces the anticancer capabilities of *C. amuricus* [79]. ***Poncirus fructus (PF)*** is an extract from the immature dry fruit of *Poncirus trifoliata*, a deciduous shrub found in South Korean islands [80]. PF shows promise as an anticancer agent, particularly against HCC. In laboratory tests, PF exhibited cell-toxic effect against HCC cells, leading to programmed cell death and a significant reduction in their ability to proliferate and form colonies. PF appears to induce cell death in HCC cells through a mitochondrial-mediated apoptosis pathway by disrupting the mitochondrial membrane potential and increasing intracellular ROS levels [80]. Furthermore, PF suppressed the migratory and invasive characteristics of HCC cells through the enhancement of the epithelial marker E-cadherin and the reduction of mesenchymal and cell cycle markers such as N-cadherin, Snail, Pin1, vimentin, cyclin D1, and a-SMA. Additionally, PF reduced the activity of MMP-9 and MMP-2, which are crucial in facilitating tumor cell invasion [80]. These findings suggest that PF may have potential in arresting the proliferation of HCC. Another whole plant extract is **Fraxini-2**, which is derived from the *Viscum album* L. mistletoe plant found on ash trees. In a clinical investigation, 12 patients with advanced HCC were administered fraxini-2 through subcutaneous injections, specifically at a dosage of 20 mg once a week for a span of 2 weeks. These patients remained on this therapeutic plan for different durations, ranging from 2.6 to 36.4 weeks. In this study, it was observed that the levels of alpha-fetoprotein (AFP), a traditionally employed serum marker for detecting HCC, appeared to balance within initial 3–4 weeks of therapy with fraxini-2. The decrease in AFP levels following the administration of fraxini-2 is an encouraging outcome, as it suggests a positive response to the treatment [81, 82].

1.3. *Alkaloids*

Coffee, which contains alkaloids like **caffeine**, has been linked to a decreased risk of HCC and chronic liver disease (Figure 2). A large-scale prospective cohort study involving over 215,000 individuals of various backgrounds revealed that coffee consumption was associated with a lower incidence of HCC and chronic liver disease. This reduced risk was consistent across different ethnicities, genders, body mass index (BMI), smoking habits, alcohol intake, and diabetes status. In an 18-year extended observational study, individuals who consumed two to three cups of coffee daily experienced a 38% lower risk of developing HCC than those who do not consume coffee. While individuals who took four or more cups per day had a 41% reduction in their risk for HCC [83]. The antioxidant properties of caffeine in the liver are linked to the transcription factor- Nrf-2 which attaches to antioxidant response elements (ARE) to activate various antioxidant

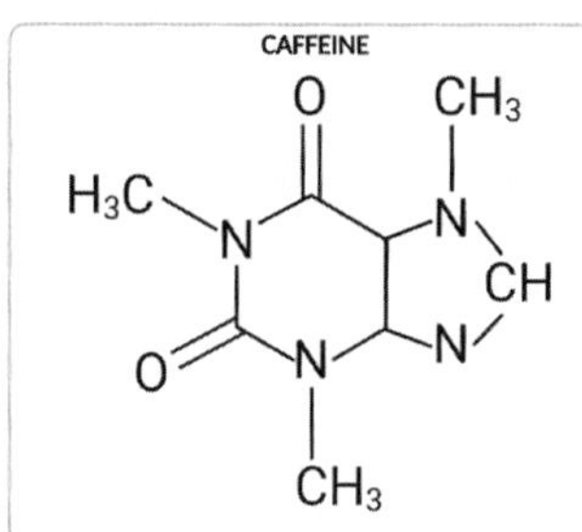

Figure 3: The afore-mentioned figure depicts the chemical structure of caffeine

genes. With rising caffeine concentration, the expression of proteins and enzymes under Nrf-2 regulation increases, leading to a decrease in overall oxidative stress [84]. **Neferine**, a bisbenzylisoquinoline alkaloid obtained from Indian Lotus (*Nelumbo nucifera*) green seed embryos, has been shown to induce programmed cell death in Hep3B cells when administered at doses exceeding 10 μM. This apoptotic effect is achieved through the downregulation of genes associated with cell proliferation, namely cyclin D3, D1, E2F-1, c-Myc, and CDK4 while also triggering endoplasmic reticulum (ER) stress [85]. Emerging evidence suggests that ***Rhizomacoptidis***, an herbal remedy, could hold promise as a potential therapeutic approach to treat HCC. The primary active compound in Rhizomacoptidis is an isoquinoline-derived alkaloid-berberine. Berberine induces apoptosis and exerts dose-dependent anti-proliferative effects (at concentrations of 10, 50, and 100 μM) on HepG2 cells. Furthermore, HepG2 cells administered with 50 μM berberine resulted in decreased expression of NF-κB-p65. This indicates that berberine could modulate the NF-κB pathway through p65 to exert its suppressive effects [86].

1.4. *Lipids*

Lipids, a category of biological compounds primarily composed of fatty acids, have demonstrated anticancer potential opposite HCC in various forms and plant derivatives. **Lipiodol**, an oil derived from poppy seeds, has a high iodine content of 38% by weight [87]. It exhibits slower clearance from liver cancer (HCC) cells than normal hepatocytes. Iodine-131-labeled lipiodol is another way to make it radioactive. This radioactive property allows it to be used as a targeted HCC treatment. Targeting cancerous cells is made easy with this medication because it gives patients approximately eight times the amount of radiation to cancerous liver tissue compared to normal liver tissue. Clinical trials have demonstrated its efficacy in improving overall survival, despite its initial use as a contrast medium in radiology for HCC patients, particularly in small tumors [87–90]. Lipiodol is a prime example of a phytochemical that contributes to HCC treatment by acting as a carrier for radiation.

1.4.1. *Isoprenoids*

Isoprenoids/terpenoids are a class of lipids present in a wide range of plants and mushrooms worldwide. They consist of varying quantities joined using isoprene units and are categorized as sesquiterpenes, triterpenes, diterpenes, monoterpenes, and so on, in accordance with the count of isoprene units in the molecule. Among the myriad classes of phytochemicals, terpenoids emerge as a sizable group with documented anticancer effects against various cancers, HCC included [91–97]. **Astrakurkurone**, derived from the consumable mushroom *Astraeus hygrometricus*, shows promise as a cell-damaging and toxic agent against HCC cells (HepG2 and Hep3B) at small doses (LD50: 58.8 μM and 122 μM). It selectively targets cancer cells, sparing normal liver cells at higher doses (250 μM). Astrakurkurone inhibits cell growth, disrupts the mitochondrial membrane, increases ROS production, and modulates apoptosis-related markers (cleaved caspase-9, Bax, and Bcl-2). This suggests astrakurkurone as a potential phytochemical for HCC treatment with anticancer properties [98]. ***Ziziphus jujuba***, a fruit like dates and belonging to the Rhamnaceae family, comprises of different bioactive substances, including multiple triterpenic acids. In a study by Kim et al., it was found that ursolic acid (UA), one of the triterpenic acids in Ziziphus jujuba, reduced cell viability and promoted apoptosis in HepG2 cells when administered at a dose of 30 μM [99]. The accurate mechanism is not fully understood; however, there is a suggestion that UA has the potential to cause cell cycle arrest by interfering with the establishment of DNA forks in the initiation phase of the cell cycle. Additionally, UA is implicated in upregulating the expression of p21/WAF1, potentially leading to cell cycle arrest and initiating apoptosis through the release of cytochrome c and activation of caspase-3 [99]. Protopanaxadiol (PPD) is a significant diol-type ginsenoside derived from ***Panax ginseng***, a traditional Chinese medicinal herb with a history of use for its anti-pathogenic, anticancer, and anti-inflammatory properties [100]. PPD has demonstrated anti-inflammatory and antioxidant effects on HCC cells (PLC/PRF/5 and HepG2) when administered at 40 and 20 μM. PPD demonstrates the ability to hinder the migration, invasion, and proliferation of these cancer cells by enhancing E-cadherin expression, an epithelial marker, and decreasing vimentin expression, a mesenchymal marker [101]. Additionally, anticancer effects of PPD involve its impact on the STAT3/Twist1 pathway, which is crucial in cancer cell proliferation, migration, and angiogenesis. PPD prevents STAT3 translocation into the nucleus and affects Twist1, a target gene of STAT3, which is known for inducing the epithelial-mesenchymal transition (EMT) in cancer cells [101]. Moreover, PPD has the potential to complement existing chemotherapies. In a study involving female BALB/C nude mice with xenografted cancer cells, a combination treatment of PPD (30 mg/kg) with the platinum anticancer drug oxaliplatin (OXA) (10 mg/kg) significantly suppressed tumor growth compared to using PPD or OXA alone [101]. **Lanatoside C**, also known as isolanid, is a triterpene cardiac glycoside derived from the *Digitalis ferruginea* plant, commonly known as "rusty foxglove." Research has demonstrated that when Mahlavu HCC cells lacking PTEN were treated with lanatoside C at a concentration of 2 μM, it led to a significant reduction in cell growth. This reduction was attributed to several factors, including the induction of G2/M cell cycle arrest, activation of the JNK pathway, initiation of apoptosis, and increased production of reactive oxygen species (ROS) *in vitro*. Furthermore, in an *in vivo* study using nude mice aged 8 to 16 weeks, the administration of lanatoside C via gavage feeding at a dosage of 6 mg/kg for 21 days resulted in a nearly 50% reduction in the size of HCC xenograft tumors, as observed through MRI imaging [102]. *Sanguisorba officinalis*, a plant in the Rosaceae family found in cooler regions of northern Europe, contains a triterpenoid saponin known as **Ziyuglycoside II**. This compound has been shown to exhibit anticancer properties in SMMC-7721 and HepG2 cancer cell lines. Ziyuglycoside II effectively increases reactive oxygen species (ROS) activity, leading to cell cycle arrest at G0/G1, ultimately resulting in apoptosis. Moreover, it reduces the migratory and infiltrative capabilities of these liver cancer cells in a dose-dependent manner. This is achieved by curtailing the expression of MMP-9 and MMP-2 and blocking the EGFR/NF-kB pathway. Notably, Ziyuglycoside II demonstrates lower toxicity to

ARTEMISININ

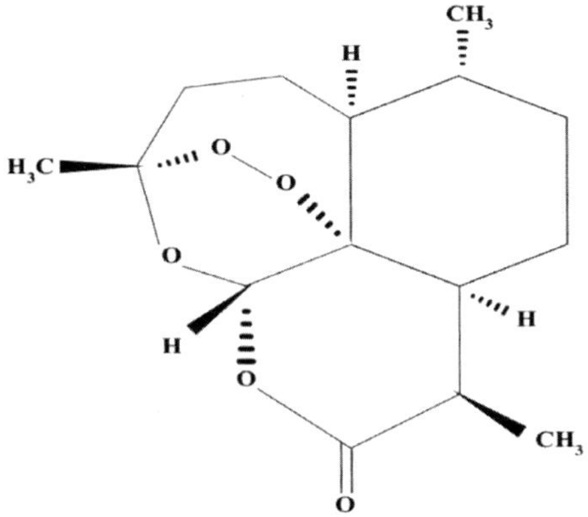

Figure 4: The figure depicts the chemical structure of Artemisinin

normal cells (BRL3A and HEK293T), highlighting its selective cell-toxicity against HCC [103]. **Artemisinin**, a sesquiterpene lactone compound found in sweet wormwood (Artemisia annua), exhibits anticancer properties (Figure 3). When administered at 100 μg/mL, artemisinin and its derivatives effectively inhibit the proliferation of HepG2 and Huh-7 liver cancer cells. This inhibition is achieved by inhibiting the mTOR and PI3K/AKT signaling pathways, which play a crucial role in regulating both angiogenesis and programmed cell death in HCC. By targeting these pathways, artemisinin regulates the growth and angiogenic potential of HCC cells. Artemisinin additionally reduces the levels of anti-apoptotic proteins such as survivin and XIAP, concurrently elevating the expression of cleaved PARP and caspase-3. These actions promote apoptosis in HepG2 and Huh7 cells [104, 105]. Furthermore, in cell adhesion assays, artemisinin enhances cell-cell adhesion in HCC cells, denoting its ability to restrict the metastatic potential of HCC [105].

Ardipusilloside I, a triterpene derived from the Chinese medicinal herb *Ardisia pusilla* A. DC, demonstrates significant anti-neoplastic properties against SMMC-7721 and HepG2 HCC cell lines when administered at a concentration of 50 μM. These effects are achieved through the prohibition of cell survival, invasion, and metastasis. The key mechanisms involve the repression of the Akt and MEK/ERK signaling pathways, leading to the curtailment of matrix metalloproteinase-2 and 9. Moreover, ardipusilloside I effectively reduces HCC cell metastasis by triggering Rac1, which then upregulates E-cadherin expression, ultimately diminishing the cells' metastatic potential [106]. ***Diospyros kaki***, commonly known as kaki persimmon, is rich in terpenoids and flavonoids. Ethanol extracts from its leaves have shown the ability to govern EMT and stemness characteristics in HCC cells by inhibiting the hepatocyte growth factor (HGF)/Met pathway. When HepG2, Hep3B, and SNU475 cell lines were administered with a 50 µg/mL ethanolic extract of *D. kaki* leaves, it resulted in reduced expression of keratin19 and CD44, as well as decreased expression of MMP-1/2/9, vimentin, and snail. Simultaneously, there was an upregulated expression of E-cadherin when HGF was added along with *D. kaki* leaf extract, indicating its capacity to inhibit cancer cell growth, even in the presence of HGF. Furthermore, the study assessed the efficiency of combining the gold standard chemotherapy treatment, sorafenib, with 50 µg/mL of *D. kaki* extract. The combination lowered the IC50 of sorafenib from 3.7 µg/mL, 5.9 µg/mL, and 9.5 µg/mL in Hep3B, HepG2, and SNU475 cell lines, respectively, to 1.8 µg/mL, 2.7 µg/mL, and 5.9 µg/mL. Notably, *D. kaki* leaf extract showed no toxicity to cancer cells at concentrations as high as 50 µg/mL, which represented the maximum dose examined [107]. ***Bruceajavanica***, a flowering shrub, has a history of traditional use in Chinese medicine for ailments such as dysentery, malaria, and cancer. The fruit of this plant is particularly abundant in quassinoids, a class of triterpene lactones known for their potent anticancer properties. One of the key quassinoids found in Bruceajavanica oil (BJO) is brusatol [108]. In a study, male Kunming mice with implanted H22 cell hepatomas were intraperitoneally injected with brusatol-enriched BJO (BE-BJO) at 610 mg/kg, regular BJO at 2000 mg/kg, and brusatol-free BJO (BF-BJO) at 2000 mg/kg. The results revealed that tumorigenesis was effectively suppressed in mice treated with BE-BJO. RNA analysis showed a significant increase in miRNA-29b and p53 expression in response to BE-BJO. Both BJO and BE-BJO were found to downregulate Bcl-2 while enhancing the expression of Bax, Bad, cytosolic cytochrome c, cleaved caspase-3, cleaved caspase-9, and cleaved PARP, ultimately inducing apoptosis in H22 xenografts in the mice. These discoveries highlight the significant capacity of brusatol, a major active compound from BJO, in causing cell death in HCC [109].

2. Phytochemicals used in Clinical Trials for Liver Cancer

Phytochemicals have gained significant attention in recent years for their potential role in liver cancer clinical trials. These natural compounds found in plants have shown promise as adjunctive therapies for managing liver cancer, opening new avenues for research and treatment approaches.

a) **Huaier granule for prevention of recurrence and metastasis of hepatocarcinoma following local ablation:** A multicentre, prospective cohort study investigating Huaier granule for the prevention of recurrence and metastasis of hepatocarcinoma following local ablation is a medical research study designed to assess the effectiveness and safety of Huaier granule as a potential treatment option for hepatocarcinoma patients who have undergone local ablation therapy. Huaier granule is a traditional Chinese medicine derived from the fungus *Trametes robiniophila* Murr. It has been researched for its potential anticancer properties, among other health benefits. The study focuses on monitoring and ensuring the safety of the treatment, including the evaluation of any adverse effects [110].
b) **Resveratrol and human hepatocyte function in cancer:** The primary objective of this research was to assess the potential therapeutic impact of resveratrol, a dietary supplement, on the cellular functionality of both healthy liver cells and diseased liver cells (specifically, cancer cells), utilizing liver tissue samples obtained during elective liver surgeries. The investigation aimed to examine three distinct metrics, with the underlying hypothesis that the

administration of resveratrol as a dietary supplement would lead to the following outcomes:

1. Enhancement of metabolic function within liver cells.
2. Suppression of cellular growth and proliferation within cancer cells.
3. Reduction of inflammatory processes in the liver.

However, it is noteworthy that the study was terminated after a duration of six months [111].

c) **Hepatocellular carcinoma on cirrhosis with child A/B7 and hepatic intra-arterial injection of idarubicin/lipiodol emulsion (LIDA-BII):** In this clinical trial, the researchers aim to assess the efficacy and safety of hepatic chemotherapy. This treatment involves the intra-arterial injection of Idarubicin, which is emulsified with Lipiodol, a lipid-based carrier, without concurrent embolization. This therapy is intended for patients with non-metastatic, unresectable HCC, specifically those diagnosed with cirrhotic livers with Child-Pugh classifications of A or B7 [112].

d) **TACE oil by TAE/TACE in patients with hepatocellular carcinoma:** The primary objective of this study is to evaluate the safety and effectiveness of TACE/TAE treatment with TACE Oil in patients diagnosed with unresectable HCC. Patients with HCC who meet the eligibility criteria will be admitted to the hospital for treatment. TAE or TACE procedures will be performed during hospitalization, and patients will be closely observed for 1 to 7 days after embolization. Phase I will involve the sequential enrollment of 12 evaluable subjects.

   The first three subjects will receive TAE treatment, regardless of their contraindications to doxorubicin. The subsequent three subjects (fourth to sixth) will undergo TACE treatment. The remaining subjects may receive either TAE or TACE treatment. For the first six subjects in Phase I, after completion of TAE or TACE treatment and a 2-week follow-up, the safety and tolerability data will be reviewed by the SRC. Approval by the SRC is required before the next subject can start treatment. For the 7th to 12th subjects in Phase I, the safety and tolerability data will be reviewed by the SRC after treatment and until discharge from the hospital. After the safety and tolerability data for all 12 evaluable subjects in Phase I have been reviewed and approved by the SRC, the study may proceed to Phase II part. Phase II will include 70 evaluable subjects who will be randomized in a 1:1 ratio. They will receive TAE/TACE treatment using either TACE oil or lipiodol for the purpose of safety and efficacy assessment. The study will involve close monitoring and follow-up of patients for a specified period after treatment to evaluate both safety and efficacy. This comprehensive approach aims to determine the potential benefits and risks associated with TACE/TAE treatment using TACE Oil for HCC [113].

e) **Lipiodol-TACE with idarubicin for hepatocellular carcinoma:** The objective of this real-world investigation is to assess the safety and effectiveness of using lipiodol-TACE in conjunction with idarubicin for the treatment of HCC. Idarubicin is a DNA topoisomerase II inhibitor that causes DNA strand breakage, leading to cell cycle arrest in the G2 phase and inducing DNA cleavage, ultimately resulting in cell apoptosis. It can also intercalate between DNA base pairs, generating free radicals that disrupt the DNA double helix structure, impeding DNA strand extension, replication, and transcription. Preclinical studies have demonstrated that idarubicin exhibits superior anti-tumor activity compared to epirubicin, particularly against SUN-449 human hepatoma cells. In recent years, both domestic and international researchers have conducted various investigations into the use of a lipiodol-idarubicin emulsion for the treatment of HCC, yielding favorable outcomes. This prospective, multicentre real-world study seeks to evaluate the effectiveness and safety of lipiodol-TACE with idarubicin in Chinese patients with HCC [114].

f) **Phase II study of viscum fraxini-2 in patients with advanced hepatocellular carcinoma:** Mistletoe extract known as viscum fraxini, derived from mistletoe (*Viscum album* L.) grown on ash trees, boasts the highest concentration of lectins. The aim of this study was to assess the safety and effectiveness of viscum fraxini-2 in individuals diagnosed with advanced HCC who had not undergone prior systemic chemotherapy. The study included 23 patients with unresectable HCC who had measurable tumors. Mistletoe extract has been found to have immunostimulatory effects attributed to low molecular weight oligosaccharides. This stimulation of natural killer (NK) cell activity seems to be linked to increased production of interferon (INF-γ) by T cells and tumor necrosis factor-α (TNF-α) by macrophages. Additionally, lectin components in mistletoe preparations play a crucial role, boosting the activity of various immune cells, such as neutrophils, NK cells, and large granular lymphocytes, and activating monocyte-macrophage and helper cell subpopulations. This is associated with elevated levels of cytokines such as interleukins IL-1, IL-6, granulocyte-macrophage colony-stimulating factor (GM-CSF), and TNF-α. Apart from their immunostimulatory effects, mistletoe extract and lectins also exhibit direct cytotoxic effects. Lectins are considered essential components responsible for apoptosis. Additionally, viscotoxins, a group of cytotoxic polypeptides, can disrupt cell membranes, enhancing cell permeability. Therefore, mistletoe extracts can induce both apoptosis and cell lysis, leading to subsequent immune stimulation. In summary, complete mistletoe extract, including membrane lipids like viscum fraxini, affects both the T-cell and B-cell components of the immune system. It initiates the proliferation and activation of immune cells and the expression of cytokines, supporting antitumor effects [115].

g) **First-in-class immune-modulating small molecule Icaritin in advanced hepatocellular carcinoma: preliminary results of safety, durable survival, and immune biomarkers:** This phase I study aimed to evaluate Icaritin as a potential oral immunotherapy in combination with immune-checkpoint inhibitors for advanced HCC, a condition with limited treatment options and a grim prognosis. Eligible patients with advanced HCC (Child-Pugh Class A or B) received a fixed oral dose of either 600 or 800 mg of Icaritin twice daily. The main objective was to assess safety, while secondary objectives included measuring time-to-progression (TTP), overall survival (OS), and clinical benefit rate (CBR).

The study also explored the impact of Icaritin on immune biomarkers and immune-modulating activities in myeloid cells. The findings revealed that Icaritin exhibited a favorable safety profile and provided preliminary, sustained survival benefits for advanced HCC patients. These benefits were associated with immune-modulating effects on Icaritin and its impact on immune biomarkers. This suggests the potential of Icaritin as an innovative oral immunotherapy for advanced HCC, when used in conjunction with antibody-based PD-1/PD-L1 blockade therapies [116].

h) **A Phase II study of irinotecan in patients with advanced hepatocellular carcinoma:** In this Phase II clinical trial, irinotecan, a water-soluble inhibitor of topoisomerase-1 derived from plant alkaloids, was evaluated for its effectiveness in patients with advanced HCC, a condition with a grim prognosis. Eligible patients had received a maximum of one prior chemotherapy regimen, displayed measurable disease, had a good performance status, and their major organs were functioning adequately. The treatment involved administering irinotecan at a starting dose of 125 mg/m^2 weekly for 4 weeks followed by a 2-week break, making up one treatment cycle. After two cycles, patients underwent radiological restaging, and dose adjustments were made if toxicity was observed. Irinotecan showed limited efficacy in advanced hepatocellular cancer, and there were significant toxicity issues, likely due to compromised liver function or difficulties in metabolizing and eliminating the drug. Despite these challenges, the study suggests that further investigation of new therapies for this disease is warranted [117].

i) **A Phase I study of continuous hepatic arterial infusion of Irinotecan in patients with locally advanced hepatocellular carcinoma:** The goal of this Phase I study was to determine the highest tolerated dose and the toxicity limits of a continuous infusion of irinotecan administered via a hepatic artery port-a-cath in patients with HCC and cirrhosis. The aim was to explore new treatment approaches for advanced HCC and assess response rates and time-to-progression (TTP). Irinotecan was given as a continuous five-day infusion every 21 days, with dose increases of

2.5 mg/m^2/day for every three patients, beginning at 7.5 mg/m^2/day. Dose-limiting toxicity was defined as one patient in each group experiencing severe (G4) hematologic or significant (G3) non-hematologic side effects, which were confirmed in two groups. Dose-limiting toxicity primarily manifested as severe diarrhea (G3) in two patients at a dose of 27.5 mg/m^2/day, leading to the recommended dose being set at 25 mg/m^2/day. Nineteen out of 30 patients faced complications related to the port-a-cath placement, and one patient succumbed to liver ischemia and sepsis. The median TTP was 11.3 months. In summary, intra-arterial infusion of irinotecan is a viable option for patients with HCC and cirrhosis, with a recommended dose of 25 mg/m^2/day. Although there were no major drug-related adverse events, concerns arose regarding the insertion and management of the intra-arterial device [118].

j) **Berberine suppresses Id-1 expression and inhibits the growth and development of lung metastases in hepatocellular carcinoma:** Berberine, a quaternary ammonium salt classified among isoquinoline alkaloids, is thought to be the primary antitumor component of Coptis Rhizome, a traditional Chinese medicinal herb. This study demonstrates effectiveness of berberine implants in preventing the spread of primary HCC into surrounding normal liver tissue, showcasing its potent anti-metastatic properties in living organisms. Berberine's antitumor effects align with previous findings in various cancers, including the suppression of cell proliferation, invasiveness, and the HIF-1α/VEGF signaling pathway. Significantly, further investigation reveals that berberine profoundly inhibits the expression of Id-1, a pivotal regulator in HCC development and metastasis. Berberine achieves this by reducing Id-1 transcription through the inhibition of its promoter activity. Specifically reducing Id-1 through RNA transcript knockdown in HCC cells leads to inhibited growth, invasion, and reduced VEGF secretion, demonstrating the functional relevance of Id-1 downregulation induced by berberine. Lastly, in HCC models, anti-proliferative and anti-invasive effects can be

Table 1: The table represents all the clinical trials which utilized phytochemicals for the treatment of hepatocellular carcinoma

Phytochemical	Study Phase	Purpose of Study	References
Huaier granule (*Trametes robiniophila* Murr)	Phase IV	Monitoring the safety and efficacy of Huaier granules in HCC	[110]
Resveratrol	Phase I and Phase II	Comparative study on the impact of resveratrol on the cell functionality on both healthy and diseased liver cells	[111]
Idarubicin	Phase II	Safety and efficacy of Idarubicin emulsified with lipiodol in hepatic chemotherapy	[112]
Poppyseed oil	Phase I and Phase II study	To evaluate the safety and effectiveness of TACE/TAE treatment with TACE oil or lipiodol in patients diagnosed with unresectable HCC	[113]
Idarubicin	Phase II and Phase III	To evaluate the effectiveness and safety of lipiodol-TACE with idarubicin in Chinese patients with hepatocellular carcinoma	[114]
Viscum fraxini-2 (*Viscum album* L.)	Phase II	To assess the safety and effectiveness of viscum fraxini-2 in individuals diagnosed with advanced HCC who had not undergone prior systemic chemotherapy	[115]
Icaritin	Phase I	To evaluate Icaritin as a potential oral immunotherapy in combination with immune-checkpoint inhibitors for advanced HCC	[116]

(*Continued*)

Table 1: (*Continued*)

Phytochemical	Study Phase	Purpose of Study	References
Irinotecan	Phase II	To evaluate effectiveness in patients with advanced hepatocellular carcinoma	[117]
Irinotecan	Phase I	To determine the highest tolerated dose and the toxicity limits of a continuous infusion of irinotecan administered via a hepatic artery port-a-cath in patients with hepatocellular carcinoma and cirrhosis	[118]
Berberine	Preclinical study	To evaluate the effectiveness of berberine implants in preventing the spread of primary HCC into surrounding normal liver tissue, showcasing its potent anti-metastatic properties in living organisms	[119]

partially reversed by overexpressing Id-1, unveiling a novel anti-cancer and anti-invasion mechanism of berberine through Id-1 suppression [119].

3. Conclusion

Phytochemicals, sourced from diverse plants, encompassing structures such as phenols, whole plant extracts, alkaloids, and lipids, display a range of biological activities suitable for intervention in liver cancer. In this chapter of clinical trial, the researchers aim to assess the efficacy and safety of hepatic chemotherapy. While there is promising evidence, many phytochemicals lack the robust scientific foundation required to progress confidently into advanced research phases, primarily due to insufficient study. Several findings underscore the anti-cancer attributes of phytochemicals, including their ability to induce apoptosis, exert anti-angiogenic effects, and modulate signaling pathways implicated in the progression of liver cancer. Clinical trials underscore the manageable safety profiles of these phytochemicals, supporting their potential as either adjunctive or standalone treatments for liver cancer. However, persistent challenges and limitations, such as variations in study designs, patient populations, and a lack of standardized protocols across trials, remain. In conclusion, despite commendable progress, a critical requirement exists for more robust and standardized clinical trials to validate the therapeutic potential of phytochemicals in liver cancer. The intricate interplay between phytochemicals and the complex molecular pathways involved demands a nuanced and comprehensive approach. Collaboration among researchers, clinicians, and pharmaceutical entities is pivotal for advancing the field and translating promising discoveries into clinically meaningful outcomes for individuals with liver cancer. The ongoing endeavor to integrate phytochemicals into mainstream liver cancer therapeutics holds the promise of introducing innovative and effective treatment modalities for this challenging disease.

References

1. Sung, H.; Ferlay, J.; Siegel, R.L.; Laversanne, M.; Soerjomataram, I.; Jemal, A.; Bray F. Global cancer statistics 2020: GLOBOCAN estimates of incidence and mortality worldwide for 36 cancers in 185 countries. *CA Cancer J. Clin.* 2021, 71, 209–249. doi: 10.3322/caac.21660.
2. Sagnelli, E.; Macera, M.; Russo, A.; Coppola, N.; Sagnelli, C. Epidemiological and etiological variations in hepatocellular carcinoma. *Infection* 2020, 48, 7–17. doi: 10.1007/s15010-019-01345-y.
3. Bray, F.; Ferlay, J.; Soerjomataram, I.; Siegel, R.L.; Torre, L.A.; Jemal, A. Global cancer statistics 2018: GLOBOCAN estimates of incidence and mortality worldwide for 36 cancers in 185 countries. *CA Cancer J. Clin.* 2018, 68, 394–424. doi: 10.3322/caac.21492.
4. Sarveazad, A.; Agah, S.; Babahajian, A.; Amini, N.; Bahardoust, M. Predictors of 5 year survival rate in hepatocellular carcinoma patients. *J. Res. Med. Sci.* 2019, 24, 86. doi: 10.4103/jrms.JRMS_1017_18.

5. Sun, W.; Fu, S.; Wu, S.; Tu, R. Growing evidence of exosomal microRNA-related metastasis of hepatocellular carcinoma. *Biomed Res. Int.* 2020, 2020, 4501454. doi: 10.1155/2020/4501454.
6. Keating, G.M. Sorafenib: A review in hepatocellular carcinoma. *Target Oncol.* 2017, 12, 243–253. doi: 10.1007/s11523-017-0484-7.
7. de Martel, C.; Maucort-Boulch, D.; Plummer, M.; Franceschi S. World-wide relative contribution of hepatitis B and C viruses in hepatocellular carcinoma. *Hepatology* 2015, 62, 1190–1200. doi: 10.1002/hep.27969.
8. Chen, D.S. Hepatitis C virus in chronic liver disease and hepatocellular carcinoma in Taiwan. *Princess Takamatsu Symp.* 1995, 25, 27–32.
9. Zhang, D.Y.; Friedman S.L. Fibrosis-dependent mechanisms of hepatocarcinogenesis. *Hepatology* 2012, 56, 769–775. doi: 10.1002/hep.25670.
10. Nordenstedt, H.; White, D.L.; El-Serag, H.B. The changing pattern of epidemiology in hepatocellular carcinoma. *Dig. Liver Dis.* 2010, 42(Suppl. 3), S206–S214. doi: 10.1016/S1590-8658(10)60507-5.
11. Gentile, D.; Donadon, M.; Lleo, A.; Aghemo, A.; Roncalli, M.; di Tommaso, L.; Torzilli, G. Surgical treatment of hepatocholangio carcinoma: A systematic review. *Liver Cancer* 2020, 9, 15–27. doi: 10.1159/000503719.
12. Spallanzani, A.; Orsi, G.; Andrikou, K.; Gelsomino, F.; Rimini, M.; Riggi, L.; Cascinu, S. Lenvatinib as a therapy for unresectable hepatocellular carcinoma. *Expert Rev. Anticancer Ther.* 2018, 18, 1069–1076. doi: 10.1080/14737140.2018.1524297.
13. Llovet, J.M.; Ricci, S.; Mazzaferro, V.; Hilgard, P.; Gane, E.; Blanc, J.F.; de Oliveira, A.C.; Santoro, A.; Raoul, J.L.; Forner, A.; et al. Sorafenib in advanced hepatocellular carcinoma. *N. Engl. J. Med.* 2008, 359, 378–390. doi: 10.1056/NEJMoa0708857.
14. Rimassa, L.; Pressiani, T.; Merle, P. Systemic treatment options in hepatocellular carcinoma. *Liver Cancer* 2019, 8, 427–446. doi: 10.1159/000499765.
15. Zheng, A.; Chevalier, N.; Calderoni, M.; Dubuis, G.; Dormond, O.; Ziros, P.G.; Sykiotis, G.P.; Widmann, C. CRISPR/Cas9 genome-wide screening identifies KEAP1 as a sorafenib, lenvatinib, and regorafenib sensitivity gene in hepatocellular carcinoma. *Oncotarget.* 2019, 10, 7058–7070. doi: 10.18632/oncotarget.27361.

16. Ao, J.; Chiba, T.; Shibata, S.; Kurosugi, A.; Qiang, N.; Ma, Y.; Kan, M.; Iwanaga, T.; Sakuma, T.; Kanzaki, H.; et al. Acquisition of mesenchymal-like phenotypes and overproduction of angiogenic factors in lenvatinib-resistant hepatocellular carcinoma cells. *Biochem. Biophys. Res. Commun.* 2021, 549, 171–178. doi: 10.1016/j.bbrc.2021.02.097.
17. Tang, W.; Chen, Z.; Zhang, W.; Cheng, Y.; Zhang, B.; Wu, F.; Wang, Q.; Wang, S.; Rong, D.; Reiter, F.P.; et al. The mechanisms of sorafenib resistance in hepatocellular carcinoma: Theoretical basis and therapeutic aspects. *Signal. Transduct. Target. Ther.* 2020, 5, 87. doi: 10.1038/s41392-020-0187-x.
18. Rodriguez, S.; Skeet, K.; Mehmetoglu-Gurbuz, T.; Goldfarb, M.; Karri, S.; Rocha, J.; Shahinian, M.; Yazadi, A.; Poudel, S.; Subramani, R. Phytochemicals as an alternative or integrative option, in conjunction with conventional treatments for hepatocellular carcinoma. *Cancers* 2021, 13(22), 5753. https://doi.org/10.3390/cancers13225753.
19. Zhou, D.D.; Luo, M.; Shang, A.; Mao, Q.Q.; Li, B.Y.; Gan, R.Y.; Li, H.B. Antioxidant food components for the prevention and treatment of cardiovascular diseases: Effects, mechanisms, and clinical studies. *Oxid. Med. Cell Longev.* 2021, 2021, 6627355. doi: 10.1155/2021/6627355.
20. Graf, B.L.; Raskin, I.; Cefalu, W.T.; Ribnicky, D.M. Plant-derived therapeutics for the treatment of metabolic syndrome. *Curr. Opin. Investig. Drugs* 2010, 11, 1107–1115.
21. Sharifi-Rad, M.; Lankatillake, C.; Dias, D.A.; Docea, A.O.; Mahomoodally, M.F.; Lobine, D.; Chazot, P.L.; Kurt, B.; Tumer, T.B.; Moreira, A.C.; et al. Impact of natural compounds on neurodegenerative disorders: From preclinical to pharmacotherapeutics. *J. Clin. Med.* 2020, 9, 1061. doi: 10.3390/jcm9041061.
22. Ganesan, K.; Xu, B. A Critical review on polyphenols and health benefits of black soybeans. *Nutrients* 2017, 9, 455. doi: 10.3390/nu9050455.
23. Dai, J.; Mumper, R.J. Plant phenolics: Extraction, analysis and their antioxidant and anticancer properties. *Molecules* 2010, 15, 7313–7352. doi: 10.3390/molecules15107313.
24. Anantharaju, P.G.; Gowda, P.C.; Vimalambike, M.G.; Madhunapantula, S.V. An overview on the role of dietary phenolics for the treatment of cancers. *Nutr. J.* 2016, 15, 99. doi: 10.1186/s12937-016-0217-2.

25. Malhotra, A.; Bath, S.; Elbarbry, F. An organ system approach to explore the antioxidative, anti-inflammatory, and cytoprotective actions of resveratrol. *Oxid Med. Cell Longev.* 2015, 2015, 803971.
26. Aja, I.; Ruiz-Larrea, M.B.; Courtois, A.; Krisa, S.; Richard, T.; Ruiz-Sanz, J.I. Screening of natural stilbene oligomers from *Vitis vinifera* for anticancer activity on human hepatocellular carcinoma cells. *Antioxidants* 2020, 9, 469.
27. Dai, H.; Li, M.; Yang, W.; Sun, X.; Wang, P.; Wang, X.; Su, J.; Hu, X.; Zhao, M. Resveratrol inhibits the malignant progression of hepatocellular carcinoma via MARCH1-induced regulation of PTEN/AKT signaling. *Aging* 2020, 12, 11717–11731.
28. Rawat, D.; Chhonker, S.K.; Naik, R.A.; Koiri, R.K. Modulation of antioxidant enzymes, SIRT1 and NF-B by resveratrol and nicotinamide in alcohol-aflatoxin B1-induced hepatocellular carcinoma. *J. Biochem. Mol. Toxicol.* 2021, 35, e22625.
29. Dai, W.; Wang, F.; Lu, J.; Xia, Y.; He, L.; Chen, K.; Li, J.; Li, S.; Liu, T.; Zheng, Y.; et al. By reducing hexokinase 2, resveratrol induces apoptosis in HCC cells addicted to aerobic glycolysis and inhibits tumor growth in mice. *Oncotarget.* 2015, 6, 13703–13717.
30. Zhang, Q.; Huang, H.; Zheng, F.; Liu, H.; Qiu, F.; Chen, Y.; Liang, C.L.; Dai, Z. Resveratrol exerts antitumor effects by downregulating CD8. *Oncoimmunology* 2020, 9, 1829346.
31. Rahman, M.; Almalki, W.H.; Afzal, O.; Alfawaz Altamimi, A.S.; Kazmi, I.; Al-Abbasi, F.A.; Choudhry, H.; Alenezi, S.K.; Barkat, M.A.; Beg, S.; et al. Cationic solid lipid nanoparticles of resveratrol for hepatocellular carcinoma treatment: Systematic optimization, *in vitro* characterization and preclinical investigation. *Int. J. Nanomed.* 2020, 15, 9283–9299.
32. Jagwani, S.; Jalalpure, S.; Dhamecha, D.; Jadhav, K.; Bohara, R. Pharmacokinetic and pharmacodynamic evaluation of resveratrol loaded cationic liposomes for targeting hepatocellular carcinoma. *ACS Biomater. Sci. Eng.* 2020, 6, 4969–4984.
33. McCormack, D.; McFadden, D. Pterostilbene and cancer: Current review. *J. Surg. Res.* 2012, 173, e53–e61.
34. Chen, R.J.; Kuo, H.C.; Cheng, L.H.; Lee, Y.H.; Chang, W.T.; Wang, B.J.; Wang, Y.J.; Cheng, H.C. Apoptotic and nonapoptotic activities of pterostilbene against cancer. *Int. J. Mol. Sci.* 2018, 19, 287.

35. Qian, Y.Y.; Liu, Z.S.; Yan, H.J.; Yuan, Y.F.; Levenson, A.S.; Li, K. Pterostilbene inhibits MTA1/HDAC1 complex leading to PTEN acetylation in hepatocellular carcinoma. *Biomed Pharmacother.* 2018, 101, 852–859.
36. Anand David, A.V.; Arulmoli, R.; Parasuraman, S. Overviews of biological importance of quercetin: A bioactive flavonoid. *Pharmacogn. Rev.* 2016, 10, 84–89.
37. Xu, D.; Hu, M.J.; Wang, Y.Q.; Cui, Y.L. Antioxidant activities of quercetin and its complexes for medicinal application. *Molecules* 2019, 24, 1123.
38. Maurya, A.K.; Vinayak, M. Anticarcinogenic action of quercetin by downregulation of phosphatidylinositol 3-kinase (PI3K) and protein kinase C (PKC) via induction of p53 in hepatocellular carcinoma (HepG2) cell line. *Mol. Biol. Rep.* 2015, 42, 1419–1429.
39. Maurya, A.K.; Vinayak, M. Modulation of PKC signaling and induction of apoptosis through suppression of reactive oxygen species and tumor necrosis factor receptor 1 (TNFR1): Key role of quercetin in cancer prevention. *Tumour Biol.* 2015, 36, 8913–8924.
40. Wu, H.; Pan, L.; Gao, C.; Xu, H.; Li, Y.; Zhang, L.; Ma, L.; Meng, L.; Sun, X.; Qin, H. Quercetin inhibits the proliferation of glycolysis-addicted HCC cells by reducing hexokinase 2 and Akt-mTOR pathway. *Molecules* 2019, 24, 1993.
41. Lincet, H.; Icard, P. How do glycolytic enzymes favour cancer cell proliferation by nonmetabolic functions? *Oncogene* 2015, 34, 3751–3759.
42. Mayer, D.; Klimek, F.; Rempel, A.; Bannasch, P. Hexokinase expression in liver preneoplasia and neoplasia. *Biochem. Soc. Trans.* 1997, 25, 122–127.
43. Delle Monache, S.; Sanità, P.; Trapasso, E.; Ursino, M.R.; Dugo, P.; Russo, M.; Ferlazzo, N.; Calapai, G.; Angelucci, A.; Navarra, M. Mechanisms underlying the anti-tumoral effects of Citrus Bergamia juice. *PLoS One* 2013, 8, e61484.
44. Ferlazzo, N.; Cirmi, S.; Russo, M.; Trapasso, E.; Ursino, M.R.; Lombardo, G.E.; Gangemi, S.; Calapai, G.; Navarra, M. NF-kB mediates the antiproliferative and proapoptotic effects of bergamot juice in HepG2 cells. *Life Sci.* 2016, 146, 81–91.

45. Arai, Y.; Watanabe, S.; Kimira, M.; Shimoi, K.; Mochizuki, R.; Kinae, N. Dietary intakes of flavonols, flavones and isoflavones by Japanese women and the inverse correlation between quercetin intake and plasma LDL cholesterol concentration. *J. Nutr.* 2000, 130, 2243–2250.
46. Sundarraj, K.; Raghunath, A.; Panneerselvam, L.; Perumal, E. Fisetin, a phytopolyphenol, targets apoptotic and necroptotic cell death in HepG2 cells. *Biofactors* 2020, 46, 118–135.
47. Dai, Q.; Yin, Q.; Wei, L.; Zhou, Y.; Qiao, C.; Guo, Y.; Wang, X.; Ma, S.; Lu, N. Oroxylin a regulates glucose metabolism in response to hypoxic stress with the involvement of hypoxia-inducible factor-1 in human hepatoma HepG2 cells. *Mol. Carcinog.* 2016, 55, 1275–1289.
48. Wei, L.; Dai, Y.; Zhou, Y.; He, Z.; Yao, J.; Zhao, L.; Guo, Q.; Yang, L. Oroxylin a activates PKM1/HNF4 alpha to induce hepatoma differentiation and block cancer progression. *Cell Death Dis.* 2017, 8, e2944.
49. Kuo, C.J.; Conley, P.B.; Chen, L.; Sladek, F.M.; Darnell, J.E.; Crabtree, G.R. A transcriptional hierarchy involved in mammalian cell-type specification. *Nature* 1992, 355, 457–461.
50. Saha, S.K.; Parachoniak, C.A.; Ghanta, K.S.; Fitamant, J.; Ross, K.N.; Najem, M.S.; Gurumurthy, S.; Akbay, E.A.; Sia, D.; Cornella, H.; et al. Mutant IDH inhibits HNF-4 to block hepatocyte differentiation and promote biliary cancer. *Nature* 2014, 513, 110–114.
51. Gu, Y.; Zhu, C.F.; Iwamoto, H.; Chen, J.S. Genistein inhibits invasive potential of human hepatocellular carcinoma by altering cell cycle, apoptosis, and angiogenesis. *World J. Gastroenterol.* 2005, 11, 6512–6517.
52. Tong, Y.; Wang, M.; Huang, H.; Zhang, J.; Huang, Y.; Chen, Y.; Pan, H. Inhibitory effects of genistein in combination with gefitinib on the hepatocellular carcinoma Hep3B cell line. *Exp. Ther. Med.* 2019, 18, 3793–3800.
53. Lee, S.R.; Kwon, S.W.; Lee, Y.H.; Kaya, P.; Kim, J.M.; Ahn, C.; Jung, E.M.; Lee, G.S.; An, B.S.; Jeung, E.B.; et al. Dietary intake of genistein suppresses hepatocellular carcinoma through AMPK-mediated apoptosis and anti-inflammation. *BMC Cancer* 2019, 19, 6.

54. Peng, W.; Hu, C.; Shu, Z.; Han, T.; Qin, L.; Zheng, C. Antitumor activity of tatariside F isolated from roots of ***Fagopyrum tataricum*** (L.) Gaertn against H22 hepatocellular carcinoma via up-regulation of p53. *Phytomedicine* 2015, 22, 730–736.
55. Jiang, F.; Mu, J.; Wang, X.; Ye, X.; Si, L.; Ning, S.; Li, Z.; Li, Y. The repressive effect of miR-148a on TGF beta-SMADs signal pathway is involved in the glabridin-induced inhibition of the cancer stem cells-like properties in hepatocellular carcinoma cells. *PLoS One* 2014, 9, e96698.
56. Hsieh, M.J.; Lin, C.W.; Yang, S.F.; Chen, M.K.; Chiou, H.L. Glabridin inhibits migration and invasion by transcriptional inhibition of matrix metalloproteinase 9 through modulation of NF-B and AP-1 activity in human liver cancer cells. *Br. J. Pharmacol.* 2014, 171, 3037–3050.
57. Abd El Maksoud, A.I.; Taher, R.F.; Gaara, A.H.; Abdelrazik, E.; Keshk, O.S.; Elawdan, K.A.; Morsy, S.E.; Salah, A.; Khalil, H. Selective regulation of B-Raf dependent K-Ras/Mitogen-activated protein by natural occurring multi-kinase inhibitors in cancer cells. *Front. Oncol.* 2019, 9, 1220.
58. Liu, H.X.; Xu, M.Q.; Li, S.P.; Tian, S.; Guo, M.X.; Qi, J.Y.; He, C.J.; Zhao, X.S. Jujube leaf green tea extracts inhibits hepatocellular carcinoma cells by activating AMPK. *Oncotarget* 2017, 8, 110566–110575.
59. Mohamed, G.A.; Al-Abd, A.M.; El-Halawany, A.M.; Abdallah, H.M.; Ibrahim, S.R.M. New xanthones and cytotoxic constituents from ***Garcinia mangostana*** fruit hulls against human hepatocellular, breast, and colorectal cancer cell lines. *J. Ethnopharmacol.* 2017, 198, 302–312.
60. Wudtiwai, B.; Pitchakarn, P.; Banjerdpongchai, R. Alpha-mangostin, an active compound in ***Garcinia mangostana***, abrogates anoikis-resistance in human hepatocellular carcinoma cells. *Toxicol. In Vitro* 2018, 53, 222–232.
61. Yang, S.; Zhou, F.; Dong, Y.; Ren, F. Mangostin induces apoptosis in human osteosarcoma cells through ROS-mediated endoplasmic reticulum stress via the WNT Pathway. *Cell Transplant.* 2021, 30, 9636897211035080.
62. Panthong, A.; Norkaew, P.; Kanjanapothi, D.; Taesotikul, T.; Anantachoke, N.; Reutrakul, V. Anti-inflammatory, analgesic and

antipyretic activities of the extract of gamboge from *Garcinia hanburyi* Hook f. *J. Ethnopharmacol.* 2007, 111, 335–340.

63. Guo, Q.L.; You, Q.D.; Wu, Z.Q.; Yuan, S.T.; Zhao, L. General gambogic acids inhibited growth of human hepatoma SMMC-7721 cells *in vitro* and in nude mice. Acta *Pharmacol. Sin.* 2004, 25, 769–774.
64. Duan, D.; Zhang, B.; Yao, J.; Liu, Y.; Sun, J.; Ge, C.; Peng, S.; Fang, J. Gambogic acid induces apoptosis in hepatocellular carcinoma SMMC-7721 cells by targeting cytosolic thioredoxin reductase. *Free Radic. Biol. Med.* 2014, 69, 15–25.
65. Chen, J.; Chen, L.; Lu, T.; Xie, Y.; Li, C.; Jia, Z.; Cao, J. ER 36 is an effective target of epigallocatechin-3-gallate in hepatocellular carcinoma. *Int. J. Clin. Exp. Pathol.* 2019, 12, 3222–3234.
66. Bimonte, S.; Albino, V.; Piccirillo, M.; Nasto, A.; Molino, C.; Palaia, R.; Cascella, M. Epigallocatechin-3-gallate in the prevention and treatment of hepatocellular carcinoma: Experimental findings and translational perspectives. *Drug Des. Devel. Ther.* 2019, 13, 611–621.
67. Zhang, Q.; Tang, X.; Lu, Q.; Zhang, Z.; Rao, J.; Le, A.D. Green tea extract and (-)-epigallocatechin-3-gallate inhibit hypoxia- and serum-induced HIF-1alpha protein accumulation and VEGF expression in human cervical carcinoma and hepatoma cells. *Mol. Cancer Ther.* 2006, 5, 1227–1238.
68. Zhang, Y.; Owusu, L.; Duan, W.; Jiang, T.; Zang, S.; Ahmed, A.; Xin, Y. Anti-metastatic and differential effects on protein expression of epigallocatechin-3-gallate in HCCLM6 hepatocellular carcinoma cells. *Int. J. Mol. Med.* 2013, 32, 959–964.
69. Chen, L.; Ye, H.L.; Zhang, G.; Yao, W.M.; Chen, X.Z.; Zhang, F.C.; Liang, G. Autophagy inhibition contributes to the synergistic interaction between EGCG and doxorubicin to kill the hepatoma Hep3B cells. *PLoS One* 2014, 9, e85771.
70. Sojoodi, M.; Wei, L.; Erstad, D.J.; Yamada, S.; Fujii, T.; Hirschfield, H.; Kim, R.S.; Lauwers, G.Y.; Lanuti, M.; Hoshida, Y.; et al. Epigallocatechin gallate induces hepatic stellate cell senescence and attenuates development of hepatocellular carcinoma. *Cancer Prev. Res.* 2020, 13, 497–508.
71. Tang, Y.; Cao, J.; Cai, Z.; An, H.; Li, Y.; Peng, Y.; Chen, N.; Luo, A.; Tao, H.; Li, K. Epigallocatechin gallate induces chemopreventive

effects on rats with diethylnitrosamine-induced liver cancer via inhibition of cell division cycle 25A. *Mol. Med. Rep.* 2020, 22, 3873–3885.

72. Liao, S.; Lin, J.; Liu, J.; Chen, T.; Xu, M.; Zheng, J. Chemoprevention of elite tea variety CFT-1 rich in EGCG against chemically induced liver cancer in rats. *Food Sci. Nutr.* 2019, 7, 2647–2665.
73. Agioutantis, P.C.; Kotsikoris, V.; Kolisis, F.N.; Loutrari, H. RNA-seq data analysis of stimulated hepatocellular carcinoma cells treated with epigallocatechin gallate and fisetin reveals target genes and action mechanisms. *Comput. Struct. Biotechnol. J.* 2020, 18, 686–695.
74. Kang, Q.; Tong, Y.; Gowd, V.; Wang, M.; Chen, F.; Cheng, K.W. Oral administration of EGCG solution equivalent to daily achievable dosages of regular tea drinkers effectively suppresses miR483-3p induced metastasis of hepatocellular carcinoma cells in mice. *Food Funct.* 2021, 12, 3381–3392.
75. Yang, H.; Wang, M.; Sun, H.; Zhu, S.; Jin, J. Synergetic effect of EP1 receptor antagonist and (-)-epigallocatechin-3-gallate in hepatocellular carcinoma. *Pharmacology* 2019, 104, 267–275.
76. Hu, Z.; Yang, A.; Su, G.; Zhao, Y.; Wang, Y.; Chai, X.; Tu, P. Huaier restrains proliferative and invasive potential of human hepatoma SK-HEP-1 cells partially through decreased lamin B1 and elevated NOV. *Sci. Rep.* 2016, 6, 31298.
77. Shan, L.; Li, Y.; Jiang, H.; Tao, Y.; Qian, Z.; Li, L.; Cai, F.; Ma, L.; Yu, Y. Huaier restrains proliferative and migratory potential of hepatocellular carcinoma cells partially through decreased yes-associated protein 1. *J. Cancer* 2017, 8, 4087–4097.
78. Chen, Q.; Shu, C.; Laurence, A.D.; Chen, Y.; Peng, B.G.; Zhen, Z.J.; Cai, J.Q.; Ding, Y.T.; Li, L.Q.; Zhang, Y.B.; et al. Effect of Huaier granule on recurrence after curative resection of HCC: A multicentre, randomised clinical trial. *Gut* 2018, 67, 2006–2016.
79. Pham, H.H.; Seong, Y.A.; Oh, C.W.; Kim, G.D. The herbal medicine *Cyperus amuricus* inhibits proliferation of human hepatocellular carcinoma Hep3B cells by inducing apoptosis and arrest at the G0/G1 cell cycle phase. *Int. J. Oncol.* 2016, 49, 2046–2054.
80. Munakarmi, S.; Chand, L.; Shin, H.B.; Hussein, U.K.; Yun, B.S.; Park, H.R.; Jeong, Y.J. Anticancer effects of Poncirus fructus on hepatocellular

carcinoma through regulation of apoptosis, migration, and invasion. *Oncol. Rep.* 2020, 44, 2537–2546.

81. Lee, R.T.; Yang, P.; Alahmadi, A.; McQuade, J.; Yuan, E.; Difeo, A.; Narla, G.; Kaseb, A. Mistletoe extract viscum fraxini-2 for treatment of advanced hepatocellular carcinoma: A case series. *Case Rep. Oncol.* 2021, 14, 224–231.
82. Galle, P.R.; Foerster, F.; Kudo, M.; Chan, S.L.; Llovet, J.M.; Qin, S.; Schelman, W.R.; Chintharlapalli, S.; Abada, P.B.; Sherman, M.; et al. Biology and significance of alpha-fetoprotein in hepatocellular carcinoma. *Liver Int.* 2019, 39, 2214–2229.
83. Setiawan, V.W.; Wilkens, L.R.; Lu, S.C.; Hernandez, B.Y.; Le Marchand, L.; Henderson, B.E. Association of coffee intake with reduced incidence of liver cancer and death from chronic liver disease in the US multiethnic cohort. *Gastroenterology* 2015, 148, 118–125.
84. Cavin, C.; Marin-Kuan, M.; Langouët, S.; Bezençon, C.; Guignard, G.; Verguet, C.; Piguet, D.; Holzhäuser, D.; Cornaz, R.; Schilter, B. Induction of Nrf2-mediated cellular defenses and alteration of phase I activities as mechanisms of chemoprotective effects of coffee in the liver. *Food Chem. Toxicol.* 2008, 46, 1239–1248.
85. Yoon, J.S.; Kim, H.M.; Yadunandam, A.K.; Kim, N.H.; Jung, H.A.; Choi, J.S.; Kim, C.Y.; Kim, G.D. Neferine isolated from *Nelumbo nucifera* enhances anti-cancer activities in Hep3B cells: Molecular mechanisms of cell cycle arrest, ER stress induced apoptosis and anti-angiogenic response. *Phytomedicine* 2013, 20, 1013–1022.
86. Li, M.; Zhang, M.; Zhang, Z.L.; Liu, N.; Han, X.Y.; Liu, Q.C.; Deng, W.J.; Liao, C.X. Induction of apoptosis by berberine in hepatocellular carcinoma HepG2 cells via downregulation of NF-κB. *Oncol. Res.* 2017, 25, 233–239.
87. Leung, W.T.; Lau, W.Y.; Ho, S.; Chan, M.; Leung, N.; Lin, J.; Ho, K.C.; Metreweli, C.; Johnson, P.J.; Li, A.K. Selective internal radiation therapy with intra-arterial iodine-131-lipiodol in inoperable hepatocellular carcinoma. *J. Nucl. Med.* 1994, 35, 1313–1318.
88. Lau, W.Y.; Lai, E.C.; Leung, T.W.; Yu, S.C. Adjuvant intra-arterial iodine-131-labeled lipiodol for resectable hepatocellular carcinoma: A prospective randomized trial-update on 5-year and 10-year survival. *Ann. Surg.* 2008, 247, 43–48.

89. Lintia-Gaultier, A.; Perret, C.; Ansquer, C.; Eugène, T.; Kraeber-Bodéré, F.; Frampas, E. Intra-arterial injection of 131I-labeled lipiodol for advanced hepatocellular carcinoma: A 7 years' experience. *Nucl. Med. Commun.* 2013, 34, 674–681.
90. Zhou, B.; Shan, H.; Zhu, K.S.; Jiang, Z.B.; Guan, S.H.; Meng, X.C.; Zeng, X.C. Chemoembolization with lobaplatin mixed with iodized oil for unresectable recurrent hepatocellular carcinoma after orthotopic liver transplantation. *J. Vasc. Interv. Radiol.* 2010, 21, 333–338.
91. Mani, J.S.; Johnson, J.B.; Hosking, H.; Ashwath, N.; Walsh, K.B.; Neilsen, P.M.; Broszczak, D.A.; Naiker, M. Antioxidative and therapeutic potential of selected Australian plants: A review. *J. Ethnopharmacol.* 2021, 268, 113580.
92. Arnesen, J.A.; Kildegaard, K.R.; Cernuda Pastor, M.; Jayachandran, S.; Kristensen, M.; Borodina, I. Strains engineered for the production of terpenoids. *Front. Bioeng. Biotechnol.* 2020, 8, 945.
93. Jiang, M.; Wu, Z.; Guo, H.; Liu, L.; Chen, S. A review of terpenes from marine-derived fungi: 2015–2019. *Mar. Drugs* 2020, 18, 321.
94. Hillier, S.G.; Lathe, R. Terpenes, hormones and life: Isoprene rule revisited. *J. Endocrinol.* 2019, 242, R9–R22.
95. Firn, R.D.; Jones, C.G. Natural products–a simple model to explain chemical diversity. *Nat. Prod. Rep.* 2003, 20, 382–391.
96. Thoppil, R.J.; Bishayee, A. Terpenoids as potential chemopreventive and therapeutic agents in liver cancer. *World J. Hepatol.* 2011, 3, 228–249.
97. Dasgupta, A.; Acharya, K. Mushrooms: An emerging resource for therapeutic terpenoids. *3 Biotech* 2019, 9, 369.
98. Dasgupta, A.; Dey, D.; Ghosh, D.; Lai, T.K.; Bhuvanesh, N.; Dolui, S.; Velayutham, R.; Acharya, K. Astrakurkurone, a sesquiterpenoid from wild edible mushroom, targets liver cancer cells by modulating Bcl-2 family proteins. *IUBMB Life* 2019, 71, 992–910.
99. Kim, D.K.; Baek, J.H.; Kang, C.M.; Yoo, M.A.; Sung, J.W.; Chung, H.Y.; Kim, N.D.; Choi, Y.H.; Lee, S.H.; Kim, K.W. Apoptotic activity of ursolic acid may correlate with the inhibition of initiation of DNA replication. *Int. J. Cancer* 2000, 87, 629–636.

100. Yang, Y.; Qiu, S.; Qian, L.; Tian, Y.; Chen, Y.; Bi, L.; Chen, W. OCF can repress tumor metastasis by inhibiting epithelial-mesenchymal transition involved in PTEN/PI3K/AKT pathway in lung cancer cells. *PLoS One* 2017, 12, e0174021.
101. Yang, L.; Zhang, X.Y.; Li, K.; Li, A.P.; Yang, W.D.; Yang, R.; Wang, P.; Zhao, Z.H.; Cui, F.; Qin, Y.; et al. Protopanaxadiol inhibits epithelial-mesenchymal transition of hepatocellular carcinoma by targeting STAT3 pathway. *Cell Death Dis.* 2019, 10, 630.
102. Durmaz, I.; Guven, E.B.; Ersahin, T.; Ozturk, M.; Calis, I.; Cetin-Atalay, R. Liver cancer cells are sensitive to lanatoside C induced cell death independent of their PTEN status. *Phytomedicine* 2016, 23, 42–51.
103. Liao, W.; Fan, L.; Zheng, Z.; Liu, H.; Deng, H.; Li, M.; Liu, F.; Yang, A. Ziyuglycoside II exerts antiproliferative and antimetastasis effects on hepatocellular carcinoma cells. *Anticancer Drugs* 2020, 31, 819–827.
104. Jung, K.H.; Rumman, M.; Yan, H.; Cheon, M.J.; Choi, J.G.; Jin, X.; Park, S.; Oh, M.S.; Hong, S.S. An ethyl acetate fraction of *Artemisia capillaris* (ACE-63) induced apoptosis and anti-angiogenesis via inhibition of PI3K/AKT signaling in hepatocellular carcinoma. *Phytother. Res.* 2018, 32, 2034–2046.
105. Weifeng, T.; Feng, S.; Xiangji, L.; Changqing, S.; Zhiquan, Q.; Huazhong, Z.; Peining, Y.; Yong, Y.; Mengchao, W.; Xiaoqing, J.; et al. Artemisinin inhibits *in vitro* and *in vivo* invasion and metastasis of human hepatocellular carcinoma cells. *Phytomedicine* 2011, 18, 158–162.
106. Lou, L.; Ye, W.; Chen, Y.; Wu, S.; Jin, L.; He, J.; Tao, X.; Zhu, J.; Chen, X.; Deng, A.; et al. Ardipusilloside inhibits survival, invasion and metastasis of human hepatocellular carcinoma cells. *Phytomedicine* 2012, 19, 603–608.
107. Chen, L.I.; Guo, Y.; Alsaif, G.; Gao, Y. Total flavonoids isolated from *Diospyros kaki* L. f. leaves induced apoptosis and oxidative stress in human cancer cells. *Anticancer Res.* 2020, 40, 5201–5210.
108. Chen, H.M.; Lai, Z.Q.; Liao, H.J.; Xie, J.H.; Xian, Y.F.; Chen, Y.L.; Ip, S.P.; Lin, Z.X.; Su, Z.R. Synergistic antitumor effect of brusatol combined with cisplatin on colorectal cancer cells. *Int. J. Mol. Med.* 2018, 41, 1447–1454.

109. Wang, T.; Dou, Y.; Lin, G.; Li, Q.; Nie, J.; Chen, B.; Xie, J.; Su, Z.; Zeng, H.; Chen, J.; et al. The anti-hepatocellular carcinoma effect of *Brucea javanica* oil in ascitic tumor-bearing mice: The detection of brusatol and its role. *Biomed Pharm.* 2021, 134, 111122.
110. https://www.clinicaltrials.gov/study/NCT03356236?cond=Hepatocellular%20Carcinoma&intr=Huaier&aggFilters=status:rec%20act&rank=1&page=1&limit=10.
111. https://www.clinicaltrials.gov/study/NCT02261844?cond=Hepatocellular%20Carcinoma&intr=Resveratrol&aggFilters=status:rec%20act%20wit%20enr%20sus&rank=1&limit=10.
112. https://www.clinicaltrials.gov/study/NCT03727633?cond=Hepatocellular%20Carcinoma&intr=Lipiodol&aggFilters=status:rec%20act%20wit%20enr%20sus&rank=2&limit=10.
113. https://www.clinicaltrials.gov/study/NCT05435014?cond=Hepatocellular%20Carcinoma&intr=Lipiodol&aggFilters=status:rec%20act%20wit%20enr%20sus&rank=3&limit=10.
114. https://www.clinicaltrials.gov/study/NCT05280444?cond=Hepatocellular%20Carcinoma&intr=Lipiodol&aggFilters=status:rec%20act%20wit%20enr%20sus&rank=5&limit=10.
115. Mabed, M.; El-Helw, L.; Shamaa, S. Phase II study of viscum fraxini-2 in patients with advanced hepatocellular carcinoma. *Br. J. Cancer* 2004, 90, 65–69.
116. Fan, Y.; Li, S.; Ding, X.; Yue, J.; Jiang, J.; Zhao, H.; Hao, R.; Qiu, W.; Liu, K.; Li, Y.; et al. First-in-class immune-modulating small molecule Icaritin in advanced hepatocellular carcinoma: Preliminary results of safety, durable survival and immune biomarkers. *BMC Cancer* 2019, 19, 279.
117. O'Reilly, E.M.; Stuart, K.E.; Sanz-Altamira, P.M.; Schwartz, G.K.; Steger, C.M.; Raeburn, L.; Kemeny, N.E.; Kelsen, D.P.; Saltz, L.B. A phase II study of irinotecan in patients with advanced hepatocellular carcinoma. *Cancer* 2001, 91, 101–105.
118. Brandi, G.; Biasco, G.; Mirarchi, M.G.; Golfieri, R.; Di Paolo, A.; Borghi, A.; Fanello, S.; Derenzini, E.; Agostini, V.; Giampalma, E.; et al. A phase I study of continuous hepatic arterial infusion of irinotecan in patients with locally advanced hepatocellular carcinoma. *Dig. Liver Dis.* 2011, 43, 1015–1021.

119. Tsang, C.M.; Cheung, K.C.; Cheung, Y.C.; Man, K.; Lui, V.W.; Tsao, S.W.; Feng, Y. Berberine suppresses Id-1 expression and inhibits the growth and development of lung metastases in hepatocellular carcinoma. *Biochim. Biophys. Acta* 2015, 1852(3), 541–551. doi: 10.1016/j.bbadis.2014.12.004.

https://doi.org/10.1142/9789811293320_0015

Chapter 15

The Emerging Role of Phytochemicals in Nanotechnology for Targeting Liver Cancer

Deiviga Murugan[1], Sweata Hanson[1], Jinsha P V[1], Raja Biswas[2], Bipin G Nair[1], Sankarprasad Bhuniya[3], and Nandita Mishra[1,*]

[1]*School of Biotechnology, Amrita Vishwa Vidyapeetham, Kollam, Kerala, India*

[2]*Amrita School of Nanosciences and Molecular Medicine, Amrita Vishwa Vidyapeetham, Kochi, Kerala, India*

[3]*Centre for Interdisciplinary Sciences, JIS Institute of Advanced Studies and Research, Kolkata, India*

Table of Contents:

*Corresponding author: E-mail: nanditamishra@am.amrita.edu

Abbreviations:

PLCs — Primary liver cancers
NNI — National Nanotechnology Initiative
CDs — Carbon-based quantum dots
NP — Nanoparticle
DDS — Drug delivery system
HCC — Hepatocellular carcinoma
CCA — Cholangiocarcinoma
ICC — Intrahepatic cholangiocarcinoma
HBV — Hepatitis B virus
HCV — Hepatitis C virus
VEGFR — Vascular endothelial growth factor receptor
PDGFR — Platelet-derived growth factor
FGFR — Fibroblast growth factor receptor
SPR — Surface plasmon resonance
PEG — Polyethylene glycol
PLGA — Poly (lactic-co-glycolic acid)
PLA — Polylactic acid
TRAF — Tumor necrosis factor receptor–associated factor
CDKs — Cyclin-dependent kinases
TNF — Tumor necrosis factor
EGF — Epidermal growth factor
FGF — Fibroblast growth factor
PKA — Protein kinase A
PKC — Protein kinase C
MAPK — Mitogen-activated protein kinase
TYK2 — Tyrosine-kinase 2

Ap-1 — Activator protein 1
NF-κB — Nuclear factor kappa B
Nrf2 — Nuclear factor erythroid 2–related factor 2
ICAM-1 — Intercellular adhesion molecule-1
VCAM-1 — Vascular cell adhesion molecule-1
ASGPR — Asialoglycoprotein receptor
GPC-3 — Glypican-3
TfR — Transferrin receptor
FR — Folic acid receptor
SR-B1 — Scavenger receptor class B type I
CSCs — Cancer stem cells
LCSCs — Liver cancer stem cells

Abstract

The treatment of liver cancer is a pressing issue owing to the limited accessibility of chemotherapy drugs and the pronounced resistance to anticancer medications. Lately, phytochemicals have garnered significant attention for their potential in cancer treatment because of their minimal toxicity and ability to target a broad spectrum of cancer pathways with anticancer properties. Still, phytochemicals have been restricted by low water solubility, poor bioavailability, poor cell penetration, hepatic disposition, a narrow therapeutic index, and quick absorption by normal tissues. Therefore, there is ongoing research into nanoparticle-based delivery systems to enhance the therapeutic effectiveness of these phytochemicals. Nanobiotechnology employs nanoparticles for the safe and efficient administration of drugs based on the tumor's unique characteristics. Further, it provides a novel approach for accurately diagnosing and treating liver cancer by adapting them to each patient's unique physiology and pathology at both genetic and proteomic levels. Nanoparticles of gold, silver, platinum, metal oxides, calcium, and selenium, along with various inorganic nanoparticles such as carbon-based nanoparticles encompassing polymeric, polysaccharide, and lipid nanoparticles, as well as carbon dots, have seen widespread application as nano-vehicles (drug delivery system [DDS]) for administering phytochemicals in the treatment of liver cancer. Many phytochemicals such as resveratrol, hesperetin, kaempferol, and EGCG conjugated to FDA-approved gold nanoparticles exert higher anti-HCC effects than the free compounds. Despite the successful application of nanobiotechnology in cancer research, the clinical translation of such approaches continues to pose a challenge due to the limited understanding of the interactions between nanomedicine/nanomaterials and biology, along with their toxicological and immunological aspects, and large-scale manufacturing of nanoparticles, which offers a future research opportunity.

1. Introduction

Hepatocellular carcinoma (HCC), the prevailing type of primary liver cancer (PLC), is an aggressive tumor commonly associated with chronic liver ailments, infections such as hepatitis B or hepatitis C, and the presence of alcoholic or non-alcoholic fatty liver disease. With an estimated 906,000 cases and 830,000 deaths in 2020, it is the sixth most common malignancy and the third leading cause of cancer mortality globally. In most locations, males have incidence and death rates two to three times greater than female (GLOBOCAN) [1].

Due to restricted therapeutic choices, the outcome frequently results in disease recurrence. Chemotherapy, involving the direct infusion of medication into the hepatic artery to minimize systemic side effects, often falls short of achieving the intended treatment outcome, as the healthy liver cells typically metabolize most of the administered dosage, leading to a decrease in the effective dose reaching the tumor cells. Despite the dose reduction in chemotherapy, the undesirable side effects persist, including hair loss, nausea, and fatigue.

In recent times, targeted therapy, which involves the inhibition of specific kinases aiding tumor growth or promoting their blood circulation, has displayed encouraging potential. Sorafenib and lenvatinib are two targeted medications that have recently been approved for the treatment of liver cancer. Immunotherapy has also emerged as a possible treatment option for liver cancer. This procedure entails targeting a protein (e.g., atezolizumab targets programmed cell death protein 1) on T cells or the equivalent binder on cancer cells to prevent the malignancy from evading immune response. In contrast to conventional chemotherapy and radiation treatments, targeted and immune therapies demonstrate superior therapeutic efficacy, although their long-term impact is limited. These therapies might even elicit undesirable autoimmune responses [2].

Phytochemicals are secondary metabolites derived from several plants [3]. Several phytochemicals, such as quercetin, epigallocatechin-3-gallate, and resveratrol, among others, have been extensively explored for their anticancer properties. While it has been shown that herbal remedies can mitigate the toxicity and drug resistance linked to conventional medicines, investigating their pharmacokinetic characteristics has presented difficulties [4].

To address this issue, many researchers have begun to explore the realm of nanotechnology. Nanotechnology, which involves the use of materials at the nano-scale (typically less than 100 nm) for various applications, has excellent potential to provide novel therapeutic strategies in cancer treatment [5–7]. In addition to serving as an optimal therapeutic choice for cancer, these nanoparticles (NPs) have also been investigated for their role in cancer diagnosis, known as cancer theranostics. For instance, magnetic nanoparticles have been utilized both as a diagnostic tool in MRI and as a nanocarrier system for drug delivery [8]. Although diverse forms of inorganic nanoparticles have had historical applications, primarily in the realm of art, a concerted scientific push for this technology did not materialize until the recent past. Within this fast-growing field, several shapes such as sheets, spheres and tubes, and a wide range of materials such as precious metals, metal oxides, various inorganic salts, and silica are being employed at a definite size of 1–100 nm as defined by the U.S. National Nanotechnology Initiative (NNI). Carbon-based nanoparticles, including liposomes, nanotubes, graphene derivatives, lipid nanoparticles, micelles, and carbon-based quantum dots (CDs), have been developed in various biomedical applications owing to their unique structural and mechanical properties [9]. Specialized nanoparticles are also in continual development, such as up-conversion NPs, metal-organic frameworks (MOFs), and Janus NP (NP in which the surface has distinct regions with differing physical properties). Nanomedicine has just recently emerged as a potential topic of nanotechnology in the twenty-first century. This rise has been particularly evident in the field of medicine where conventional approaches are less than optimal, such as cancer therapy, or where illness is outpacing therapies, as is the situation with antibiotic-resistant bacteria. Most NP types can serve as carriers in a drug delivery system (DDS), and some NPs have built-in therapeutic benefits. These characteristics have sparked a boom in research on using NPs as a DDS for cancer treatment. DDSs are being continuously explored these years due to the increase in the use of nanotechnology for therapeutics. The designing of these systems can be exclusive based on the targets or diseases. These systems have exhibited considerable advantages in the context of liver cancer by reducing adverse effects and potentially facilitating targeted treatment of the affected region [10].

Nanotechnology-based techniques can be used by precisely targeting and delivering the molecules to the tumor, keeping a constant concentration throughout their range of action, and overcoming the drawbacks of plant-based treatments. Even with the ever-expanding therapeutic strategies in liver cancer, especially concerning nanomedicine, understanding tumor biology and its application in nanotechnology becomes imperative.

2. Liver Cancer and Its Therapeutic Challenges

PLCs predominantly consist of HCC, intrahepatic cholangiocarcinoma (ICC), and combined hepatocellular-cholangiocarcinoma (cHCC-ICC), with hepatic angiosarcoma, hepatic hemangiosarcoma and hepatoblastoma as minor subtypes (Figure 1) [11]. HCC, the most common type of PLC, arises from the hepatocytes and its development is mainly attributed to chronic liver injury and inflammation, with the main contributing factor being hepatitis B (HBV) and hepatitis C (HCV) viral infection. Etiological factors of HCC are not limited to HBV and HCV infection but also include other factors such as food contaminants such as aflatoxins, alcohol consumption,

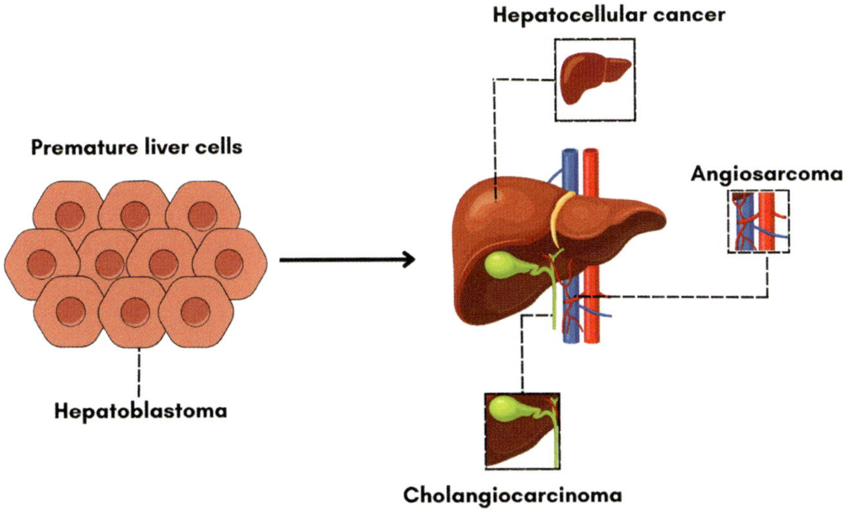

Figure 1: Different types of liver cancer based on the anatomical origin. The figure was generated using Canva (www.canva.com)

tobacco smoking, fatty liver, obesity, and diabetes [12]. Intrahepatic cholangiocarcinoma (ICC), the second most common form of liver cancer, originates from the biliary tract epithelium. The risk factors for ICC include biliary tract diseases, such as cholelithiasis, choledocholithiasis, congenital anomalies, such as choledochal cysts, infections such as liver flukes or viral hepatitis, metabolic disorders, tobacco and alcohol consumption [13]. The third type, cHCC-ICC, presents with complex pathologies as they comprise both hepatocytic and cholangiocytic differentiation. Appearance and clinical presentations may change based on the tumor's proportion of both components, which also affects how they appear. For instance, the tumor exhibits more imaging and clinical characteristics of HCC if the hepatocytic component Is more prominent and presents as ICC if the cholangiocytic components are dominant [14].

Other rare types of liver cancer include hepatic angiosarcoma or hemangiosarcoma (cancer that arises from the endothelial cells lining the blood vessels of the liver) and hepatoblastoma (cancers that originate from the liver precursor cells) [11].

The conventional chemotherapeutic strategies for HCC are limited owing to its lower response and survival rates with higher relapse rates. The first-line medication the FDA recognizes for treating HCC is sorafenib [15]. This drug is a potent multi-kinase inhibitor with significant anticancer and anti-angiogenic properties. By 2019, the FDA had approved several additional medications as first- and second-line therapies such as lenvatinib (targeting vascular endothelial growth factor receptor (VEGFR1-3), platelet-derived growth factor (PDGFRα), fibroblast growth factor receptor (FGFR), and the KIT and RET tyrosine kinases), regorafenib (targeting VEGFR1-3, PDGFR-β, FGFR, and oncogenic receptor tyrosine kinases (KIT, RET, and RAF)), cabozantinib (targeting vascular endothelial growth factor receptors (VEGFR1-3), the TAM kinase family (TYRO3, AXL and MER), KIT, RET, FLT3, and MET receptor tyrosine kinases), and ramucirumab (targeting VEGFR2 pathway) [16]. Considerations for immunotherapy treatments for HCC include the use of the antibodies pembrolizumab and nivolumab [17]. Early-stage HCCs have a reasonable recurrence rate and can be managed with a few carefully chosen resections performed either conventionally or laparoscopically [18]. The use of combination medications such as gemcitabine and cisplatin, a platinum-based medicine, is typically the first line of therapy for ICC. The survival and prognosis rates for ICC are frequently low because of the lack of effective therapies, and clinical studies are currently being conducted for further combinations of medications, such as gemcitabine and oxaliplatin [19]. In cHCC-ICC, chemotherapeutic combinations along with surgery-based treatments are yet to be fully explored [20].

Such therapeutic restrictions for liver cancer are potentially due to the convoluted portal circulation and tumor heterogeneity. In HCC, the maximum blood supply to the liver tissues is received by the hepatic artery as opposed to the normal liver tissues, which receive upto 80% of their blood supply from the portal vein. This alteration affects the delivery of the drugs to the tumor site via systemic circulation [21]. Thus, a more targeted approach to drug delivery becomes essential. Apart from the circulation, a heterogeneous cell population within the tumor microenvironment due to several genetic and epigenetic influences causes the tumor to be drug-resistant. Appropriate diagnosis, administration of combinatorial therapies and a more focused drug delivery strategy, such as nanoparticles, may help combat such limitations in treating liver cancer [22].

3. Nanoparticles in Liver Cancer

In the treatment of liver cancer, nanoparticle-mediated DDSs aim to administer drugs at potent concentrations, circumventing harsh biological conditions like the acidic pH of the stomach, ensuring optimal effectiveness, precise drug release at the specific site, and facilitating the simultaneous delivery of multiple drugs [23, 24]. Nanoparticles with various physicochemical and biological characteristics have been continually explored for their drug or gene delivery applications. Several factors, such as the biocompatibility of the nanoparticles, mechanism and the site of action, the interaction of the nanoparticles with the target cells and their receptors, the delivery of the drug to the desired site, and the drug retention are to be considered carefully before selecting suitable nanoparticles [25].

3.1. *Types of nanoparticles used in liver cancer*

3.1.1. *Inorganic nanoparticles*

Inorganic nanoparticles mainly comprise metallic and ceramic materials for drug delivery applications. Because of their unique optical characteristics, such as surface plasmon resonance (SPR), which allows them to regulate the optical field, metallic nanoparticles are of tremendous interest in biological applications. The substantial surface area, variable hole size, high pore volume, and surface modulation of the metallic nanoparticles make them appropriate for DDSs [26]. Ceramic nanoparticles, consisting of carbonates, phosphates, oxides of metals and metalloids such as calcium and titanium, respectively, are also used in biomedical applications, owing to their higher stability and loading capacity [27].

3.1.2. *Organic nanoparticles*

This category of nanoparticles is derived from organic compounds such as carbohydrates, proteins, and lipids. Liposomes (spherical vesicles with aqueous core enclosed by phospholipid layers [28]), dendrimers (macromolecules with symmetric branching units around a polymer core [29]), micelles (spherical amphiphilic molecules that can deliver hydrophobic drugs [30]), and protein complexes are the commonly used nanoparticles in this class. In contrast to metallic nanoparticles, these organic substances are non-harmful and resistant to degradation. Owing to their unstable structure formed through non-covalent intermolecular interactions, they can be easily excreted from the body [31]. A separate class of organic nanoparticles, solely made from carbon atoms, is used in a wide range of drug delivery due to their unique electrical conductivity, electron affinity, high strength, optical, thermal, and adsorption/absorption properties. These carbon-based nanoparticles mainly include the fullerenes C_{60} carbon allotropes [32], carbon black nanoparticles, and carbon quantum dots (relatively smaller nanoparticles, about 1–10 nm, with tunable emission properties) [33].

The types of nanoparticles are represented schematically in Figure 2.

3.2. *Nanoparticles as drug delivery systems in liver cancer*

Though nanoparticles may possess inherent therapeutic properties, they mainly act as vehicles of drugs, known as DDS. A typical DDS comprises a carrier, a target ligand, and a therapeutic component [34]. The ligand helps in the drug delivery to the desired specific target, which could either be active or passive targeting (Figure 3). Active targeting entails delivering the medication component directly to the target region. For example, folic acid has been commonly employed as a cancer cell target in several tumors since many malignancies, including breast, colorectal, and liver, have been shown to overexpress folic acid receptors in their cell membrane. Passive targeting refers to

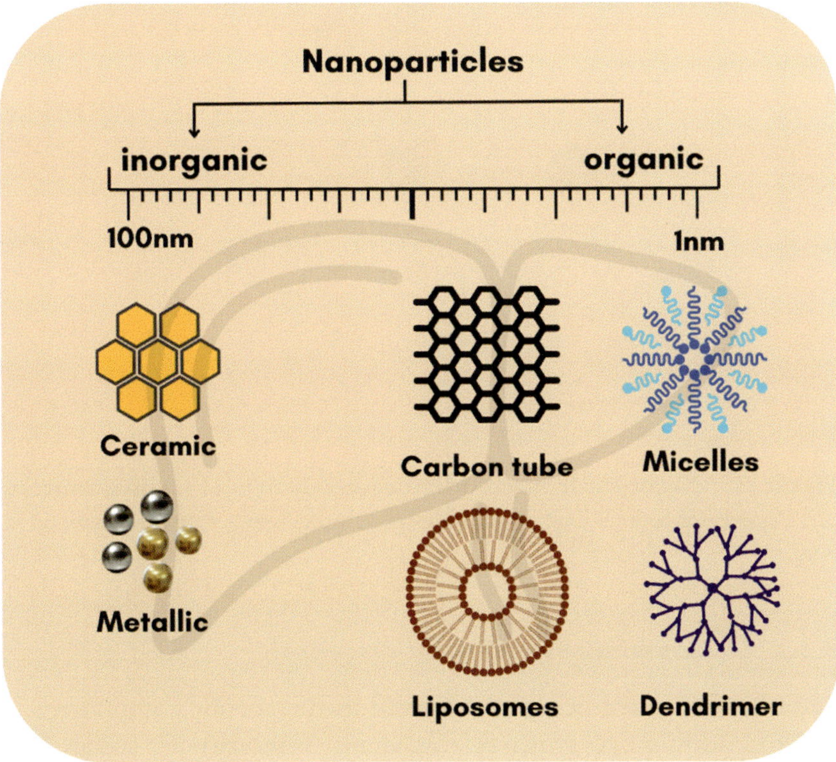

Figure 2: Classification of nanoparticles based on their composition. The figure was generated using Canva (www.canva.com)

medication delivery through the bloodstream to distant areas. Occasionally, a method employed involves applying a polyethylene glycol (PEG) coating to reduce the likelihood of the DDS being identified as a foreign substance by the body's immune system [35].

Several pharmacological components are exploited as therapeutic species in nanoparticle-based liver cancer delivery. Doxorubicin, docetaxel, sorafenib, paclitaxel, 5-fluorouracil, and gemcitabine have all been encapsulated into nanoparticles. In preclinical models of HCC, this method was demonstrated to improve retention time within tumor cells and significantly suppress tumor development [36].

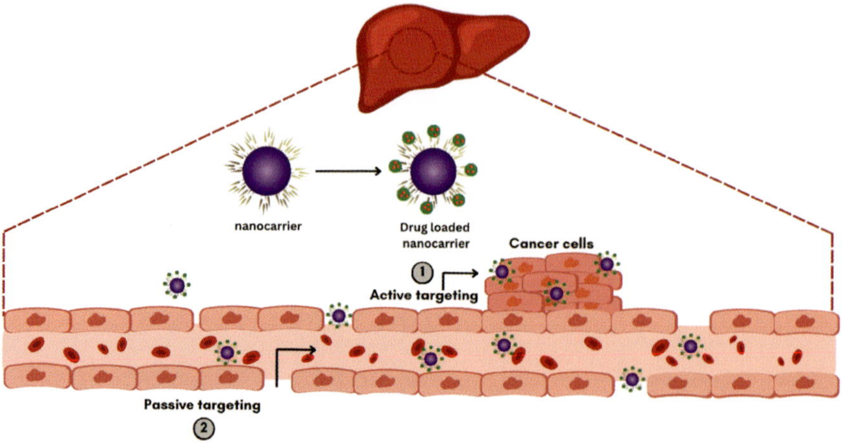

Figure 3: Nanoparticle-based drug delivery system. (1) Active targeting (2) Passive targeting. The figure was generated using Canva (www.canva.com)

3.2.1. *Phytochemicals as therapeutic components*

Plant bioactives are being investigated as therapeutic components in DDS in addition to synthetic medicines. Nanoparticles-based drug delivery may be able to overcome the limitations of phytochemicals by improving solubility, increasing bioavailability, targeting tumor cells or tissues but not healthy cells, improving cellular uptake, lowering doses, and achieving steady-state therapeutic concentrations of phytochemicals over an extended period [37]. Multi-drug resistance is another major constraint in phytochemical-based cancer therapy, owing to the restricted blood flow to deep regions of the tumor, which might impair drug delivery. Nanoparticle-based drug delivery can help bypass this obstacle by targeted delivery of the drug molecules to the tumor site [38]. Apart from being less toxic *in vivo*, these plant-mediated NP syntheses have also proven to be ecologically favorable owing to their fast, renewable method with low-cost consumption and low-hazard yields compared to conventional methods.

4. Phytochemicals in Liver Cancer

It is well studied that the plant bioactives exert their anticancer effects through several mechanisms including apoptosis induction, regulation of oncogenes and tumor-suppressor genes, cell proliferation inhibition, interference in cell signaling pathways, anti-angiogenic action, and anti-metastatic action [39]. An understanding of how the phytochemicals elicit their anticancer effects introduces diverse targets which include pro-apoptotic proteins (caspases and Bax), anti-apoptotic proteins (Bcl-2, TRAF1, and survivin), cell cycle proteins (cyclin D, CDK1, CDK2, p27, and p21), growth factors (TNF, EGF, FGF, and PDGF), protein kinases (PKA, PKC, MAPK, and TYK2), transcription factors (Ap1, NF-κB, Nrf2, and p53), and cell adhesion molecules (ICAM-1 and VCAM-1).

4.1. *Hepatocellular carcinoma*

Several studies have reported the anticancer effects of several plant metabolites in HCC. Numerous phytochemicals are now undergoing clinical trials to treat HCC, suggesting a potential clinical therapeutic agent in the future. Several classes of plant metabolites are known to have anticancer potency against HCC (Figure 4).

4.1.1. *Terpenoids*

Terpenoids (cyclic structures containing oxygen) are simple lipids derived from isoprene. Previous studies demonstrate several terpenoid-rich sources against HCC. Astrakurkurone, a terpene from mushroom *Astraeus hygrometricus*, has been shown to possess anticancer activity against liver cancer cell lines HepG2 and Hep3B [40]. A triterpene from *Ardisia pusilla* was also studied for its anticancer properties against HepG2 and SMMC-7721 cell lines. The compound exerted its anticancer effects by the suppression of MEK/ERK and Akt signaling pathways and activation of Rac1 [41].

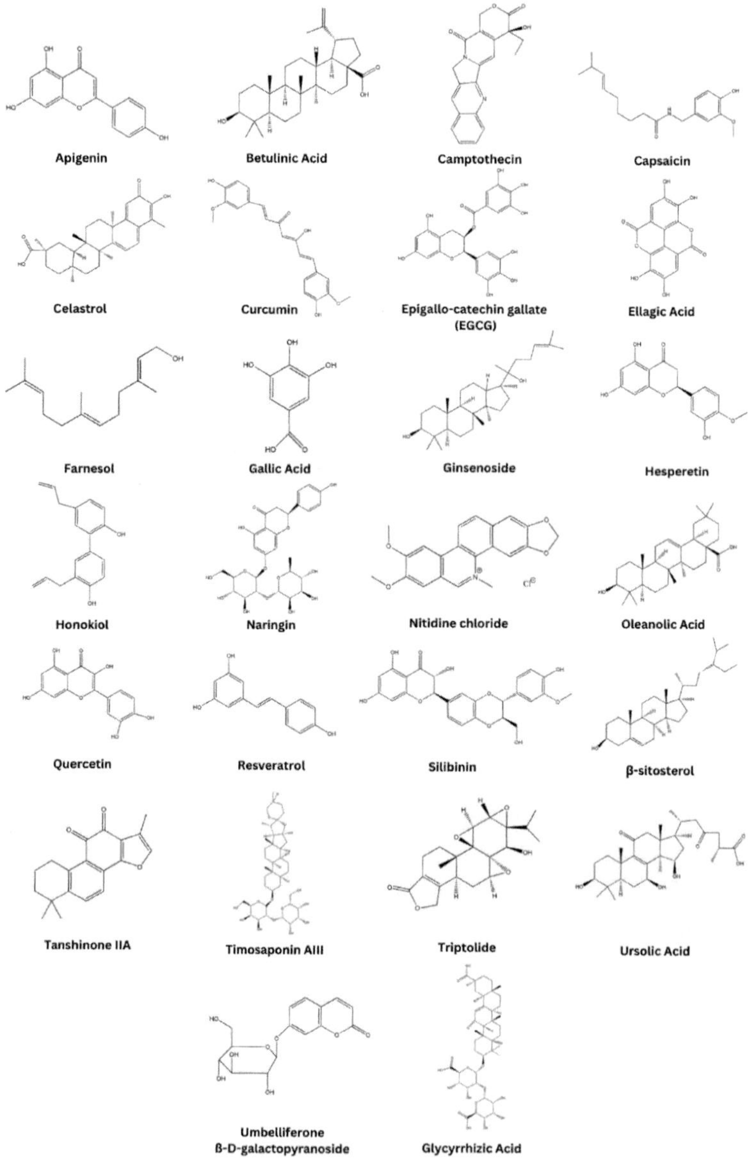

Figure 4: Some important phytochemicals incorporated into nanoparticles for hepatocellular cancer treatment. The structures were drawn using ChemDraw (https://perkinelmerinformatics.com/products/research/chemdraw), and the figure was generated using Canva (www.canva.com)

4.1.2. *Phenols (Flavonoids)*

Phenols are a class of aromatic compounds with one or more hydroxyl groups. Flavonoids are an important class of phenols that are known to possess anti-inflammatory, antioxidant, anti-bacterial, and anti-viral properties apart from anticancer properties. Several flavonoids have been reported to have anticancer effects on HCC cell lines. A study showed that a flavonoid, Oroxylin A, from *Scutellariae radix*, inhibited the growth of HepG2 cells through the inhibition of HIF-1α expression [42]. Another research showed that quercetin, a flavonoid present in many fruits and vegetables, suppressed glycolysis in Bel-7402 and SMMC-7721 cells by lowering levels of HK-2, a critical enzyme involved in glycolysis that is overexpressed in HCC [43].

4.1.3. *Alkaloids*

Alkaloids are a class of organic nitrogenous compounds known to have essential physiological effects on humans. The alkaloid-containing substances have long been investigated for anticancer properties. Berberine, an element present in *Rhizoma coptidis*, exhibited anticancer properties on HepG2 cells by inhibiting the NF-κB pathway and promoting apoptosis [44]. Another study found that irinotecan, a chemical derived from *Camptotheca acuminata*, improved the condition in individuals with HCC after therapy. This compound is recognized for its interference with DNA synthesis by inhibiting the activity of topoisomerase I [45].

4.2. *Cholangiocarcinoma*

There have been few investigations to identify phytochemicals with potential anticancer effects against Cholangiocarcinoma (CCA). A study showed that capsaicin from *Capsicum annum* exerts anticancer properties primarily through NF-κB signaling pathway interference, which interferes with the transcription of matrix metalloproteinase-9 [46]. Similarly, the flavonoid luteolin has been demonstrated to inhibit cell cycle proteins, cyclin A and Cdc25A, and reduce anti-apoptotic proteins (Bcl-2 family) [47]. Other key bioactives produced from *Zingiber officinale* and *Atractylodes lancea* are also tested against CCA in preclinical studies [48, 49].

4.3. *Hepatoblastoma*

Based on a particular study, Korean *Citrus aurantium* harbors various flavonoids that hinder the proliferation of hepatoblastoma HepG2 cell lines. Reduced levels of p-Akt, Bcl-2, and Bcl-XL were linked to the mechanism of action, as are elevated levels of pro-apoptotic proteins such as caspase 3, Bax, and Bak [50]. Similarly, theanine, from *Camellia sinensis*, was studied for its anti-tumor potential against human hepatoblastoma cells HepG2, targeting the mitochondrial pathway [51].

5. Studies of Phytochemicals Incorporated Nanoparticles for Liver Cancer Treatment

Despite a rise in preclinical studies of plant medicines for treating liver cancer, many pharmacokinetic restrictions often pose a challenge in the clinical translation of these natural agents. Consequently, multiple research studies are underway to develop diverse nanoparticle formulations (NP) aimed at overcoming these challenges and facilitating improved delivery of the bioactive components found in plants.

5.1. *Synthesis of nanoparticles*

Synthesis of NPs usually involves two approaches, namely the top-down and bottom-up [52]. The top-down approach involves the synthesis of nano-sized particles through the transformation of bulk materials. This primarily entails cutting, grinding, and shaping the materials for the desired pattern and shape. Top-down approaches are simple but not very useful as they form extremely tiny and irregularly shaped particles. The most significant disadvantage of this method is achieving optimal particle size and shape. In the bottom-up approach, on the other hand, NPs are formed from the bottom-up self-assembly of atoms, molecules, or clusters. The bottom-up technique has shown to be advantageous since it produces particles with homogenous size, shape, and chemical composition. This method is also less expensive. There are different classes of nanoparticles based on their composition, as described below.

5.1.1. *Metallic nanoparticles*

The plant-based NP synthesis, often known as the "green synthesis" of NP, primarily uses inorganic metallic nanoparticles and is generally accomplished by the chemical reduction process. This process is characterized by the reduction of metal ions, followed by nucleation of the reduced metal ions. The secondary metabolites present in the plants, such as terpenoids, flavonoids, and alkaloids, are responsible for the bio-reduction of these metal ions. These plant molecules further help in the aggregation and stabilization of these nanoparticles, which can be characterized by several spectroscopic and microscopic techniques [53]. These plant-based metallic nanoparticles are being explored for treating liver cancer, but the translation to preclinical studies has been limited. Zhang et al. performed *in vitro* as well as *in vivo* anti-HCC studies using resveratrol-Au nanoparticles in liver cancer cells (HepG2) and tumor xenografts [54]. In a more recent research endeavor, the efficacy of genistein-fortified zinc ferrite nanoparticles was examined both *in vitro* and *in vivo* as a potential treatment for hepatic cancer [55].

5.1.2. *Lipid-based nanoparticles*

Lipid-based nanoparticles, especially liposomes, are commonly employed as carriers for drug delivery. The Bangham technique was the first widely used method for liposomal synthesis. The process briefly involves using an organic solvent to dissolve lipids and removing the organic solvent to get a thin lipid film. The thin lipid film is then hydrated in an aqueous medium by continuous agitation for up to 2 hours at 60°C–70°C, where it expands to form spherical closed liposomes [56]. The synthesis of plant-based liposomes for liver cancer treatment involves the integration of specific bioactive molecules with lipids, facilitating the development of liposomes tailored for this purpose. For instance, in a study, resveratrol-loaded cationic liposomes were developed against HCC, which exhibited better anticancer properties than free resveratrol [57]. In a separate study involving celastrol, its limitations were effectively addressed through the creation of galactosylated liposomes that were loaded with celastrol, thereby enhancing its potential for treating HCC [58]. Another class of lipid nanoparticles is the solid lipid nanoparticles as drug carriers. Characterized by a robust lipid core consisting of fatty acids, waxes, and triglycerides, these liposomes possess a size range of 50–200 nm. These are usually synthesized by several methods, which include high-weight homogenization, ultrasonication, solvent evaporation, micro-emulsion, precipitation and film-ultrasound dispersion techniques [59]. Plant-based solid lipid nanoparticles are being studied in preclinical phases to treat liver cancer. The efficacy of capsaicin against HCC was enhanced using solid lipid nanoparticles, which improved the release of the drug as well as its anticancer activity [60].

5.1.3. *Polymer-based nanoparticles*

Polymers such as poly(lactic-co-glycolicacid) (PLGA), polylactic acid (PLA), polyethylene glycol (PEG), and chitosan are also being explored for the development of phytochemical-based nanoparticles, owing to their easy manipulation of size and surface properties. Some desired methods for synthesizing polymeric nanoparticles include nanoprecipitation, emulsification, ionic gelation, and microfluidics. Polymeric nanoparticles may be readily designed with phytochemicals by physically or chemically entrapping inside the polymeric molecules or by binding to the polymer's surface, and these tailored nanoparticles have shown promising effects for the treatment of HCC. In a study, apigenin-loaded PLGA nanoparticles were used for prolonged drug release and a suitable target against HCC in both *in vitro* and *in vivo* settings [61].

While these studies are in the preclinical phase, it becomes crucial to consider the methods of administration and *in vivo* targets as they progress into the clinical stage.

6. Strategies for Targeting Liver Cancer *In Vivo*

The intricacy of these nanoparticle-based therapies grows as they transit from *in vitro* to *in vivo* systems. The most common methods for nanoparticle distribution include oral, olfactory, transdermal, and intravenous. The oral route is the most preferred route of any drug due to its convenience. However, it deals with several drawbacks such as poor drug bioavailability and absorption, rapid metabolism due to the variety of pH conditions, and the breakdown of peptide medicines by proteolytic enzymes present in the colon [62]. Hence, other modes, such as olfactory, transdermal, and intravenous, are gaining perspective.

Several physiological factors within the living system directly or indirectly affect nanoparticle drug delivery. Nanoparticles are exposed to various circulatory proteins, including immunoglobulins, transferrin, fibrinogen, and albumin, which affects the therapeutic activity of these nanoparticles owing to the binding or adsorption of these proteins onto the NP surface [63]. Along with these proteins, it is essential for these nanoparticles to escape the liver resident phagocytic cells (Kupffer cells), which are responsible for drug clearance. Also, the nanoparticles with varying physiochemical characteristics may interact differently with cancer cell membranes. The surface charge, for example, has been shown to influence nanoparticle internalization through changing membrane potential. Modifying the surface of nanoparticles with a positively charged ligand might, therefore, hypothetically increase HCC cell membrane penetration [64].

Several strategies are being employed for improving the nanoparticles targeting liver cancer *in vivo*. Surface biomarkers are commonly employed to target liver cancer, especially HCC. Receptors such as asialoglycoprotein receptor (ASGPR), glypican-3 (GPC-3), transferrin receptor (TfR), folic acid receptor (FR), and scavenger receptor class B type I (SR-B1) are being utilized for nanoparticles-based targeted drug delivery (Figure 5) [65]. ASGPR is a transmembrane molecule found abundantly in hepatic cell membranes that has been investigated as a target for galactose-mediated nanoparticle delivery [66].

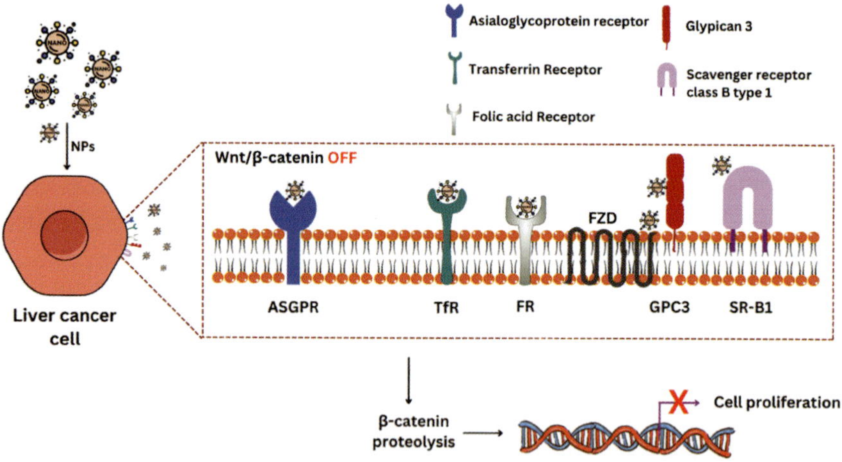

Figure 5: Surface receptors for nanoparticle-based drug delivery in liver cancer (hepatocellular carcinoma) therapy. The figure was generated using Canva (www.canva.com)

The GPC3 protein receptor, which controls the cell proliferation activity by targeting the Wnt pathway, is successfully targeted for drug delivery to HCC due to its overexpression in the tumor as opposed to normal and cirrhotic livers [67]. Research has indicated promising results in targeting HCC through GPC3 monoclonal antibodies, resulting in the suppression of HepG2 cell proliferation [68, 69]. The utilization of TfR1 receptors as targets for HCC is being explored, considering the liver's active role in iron storage and metabolism, alongside their heightened expression in HCC [70]. The use of transferrin (Tf) as targeting ligands has been studied but with the limitations of endogenous Tf blockage that may inhibit the drug delivery [71]. The folic acid receptor is also overexpressed in several cancers, including HCC, making it an ideal target for folic acid-mediated drug delivery [72]. Moreover, the SR-B1 receptor, critical in maintaining cholesterol balance, is identified for its overexpression in HCC attributable to amplified HDL metabolism in tumor cells, rendering it a suitable candidate for HCC targeting through ApoA-1 ligands [73].

In addition to targeting surface receptors, phytochemical nanoparticles can also target cancer stem cells (CSCs), the circulating precursor cells, preventing recurrence and metastasis [74]. These phytochemical-based nanoparticles target the CSCs via their surface markers, receptors, signaling pathways, and epigenetic alterations. Though nanoparticles targeting liver cancer stem cells (LCSC) have been well studied [75], developing phytochemical nanoparticles for such LCSCs would be a promising study in the future.

Though many phytochemicals have been investigated *in vitro* for anticancer activities against liver cancer, specific phytochemicals are being tested preclinically incorporated into nanoparticles, as summarized in Table 1.

7. Conclusion and Prospects

Due to the cutting-edge advancements in HCC nanomedicine, it is now feasible to precisely target specific tumors more effectively than conventional methods. Even though nanoparticles have been extensively explored for cancer therapies, the key to the development of clinical medicine would entail optimal nanoparticle design as well as an in-depth understanding of their toxicity and pharmacokinetic properties. Furthermore, the use of phytochemicals attempts to address the limitations associated with conventional chemotherapeutics, such as drug resistance. The vast literature on the use of phytochemical-based nanoparticles for liver cancer treatment shows its potential toward an excellent anticancer therapy. To develop an ideal anti-liver cancer therapy, it becomes imperative to take into account some critical factors, including the stability of plant bioactives, designing a compatible nanocarrier, and their uptake and metabolism *in vivo*. In light of the growing number of studies on nanoparticle-based drug delivery, this appears plausible.

Table 1: Phytochemical-based nanoparticles for HCC treatment in preclinical studies

S.No	Phytochemical and Class	Biological Sources	Nanoparticle and Class	*In Vitro* Mechanism	*In Vivo* Model	Refs.
1.	Apigenin (Flavonoid)	*Matricaria chamomilla*	Galactose-PLGA[1] (Polymer)	Increased expression of pro-apoptotic factors (Bax and p53) and suppressed anti-apoptotic factors (Bcl-xL and Bcl-2) (*in vivo*)	Male Wistar rats	[76]
2.	Berberine (Alkaloid) and Diosmin (Flavonoid)	*Berberine: Berberis vulgaris; Diosmin: Citrus limon*	Casein micelles (Lipid)	Downregulation of cell necrosis markers (NF-κB and TNF-α), inflammatory marker COX2; inhibition of angiogenesis (*in vivo*)	BALB/c male mice	[77]
3.	Betulinic acid (Terpenoid)	*Betula pendula*	PLGA (Polymer)	Overexpression of anti-apoptotic caspases 3 & 8	Albino Wistar rats	[78]
4.	Camptothecin (Alkaloid)	Bark and stem of *Camptotheca acuminata*	PEG[2] (Polymer)	—	Female BALB/c mice	[79]
5.	Celastrol (Terpenoid)	*Tripterygium wilfordii*	PSN-LMWH[3] (Polymer)	Inactivation of PI3K/Akt/mTOR signaling pathway and ROS-mediated mitochondrial dysfunction	C57BL/6 mice, BALB/c mice, nude mice	[80]
6.	Curcumin (Alkaloid)	*Curcuma longa*	PLL[4] (Polymer)	—	BALB/c nude mice	[81]

7.	Epigallocatechin gallate (EGCG) and Honokiol (Polyphenols)	*EGCG: Camellia sinensis* *Honokiol: Magnolia dealbata*	Chitin (Polymer)	Inhibition of cell proliferation in the G2/M phase and decrease in mitochondrial membrane potential	Male BALB/c Nude	[82]
8.	Gallic acid (Polyphenol)	*Quercus spp. and Punica spp.*	Gallium (Metal)	Increased ROS production	Adult male Swiss albino rats	[83]
9.	Ginsenoside (Terpenoid)	*Panax ginseng*	Iron and iron oxide (Metal)	Increased in tumor inhibitory cytokines such as tumor necrosis factor (TNF-α), interferon-γ (IFN-γ), interleukin-1β (IL-1β), IL-12 (p70), IL-17, IL-15, and granulocyte colony-stimulating factor (G-CSF)	C57BL/6 mice	[84]
10.	Naringin (Flavonoid)	*Citrus sinensis*	Solid lipid nanoparticles (Lipid)	—	Male Wistar rats	[85]
11.	Nitidine chloride (Alkaloid)	*Zanthoxylum nitidum*	TPGS[5] (Polymer)	Reduced expression of AQP3 and STAT3	BALB/c nude mice	[86]
12.	Oleanolic acid (Terpenoid)	*Olea europaea*	PLGA-TPGS (Polymer)	Reduced expression level of intercellular adhesion molecule-1 and VEGF in liver cancer	Male mice	[87]

(*Continued*)

Table 1: (*Continued*)

S.No	Phytochemical and Class	Biological Sources	Nanoparticle and Class	*In Vitro* Mechanism	*In Vivo* Model	Refs.
13.	Quercetin (Flavonoid)	*Allium cepa*	PLGA-TPGS (Polymer)	—	Kunming male mice	[88]
14.	Resveratrol (Polyphenol)	*Polygonum cuspidatum*	Gold (Metal)	Down regulation of pro-caspase-9, pro-caspase-3, PI3K and Akt and upregulating caspase-8 and Bax	BALC/c nude mice	[54]
15.	β-sitosterol (Terpenoid)	*Oryza sativa*	PEG-Niosomes (Polymer-Lipid)	Increased expression of caspases i.e. caspase 3 and 9	Male albino wistar rats	[89]
16.	Tanshinone II A (Terpenoid)	*Salvia miltiorrhiza*	Niosomes (Lipid)	Apoptosis induction, inhibition of cell proliferation, reduction in phosphorylation of p38/MAPK and AKT	Sprague-Dawley rats	[90]
17.	Triptolide (Terpenoid)	T*ripterygium wilfordii*	Liposomes (Lipid)	Inhibition of cell proliferation and induction of apoptosis through the mitochondrial pathway, induces necroptosis through RIPK1/RIPK3/MLKL signaling	BALB/C nude mice	[91]
18.	Ursolic acid (Terpenoid)	*Mirabilis jalapa*	Polymeric micelles (Polymer-Lipid)	—	Male Kunming mice	[92]

Note: 1PLGA: poly lactic-co-glycolic acid; 2PEG: polyethylene glycol; 3PSN-LMWH: P-selectin targeting peptide-low molecular weight heparin; 4PLL: poly-l-lysine; 5TPGS: d-alpha-tocopheryl polyethylene glycol 1000 succinate

References

1. Sung, H., et al., Global cancer statistics 2020: GLOBOCAN estimates of incidence and mortality worldwide for 36 cancers in 185 countries. *CA: A Cancer Journal for Clinicians*, 2021. **71**(3): p. 1–41.
2. Mintz, K. J. and Leblanc, R. M., The use of nanotechnology to combat liver cancer: Progress and perspectives. *Biochimica et Biophysica Acta (BBA)-Reviews on Cancer*, 2021. **1876**(2): p. 188621.
3. Davidson, K. T., Zhu, Z. and Fang, Y., Phytochemicals in the fight against cancer. *Pathology & Oncology Research*, 2016. **22**: p. 655–660.
4. Abotaleb, M., et al., Therapeutic potential of plant phenolic acids in the treatment of cancer. *Biomolecules*, 2020. **10**(2): p. 1–22.
5. Wang, M. and Thanou, M., Targeting nanoparticles to cancer. *Pharmacological Research*, 2010. **62**(2): p. 90–99.
6. Brigger, I., Dubernet, C. and Couvreur, P., Nanoparticles in cancer therapy and diagnosis. *Advanced Drug Delivery Reviews*, 2012. **64**: p. 24–36.
7. Gao, Y., et al., Multifunctional nanoparticle for cancer therapy. *MedComm*, 2023. **4**(1): p. e187.
8. Singh, A. and Sahoo, S.K., Magnetic nanoparticles: A novel platform for cancer theranostics. *Drug Discovery Today*, 2014. **19**(4): p. 474–481.
9. Patel, K. D., Singh, R. K. and Kim, H. W., Carbon-based nanomaterials as an emerging platform for theranostics. *Material Horizons*, 2019. **6**(3): p. 434–469.
10. Basu, A., Namporn, T. and Ruenraroengsak, P., Critical review in designing plant-based anticancer nanoparticles against hepatocellular carcinoma. *Pharmaceutics*, 2023. 15(6): p. 1611.
11. Ponomarkov, V. and Mackey, L. J., Tumors of the liver and biliary system. *Bulletin of the World Health Organization*, 1976. **53**(2–3): p. 187–194.
12. Chuang, S. C., La Vecchia, C. and Boffetta, P., Liver cancer: Descriptive epidemiology and risk factors other than HBV and HCV infection. *Cancer Letters*, 2009. **286**(1): p. 9–14.
13. Clements, O., et al., Risk factors for intrahepatic and extrahepatic cholangiocarcinoma: A systematic review and meta-analysis. *Journal of Hepatology*, 2020. **72**(1): p. 95–103.

14. Komuta, M., Histological heterogeneity of primary liver cancers: Clinical relevance, diagnostic pitfalls and the pathologist's role. *Cancers*, 2021. **13**(12): p. 2871.
15. Lang, L., FDA approves sorafenib for patients with inoperable liver cancer. *Gastroenterology*, 2008. **134**(2): p. 379.
16. Nault, J. C., Galle, P. R. and Marquardt, J. U., The role of molecular enrichment on future therapies in hepatocellular carcinoma. *Journal of Hepatology*, 2018. **69**(1): p. 237–247.
17. Dyhl-Polk, A., et al., Clinical trials of immune checkpoint inhibitors in hepatocellular carcinoma. *Journal of Clinical Medicine*, 2021. **10**(12): p. 2662.
18. Vogel, A., et al., Correction to: "Hepatocellular carcinoma: ESMO Clinical Practice Guidelines for diagnosis, treatment and follow-up." *Annals of Oncology*, 2019. **30**(5): p. 871–873.
19. Andre, T., et al., Gemcitabine combined with oxaliplatin (GEMOX) in advanced biliary tract adenocarcinoma: A GERCOR study. *Annals of Oncology*, 2004. **15**(9): p. 1339–1343.
20. Kobayashi, S., et al., Multicenter retrospective analysis of systemic chemotherapy for unresectable combined hepatocellular and cholangiocarcinoma. *Cancer Science*, 2018. **109**(8): p. 2549–2557.
21. Cabrera, R. and Nelson, D. R., The management of hepatocellular carcinoma. *Alimentary Pharmacology & Therapeutics*, 2010. **31**(4): p. 461–476.
22. Zhang, A., et al., Tumor heterogeneity reshapes the tumor microenvironment to influence drug resistance. *International Journal of Biological Sciences*, 2022. **18**(7): p. 3019–3033.
23. Farokhzad, O. C. and Langer, R., Impact of nanotechnology on drug delivery. *ACS Nano*, 2009. **3**(1): p. 16–20.
24. Metkar, S. P., Nanoparticle drug delivery systems in hepatocellular carcinoma: A focus on targeting strategies and therapeutic applications. *OpenNano*, 2023. **12**: p. 100159.
25. Yokoyama, M., Drug targeting with nano-sized carrier systems. *Journal of Artificial Organs*, 2005. **8**: p. 77–84.
26. Chandrakala, V., Aruna, V. and Angajala, G., Review on metal nanoparticles as nanocarriers: Current challenges and perspectives in drug delivery systems. *Emergent Materials*, 2022. **5**(6): p. 1593–1615.

27. Moreno-Vega, A. I., et al., Polymeric and ceramic nanoparticles in biomedical applications. *Journal of Nanotechnology*, 2012. **2012**: p. 936041.
28. Guimarães, D., Cavaco-Paulo, A. and Nogueira, E., Design of liposomes as drug delivery system for therapeutic applications. *International Journal of Pharmaceutics*, 2021. **601**: p. 120571.
29. Abbasi, E., et al., Dendrimers: Synthesis, applications, and properties. *Nanoscale Research Letters*, 2014. **9**: 1–10.
30. Husseini, G. A. and Pitt, W. G., Micelles and nanoparticles for ultrasonic drug and gene delivery. *Advanced Drug Delivery Reviews*, 2008. **60**(10): p. 1137–1152.
31. Ng, K. K. and Zheng, G., Molecular interactions in organic nanoparticles for phototheranostic applications. *Chemical Reviews*, 2015. **115**(19): p. 11012–11042.
32. Bakry, R., et al., Medicinal applications of fullerenes. *International Journal of Nanomedicine*, 2007. **2**(4): p. 639–649.
33. Wang, Y. and Hu, A., Carbon quantum dots: Synthesis, properties and applications. *Journal of Materials Chemistry C*, 2014. **2**(34): p. 6921–6939.
34. Jain, K. K., Drug delivery systems-an overview. *Drug Delivery Systems*, 2008. p. 1–50.
35. Torchilin, V. P., Passive and active drug targeting: Drug delivery to tumors as an example. *Drug Delivery*, 2010. **197**: p. 3–53.
36. Bakrania, A., Zheng, G. and Bhat, M., Nanomedicine in hepatocellular carcinoma: A new frontier in targeted cancer treatment. *Pharmaceutics*, 2021. **14**(1): p. 41.
37. Bhadoriya, S. S., et al., Bioavailability and bioactivity enhancement of herbal drugs by "Nanotechnology": A review. *Journal of Current Pharmaceutical Research*, 2011. **8**(1): 1–7.
38. Patel, N. R., et al. Nanopreparations to overcome multidrug resistance in cancer. *Advanced Drug Delivery Reviews*, 2013. **65**(13–14): p. 1748–1762.
39. Shukla, S. and Mehta, A., Anticancer potential of medicinal plants and their phytochemicals: A review. *Brazilian Journal of Botany*, 2015. **38**: p. 199–210.
40. Dasgupta, A., et al., Astrakurkurone, a sesquiterpenoid from wild edible mushroom, targets liver cancer cells by modulating bcl-2 family proteins. *IUBMB Life*, 2019. **71** (7): p. 992–1002.

41. Lou, L., et al., Ardipusilloside inhibits survival, invasion and metastasis of human hepatocellular carcinoma cells. *Phytomedicine*, 2012. **19**(7): p. 603–608.
42. Dai, Q., et al., Oroxylin A regulates glucose metabolism in response to hypoxic stress with the involvement of hypoxia-inducible factor-1 in human hepatoma HepG2 cells. *Molecular Carcinogenesis*, 2016. **55**(8): p. 1275–1289.
43. Wu, H., et al., Quercetin inhibits the proliferation of glycolysis-addicted HCC cells by reducing hexokinase 2 and Akt-mTOR pathway. *Molecules*, 2019. **24**(10): p. 1993.
44. Li, M., et al., Induction of apoptosis by berberine in hepatocellular carcinoma HepG2 cells via downregulation of NF-κB. *Oncology Research Featuring Preclinical and Clinical Cancer Therapeutics*, 2017. **25**(2): p. 233–239.
45. Reyhanoglu, G. and Smith, T., *Irinotecan*. StatPearls Publishing, 2023.
46. Lee, G. R., et al., Capsaicin suppresses the migration of cholangiocarcinoma cells by down-regulating matrix metalloproteinase-9 expression via the AMPK–NF-κB signaling pathway. *Clinical & Experimental Metastasis*, 2014. **31**: p. 897–907.
47. Aneknan, P., et al., Luteolin arrests cell cycling, induces apoptosis and inhibits the JAK/STAT3 pathway in human cholangiocarcinoma cells. *Asian Pacific Journal of Cancer Prevention*, 2014. **15**(12): p. 5071–5076.
48. Plengsuriyakarn, T., et al., Preclinical studies of toxicity and anti-cholangiocarcinoma activity of the standardized capsule formulation of *Atractylodes lancea* (Thunb.) DC. *BMC Complementary Medicine and Therapies*, 2023. **23**(1). p. 1–15.
49. Plengsuriyakarn, T. and Na-Bangchang, K., Preclinical toxicology and anticholangiocarcinoma activity of oral formulation of standardized extract of *Zingiber officinale. Planta Medica*, 2020. **86**(02): p. 104–112.
50. Lee, S. H., et al., Flavonoids of Korean *Citrus aurantium* L. induce apoptosis via intrinsic pathway in human hepatoblastoma HepG2 cells. *Phytotherapy Research*, 2015. **29**(12): p. 1940–1949.
51. Xin, Y., et al., Theanine, an antitumor promoter, induces apoptosis of tumor cells via the mitochondrial pathway. *Molecular Medicine Reports*, 2018. **18**(5): p. 4535–4542.

52. Nadaf, S. J., et al., Green synthesis of gold and silver nanoparticles: Updates on research, patents, and future prospects. *OpenNano*, 2022. **8**: p. 100076.
53. Khan, F., et al., Green nanotechnology: Plant-mediated nanoparticle synthesis and application. *Nanomaterials*, 2022. **12**(4): p. 673.
54. Zhang, D., et al., Nano-gold loaded with resveratrol enhance the anti-hepatoma effect of resveratrol *in vitro* and *in vivo*. *Journal of Biomedical Nanotechnology*, 2019. **15**(2): p. 288–300.
55. Otuechere, C. A., et al., Green synthesis of genistein-fortified zinc ferrite nanoparticles as a potent hepatic cancer inhibitor: Validation through experimental and computational studies. *Chemistry & Biodiversity*, 2023. **20**: p. e202300719.
56. Bangham, A., Standish, M. and Watkens, J., Liposomes by film hydration technique. *JC Journal of Molecular Biology*, 1965. **13**(238): p. 80093–80096.
57. Jagwani, S., et al., Pharmacokinetic and pharmacodynamic evaluation of resveratrol loaded cationic liposomes for targeting hepatocellular carcinoma. *ACS Biomaterials Science & Engineering*, 2020. **6**(9): p. 4969–4984.
58. Chen, X., et al., Celastrol-loaded galactosylated liposomes effectively inhibit AKT/c-Met-triggered rapid hepatocarcinogenesis in mice. *Molecular Pharmaceutics*, 2020. **17**(3): p. 738–747.
59. Lingayat, V. J., Zarekar, N. S. and Shendge, R. S., Solid lipid nanoparticles: A review. *Nanoscience and Nanotechnology Research*, 2017. **4**(2): p. 67–72.
60. Kunjiappan, S., et al., Capsaicin-loaded solid lipid nanoparticles: Design, biodistribution, *in silico* modeling and *in vitro* cytotoxicity evaluation. *Nanotechnology*, 2020. **32**(9): p. 95101.
61. Bhattacharya, S., et al., Apigenin loaded nanoparticle delayed development of hepatocellular carcinoma in rats. *Nanomedicine: Nanotechnology, Biology and Medicine*, 2018. **14**(6): p. 1905–1917.
62. Bose, T., et al., Overview of nano-drugs characteristics for clinical application: The journey from the entry to the exit point. *Journal of Nanoparticle Research*, 2014. **16**: p. 1–25.
63. Nguyen, V. H. and Lee, B. J., Protein corona: A new approach for nanomedicine design. *International Journal of Nanomedicine*, 2017. **12**: p. 3137–3151.

64. Rothbard, J. B., Jessop, T. C. and Wender, P. A., Adaptive translocation: The role of hydrogen bonding and membrane potential in the uptake of guanidinium-rich transporters into cells. *Advanced Drug Delivery Reviews.* 2005. **57**(4): p. 495–504.
65. Bakrania, A., Zheng, G. and Bhat, M., Nanomedicine in hepatocellular carcinoma: A new frontier in targeted cancer treatment. *Pharmaceutics*, 2022. **14**(1): p. 1–25.
66. Pranatharthiharan, S., Asialoglycoprotein receptor targeted delivery of doxorubicin nanoparticles for hepatocellular carcinoma. *Drug Delivery*, 2017. 24(1): p. 20–29.
67. Ho, M. and Kim, H., Glypican-3: A new target for cancer immunotherapy. *European Journal of Cancer*, 2011. **47**(3): p. 333–338.
68. Park, J. O., et al., Glypican-3 targeting of liver cancer cells using multifunctional nanoparticles. *Molecular Imaging*, 2011. **10**(1): p. 2010–7290.
69. Li, Z., Glypican-3 antibody functionalized Prussian blue nanoparticles for targeted MR imaging and photothermal therapy of hepatocellular carcinoma. *Journal of Materials Chemistry B*, 2014. **2**(23): p. 3686–3696.
70. Holmström, P., et al., Expression of iron regulatory genes in a rat model of hepatocellular carcinoma. *Liver International*, 2006. **26**(8): p. 976–985.
71. Tang, J., et al., A stabilized retro-inverso peptide ligand of transferrin receptor for enhanced liposome-based hepatocellular carcinoma-targeted drug delivery. *Acta Biomaterialia*, 2019. **83**: p. 379–389.
72. Ghalehkhondabi, V., Soleymani, M. and Fazlali, A., Folate-targeted nanomicelles containing silibinin as an active drug delivery system for liver cancer therapy. *Journal of Drug Delivery Science and Technology*, 2021. **61**: p. 102157.
73. Cruz, W., et al., Lipoprotein-like nanoparticle carrying small interfering RNA against spalt-like transcription factor 4 effectively targets hepatocellular carcinoma cells and decreases tumor burden. *Hepatology Communications*, 2020. **4**(5): p. 769–782.
74. Koklesova, L., et al., Phytochemical-based nanodrugs going beyond the state-of-the-art in cancer management — Targeting cancer stem cells in the framework of predictive, preventive, personalized medicine. *Frontiers in Pharmacology*, 2023. **14**: p. 1121950.

75. Ishiguro, K., et al., Targeting liver cancer stem cells using engineered biological nanoparticles for the treatment of hepatocellular cancer. *Hepatology Communications*, 2020. **4**(2): p. 298–313.
76. Ganguly, S., et al., Apigenin-loaded galactose tailored PLGA nanoparticles: A possible strategy for liver targeting to treat hepatocellular carcinoma. *Colloids and Surfaces B: Biointerfaces*, 2021. **204**: p. 111778.
77. Abdelmoneem, M. A., et al., Dual-targeted casein micelles as green nanomedicine for synergistic phytotherapy of hepatocellular carcinoma. *Journal of Controlled Release*, 2018. **287**: p. 78–93.
78. Kumar, P., et al., Poly(lactic-co-glycolic acid)-loaded nanoparticles of betulinic acid for improved treatment of hepatic cancer: Characterization, *in vitro* and *in vivo* evaluations. *International Journal of Nanomedicine*, 2018. **13**: p. 975–990.
79. Zhou, R., et al., Functional cRGD-conjugated polymer prodrug for targeted drug delivery to liver cancer cells. *ACS Omega*, 2022. 7(24): p. 21325–21336.
80. Zhou, M., et al., A celastrol-based nanodrug with reduced hepatotoxicity for primary and metastatic cancer treatment. *EBioMedicine*, 2023. **94**: p. 104724.
81. Yang, D. H., et al., Preparation of poly-l-lysine-based nanoparticles with pH-sensitive release of Curcumin for targeted imaging and therapy of liver cancer *in vitro* and *in vivo*. *Drug Delivery*, 2018. **25**(1): p. 950–960.
82. Tang, P., et al., Honokiol nanoparticles based on epigallocatechin gallate functionalized chitin to enhance therapeutic effects against liver cancer. *International Journal of Pharmaceutics*, 2018. **545**(1–2): p. 74–83.
83. Mostafa, N., et al., Rationale for tailoring an alternative oncology trial using a novel gallium-based nanocomplex: Mechanistic insights and preclinical challenges. *Technology in Cancer Research & Treatment*, 2022. **21**: p. 15330338221085376.
84. Ren, Z., et al., Nanoparticle conjugation of ginsenoside Rg3 inhibits hepatocellular carcinoma development and metastasis. *Small*, 2020. **16**(2): p. 1905233.
85. Wang, W., et al., Protective role of naringin loaded solid nanoparticles against aflatoxin B1 induced hepatocellular carcinoma. *Chemico-Biological Interactions*, 2022. **351**: p. 109711.

86. Li, D., et al., A novel nitidine chloride nanoparticle overcomes the stemness of CD133+EPCAM+ Huh7 hepatocellular carcinoma cells for liver cancer therapy. *BMC Pharmacology and Toxicology*, 2022. **23**(1): p. 1–10.
87. Bao, X., et al., A novel oleanolic acid-loaded PLGA-TPGS nanoparticle for liver cancer treatment. *Drug Development and Industrial Pharmacy*, 2015. **41**(7): p. 1193–1203.
88. Guan, X., et al., Quercetin-loaded poly (lactic-co-glycolic acid)-d-α-tocopheryl polyethylene glycol 1000 succinate nanoparticles for the targeted treatment of liver cancer. *Drug Delivery*, 2016. **23**(9): p. 3307–3318.
89. Nisha, R., et al., Assessments of *in vitro* and *in vivo* antineoplastic potentials of β-sitosterol-loaded PEGylated niosomes against hepatocellular carcinoma. *Journal of Liposome Research*, 2020. **31**(3): p. 304–315.
90. Hu, X., et al. Galactose-modified PH-sensitive niosomes for controlled release and hepatocellular carcinoma target delivery of tanshinone IIA. *AAPS PharmSciTech*, 2021. **22**: p. 1–14.
91. Zheng, Y., et al., Membrane protein-chimeric liposome-mediated delivery of triptolide for targeted hepatocellular carcinoma therapy. *Drug Delivery*, 2021. **28**(1): p. 2033–2043.
92. Zhou, M., et al., Polymeric micelles loading with ursolic acid enhancing anti-tumor effect on hepatocellular carcinoma. *Journal of Cancer*, 2019. **10**(23): p. 5820.

https://doi.org/10.1142/9789811293320_bmatter

Index